REGIONAL CANCER THERAPY

Edited by

PETER M. SCHLAG, MD

*Professor and Head of Surgical Oncology, Robert-Rössle-Hospital
and Tumor Institute, Charité University of Medicine, Berlin,
and Max-Delbrück-Center for Molecular Medicine, Berlin, Germany*

ULRIKE STEIN, PhD

*Assistant Professor, Tumor Metastasis and Therapy Response Program,
Robert-Rössle-Hospital and Tumor Institute, Charité University
of Medicine, Berlin, and Max-Delbrück-Center for Molecular
Medicine, Berlin, Germany*

Foreword by

ALEXANDER M. M. EGGERMONT, MD, PhD

*Professor and Head of Surgical Oncology
Erasmus University MC—Daniel den Hoed Cancer Center
Rotterdam, The Netherlands*

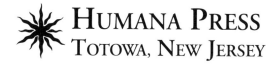
HUMANA PRESS
TOTOWA, NEW JERSEY

© 2007 Humana Press Inc.
999 Riverview Drive, Suite 208
Totowa, New Jersey 07512
www.humanapress.com

Due diligence has been taken by the publishers, editors, and authors of this book to assure the accuracy of the information published and to describe generally accepted practices. The contributors herein have carefully checked to ensure that the drug selections and dosages set forth in this text are accurate and in accord with the standards accepted at the time of publication. Notwithstanding, as new research, changes in government regulations, and knowledge from clinical experience relating to drug therapy and drug reactions constantly occurs, the reader is advised to check the product information provided by the manufacturer of each drug for any change in dosages or for additional warnings and contraindications. This is of utmost importance when the recommended drug herein is a new or infrequently used drug. It is the responsibility of the treating physician to determine dosages and treatment strategies for individual patients. Further it is the responsibility of the health care provider to ascertain the Food and Drug Administration status of each drug or device used in their clinical practice. The publisher, editors, and authors are not responsible for errors or omissions or for any consequences from the application of the information presented in this book and make no warranty, express or implied, with respect to the contents in this publication.

Cover design by Carlotta L. C. Craig

Cover illustration: Taken from Fig. 1 in Chapter 16. The illustration depicts stromal invasion by malignant peritoneal mesothelioma," by D. P. Mangiameli et al.

This publication is printed on acid-free paper. ∞
ANSI Z39.48-1984 (American National Standards Institute)
Permanence of Paper for Printed Library Materials

For additional copies, pricing for bulk purchases, and/or information about other Humana titles, contact Humana at the above address or at any of the following numbers: Tel.:973-256-1699; Fax: 973-256-8341; Email: orders@humanapr.com; or visit our Website: http://humanapress.com

Printed in the United States of America. 10 9 8 7 6 5 4 3 2 1

E-ISBN 1-59745-225-4 ISBN13 978-1-58829-672-6 EISBN13 978-1-59745-225-0
Library of Congress Cataloging-in-Publication Data
Regional cancer therapy / edited by Peter M. Schlag, Ulrike Stein ; foreword by Alexander M.M. Eggermont.
p. ; cm. — (Cancer drug discovery and development)
Includes bibliographical references and index.
ISBN 1-58829-672-5 (alk. paper)
1. Cancer—Chemotherapy. 2. Drug targeting. 3. Infusion therapy. 4. Antineoplastic agent—Administration. I. Schlag, P. (Peter), 1948- II. Stein, Ulrike. III. Series.
[DNLM: 1. Neoplasms—therapy. 2. Chemotherapy, Cancer, Regional Perfusion. 3. Combined Modality Therapy—methods. 4. Drug Resistance, Multiple. 5. Drug Resistance, Neoplasm. QZ 266 R3356 2007]
RC271.C5R44 2007
616.99'4061—dc22   2006015503

REGIONAL CANCER THERAPY

CANCER DRUG DISCOVERY AND DEVELOPMENT

BEVERLY A. TEICHER, SERIES EDITOR

FOREWORD

Regional cancer therapies remain important options in the management of malignant disease, in spite of the venue of more targeted agents for systemic therapies. New technologies and better guidance systems for radiofrequency ablation and intrastitial laser therapies, highly selective intravascular approaches with improved catheters and guidance systems, improved agents for embolizations, and new vasoactive drugs for isolated limb and liver perfusions are just a few of the new developments in a field that is alive and progressing.

Regional Cancer Therapy, so well put together by the editors Peter M. Schlag and Ulrike S. Stein, presents an overview of today's realities and tomorrow's possibilities. Regional cancer therapy models provide ways to make new discoveries about tumor biology and new agents that may be used regionally as well as systemically. This book should therefore be of interest to all clinicians and scientists with an interest in tumor biology as well as clinical advances.

Alexander M. M. Eggermont, MD, PhD
Professor and Head of Surgical Oncology
Erasmus University MC—Daniel den Hoed Cancer Center
Rotterdam, the Netherlands

PREFACE

The treatment of malignant tumors has been substantially improved in recent years due to developments in clinical medicine and technology as well as by advances in molecular biological research. Modern molecular and genetic techniques allow the characterization of molecules that are decisive for tumor development and progression. Considerable success has been achieved in selected solid tumors using molecular-targeted therapies, e.g., for GIST treated with Gleevec or breast cancer treated with Herceptin. These remain, perhaps, the most successful examples of molecular-targeted systemic cancer therapies. Avastin, acting to inhibit VEGF signaling, is another example with apparently wider utility, owing to the more general importance of angiogenesis in tumor biology. Therapies directed against the process of metastasis could potentially provide an additional dimension to therapeutic regimens in the future.

Curative treatment requires control of both local and systemic disease. Advances in diagnostic procedures have made it possible to more accurately assess the distribution and extent of malignant disease and define a role for both surgery and regional therapy in modern cancer treatment. The concept of regional cancer therapy aims at a targeted destruction of a tumor disease that is not accessible by classical surgical tumor resection or radiotherapeutic ablation. Modern regional tumor therapy, based on progress in technology and research, will contribute to new dimensions in this exciting field of oncology.

Regional Cancer Therapy describes findings and technical features of regional tumor therapy with diverse facets considered for various tumor entities and locations. New developments and conceptual formulations are presented with respect to both tumor biology and technical aspects. Clinical trial concepts and treatment protocols currently employed to improve regional tumor therapy are discussed in this book in detail. Thus, the book represents not only a therapeutic vade mecum for the current possibilities for effective regional tumor therapy, but also provides numerous suggestions for future advances. The book will be of value not only for clinical oncologists, but also for scientists who are interested in the fundamentals of regional tumor therapy as it relates to optimizing translational approaches.

Regional tumor therapy, in general, is an excellent example of an interdisciplinary strategy. Thus, not only the classical oncological disciplines, such as surgical oncology, radiotherapy, and medical oncology, but also interventional radiology and nuclear medicine, and medical students and other medical support staff will benefit from reading *Regional Cancer Therapy*.

The editors are very thankful to all authors for their valuable contributions, which provide a thorough description of the concepts of regional cancer therapy. This enabled us to bring the reader a balanced book where all sides of the regional cancer therapy issues are covered fairly. We hope that *Regional Cancer Therapy* will stimulate interest and rapid advances in the important field of regional cancer therapy for the improved treatment of patients.

Peter M. Schlag, MD, PhD
Ulrike S. Stein, PhD

Contents

CONTRIBUTORS

TAKAYUKI AIMOTO • *Department of Surgery, Nippon Medical School, Tokyo, Japan*

H. RICHARD ALEXANDER • *National Cancer Institute, Bethesda MD*

GIANFRANCO AMICUCCI • *Department of Surgical Sciences, University of L'Aquila, Italy*

EREN BERBER • *Department of General Surgery, The Cleveland Clinic Foundation, Cleveland, OH*

DAVID P. BERRY • *Department of Hepatobiliary and Pancreatic Surgery, The Leicester General Hospital, Leicester, UK*

MANOOP S. BHUTANI • *Department of Internal Medicine, Division of Gastroenterology, University of Texas Medical Branch, Galveston TX*

FLAVIA BRUNSTEIN • *Department of Surgical Oncology, Erasmus University Medical Center-Daniel den Hoed Cancer Center, Rotterdam, The Netherlands*

MAURIZIO CANTORE • *Department of Oncology, AUSL-Carrara, Italy*

MARCO CLEMENTI • *Department of Surgical Sciences, University of L'Aquila, Italy*

TIMM DENECKE • *Clinic for Radiation Oncology and Radiation Medicine, Charité Campus Virchow-Klinkum, Berlin, Germany*

MARCELLO DERACO • *Department of Surgery, Melanoma and Sarcoma Unit, National Cancer Institute of Milan, Italy*

THOMAS J. DOUGHERTY • *Photodynamic Therapy Center, Roswell Park Cancer Institute, Buffalo, NY*

ALEXANDER M. M. EGGERMONT • *Department of Surgical Oncology, Erasmus University Medical Center–Daniel den Hoed Cancer Center, Rotterdam, The Netherlands*

GIAMMARIA FIORENTINI • *Department of Oncology, AUSL-Empoli, Italy*

GIUSEPPE GARCEA • *The Robert Kilpatrick Clinical Sciences Building, The Leicester Royal Infirmary, Leicester, UK*

HANS GELDERBLOM • *Department of Clinical Oncology, Leiden University Medical Center, Leiden, The Netherlands*

JOHANNA GELLERMANN • *Clinic for Radiation Oncology and Radiation Medicine, Charité University of Medicine, Berlin, Germany*

SVETLANA GELPERINA • *Research Center for Molecular Diagnostics and Therapy, Moscow, Russia*

AMANJIT S. GILL • *Department of Radiology, University of Texas Medical Branch, Galveston, TX*

SANDRA GRÜNBERG • *Department of Surgical Oncology, Robert-Rössle-Hospital and Tumor Institute, Charité University of Medicine, Berlin, Germany*

DIRK J. GRÜNHAGEN • *Department of Surgical Oncology, Erasmus University Medical Center-Daniel den Hoed Cancer Center, Rotterdam, The Netherlands*

STEFANO GUADAGNI • *Department of Surgical Sciences, University of L'Aquila, Italy*

HENK-JAN GUCHELAAR • *Department of Clinical Pharmacy and Toxicology, Leiden University Medical Center, Leiden, the Netherlands*

TIMO L. M. TEN HAGEN • *Department of Surgical Oncology, Erasmus University Medical Center–Daniel den Hoed Cancer Center, Rotterdam, The Netherlands*

ENRIQUE LOPEZ HÄNNINEN • *Clinic for Radiation Oncology and Radiation Medicine, Charité University of Medicine, Berlin, Germany*

CLAUS-DIETER HEIDECKE • *Department of Surgery, Ernst-Moritz-Arndt-University, Greifswald, Germany*

THOMAS OLIVER HENKEL • *Urologische Gemeinschaftspraxis, Berlin, Germany*

NORBERT HOSTEN • *Department of Radiology, Ernst-Moritz-Arndt-University, Greifswald, Germany*

DIETER JOCHAM • *Department of Urology, University of Lübeck, Medical School, Lübeck, Germany*

ANDREAS JORDAN • *Center of Biomedical Nanotechnology, Department of Radiology, Charité University of Medicine, Berlin, Germany*

FRANK KAHMANN • *Urologische Gemeinschaftspraxis, Berlin, Germany*

EVANGELOS KANAVOS • *Department of Surgical Sciences, University of L'Aquila, Italy*

INGO KAUSCH • *Department of Urology, University of Lübeck, Medical School, Lübeck, Germany*

NANCY KEMENY • *Department of Medical Oncology, Memorial Sloan-Kettering Cancer Center, New York, NY*

SHIGEKI KUSAMURA • *Department of Surgery, Melanoma and Sarcoma Unit, National Cancer Institute of Milan, Italy*

CLAUDIO LELY • *Department of Surgical Sciences, University of L'Aquila, Italy*

STEVEN K. LIBUTTI • *National Cancer Institute, Bethesda, MD*

KLAUS MAIER-HAUFF • *Department of Neurosurgery, Bundeswehrkrankenhaus, Berlin, Germany*

YASUHIRO MAMADA • *Department of Surgery, Nippon Medical School, Tokyo, Japan*

DAVID P. MANGIAMELI • *National Cancer Institute, Bethesda, MD*

YOSHIAKI MIZUGUCHI • *Department of Surgery, Nippon Medical School, Tokyo, Japan*

DAVID L. MORRIS • *Department of Surgery, University of New South Wales, St. George Hospital, Sydney, Australia*

YOSHIHARU NAKAMURA • *Department of Surgery, Nippon Medical School, Tokyo, Japan*

MOSHE Z. PAPA • *Department of Surgery and Surgical Oncology and the Breast Service, Chaim Sheba Medical Center, Tel Hashomer, Israel*

JAMES F. PINGPANK • *National Cancer Institute, Bethesda, MD*

FRANCESCO RASPAGLIESI • *Department of Surgery, Gynecology Unit, National Cancer Institute of Milan, Italy*

FARUQUE RIFFAT • *Department of Surgery, University of New South Wales, St. George Hospital, Sydney, Australia*

JOOST ROTHBARTH • *Department of Surgery, Leiden University Medical Center, Leiden, The Netherlands*

CRISTINA RUSCITTI • *Department of Surgical Sciences, University of L'Aquila, Italy*

SIEGEL SADETZKI • *Cancer and Radiation Epidemiology Unit, Gertner Institute, Chaim Sheba Medical Center, Tel Hashomer, Israel*

MARIO SCHIETROMA • *Department of Surgical Sciences, University of L'Aquila, Italy*

PETER M. SCHLAG • *Department of Surgical Oncology, Robert-Rössle-Hospital and Tumor Institute, Charité Univerisyt of Medicine, Berlin, and Max-Delbrück-Center for Molecular Medicine, Berlin, Germany*

TETSUYA SHIMIZU • *Department of Surgery, Nippon Medical School, Tokyo, Japan*

ALLAN E. SIPERSTEIN • *Department of General Surgery, The Cleveland Clinic Foundation, Cleveland, OH*

YEHUDA SKORNICK • *Washington Cancer Institute, Washington Hospital Center, Washington, DC*

ULRIKE S. STEIN • *Department of Surgical Oncology, Robert-Rössle-Hospital and Tumor Institute, Charité University of Medicine, Berlin, and Max-Delbrück-Center for Molecular Medicine, Berlin, Germany*

PAUL H. SUGARBAKER • *Washington Cancer Institute, Washington Hospital Center, Washington, DC*

TAKASHI TAJIRI • *Department of Surgery, Nippon Medical School, Tokyo, Japan*

NOBUHIKO TANIAI • *Department of Surgery, Nippon Medical School, Tokyo, Japan*

REBECCA TAYLOR • *Memorial Sloan-Kettering Cancer Center, New York, NY*

JAMES TOMLINSON • *Memorial Sloan-Kettering Cancer Center, New York, NY*

PER-ULF TUNN • *Department of Surgical Oncology, Robert-Rössle-Hospital and Tumor Institute, Charité University of Medicine, Berlin, Germany*

EIJI UCHIDA • *Department of Surgery, Nippon Medical School, Tokyo, Japan*

CORNELIUS J. H. VAN DE VELDE • *Department of Surgery, Leiden University Medical Center, Leiden, The Netherlands*

SERGE VAN RUTH • *Department of Dermatology, University Medical Center Utrecht, Utrecht, The Netherlands*

WOLFGANG WALTHER • *Department of Surgical Oncology, Robert-Rössle-Hospital and Tumor Institute, Charité University of Medicine, and Max-Delbrück-Center for Molecular Medicine, Berlin, Germany*

CHRISTIANE WEIGEL • *Department of Radiology, Ernst-Moritz-Arndt-University Greifswald, Germany*

ROBERT F. WONG • *Department of Internal Medicine, Division of Gastroenterology, University of Utah School of Medicine, Salt Lake City, UT*

PETER WUST • *Clinic for Radiation Oncology and Radiation Medicine, Charité University of Medicine, Berlin, Germany*

TRISTAN D. YAN • *Department of Surgery, University of New South Wales, St. George Hospital, Sydney, Australia*

HIROSHI YOSHIDA • *Department of Surgery, Nippon Medical School, Tokyo, Japan*

FRANS A. N. ZOETMULDER • *Department of Surgical Oncology, Netherlands Cancer Institute-Antoni van Leeuwenhoek Hospital, Amsterdam, The Netherlands*

I BACKGROUND

1

Biological Background

Multidrug Resistance—Clinical Implications

Ulrike S. Stein*, PhD, Wolfgang Walther, PhD, and Peter M. Schlag, MD, PhD

CONTENTS

SUMMARY

Drug resistance of human tumors to a variety of chemotherapeutic agents remains the major cause of cancer treatment failure. Although multiple mechanisms of drug resistance may occur in parallel or sequentially at all different levels of drug action, one resistance mechanism was identified within the last two decades that very likely represents the most frequent cause for the development of drug resistance in cancer cells: the phenomenon of multidrug resistance (MDR). MDR, the simultaneous resistance toward structurally and functionally unrelated cytostatic drugs, depends mainly on the presence of different transporter proteins, their genetic polymorphisms, and their regulation/deregulation. Thus, decreased uptake and/or increased efflux, lowered net accumulation, and, in consequence, less efficiency of anticancer drugs is the clinical hurdle.

The biology of the most prominent members of the MDR-associated, membrane-spanning ATP-binding cassette (ABC) transporter proteins (MDR1, MRP1, and BCRP), their transport mechanisms, and the spectra of cytostatic drugs are summarized in this chapter. The clinical importance of these MDR-associated molecules (their basal and therapy-induced expression) is discussed for different solid tumors with respect to clinical outcome parameters. Resistance profiling and response prediction as essential prerequisites for tailor-made, patient-individual MDR reversal as

From: *Cancer Drug Discovery and Development: Regional Cancer Therapy*
Edited by: P. M. Schlag and U. S. Stein © Humana Press Inc., Totowa, NJ

well as intervention strategies targeting functional, translational, and transcriptional levels are evaluated.

Key Words: Multidrug resistance; MDR1; MRP1; BCRP; prediction; reversal; inhibitors.

1. INTRODUCTION: DRUG RESISTANCE AND CANCER

Treatment of most locally confined malignant tumors is presently based on surgical and radiotherapeutic approaches. For advanced and metastatic tumors, chemotherapy is the most effective treatment, with clinical success differing from patient to patient. Some patients are cured, others respond transiently, and a third group has incomplete responses. Furthermore, clinical oncologists have noted that cancer patients treated with multiple anticancer drugs developed cross-resistance to many other chemotherapeutics to which they had never been exposed. As a consequence, the possibility of curing these patients with chemotherapy is dramatically reduced *(1,2)*.

Multiple mechanisms of drug resistance may occur in parallel or sequentially at all different levels of drug action, leading to intrinsic (without any treatment) or acquired (therapy-induced) resistance toward cytotoxic drugs. Anticancer drugs have different ways to enter the cell. Uptake of hydrophilic drugs into the cell depends on transporters, carriers, or channels, since these drugs are not able to cross the cell membrane by themselves. Defects in drug uptake proteins lead to reduced influx, resulting in lowered intracellular drug concentration, and the cell becomes resistant to a single drug. Natural anticancer products such as anthracyclines, vinca alkaloids, epipodophyllotoxins, and taxanes are hydrophobic and enter the cell by diffusion across the cell membrane. Resistance toward these drugs develops by increased drug efflux depending on the activity of efflux pumps, such as transmembrane energy (ATP)-dependent transporter proteins. Thus, intracellular drug concentration is reduced; the cell becomes resistant to a panel of hydrophobic drugs. Furthermore, activation of proteins that are involved in metabolism or detoxification of drugs may cause drug resistance without affecting drug accumulation. Intracellular drug redistribution, e.g., the nucleocytoplasmic drug transport by vaults, may contribute to drug resistance. Moreover, cytostatic-induced activation of nuclear proteins such as mismatch repair genes involved in enhanced repair of drug-induced DNA damage may lead to drug resistance. Cells may also become resistant to drug-induced cell death by activation of anti-apoptotic proteins and by affecting the cell cycle and checkpoints *(1–3)*.

Although several mechanisms might be able to contribute to a drug resistance phenotype, one resistance mechanism was identified within the last two decades that very likely represents the most frequent cause for the development of drug resistance in cancer cells: the phenomenon of multidrug resistance (MDR). MDR reflects the ability of a tumor cell to resist typically lethal or sublethal doses of multiple usually cytotoxic drugs. MDR is defined as the simultaneous resistance to structurally and functionally unrelated natural product anticancer drugs. To date, MDR of human tumors to a variety of chemotherapeutic agents still represents the major cause of failure of cancer chemotherapy. Therefore, the need to identify those tumors with high intrinsic and/or therapy-inducible MDR is desired. Patient-individual response prediction and tailor-made reversal of MDR are the ultimate goals to improve cancer chemotherapy.

2. MULTIDRUG RESISTANCE, ABC TRANSPORTERS, AND DRUG TRANSPORT

The development of the MDR phenotype is dependent on expression of MDR-associated genes encoding energy-dependent transmembrane transporter proteins *(4)*. They act as drug efflux pumps, thereby lowering the intracellular concentration of cytotoxic drugs through increased drug efflux. These drug efflux pumps belong to the intensively studied protein superfamily of ATP-binding cassette (ABC) transporter proteins representing the largest gene family of transmembrane proteins *(5)*. The normal physiological functions of these transporters are the protection of epithelial cells (e.g., those of the gastrointestinal tract, liver and kidney) and brain capillaries for the uptake of xenobiotics and the promotion of their excretion in the bile and urine. They also transport multiple classes of anticancer drugs such as anthracyclines, vinca alkaloids, epipodophyllotoxins, taxanes, and others out of the cell, making it multidrug resistant. ABC transporter-mediated drug transport is energy dependent, driven by hydrolysis of ATP *(4)*.

In the human genome, 48 ABC transporters have been identified so far *(5)*. Based on sequence similarities—they share common features such as nucleotide binding sites and transmembrane domains—they have been classified into seven subfamilies by phylogenetic analysis. Important ABC transporters associated with the MDR phenotype are encoded by the following genes:

1. The multidrug resistance gene 1 (MDR1, or ABCB1; subfamily ABCB) encodes P-glycoprotein, causing the so-called classical, P-glycoprotein-mediated MDR.
2. The genes for the multidrug resistance-associated proteins 1, 2, and 3 (MRP1–3, or ABCC1–3; subfamily ABCC) as well as the gene for the breast cancer resistance protein (BCRP); also called ABC transporter in placenta [ABCP] and mitoxantrone resistance gene [MXR or ABCG2; subfamily ABCG] lead to the so-called atypical, non-P-glycoprotein-mediated MDR.

For some of these MDR-associated ABC transporters, a causal role for generation of the MDR phenotype has been demonstrated, e.g., MDR1, MRP1, BCRP; for others, an ability to transport multiple cytotoxic compounds has been shown. The spectrum of anticancer drugs transported by the ABC transporters includes anthracyclines such as doxorubicin, daunorubicin, epirubicin, and mitoxantrone, vinca alkaloids such as vincristine and vinblastine, epipodophyllotoxins such as etoposide and tenoposide, and taxanes such as paclitaxel and docetaxel. Interestingly, the drug spectra of single MDR-associated ABC transporters are overlapping but not identical. Moreover, it has been shown for several transporters that their substrate specificities might vary owing to defined point mutations within their genes.

2.1. MDR1/P-Glycoprotein

The ABCB subfamily of ABC transporters harbors 12 members, with the most prominent being, the MDR1 gene, which was first described about three decades ago *(6,7)*. MDR1/P-glycoprotein is the first cloned human ABC transporter, for which direct generation of the MDR phenotype was shown by gene transduction *(8,9)*. The MDR1 gene encodes P-glycoprotein, a multidrug efflux pump with two nucleotide binding sites and two transmembrane domains each consisting of 12 membrane-spanning α-helices that is believed to determine the substrate specificity of the drug transported. P-glycoprotein is able to bind a wide spectrum of hydrophobic, neutral, or positively charged substrates, such as anthracyclines, vinca alkaloids, epipodophyllotoxins, and taxanes. After binding of the drug, ATP hydrolysis leads to conformational changes in the protein as an essential prerequisite for release of the substrate out of the cell. Then ATP hydrolysis is necessary for resetting of the transporter molecule *(4,5)*.

MDR1 gene expression has been analyzed in an enormous number of studies. In humans, high expression levels have been repeatedly detected in normal tissues with excretory or secretory functions, such as on the apical surface of columnar epithelial cells of small and large intestines, the biliary canalicular membrane of hepatocytes, the apical surface of epithelial cells of the proximal tubules of the kidney, the apical surface of epithelial cells of the placenta, and the apical surface of endothelial cells in blood capillaries of the brain *(10,11)*. Interestingly, MDR1 expression appears to increase progressively over the total length of the gastrointestinal tract, with low levels in the stomach, intermediate levels in the jejunum, and high levels in the colon *(12)*.

In tumors of these tissues, such as colon, kidney, adrenocortical, and hepatocellular cancers, P-glycoprotein expression is inherently overexpressed, making them primarily chemotherapy-resistant toward a wide panel of anticancer drugs *(12)*. This basically is a major reason for the limited selection of chemotherapeutics to tumors of these organs, e.g., for therapy of gastrointestinal cancer *(1,12–15)*.

Furthermore, in addition to basal expression levels of MDR1, external factors such as components of multimodal cancer therapy are able to induce expression of the MDR1 gene. Thus, cytostatics, but also heat or radiation, might lead to elevation of MDR1 gene expression (e.g., refs. *16–20*). Several studies have shown that in approx 50% of all treated tumors, induction of MDR1 expression has been observed *(21)*. By identification of the MDR1 gene promoter and generation of promoter deletion mutants, drug- and heat-responsive elements have been identified, mediating therapy-caused stress signals into transcriptional activation of the MDR1 gene *(22)*. This is in agreement with the chemotherapy- or hyperthermia-induced elevation of MDR1 gene expression that have been detected in patients. However, single-nucleotide polymorphisms, either of the MDR1 promoter *(23,24)* or of the MDR1 gene *(25)* may alter basal expression levels as well as drug inducibility. Mutations mainly affecting positions 2677 and 3435 of the MDR1 gene were associated with altered P-glycoprotein expression and function. Thus, MDR1 gene polymorphisms may also play a role in patients who do not respond to drug treatment.

Tumors that are more sensitive to chemotherapy show low or intermediate basal MDR1 expression but develop upregulation of MDR1 expression following chemotherapy, which results in the acquired type of drug resistance *(26,27)*. For example, expression of P-glycoprotein was increased after treatment in myeloma (pretreatment/posttreatment 6%/43%), in breast cancer (14%/43% and 11%/30%), and in ovarian (15%/48%) and cervical cancer (39%/88%) *(29–32)*. Moreover, in patients with unresectable pulmonary sarcoma metastases, who underwent isolated single lung perfusion with doxorubicin, relative MDR1 expression was measured in metastastic tumor nodules after initiation of chemoperfusion. Increases in MDR1 expression (up to 15-–fold) were detected 50 min after administration of doxorubicin. This observation demonstrates that MDR1 expression can be activated very rapidly in human tumors after transient exposure to chemotherapy *(33)*. Heat, as an external stress factor, may also induce MDR1 gene expression. However, hyperthermic isolated limb perfusion of sarcoma and melanoma patients did not lead to induction of ABC transporters, probably because of the mild temperatures applied. Interestingly, expression of the major vault protein, a component of vault-mediated drug resistance, was induced *(34,35)*. On the other hand, regional cancer therapy techniques for organ-specific administration of drugs, such as lung perfusion, isolated limb perfusion, hepatic arterial infusion, intrathecal therapy, hyperoxygenation, and hyperthermia, are all strategies aiming at increasing drug delivery. However, this goal of an elevated drug accumulation at the tumor site must be evaluated in the context of the treatment modalities/external stress factors such as radiation, hyperthermia, or chemotherapy itself, balancing the increased organ-site drug accumulation with risk of MDR induction.

For nonsolid cancers, e.g., acute myelogenous leukemia, the most reproducible results on MDR1 expression levels, treatment-caused inductions, and correlations to clinical outcome have been reported (e.g., ref. *36*). Although the prognostic implications of MDR1 expression are controversial, the value of P-glycoprotein as marker for poor prognosis has been repeatedly supported (e.g., ref. *37*). For a variety of solid tumors, in particular for those more chemosensitive to drug treatment, acquired chemoresistance was accompanied with upregulated levels of MDR1 after exposure to chemotherapy. Correlation of clinical outcome parameters with MDR1 expression have been reported for bone and soft tissue sarcomas *(38–40)*, breast cancer *(41,42)*, and others.

2.2. The MRP Family

The ABCC subfamily of ABC transporters consists of 11 members with 9 MRP-related gene-associated proteins (MRP1–9 or ABCC1–6 and ABCC10–12). The most studied member, MRP1, was identified more than a decade ago in a non-P-glycoprotein-expressing, but multidrug-resistant human tumor cell line *(43)*. MRP1 is structurally similar to P-glycoprotein, however, with an amino-terminal extension of five membrane spanning α-helices. Like MRP1, MRP2, MRP3, and MRP6 harbor these extra amino-terminal transmembrane domains when compared with P-glycoprotein.

The spectrum of transported hydrophobic natural anticancer drugs overlap those transported by P-glycoprotein and also includes compounds of anthracyclines, vinca alkaloids, and epipodophyllotoxins. Like P-glycoprotein, the substrate specificity of MRP1 is altered owing to single amino acid substitutions within the respective transporter protein. However, the mechanism of drug transport is different. The MRPs transport anionic and neutral drugs conjugated to acidic ligands, such as glutathione, glucuronate, or sulfate. Alternatively, they can cause resistance to neutral drugs without conjugation but by cotransporting these drugs with free glutathione *(3,44–46)*. MRP4, MRP5, and MRP7 lack the additional helical regions but show higher sequence similarities to MRP1 than to P-glycoprotein or other ABC transporters. Both MRP4 and MRP5, are also organic anion transporters, like MRP1, -2, and -3, which have been identified to pump nucleotide analogs.

Gene transduction has shown that MRP1 plays a causal role in conferring the MDR phenotype on previously chemosensitive cells. Basal expression of MRP1 has been found to be ubiquitous in human tissues. Moreover, in almost all malignant tissues, basal MRP1 expression levels have been determined *(47)*, as reported, for example, in myeloma (in 100% of the tumors analyzed), breast cancer (100%), lung cancer (88% for small cell lung cancer [SCLC], 100% for non-small cell lung cancer [NSCLC]), sarcomas (80%) *(48–51)*. High MRP1 expression levels have been observed for lung, breast, and ovarian cancer *(26)*. Moreover, for several tumor entities, correlations of high MRP1 expression with clinical outcome parameters such as response to chemotherapy and disease-free survival have been reported, e.g., for mammary, lung, and ovarian carcinomas, as well as for leukemias; in refractory hematological malignancies, increases in MRP1 have also been observed *(52)*. Moreover, a prognostic significance of MRP1 expression has been reported for primary breast cancer *(53)*. However, the clinical importance of MRP1 is still a matter of discussion, since studies have both confirmed and rejected a correlation of MRP1 expression level and outcome.

2.3. BCRP

BCRP (also called ABCP and MXR) was originally identified in a mitoxantrone-resistant, but P-glycoprotein and MRP1-negative human carcinoma cell line and was given three names because of its almost simultaneous discovery by three independent groups *(54–56)*. BCRP also encodes an ABC transporter and, together with four additional members, constitutes the ABCG subfamily. By contrast, this so-called half-transporter harbors only one nucleotide binding site and only one transmembrane domain with six membrane-spanning α-helices; full transporters such as P-glycoprotein and the MRPs contain two nucleotide binding sites and two transmembrane domains, suggesting BCRP homodimerization to gain full transport activity *(55)*.

Transduction of BCRP cDNA also caused the resistance phenotype. The drug spectra of BCRP considerably overlap with those of P-glycoprotein, including mitoxantrone, topotecan, and doxorubicin, with differing efficiences, however. High levels of BCRP were mainly detected in several mitoxantrone-resistant mammary, colon, ovarian, and gastric human cell lines *(57–61)*. Thus, BCRP showed high affinities for mitoxantrone, representing the long-sought transporter for this cytotoxic compound. Further BCRP substrates are methotrexate and flavopiridol. Tyrosine kinase inhibitors such as imatinib and gefitinib are also transported by BCRP (and also by P-glycoprotein). Vincristine and taxanes, typical P-glycoprotein substrates, are not included in the BCRP drug spectrum. It has been shown for P-glycoprotein and MRP1 that defined point mutations leading to amino acid substitutions, particularly within the transmembrane domains, alter substrate specificity and transport efficiency. This has also been confirmed for BCRP, e.g., for substitutions of arginine at position 482 for threonine or glycine, occurring during drug selection *(62,63)*.

BCRP was mainly detected in human tissues such as intestine, colon, mammary, liver canaliculi, and renal tubules and is highly expressed in placenta and the blood-brain barrier *(1,2,13)*. Intrinsic BCRP expression was frequently observed in human tumors of different entities. So far, high BCRP expression levels have been published for carcinomas of the digestive tract, for lung carcinomas, and for melanomas *(64)*. Its clinical relevance of high and/or therapy-induced BCRP expression in the context of clinical parameters such as response to chemotherapy and survival remains to be elucidated.

3. PREDICTION OF CHEMOSENSITIVITY AND TREATMENT RESPONSE

Different mechanisms and genes contribute to intrinsic and/or acquired drug resistance. For patients to qualify for a respective treatment regime, and for tailor-made patient-individual therapies, knowledge of the expression and function of genes and proteins related to drug resistance represents an essential prerequisite. Since single individual markers have shown limited predictive value, the simultaneous analysis of a panel of resistance-associated genes is desired.

However, up to now clinical tests for predicting cancer chemotherapy response are not available. So far, several reports have described the generation of expression profiles for the prediction of chemosensitivity. For three human cell lines, expression profiles of 38 ABC transporters have been generated by using low-density microarrays combined with quantitative real-time polymerase chain reaction (PCR) *(65)*. For the 60-cell line panel of the National Cancer Institute (NCI), expression profiles of the known 48 ABC transporters have been created by means of quantitative real-time reverse transcription (RT)-PCR *(66)*. Furthermore, doxorubicin sensitivity in human breast tumors was predicted on the basis of microarray-generated and quantitative real-time RT-PCR-validated expression profiles and correlated with patient survival *(67)*. These approaches demonstrate the significance of in vitro experiments and may serve for the development of diagnostic tools for cancer response prediction in clinical samples.

4. INTERVENTION STRATEGIES FOR REVERSAL OF MDR

The failure of certain cancer chemotherapies was primarily linked to basal and/or induced expression of P-glycoprotein. The identification of MDR1/P-glycoprotein and its correlation with parameters of clinical outcome gave rise to the following optimistic assumption: "The high hope of P-glycoprotein was that here was a single protein that confers resistance to a whole array of structurally unrelated anticancer drugs. That was a very attractive idea. It raised the possibility that drug resistance could be overcome, because if a single mechanism is responsible, all you have to do is learn to understand that mechanism, find strategies to overcome it, and you could cure people of cancer" *(68)*. Thus, the inhibition of P-glycoprotein aiming at reversal of the MDR phenotype has been extensively studied for more than two decades. Several approaches have been made to target the function and the expression of MDR-associated genes and proteins, such as the employment of specific antibodies, inhibiting drug transport, the introduction of antisense oligonucleotides and ribozymes, or, one of the newest developments, the transduction of small interfering RNA (siRNA) molecules. However, the most promising attempts to reverse the MDR phenotype have been made with inhibitory compounds targeting P-glycoprotein function.

4.1. Approaches Targeting the Function of MDR-Associated ABC Transporters

4.1.1. INHIBITORS

Based on this early optimism, numerous approaches have been made with so-called first-generation inhibitors of P-glycoprotein representing antagonists that have already been used for other indications, such as the calcium channel blocker verapamil and the immunosuppressive agent cyclosporine A. First-generation inhibitors are themselves substrates for P-glycoprotein and compete with the cytotoxic drug for binding and efflux by the P-glycoprotein pump, thereby limiting the efflux of the drug. As a consequence, intracellular drug concentrations increase, leading to elevated cytotoxicity; the cell becomes chemosensitive. These inhibitors worked with great success on cultured cells to overcome MDR. In the clinic, however, they produced disappointing results. A variety of problems slowed down the optimism of the early years: different intrinsic and/or therapy-induced expression profiles in certain tumors/tissues, or varying correlations of expression and clinical response in certain cancers following chemotherapy. Both might be owing to nonstandardized techniques for expression analysis. Moreover, sequence polymorphisms may also have led to modulated drug transport. In particular, in order to reverse MDR, extremely high inhibitor concentrations were needed, causing unacceptable toxicity. Furthermore, these inhibitors are not transported exclusively by P-glycoprotein, resulting in unpredictable pharmacokinetic interactions when coadministered with the drug.

In addition to the major player, P-glycoprotein, a variety of further MDR-associated genes/proteins have been identified in recent years, mainly the discovery of MRP1 with its family members, or the discovery of BCRP, and, of course, relatives of P-glycoprotein itself *(69)*. The phenotype of MDR could nolonger be attributed to a sole, even well-characterized protein but had to be understood as the net effect of a multifactorial process of an entire panel of resistance genes controlling an array of alternative resistance mechanisms.

Second-generation P-glycoprotein inhibitors, also acting as competitive substrates, were created with the aim of overcoming specifically the P-glycoprotein-mediated resistance. Compared with first-generation inhibitors, they showed less toxicity and greater potency for inhibition of P-glycoprotein. Examples of second-generation inhibitors are valspodar (PSC833, Novartis), a nonimmunosuppressive cyclosporine analog, and biricodar (VX710, Vertex Pharmaceuticals), both designed to restore the effectiveness of chemotherapeutic agents in multidrug resistant tumors. Clinical trials have demonstrated that administration of second-generation inhibitors together with the anticancer drug might lead to reversal of the MDR phenotype, e.g., when one is treating refractory cancers *(26,70)*. However, certain limitations, as seen with the early inhibitors, could not be resolved, such as unacceptable toxicity and interaction with additional transporter molecules.

Third-generation inhibitors were developed based on structure-activity relationships *(70)*. These newly generated compounds inhibit P-glycoprotein more specifically and with greater potency and do usually not interact with other transporter molecules. They are not substrates for a defined ABC transporter, as is described for first- and second-generation inhibitors. Inhibitors of the third-generation bind noncompetitively to the pump. Thereby conformational changes of the transporter protein are caused, hindering ATP hydrolysis. Consequently, drug transport out of the cell is prevented, leading to increased intracellular concentration of the cytotoxic drug and enhanced cytotoxicity. For example, the chemosensitizer zosuquidar (LY335979, Eli Lilly) reversed mitoxantrone resistance in part and vinorelbine resistance completely in P-glycoprotein-overexpressing cells; in MRP1- or BCRP-overexpressing cells, however, drug resistance was not modulated *(71)*. To date, tariquidar has been one of the most potent MDR-modulating agents (XR-9576, Xenova Group plc/QLT Inc). It was applied very successfully, achieving complete MDR reversal at low concentrations, and it holds a long duration of activity in a panel of resistant tumor cells. Tariquidar is now under evaluation in several clinical trials (*see* **Subheading 4.1.2.**).

These results demonstrate the specificity of third-generation inhibitors with respect to the ABC transporter P-glycoprotein. Moreover, it was demonstrated for several newly created inhibitors that the pharmacokinetics of classical MDR-associated drugs such as doxorubicin, vincristine, etoposide, and paclitaxel were not affected in patients. Based on these first findings obtained with the third-generation inhibitors, MDR of cancer cells might be overcome. If the mechanisms of resistance can be overcome, the spectrum of traditional agents and of treatable tumor entities will certainly be extended.

4.1.2. CLINICAL TRIALS

So far, nine randomized clinical studies have been conducted to evaluate the impact of P-glycoprotein inhibitors *(72)*. However, only three of these have shown statistically significant differences in overall survival, those performed in acute myeloid leukemia (AML) *(73)*, breast cancer *(74)*, and lung cancer patients *(75)*. One reason for the disappointing results has been the need for dose reduction of the chemotherapeutic drug in the context of the inhibitor. At present, the U.S. National Institutes of Health (NIH) is recruiting patients for three clinical phase I and II trials to evaluate the impact of the third-generation P-glycoprotein inhibitor tariquidar in solid tumors such as brain tumors, Ewing sarcomas, neuroblastomas, and rhabdomyosarcomas in children, in adrenal cortex neoplasms, as well as in lung, ovarian, and cervical neoplasms, with respect to the anticancer drugs doxorubicin, vinorelbine, vincristine, docetaxel, and etoposide (www.ClinicalTrials.gov). Most of these studies use Tc-99m sestamibi for expressional and functional control of P-glycoprotein.

4.1.3 SURROGATE ASSAY: TC-99M SESTAMIBI

To evaluate the expression and, in particular, the function of MDR1/P-glycoprotein with respect to clinical settings, Tc-99m sestamibi is employed. Tc-99m sestamibi harbors two main features in that context: it is a radionucleotide imaging agent, already in clinical use to determine cardiac dysfunction. Moreover, it is also a substrate and thus is transported by P-glycoprotein. Using this imaging agent, normal tissues and tumor areas with high P-glycoprotein expression can be identified; furthermore, the impact of P-glycoprotein inhibitors, measured as increased intratumoral drug accumulation, can be evaluated. It has been observed, e.g., in normal liver and kidney, that the uptake of Tc-99m sestamibi is increased following treatment with the inhibitors valspodar, biricodar, and tariquidar *(76–78)*. For hepatocellular carcinoma, a correlation of Tc-99m liver imaging with P-glycoprotein expression was reported *(79)*. Furthermore, increased Tc-99m sestamibi accumulation was reported for metastastic cancers following treatment with tariquidar *(78)*. For NSCLC, Tc-99m was used to predict the response to paclitaxel-based chemotherapy on the basis of P-glycoprotein detection, as demonstrated by chest images *(80)*. These findings confirm that MDR inhibitors are able to increase the accumulation of the respective substrate in P-glycoprotein-expressing normal and tumor tissues of patients. Moreover, the inhibitor concentrations achieved at the tumor site are sufficient to modulate P-glycoprotein function and thereby the MDR phenotype *(72,81)*.

At present, the NIH is recruiting patients for a clinical phase II trial to evaluate the use of sestamibi for imaging drug resistance in solid tumors (www.ClinicalTrials.gov). Patients are also being recruited for clinical trials to evaluate the impact of third-generation P-glycoprotein inhibitors in combination with chemotherapy; the monitoring of P-glycoprotein expression and function is carried out by administration of Tc-99m sestamibi. In addition, a correlation of Tc-99m imaging with expression of MRP1 in patients with hepatocellular carcinoma has been shown recently, possibly extending the use of imaging agents to MRP1-mediated MDR *(82)*.

4.1.4. Tyrosine Kinase Inhibitors

Several new molecular cancer therapeutics have been developed in recent years, such as a large variety of tyrosine kinase inhibitors. These agents are known to inhibit malignant cell growth and metastasis. Their therapeutic potential, however, depends on their access to the intracellular target, which might be disturbed by MDR-associated ABC transporters. Iressa (gefitinib), an epidermal growth factor tyrosine kinase inhibitor, as well as Gleevec (imatinib), a BCR-Abl, platelet-derived growth factor receptor (PDGFR) and c-kit tyrosine kinase inhibitor, belong to these recently developed compounds. Both Iressa and Gleevec might interact with MDR1 and also with BCRP as competitive ATP inhibitors; for both, the reversal of chemotherapy resistance has been demonstrated *(83,84)*.

4.1.5. MRP1 and BCRP Inhibitors

Although MDR1/P-glycoprotein is the central molecule in the context of MDR, the aforementioned P-glycoprotein inhibitors may also target additional ABC transporters with different affinities, e.g., biricodar also targeting MRP and BCRP and tariquidar also targeting BCRP in addition to P-glycoprotein *(85,86)*. Specific inhibitors, e.g., MK-571 for MRP1 *(61,87)* or fumitremorgin C for BCRP *(61,88)*, were used in experimental studies and worked successfully in terms of the respective transporter. However, their ability to increase accumulation of anticancer drugs associated with the MRP1- or BCRP-mediated MDR must be determined in a clinical setting.

4.1.6. Antibodies and Immunotoxins

Antibody-directed approaches might represent alternative strategies for reversal of MDR. Monoclonal P-glycoprotein-specific antibodies have been shown to affect the proliferation of P-glycoprotein-expressing tumor cells *(89,90)*. However, the best chemosensitizing results were achieved when the monoclonal antibodies were applied in combination with inhibitors *(91,92)*. An interesting approach is the use of immunotoxins, consisting of monoclonal antibodies coupled to cytotoxic agents. After binding to the antigen and internalization, cytotoxic activity toward P-glycoprotein-expressing cells was demonstrated *(93,94)*.

4.2. Approaches Targeting Transcription, Posttranscription, and Posttranslation

Further interventional strategies affect the control of expression of MDR-associated genes. Several approaches have been used to prevent or disturb transcription of the MDR1 gene, e.g., by using MDR1-specific transcriptional repressors, by cytostatic blocking of induced but not constitutive MDR1 expression, or by targeting MDR1 transcription factors *(86,95–97)*. Moreover, alternative approaches interfere with translational expression by targeting the MDR1 or MRP1 mRNA. These intervention strategies use, e.g., complementary oligodeoxyribonucleotides to form complexes with the target mRNA, so-called antisense RNAs *(98–101)*. Catalytic RNAs, so-called ribozymes, hybridize to a complementary mRNA, thereby catalyzing site-specific cleavage of the substrate. A panel of ribozymes specific for several MDR-associated ABC transporters (MDR1, MRP1, and BCRP) has been successfully applied, leading to reduced expression and reversal of MDR in vitro *(102–104)*. One of the most interesting approaches is the employment of siRNA, also known as posttranscriptional gene silencing. For MDR1 and

BCRP, some promising reports have been published, demonstrating specific expression inhibition by degradation of the complementary mRNA using siRNA as well as by vector-based transfection in vitro and in vivo *(105–108)*.

N-glycosylation and phosphorylation are posttranslational modifications for P-glyco-protein, as well as for other MDR-associated ABC transporters. With the use of glycosylation inhibitors, such as tunicamycin, it turned out that N-glycosylation may contribute to correct folding and/or stabilization of P-glycoprotein; the MDR transport function, however, was not affected *(109)*. Since the phosphorylation of P-glycoprotein is an essential prerequisite for its transporter function, protein kinases represent a potential target for overcoming MDR. Because protein kinase C is known to phosphorylate and thereby activate P-glycoprotein, inhibitors of that enzyme have been used to reverse MDR *(110)*. More selective inhibitors targeting P-glycoprotein directly will certainly improve this approach *(111)*. Although all expression-based intervention approaches work well in experimental settings, we have no data so far for clinical application.s

5. PROSPECTS

MDR, caused by ABC transporter molecules, remains the major cause of inadequate responses in cancer chemotherapy. Forty-eight ABC transporters have been identified through the Human Genome Project. Sixteen of them have known functions, and 14 are discussed in the context of human diseases. Physiological functions are mainly the transport of lipids, bile acids, toxic compounds, and peptides for antigen presentation. Since it is unlikely that many new ABC transporters will be discovered, the phenotype and development of MDR must be elucidated further in the context of the about 10 already known MDR-associated ABC transporters.

Detailed knowledge of these transporter molecules, their sequence polymorphisms, their transcriptional, translational, and posttranslational regulation, and functional features of substrate binding and transport represent the basis for the development of specific and thus successful intervention strategies for MDR reversal in the clinic. Moreover, a patient-individual resistance profiling is desired that will provide the scientific basis for selection and application of specific chemotherapeutic drugs in defined therapy regimes; it would also provide the rationale and essential prerequisite for tailor-made approaches to overcome drug resistance. Therefore, patient-individual response prediction, MDR reversal, and possibly MDR prevention strategies are the ultimate goals to improve chemotherapy, in particular when applied as regional cancer therapy.

REFERENCES

1. Gottesman MM, Fojo T, Bates SE. Multidrug resistance in cancer: role of ATP-dependent transporters. Nat Rev 2002;2:48–58.
2. Borst P, Oude Elferink R. Mammalian ABC transporters in health and diesease. Annu Rev Biochem 2002;71:537–592.
3. Gottesman MM. Mechanisms of cancer drug resistance. Annu Rev Med 2002;53:615–627.
4. Ambudkar SV, Dey S, Hrycyna CA, Ramachandra M, Pastan I, Gottesman MM. Biochemical, cellular, and pharmacological aspects of the multidrug transporter. Annu Rev Pharmacol Toxicol 1999;39:361–398.
5. Dean M, Rzhetsky A, Alleikmets R. The human ATP-binding cassette (ABC) transporter superfamily. Genome Res 2001;11:1156–1166.
6. Juliano RL, Ling V. A surface glycoprotein modulating drug permeability in Chinese hamster ovary cell mutants. Biochim Biophys Acta 1976;455:152–162.

7. Riordan JR, Ling V. Purification of P-glycoprotein from plasma membrane vesicles of Chinese hamster ovary cell mutants with reduced colchicine permeability. J Biol Chem 1979;254:12701–12705.

8. Ueda K, Cornwell MM, Gottesman MM, et al. The mdr1 gene, responsible for multidrug-resistance, codes for P-glycoprotein. Biochem Biophys Res Commun 1986;141:956–962.

9. Ueda K, Cardarelli C, Gottesman MM, Pastan I. Expression of a full-length cDNA for the human MDR1 gene confers resistance to colchicine, doxorubicin, and vinblastine. Proc Natl Acad Sci U S A 1987;84:3004–3008.

10. Thiebaut F, Tsuruo T, Hamada H, Gottesman MM, Pastan I, Willingham MC. Cellular localization of the multidrug-resistance gene product P-glycoprotein in normal human tissues. Proc Natl Acad Sci U S A 1987;84:7735–7738.

11. Cordon-Cardo C, O'Brien JP, Boccia J, Casals D, Bertino JR, Melamed MR. Expression of the multidrug resistance gene product (P-glycoprotein) in human normal and tumor tissues. J Histochem Cytochem 1990;38:1277–1287.

12. Fojo AT, Ueda K, Slamon DJ, Poplack DG, Gottesman MM, Pastan I. Expression of a multidrug-resistance gene in human tumors and tissues. Proc Natl Acad Sci U S A 1987;84:265–269.

13. Litman T, Druley TE, Stein WD, Bates SE. From MDR to MXR: new understanding of multidrug resistance systems, their properties and clinical significance. Cell Mol Life Sci 2001;58:931–959.

14. Goldstein LJ, Galski H, Fojo A, et al. Expression of a multidrug resistance gene in human cancers. J Natl Cancer Inst 1989;81:116–124.

15. Ho GT, Moodie FM, Satsangi J. Multidrug resistance 1 gene (P-glycoprotein 170): an important determinant in gastrointestinal disease? Gut 2003;52:759–766.

16. Kohno K, Sato S, Takano H, Matsuo K, Kuwano M. The direct activation of human multidrug resistance gene (MDR1) by anticancer agents. Biochem Biophys Res Commun 1989;165:1415–1421.

17. Chin KV, Tanaka S, Darlington G, Pastan I, Gottesman MM. Heat shock and arsenite increase expression of the multidrug resistance (MDR1) gene in human renal carcinoma cells. J Biol Chem 1990;265:221–226.

18. Chaudhary PM, Roninson IB. Induction of multidrug resistance in human cells by transient exposure to different chemotherapeutic drugs. J Natl Cancer Inst 1993;85;632–636.

19. Stein U, Walther W, Lemm M, Naundorf H, Fichtner I. Development and characterisation of novel human multidrug resistant mammary carcinoma lines in vitro and in vivo. Int J Cancer 1997;72:885–891.

20. Stein U, Jurchott K, Walther W, Bergmann S, Schlag PM, Royer HD. Hyperthermia-induced nuclear translocation of transcription factor YB-1 leads to enhanced expression of multidrug resistance-related ABC transporters. J Biol Chem 2001;276:28562–28569.

21. Hrycyna CA. Molecular genetic analysis and biochemical characterization of mammalian P-glycoproteins involved in multidrug resistance. Semin Cell Dev Biol 2001;12:247–256.

22. Scotto KW. Transcriptional regulation of ABC drug transporters. Oncogene 2003;22:7496–7511.

23. Stein U, Walther W, Wunderlich V. Point mutations in the mdr1 promoter of human osteosarcomas are associated with in vitro responsiveness to multidrug resistance relevant drugs. Eur J Cancer 1994;30A:1541–1545.

24. Stein U, Walther W, Shoemaker RH. Vincristine induction of mutant and wild-type human multidrug-resistance promoters is cell-type-specific and dose-dependent. J Cancer Res Clin Oncol 1996;122:275–282.

25. Brinkmann U, Eichelbaum M. Polymorphisms in the ABC drug transporter gene MDR1. Pharmacogenomics J 2001;1:59–64.

26. Leonard GD, Fojo T, Bates SE. The role of ABC transporters in clinical practice. Oncologist 2003;8:411–424.

27. Di Nicolantonio F, Mercer SJ, Knight LA, et al. Cancer cell adaptation to chemotherapy. BMC Cancer 2005;5:78–94.

28. Grogan TM, Spier CM, Salmon SE, et al. P-glycoprotein expression in human plasma cell myeloma: correlation with prior chemotherapy. Blood 1993;81:490–495.

29. Chevillard S, Pouillart P, Beldjord C, et al. Sequential assessment of multidrug resistance phenotype and measurement of S-phase fraction as predictive markers of breast cancer response to neoadjuvant chemotherapy. Cancer 1996;77:292–300.

30. Mechetner E, Kyshtoobayeva A, Zonis S, et al. Levels of multidrug resistance (MDR1) P-glycoprotein expression by human breast cancer correlate with in vitro resistance to taxol and doxorubicin. Clin Cancer Res 1998;4:389–398.

31. van der Zee AG, Hollema H, Suurmeijer AJ, et al. Value of P-glycoprotein, glutathione S-transferase pi, c-erbB-2, and p53 as prognostic factors in ovarian carcinomas. J Clin Oncol 1995;13:70–78.

32. Riou GF, Zhou D, Ahomadegbe JC, Gabillot M, Duvillard P, Lhomme C. Expression of multidrug-resistance (MDR1) gene in normal epithelia and in invasive carcinomas of the uterine cervix. J Natl Cancer Inst 1990;82:1493–1496.

33. Abolhoda A, Wilson AE, Ross H, Danenberg PV, Burt M, Scotto KW. Rapid activation of MDR1 expression in human metastatic sarcoma following in vivo exposure to doxorubicin. Clin Cancer Res 1999;5:3352–3356.

34. Stein U, Jurchott K, Schlafke M, Hohenberger P. Expression of multidrug resistance genes MVP, MDR1, and MRP1 determined sequentially before, during, and after hyperthermic isolated limb perfusion of soft tissue sarcoma and melanoma patients. J Clin Oncol 2002;20:3282–3292.

35. Scheffer GL, Schroeijers AB, Izquierdo MA, Wiemer EA, Scheper RJ. Lung resistance-related protein/major vault protein and vaults in multidrug-resistant cancer. Curr Opin Oncol 2000;12:550–556.

36. Leith CP, Kopecky KJ, Chen IM, et al. Frequency and clinical significance of the expression of the multidrug resistance proteins MDR1/P-glycoprotein, MRP1, and LRP in acute myeloid leukemia: a Southwest Oncology Group Study. Blood 1999;943:1086–1099.

37. Broxterman HJ, Sonneveld P, van Putten WJ, et al. P-glycoprotein in primary acute myeloid leukemia and treatment outcome of idarubicin/cytosine arabinoside-based induction therapy. Leukemia 2000;14:1018–1024.

38. Chan HS, Thorner PS, Haddad G, Ling V. Immunohistochemical detection of P-glycoprotein: prognostic correlation in soft tissue sarcoma of childhood. J Clin Oncol 1990;4:689–704.

39. Baldini N, Scotlandi K, Barbanti-Brodano G, et al. Expression of P-glycoprotein in high-grade osteosarcomas in relation to clinical outcome. N Engl J Med 1995;333:1380–1385.

40. Stein U, Shoemaker RH, Schlag PM. MDR1 gene expression: evaluation of its use as a molecular marker for prognosis and chemotherapy of bone and soft tissue sarcomas. Eur J Cancer 1996;32A:86–92.

41. Trock BJ, Leonessa F, Clarke R. Multidrug resistance in breast cancer: a meta-analysis of MDR1/gp170 expression and its possible functional significance. J Natl Cancer Inst 1997;89:917–931.

42. Chintamani, Singh JP, Mittal MK, et al. Role of P-glycoprotein expression in predicting response to neoadjuvant chemotherapy in breast cancer—a prospective clinical study. World J Surg Oncol 2005;3:61.

43. Cole SPC, Deeley RG. Multidrug resistance mediated by the ATP-binding cassette transporter MRP. BioEssays 1998;20:31–940.

44. Loe DW, Deeley RG, Cole SP. Characterization of vincristin transport by the (M)r 190,000 multidrug resistance protein (MRP): evidence for cotransport with reduced glutathione. Cancer Res 1998;58:5130–5136.

45. Borst P, Evers R, Kool M, Wijnholds J. A family of drug transporters: the multidrug resistance-associated proteins. J Natl Cancer Inst 2000;92:1295–1302.

46. Deeley RG, Cole SP. Substrate recognition and transport by multidrug resistance protein 1 (ABCC1). FEBS Lett 2006;580:1103–1111.

47. Nooter K, Westerman AM, Flens MJ, et al. Expression of the multidrug resistance-associated protein (MRP) gene in human cancers. Clin Cancer Res 1995;1:1301–1310.

48. Abbaszadegan MR, Futscher BW, Klimecki WT, List A, Dalton WS. Analysis of multidrug resistance-associated protein (MRP) messenger RNA in normal and malignant hematopoietic cells. Cancer Res 1994;54:4676–4679.

49. Filipits M, Suchomel RW, Dekan G, et al. MRP and MDR1 gene expression in primary breast carcinomas. Clin Cancer Res 1996;2:1231–1237.

50. Young LC, Campling BG, Voskoglou-Nomikos T, Cole SP, Deeley RG, Gerlach JH. Expression of multidrug resistance protein-related genes in lung cancer: correlation with drug response. Clin Cancer Res 1999;5:673–680.

51. Oda Y, Dockhorn-Dworniczak B, Jurgens H, Roessner A. Expression of multidrug resistance-associated protein gene in Ewing's sarcoma and malignant peripheral neuroectodermal tumor of bone. J Cancer Res Clin Oncol 1997;123:237–239.

52. Kruh GD, Belinsky MG. The MRP family of drug efflux pumps. Oncogene 2003;22:7537–7552.

53. Nooter K, Brutel de la Riviere G, Look MP, et al. The prognostic significance of expression of the multidrug resistance-associated protein (MRP) in primary breast cancer. Br J Cancer 1997;76:486–493.

54. Allikmets R, Schriml LM, Hutchinson A, Romano-Spica V, Dean M. A human placenta-specific ATP-binding cassette gene (ABCP) on chromosome 4q22 that is involved in multidrug resistance. Cancer Res 1998;58:5337–5339.

55. Doyle LA, Yang W, Abruzzo LV, et al. A multidrug resistance transporter from human MCF-7 breast cancer cells. Proc Natl Acad Sci U S A 1998;95:15665–15670.

56. Miyake K, Mickley L, Litman T, et al. Molecular cloning of cDNAs which are highly overexpressed in mitoxantrone-resistant cells: demonstration of homology to ABC transport genes. Cancer Res 1999;59:8–13.

57. Ross DD, Yang W, Abruzzo LV, et al. Atypical multidrug resistance: breast cancer resistance protein messenger RNA expression in mitoxantrone-selected cell lines. J Natl Cancer Inst 1999;91:429–433.

58. Maliepaard M, van Gastelen MA, de Jong LA, et al. Overexpression of the BCRP/MXR/ABCP gene in a topotecan-selected ovarian tumor cell line. Cancer Res 1999;59:4559–4563.

59. Allen JD, Brinkhuis RF, Wijnholds J, Schinkel AH. The mouse Bcrp/Mxr/Abcp gene: amplification and overexpression in cell lines selected for resistance to topotecan, mitoxantrone, or doxorubicin. Cancer Res 1999;59:4237–4241.

60. Litman T, Brangi M, Hudson E, et al. The multidrug-resistant phenotype associated with overexpression of the new ABC half-transporter, MXR (ABCG2). J Cell Sci 2000;113:2011–2021.

61. Stein U, Lage H, Jordan A, et al. Impact of BCRP/MXR, MRP1, and MDR1/P-glycoprotein on thermoresistant variants of atypical and classical multidrug resistant cancer cells. Int J Cancer 2002;97:751–760.

62. Honjo Y, Hrycyna CA, Yan QW, et al. Acquired mutations in the MXR/BCRP/ABCP gene alter substrate specificity in MXR/BCRP/ABCP-overexpressing cells. Cancer Res 2001;61:6635–6639.

63. Allen JD, Jackson SC, Schinkel AH. A mutation hot spot in the Bcrp1 (Abcg2) multidrug transporter in mouse cell lines selected for doxorubicin resistance. Cancer Res 2002;62:2294–2299.

64. Diestra JE, Scheffer GL, Catala I, et al. Frequent expression of the multi-drug resistance associated protein BCRP/MXR/ABCP/ABCG2 in human tumors detected by the BXP-21 monoclonal antibody in paraffin-embedded material. J Pathol 2002;198:213–219.

65. Gillet JP, Efferth T, Steinbach D, et al. Microarray-based detection of multidrug resistance in human tumor cells by expression profiling of ATP-binding cassette transporter genes. Cancer Res 2004;64:8987–8993.

66. Szakacs G, Annereau JP, Lababidi S, et al. Predicting drug sensitivity and resistance: profiling ABC transporter genes in cancer cells. Cancer Cell 2004;6:129–137.

67. Gyorffy B, Serra V, Jurchott K, et al. Prediction of doxorubicin sensitivity in breast tumors based on gene expression profiles of drug-resistant cell lines correlates with patient survival. Oncogene 2005;24:7542–7551.

68. Reynolds T. Research on drug resistance unearths many molecules, many mechanisms. J Natl Cancer Inst 1998;20:1120–1122.

69. Klein I, Sarkadi B, Varadi A. An inventory of the human ABC proteins. Biochim Biophys Acta 1999;1461:237–262.

70. Thomas H, Coley HM. Overcoming multidrug resistance in cancer: an update on the clinical strategy of inhibiting P-glycoprotein. Cancer Control 2003;10:159–165.

71. Shepard RL, Cao J, Starling JJ, Dantzig AH. Modulation of P-glycoprotein but not MRP1– or BCRP-mediated drug resistance by LY335979. Int J Cancer 2003;103:121–125.

72. Mahadevan D, Shirahatti N. Strategies for targeting the multidrug resistance-1 (MDR1)/P-gp transporter in human malignancies. Curr Cancer Drug Targets 2005;5:445–455.

73. List AF, Kopecky KJ, Willman CL, et al. Benefit of cyclosporine modulation of drug resistance in patients with poor-risk acute myeloid leukemia: a Southwest Oncology Group study. Blood 2001;98:3212–3220.

74. Belpomme D, Gauthier S, Pujade-Lauraine E, et al. Verapamil increases the survival of patients with anthracycline-resistant metastatic breast carcinoma. Ann Oncol 2000;11:1471–1476.

75. Millward MJ, Cantwell BM, Munro NC, Robinson A, Corris PA, Harris AL. Oral verapamil with chemotherapy for advanced non-small cell lung cancer: a randomised study. Br J Cancer 1993;67:1031–1035.

76. Chen CC, Meadows B, Regis J, et al. Detection of in vivo P-glycoprotein inhibition by PSC 833 using Tc-99m sestamibi. Clin Cancer Res 1997;3:545–552.

77. Peck RA, Hewett J, Harding MW, et al. Phase I and pharmacokinetic study of the novel MDR1 and MRP1 inhibitor biricodar administered alone and in combination with doxorubicin. J Clin Oncol 2001;19:3130–3141.

78. Agrawal M, Abraham J, Balis FM, et al. Increased 99mTc-sestamibi accumulation in normal liver and drug-resistant tumors after the administration of the glycoprotein inhibitor, XR9576. Clin Cancer Res 2003;9:650–656.

79. Chang CS, Yang SS, Yeh HZ, Kao CH, Chen GH. Tc-99m MIBI liver imaging for hepatocellular carcinoma: correlation with P-glycoprotein-multidrug-resistance gene expression. Hepatogastroenterology 2004;51:211–214.

80. Shiau YC, Tsai SC, Wang JJ, Ho YJ, Ho ST, Kao CH. Technetium-99m tetrofosmin chest imaging related to P-glycoprotein expression for predicting the response with paclitaxel-based chemotherapy for non-small cell lung cancer. Lung 2001;179:197–207.

81. Bates SE, Chen C, Robey R, Kang M, Figg WD, Fojo T. Reversal of multidrug resistance: lessons from clinical oncology. Novartis Found Symp 2002;243:83–96.

82. Wang H, Chen XP, Qiu FZ. Correlation of expression of multidrug resistance protein and messenger RNA with 99mTc-methoxyisobutyl isonitrile (MIBI) imaging in patients with hepatocellular carcinoma. World J Gastroenterol 2004;10:1281–1285.

83. Yang CH, Huang CJ, Yang CS, et al. Gefitinib reverses chemotherapy resistance in gefitinib-insensitive multidrug resistant cancer cells expressing ATP-binding cassette family protein. Cancer Res 2005;65:6943–6949.

84. Yeheskely-Hayon D, Regev R, Eytan GD, Dann EJ. The tyrosine kinase inhibitors imatinib and AG957 reverse multidrug resistance in a chronic myelogenous leukemia cell line. Leuk Res 2005;29:793–802.

85. Polgar O, Bates SE. ABC transporters in the balance: is there a role in multidrug resistance? Biochem Soc Trans 2005;33:241–245.

86. Borowski E, Bontemps-Gracz MM, Piwkowska A. Strategies for overcoming ABC-transporters-mediated multidrug resistance (MDR) of tumor cells. Acta Biochim Pol 2005;52:609–627.

87. Gekeler V, Ise W, Sanders KH, Ulrich WR, Beck J. The leukotriene LTD4 receptor antagonist MK571 specifically modulates MRP associated multidrug resistance. Biochem Biophys Res Commun 1995;208:345–352.

88. Allen JD, van Loevezijn A, Lakhai JM, et al. Potent and specific inhibition of the breast cancer resistance protein multidrug transporter in vitro and in mouse intestine by a novel analogue of fumitremorgin C. Mol Cancer Ther 2002;1:417–425.

89. Tsuruo T, Hamada H, Sato S, Heike Y. Inhibition of multidrug-resistant human tumor growth in athymic mice by anti-P-glycoprotein monoclonal antibodies. Jpn J Cancer Res 1989;80:627–631.

90. Mechetner EB, Roninson IB. Efficient inhibition of P-glycoprotein-mediated multidrug resistance with a monoclonal antibody. Proc Natl Acad Sci U S A 1992;89:5824–5828.

91. Naito M, Tsuge H, Kuroko C, et al. Enhancement of cellular accumulation of cyclosporine by anti-P-glycoprotein monoclonal antibody MRK-16 and synergistic modulation of multidrug resistance. J Natl Cancer Inst 1993;85:311–316.

92. Watanabe T, Naito M, Kokubu N, Tsuruo T. Regression of established tumors expressing P-glycoprotein by combinations of Adriamycin, cyclosporin derivatives, and MRK-16 antibodies. J Natl Cancer Inst 1997;89:512–518.

93. FitzGerald DJ, Willingham MC, Cardarelli CO, et al. A monoclonal antibody-Pseudomonas toxin conjugate that specifically kills multidrug-resistant cells. Proc Natl Acad Sci U S A 1987;84:4288–4292.

94. Efferth T, Volm M. Antibody-directed therapy of multidrug-resistant tumor cells. Med Oncol Tumor Pharmacother 1992;9:11–19.

95. Jin S, Gorfajn B, Faircloth G, Scotto KW. Ecteinascidin 743, a transcription-targeted chemotherapeutic that inhibits MDR1 activation. Proc Natl Acad Sci U S A 2000;97:6775–6779.

96. Tanaka H, Ohshima N, Ikenoya M, Komori K, Katoh F, Hidaka H. HMN-176, an active metabolite of the synthetic antitumor agent HMN-214, restores chemosensitivity to multidrug-resistant cells by targeting the transcription factor NF-Y. Cancer Res 2003;63:6942–6947.

97. Xu D, Ye D, Fisher M, Juliano RL. Selective inhibition of P-glycoprotein expression in multidrug-resistant tumor cells by a designed transcriptional regulator. J Pharmacol Exp Ther 2002;302:963–971.

98. Garcia-Chaumont C, Seksek O, Grzybowska J, Borowski E, Bolard J. Delivery systems for antisense oligonucleotides. Pharmacol Ther 2000;87:255–277.

99. Pakunlu RI, Cook TJ, Minko T. Simultaneous modulation of multidrug resistance and antiapoptotic cellular defense by MDR1 and BCL-2 targeted antisense oligonucleotides enhances the anticancer efficacy of doxorubicin. Pharm Res 2003;20:351–359.

100. Matsumoto Y, Miyake K, Kunishio K, Tamiya T, Seigo N. Reduction of expression of the multidrug resistance protein (MRP)1 in glioma cells by antisense phosphorothioate oligonucleotides. J Med Invest 2004;51:194–201.
101. Kang H, Fisher MH, Xu D, et al. Inhibition of MDR1 gene expression by chimeric HNA antisense oligonucleotides. Nucleic Acids Res 2004;32:4411–4419.
102. Kobayashi H, Takemura Y, Wang FS, Oka T, Ohnuma T. Retrovirus-mediated transfer of anti-MDR1 hammerhead ribozymes into multidrug-resistant human leukemia cells: screening for effective target sites. Int J Cancer 1999;81:944–950.
103. Nagata J, Kijima H, Hatanaka H, Aet al. Reversal of drug resistance using hammerhead ribozymes against multidrug resistance-associated protein and multidrug resistance 1 gene. Int J Oncol 2002;21:1021–1026.
104. Kowalski P, Stein U, Scheffer GL, Lage H. Modulation of the atypical multidrug-resistant phenotype by a hammerhead ribozyme directed against the ABC transporter BCRP/MXR/ABCG2. Cancer Gene Ther 2002;9:579–586.
105. Wu H, Hait WN, Yang JM. Small interfering RNA-induced suppression of MDR1 (P-glycoprotein) restores sensitivity to multidrug-resistant cancer cells. Cancer Res 2003;63:1515–1519.
106. Li WT, Zhou GY, Song XR, Chi WL, Ren RM, Wang XW. Modulation of BCRP mediated atypical multidrug resistance phenotype by RNA interference. Neoplasma 2005;52:219–224.
107. Pichler A, Zelcer N, Prior JL, Kuil AJ, Piwnica-Worms D. In vivo RNA interference-mediated ablation of MDR1 P-glycoprotein. Clin Cancer Res 2005;11:4487–4494.
108. Shi Z, Liang YJ, Chen ZS, Wang XW, et al. Reversal of MDR1/P-glycoprotein-mediated multidrug resistance by vector-based RNA interference in vitro and in vivo. cancer biol ther 2006;5:39–47.
109. Schinkel AH, Kemp S, Dolle M, Rudenko G, Wagenaar E. N-glycosylation and deletion mutants of the human MDR1 P-glycoprotein. J Biol Chem 1993;268:7474–7481.
110. Sato W, Yusa K, Naito M, Tsuruo T. Staurosporine, a potent inhibitor of C-kinase, enhances drug accumulation in multidrug-resistant cells. Biochem Biophys Res Commun 1990;173:1252–1257.
111. Gupta KP, Ward NE, Gravitt KR, Bergman PJ, O'Brian CA. Partial reversal of multidrug resistance in human breast cancer cells by an N-myristoylated protein kinase C-alpha pseudosubstrate peptide. J Biol Chem 1996;271:2102–2111.

2   Pharmacological Background

Hans Gelderblom, MD, Joost Rothbarth, MD, Cornelius J. H. van de Velde, MD, and Henk-Jan Guchelaar, PharmD

CONTENTS:

SUMMARY

The pharmacological rational for regional cancer therapy is based on delivering a high dose intensity of the chemotherapeutic drug, resulting in an advantageous tumor cure/normal tissue complication differential (high therapeutic ratio). Only patients with an anatomically confined tumor and technical feasibility of antitumor therapy administration are expected to reach clinical benefit. Specific pharmacological characteristics of the delivered drug are of potential additional benefit. The pharmacological background of intraperitoneal chemotherapy, isolated hepatic perfusion, and isolated extremity perfusion are given as an example of the advantages and opportunities of regional anticancer therapy.

Key Words: Intraperitoneal; chemotherapy; isolated hepatic perfusion; extremity perfusion; pharmacology; regional cancer therapy.

1. INTRODUCTION

Regional cancer therapy is based on the concept of delivering a high dose intensity to an anatomically confined tumor site. The effectiveness of the procedure depends on the biology of the tumor (*see* Chapter 1), the technique (*see* Chapter 3), and the pharmacology

From: *Cancer Drug Discovery and Development: Regional Cancer Therapy*
Edited by: P. M. Schlag and U. S, Stein © Humana Press Inc., Totowa, NJ

of the administered antitumor drug. This chapter will mainly focus on the pharmacological background of drugs used in the setting of regional therapy using examples of intraperitoneal chemotherapy, isolated hepatic perfusion, and isolated extremity perfusion.

2. THE IDEAL DRUG FOR REGIONAL CANCER THERAPY

Not every available cytotoxic drug is appropriate for use in regional cancer therapy. Important features of a drug making it a good candidate for regional therapy are discussed in this paragraph.

An important aim of regional cancer therapy is exposing the tumor to a high dose of the chemotherapeutic drug for a period long enough to exerts its antitumor effect. To reach this, several physical characteristics of the drug molecule may be of influence. Drugs with a high molecular weight are expected to give a prolonged retention time at the tumor site. However, drugs with a molecular weight over 5000 Daltons cannot diffuse across membranes of vessels and cells and may therefore be unable to reach the microenvironment of the tumor. Moreover, lipophilic compounds more easily diffuse across the lipid bilayers of membranes than hydrophilic compounds and may therefore penetrate the tumor. In contrast to passive diffusion, it is known that active transporters such as multidrug resistance-associated protein 1 (MRP1), breast cancer resistance protein (BRCP), and multidrug resistance protein 1 (MDR1), all now known as the ATP-binding cassette transporters (ABC transporters), play an important role in drug exposure at the individual tumor cells (1). Since these active transporters act as efflux pumps essentially for so-called naturally occurring chemotherapeutic drugs such as vinca alkaloids, paclitaxel, methotrexate, and etoposide, they are associated with drug resistance. Moreover, germline mutations in the genes encoding for these transporters are described and can be of influence on transporter function. Therefore, microdistribution of chemotherapeutic drugs may be associated with individual genotype and may influence tumor exposure. The pharmacological impact of these genetic factors may even be more important than the achieved high local drug concentrations as a result of regional drug delivery.

Obviously, to allow administration of high drug doses, a high water solubility is essential. Drugs are usually bound to proteins (albumin) in the plasma or perfusate to some extent. Since the unbound fraction of the drug is capable of distributing and exerting its cytotoxic action, low protein binding is a favorable characteristic for a drug used in regional cancer therapy. In regional therapy techniques using perfusates or other nonblood volumes, the extent of protein binding may be different from that in blood. Indeed, in a study of cisplatin in hyperthermic isolated limb perfusion, using a perfusate consisting of dextran solution, plasma, red blood cells, sodium bicarbonate, and heparin, a free drug fraction was found varying from 100% at the start of perfusion to 40% at the end of the 60-min perfusion period (2), which is very high and favorable compared with 5 to 10% at normal intravenous infusion.

Some chemotherapeutic drugs, such as cyclophosphamide and irinotecan, are prodrugs and need metabolic activation before the cytotoxic specimen is available. Generally, these types of drugs are not used in regional cancer therapy since their application is confined to a local region, and organs involved in metabolic activation are not reached. Drugs applied in hepatic perfusion and that need hepatic activation may form an exception.

After administration the drug is cleared from its local site. Preferably, local drug clearance is lower compared with systemic drug clearance. If so, this leads to prolonged drug retention at the local site, whereas systemic exposure, and thus expected systemic toxicity, is minimal.

Several mechanisms of action of chemotherapeutic drugs are known, such as DNA alkylating agents and antimetabolites, ultimately resulting in apoptotic or necrotic cell death. For a drug to be used in regional therapy, several features regarding mechanism of action are important. The drug should have a cytotoxic rather than a cytostatic mechanism of action, because the latter may require longer exposure time. Moreover, a steep concentration-effect relationship is essential since this is the basic rationale for delivering high dose intensity. Also, the drug should exert its antitumor effect after a relatively short exposure time.

Theoretically, beneficial effects of regional therapy are anticipated, especially in the treatment of poorly vascularized tumors, such as sarcoma, because in these tumors the drug concentration may be rate limiting for exposure to the drug. Therefore, drugs characterized by good penetration into and binding to tumor tissue and tumor cells are thought to be good candidates. Selective drug accumulations in malignant cells or tissues may be favorable for drug toxicity in normal cells exposed in the local region.

Finally, drugs with specific toxicity toward organs or tissues at the site of administration may cause (expected) toxicity when applied in regional therapy at high doses. For example, drugs with known hepatotoxic potential are not good candidates for hepatic perfusion.

3. PHARMACOLOGICAL BACKGROUND OF INTRAPERITONEAL CHEMOTHERAPY

Although intraperitoneal (i.p.) chemotherapy is hampered by poor drug distribution from surgical adhesions, inadequate drug penetration into tumor nodules or tumor entrapped in scar tissue, and repeated failures with long-term peritoneal access, survival advantages in several perioperative i.p. chemotherapy phase III studies have been reported *(3)*. In perioperative i.p. chemotherapy, these logistical problems may no longer occur. Much of the success of i.p. chemotherapy is related to exposure of the tumors within the peritoneal cavity to the higher concentrations of antineoplastic agents for longer periods that can be achieved with systemic drug administration. The antitumor effect is dependent on duration of exposure and on the drug concentration in contact with the tumor. As with other nonhepatic regional therapies, it is important that the drug does not need hepatic metabolism to its active form. Also, high molecular weight improves dwelling time and thus local anticancer effects. The solvent used to administer the drug is of importance since it can increase local drug concentrations *(4)*. For instance, the unique and favorable pharmacokinetic profile of paclitoxel (Taxol) for regional therapy is a result of paclitaxel's solvent vehicle CremophorEL (CrEL), a nonionic castor oil derivative *(5)*.

It has been demonstrated that at high local concentrations, which can be reached especially by i.p. administration, paclitaxel is entrapped in CrEL micelles *(6)*. This phenomenon may account for the prolonged (peritoneal) activity at high concentrations such as that reported for intravesical treatment *(7)*; thus paclitaxel distribution will depend on CrEL pharmacokinetics. It is also important to study drug disposition when chemotherapy is administered to confined spaces such as the peritoneal cavity. In other words, what is the systemic exposure, and consequently the risk for systemic side effects after local therapy? This has been studied in an i.p. bioavailability study measuring i.p. and i.v.

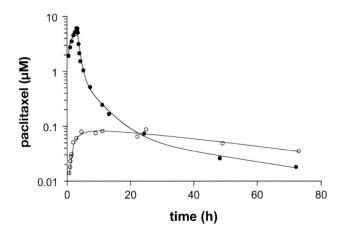

Fig. 1. Representative plasma concentration-time profiles of total paclitaxel after i.p. (open symbols) and i.v. (closed symbols) delivery of paclitaxel formulated in a mixture of CrEL-ethanol USP (1:1, v/v). (Data from Gelderblom et al., with permission *[4]*.)

concentrations of paclitaxel after administration of Taxol *(4)*. Following i.p. administration, paclitaxel concentrations in plasma were initially less than those following i.v. administration, and several hours were required for equilibrium to be attained between the peritoneal cavity and the systemic circulation. The limited surface area for paclitaxel diffusion relative to the volumes of fluid, and the fact that the peritoneal fluids are not well stirred, likely contributed to the slow equilibrium kinetics. Nevertheless, concentrations in plasma equivalent to that after i.v. administration were achieved after approximately 20 h in all patients, and paclitaxel appeared to be more slowly eliminated from the peritoneal cavity than from plasma (Fig. 1). This indicates slow peritoneal clearance of paclitaxel and high peritoneal-plasma concentration ratios of >1000 after i.p. drug administration *(8)*. These authors also documented the persistence of significant peritoneal paclitaxel levels even at 1 wk after initial i.p. drug administration, already suggesting very slow peritoneal clearance and continuous exposure of the peritoneal cavity to active concentrations of paclitaxel *(9)*.

4. PHARMACOLOGICAL BACKGROUND OF ISOLATED HEPATIC INFUSION

Isolated hepatic perfusion (IHP) involves a method of complete vascular isolation of the liver to allow regional chemotherapeutic treatment of liver tumors. IHP has been proposed as treatment modality for different kinds of nonresectable liver tumors, but most experience has been obtained with colorectal liver metastases. During the procedure the blood circulation of the liver is temporarily isolated from the systemic circulation and the liver is perfused through a recirculating perfusion circuit.

The major advantage of isolated perfusion is the possibility of treating tumors with drug levels that would be highly toxic if applied systemically. Furthermore, antitumor agents that cannot be administered systemically at therapeutical dose levels because of their toxicity, such as tumor necrosis factor-α (TNF-α), can be used. Finally, hyperther-

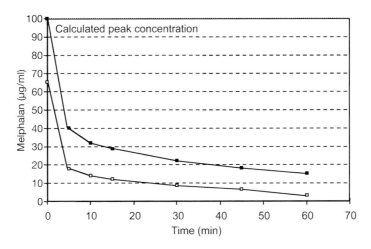

Fig. 2. Concentration of melphalan in perfusate during 1-h perfusion after addition of either 1.5 mg/kg (open symbols) or 3.0 mg/kg (closed symbols) melphalan to the isolated circuit. The calculated melphalan peak concentration is indicated. (Data from Vahrmeijer et al., with permission [12].)

mia, which is known to increase the efficacy of several drugs, can be applied by heating the circulating perfusate.

Several drugs have been used in IHP studies, including 5-fluorouracil (5-FU), mitomycin C, cisplatin, and melphalan with or without TNF-α (10). The recent clinical studies mainly employed IHP with melphalan with or without TNF-α. Melphalan is an alkylating agent with a steep dose-response curve that is effective against colorectal cancer after a relatively short exposure time and, therefore, is highly suitable for application in IHP (11). A phase I study revealed a maximally tolerated melphalan dose of 3.0 mg/kg, which is approximately fourfold the maximum systemically tolerated dose of melphalan (12). Since melphalan combined with TNF-α has shown synergistic antitumor effects in experimental studies and hyperthermia enhances the cytotoxic effect of several alkylating agents such as melphalan, melphalan treatment is combined with moderate hyperthermia (38.5–40°C) and/or TNF-α in most IHP regimens (10). When melphalan is combined with TNF-α its maximum tolerated dose (MTD) is reduced to 1.5 mg/kg .

Different procedures of drug administration during IHP have been used: bolus or continuous infusion, to the whole perfusate or in the hepatic artery (HA). The pharmacokinetic consequences of these modes of administration are expected to affect antitumor efficacy and hepatotoxicity. As shown by Vahrmeijer et al. (12), the concentration of bolus-administered melphalan in this perfusate rapidly declines in the first 5 to 10 min of its circulation, indicating a rapid uptake of melphalan by the (tumor.bearing) liver (Fig. 2). As a result, tumor exposure to high concentrations of melphalan is relatively short.

Based on the obvious advantage of intraarterial melphalan infusion in terms of prolonged high tumor exposure to cytostatics, it might be preferable to administer melphalan by continuous infusion in the HA instead of by a single bolus administered in the whole perfusate: infusing melphalan in the HA directly over a certain period would, theoretically, lead to more selective tumor exposure to melphalan and also to prolonged exposure of the tumors to high melphalan concentrations.

However, the optimum conditions (duration, concentration) of the intraarterial melphalan infusion in relation to its antitumor effect and safety have not yet been clarified. For instance, should the melphalan dose be infused over a short or long period during the vascular isolation of the liver? Obviously, a short infusion time of the cytostatic compound in a clinical setting leads to a shorter duration of the procedure and is therefore preferable. However, this can only be justified when the antitumor effect is equal or better and the (hepato)toxicity is not increased. In an in vivo rat model for liver tumors, the difference in tumor and liver uptake, antitumor effect, and hepatotoxicity of 5- and 20-min arterial melphalan infusion of a fixed melphalan dose was studied *(13)*. No difference in melphalan content of tumor/liver tissue and tumor response was found between the two treatment schedules. However, hepatotoxicity was strongly affected by the perfusion duration and thus melphalan concentration: severe cholangiofibrosis occurred in eight of nine rats treated with a 5-min infusion, but in only one of eight rats treated with a 20-min infusion of the same dose of melphalan. These results showed that tumor response was not affected by melphalan *concentration* as long as the tumors were exposed to the same *total dose* of melphalan. However, for toxicity, the concentration-toxicity curve appeared to be very steep, indicating that once the toxicity threshold concentration is reached, a small increase in melphalan concentration leads to a large increase in hepatotoxicity.

Complete vascular isolation of the liver during IHP offers the unique opportunity to control fully the perfusion flow and direction through the liver. Both may affect drug delivery to both tumors and liver tissue and thus antitumor efficacy and hepatotoxicity. Changing the perfusion direction could theoretically reduce liver toxicity without affecting antitumor efficacy. Liver tumors are almost exclusively perfused by the HA *(14)* and, therefore, the reversion of the venous blood stream through the liver should not affect the tumor exposure to arterially administered chemotherapy. Liver parenchyma, however, is perfused by both the portal vein and the HA. Studies of the blood supply of the liver show that the hepatic arterioles terminate in the first third of the sinusoids (zone 1) via an indirect or direct pathway *(15,16)*. As a result, the arterial blood reaches all three zones during normal (orthograde) single-pass perfusion, but only zone 1 of the liver sinusoids during retrograde perfusion. Thus, liver exposure to arterially infused drugs should be reduced during retrograde perfusion. An experimental study using a rat model for colorectal liver tumors indeed showed that melphalan content in tumor tissue was unaffected by retrograde IHP, but liver uptake was reduced by 80% *(17)*. These results suggest that retrograde liver perfusion may decrease hepatotoxicity while maintaining antitumor efficacy.

As mentioned before, several drugs have been applied in IHP including 5-FU, mitomycin C, cisplatin, and melphalan, but in the past 10 yr melphalan has been the only drug used in major clinical studies *(10)*. Despite the encouraging results with melphalan in recent studies, its efficacy is still limited; therefore, other drugs, such as irinotecan and oxaliplatin, might also be considered for application in IHP, as they might further increase the treatment efficacy or safety of IHP.

For successful application in IHP, a drug has to fulfil several conditions. As isolated perfusion is a short treatment, it is essential that the drug cause rapid, irreversible tumor cell cytotoxicity. In case of unexpected leakage, ideally, an agent to protect against systemic toxicity should be available. For instance, granulocyte colony-stimulating factor is used to prevent leukopenia after melphalan treatment.

Several drugs are of interest for application in IHP. In the past few years new agents, such as irinotecan and oxaliplatin, have been introduced in the systemic treatment of colorectal metastases. They resulted in increased response rates, disease-free survival, and overall survival *(18–20)*, also in patients resistant to fluoropyrimidines *(21)*. Irinotecan is a prodrug that requires activation by carboxylesterases to the active metabolite, 7-ethyl-10-hydroxy-camptothecin (SN-38), an inhibitor of topoisomerase I, which is approximately 100- to 1000-fold more active than the parent drug *(22)*; it has proved to be highly effective in the treatment of metastatic colorectal cancer. However, it may not be applicable in IHP, because it is not a direct acting agent, and the bioactivation to its active metabolite is slow: phase I trials on the pharmacokinetics and pharmacodynamics of irinotecan and SN-38 show that maximum concentrations of SN-38 are only reached about 1 h after the beginning of a 30-min intravenous irinotecan infusion *(23)*. It might be worthwhile to test the active metabolite SN-38 directly.

Oxaliplatin is rapidly absorbed and transformed by nonenzymatic pathways to its biologically active species *(24)*. It mainly exerts its cytotoxic effect by formation of DNA intra- and interstrand crosslinks, hampering DNA replication *(29)*. Substantial dose-dependent DNA adduct formation occurs within 1 h. In most studies in which oxaliplatin is administered systemically, hematological toxicity and nephrotoxicity are dose limiting, whereas hepatotoxicity is rarely mentioned. This suggests that treatment with a much higher dose of oxaliplatin might be feasible in IHP. To improve IHP treatment, experimental efficacy studies with new drugs, such as oxaliplatin, should be and are currently being conducted.

5. PHARMACOLOGICAL BACKGROUND OF ISOLATED EXTREMITY PERFUSION

Isolated extremity perfusion, such as isolated limb perfusion (ILP), is a technique that offers the opportunity to deliver high drug doses to the tumor-invaded region, while protecting the rest of the body by vascular isolation. The technique was first introduced by Creech et al. in 1958 *(26)*. Stehlin *(27)* added hyperthermia to this technique and made hyperthermic isolated limb perfusion an interesting method in the treatment of malignancies of the extremities. The technique can allow extremity-saving procedures and thus decrease patient morbidity. Advantages of ILP are the fact that the tumor is locally exposed to high concentrations of the chemotherapeutic drug, whereas only low drug concentrations are reached in the systemic circulation. Minor or no systemic side effects attend this. A case has even been described in which ILP was performed because of a contraindicative renal impairment in the treatment with the nephrotoxic drug cisplatin *(28)*. Theoretically, beneficial effects of ILP are anticipated, especially in the treatment of poorly vascularized tumors (such as osteosarcoma) because in these tumors the drug concentration may be rate limiting for exposure to the drug.

The use of extracorporeal circulation allows hyperthermic treatment. With several drugs, such as cisplatin, this can be of advantage since hyperthermia is known to enhance its cytotoxicity. Enhanced blood flow, owing to vasodilatation *(29,30)*, enhanced cellular drug uptake *(31,32)*, enhanced tissue extraction, enhanced DNA crosslinking *(33,34)*, and decreased DNA repair *(35)* are postulated to explain the phenomenon of hyperthermic potentiation. Hyperthermia may introduce some selectivity of treatment, because malignant cells have been shown to be more sensitive to heat than normal cells *(36,37)*.

Although several studies on isolated regional perfusion with a variety of drugs have been reported in recent years, relatively little is known about the pharmacokinetics and tissue distribution in these circumstances. In a pharmacokinetic study in nine patients with melanoma alone, who were treated by hyperthermic ILP with cisplatin, a decrease of 54, 80, and 80% of, respectively, total platinum, free platinum and cisplatin in the perfusate was observed after 60 min of perfusion (2). The drug elimination was characterized by first-order kinetics, resulting in an elimination half-life of 51, 28, and 27 min for, respectively, total platinum, free platinum, and cisplatin. Drug concentrations were determined in tissue biopsies taken from tumor and surrounding tissues and showed a wide variation within patients and tissues, but especially high total platinum concentrations were found in skin. This observation is particularly relevant since perfusate drug concentrations varied minimally among individuals, underscoring the importance of microenvironment distribution.

The aforementioned study and others have shown that isolated extremity perfusion with cisplatin can be safely performed but that irreversible local peripheral sensory and motor neuropathy is a relatively common side effect. Even though the second-generation platinum analog carboplatin is known for its milder neurotoxicity upon systemic administration, it appeared to cause persistent and severe local neuropathy when used in hyperthermic isolated limb perfusion that precluded its further research in this field.

6. CONCLUSIONS

The pharmacological advantage of regional cancer therapy is based on high dose intensity, resulting in a high therapeutic ratio. A high therapeutic ratio is defined by an advantageous tumor cure/normal tissue complication differential. Only patients with an anatomically confined tumor and technical feasibility of antitumor therapy administration are expected to reach clinical benefit. Specific pharmacological characteristics of the delivered drug are of potential additional benefit, as shown in this chapter with examples for intraperitoneal chemotherapy, isolated hepatic perfusion, and isolated extremity perfusion.

REFERENCES

1. Sparreboom A, Danesi R, Ando Y, Chan J, Figg WD. Pharmacogenomics of ABC transporters and its role in cancer chemotherapy. Drug Resistance Updates 2003;6:71–84.
2. Guchelaar HJ, Hoekstra HJ, Devries EGE, Uges DRA, Oosterhuis JW, Koops HS. Cisplatin and platinum pharmacokinetics during hyperthermic isolated limb perfusion for human tumors of the extremities. Br J Cancer 1992;65:898–902.
3. Sugarbaker PH, Mora JT, Carmignani P, Stuart OA, Yoo D. Update on chemotherapeutic agents utilized for perioperative intraperitoneal chemotherapy. Oncologist 2005;10:112–122.
4. Gelderblom H, Verweij J, van Zomeren DM, et al. Influence of Cremophor EL on the bioavailability of intraperitoneal paclitaxel. Clin Cancer Res 2002;8:1237–1241.
5. Gelderblom H, Verweij J, Nooter K, Sparreboom A. Cremophor EL: the drawbacks and advantages of vehicle selection for drug formulation. Eur J Cancer 2001;37:1590–1598.
6. Sparreboom A, Van Zuylen L, Brouwer E, et al. Cremophor EL-mediated alteration of paclitaxel distribution in human blood: clinical pharmacokinetic implications. Cancer Res 1999;59:1454–1457.
7. Knemeyer I, Wientjes MG, Au JLS. Cremophor reduces paclitaxel penetration into bladder wall during intravesical treatment. Cancer Chemother Pharmacol 1999;44:241–248.
8. Markman M, Rowinsky E, Hakes T, et al. Phase-I trial of intraperitoneal taxol—a Gynecologic Oncology Group Study. J Clin Oncol 1992;10:1485–1491.

9. Francis P, Rowinsky E, Schneider J, Hakes T, Hoskins W, Markman M. Phase-I feasibility and pharmacological study of weekly intraperitoneal paclitaxe—a Gynecologic-Oncology-Group Pilot-Study. J Clin Oncol 1995;13:2961–2967.

10. Rothbarth J, Tollenaar RA, Schellens JH, et al. Isolated hepatic perfusion for the treatment of colorectal metastases confined to the liver: recent trends and perspectives. Eur J Cancer 2004;40:1812–1824.

11. Rothbarth J, Vahrmeijer AL, Mulder GJ. Modulation of cytostatic efficacy of melphalan by glutathione: mechanisms and efficacy. Chem Biol Interact 2002;140:93–107.

12. Vahrmeijer AL, van Dierendonck JH, Keizer HJ, et al. Increased local cytostatic drug exposure by isolated hepatic perfusion: a phase I clinical and pharmacologic evaluation of treatment with high dose melphalan in patients with colorectal cancer confined to the liver. Br J Cancer 2000;82:1539–1546.

13. Rothbarth J, Woutersen RA, Sparidans RW, van de Velde CJ, Mulder GJ. Melphalan antitumor efficacy and hepatotoxicity: the effect of variable infusion duration in the hepatic artery. J Pharmacol Exp Ther 2003;305:1098–1103.

14. Sigurdson ER, Ridge JA, Kemeny N, Daly JM. Tumor and liver drug uptake following hepatic artery and portal vein infusion. J Clin Oncol 1987;5:1836–1840.

15. Rappaport AM. Hepatic blood flow: morphologic aspects and physiologic regulation. Int Rev Physiol 1980;21:1–63.

16. Watanabe Y, Puschel GP, Gardemann A, Jungermann K. Presinusoidal and proximal intrasinusoidal confluence of hepatic artery and portal vein in rat liver: functional evidence by orthograde and retrograde bivascular perfusion. Hepatology 1994;19:1198–1207.

17. Rothbarth J, Sparidans RW, Beijnen JH, et al. Reduced liver uptake of arterially infused melphalan during retrograde rat liver perfusion with unaffected liver tumor uptake. J Pharmacol Exp Ther 2002;303:736–740.

18. Saltz LB, Cox JV, Blanke C, et al. Irinotecan plus fluorouracil and leucovorin for metastatic colorectal cancer. Irinotecan Study Group. N Engl J Med 2000;343:905–914.

19. Tournigand C, Andre T, Achille E, et al. FOLFIRI Followed by FOLFOX6 or the reverse sequence in advanced colorectal cancer: a randomized GERCOR study. J Clin Oncol 2004;22:229–237.

20. Cunningham D, Pyrhonen S, James RD, et al. Randomised trial of irinotecan plus supportive care versus supportive care alone after fluorouracil failure for patients with metastatic colorectal cancer. Lancet 1998;352:1413–1418.

21. Raymond E, Chaney SG, Taamma A, Cvitkovic E. Oxaliplatin: a review of preclinical and clinical studies. Ann Oncol 1998;9:1053–1071.

22. Hertzberg RP, Caranfa MJ, Holden KG, et al. Modification of the hydroxy lactone ring of camptothecin: inhibition of mammalian topoisomerase I and biological activity. J Med Chem 1989;32:715–720.

23. Chabot GG, Abigerges D, Catimel G, et al. Population pharmacokinetics and pharmacodynamics of irinotecan (CPT-11) and active metabolite SN-38 during phase I trials. Ann Oncol 1995;6:141–151.

24. Extra JM, Marty M, Brienza S, Misset JL. Pharmacokinetics and safety profile of oxaliplatin. Semin Oncol 1998;25(2 Suppl 5):13–22.

25. Raymond E, Faivre S, Woynarowski JM, Chaney SG. Oxaliplatin: mechanism of action and antineoplastic activity. Semin Oncol 1998;25(2 Suppl 5):4–12.

26. Creech O, Krementz ET, Ryan RF, Winblad JN. Chemotherapy of cancer—regional perfusion utilizing an extracorporeal circuit. Ann Surg 1958;148:616–632.

27. Stehlin JS. Hyperthermic perfusion with chemotherapy for cancers of extremities. Surg Gynecol Obstet Int Abstr Surg 1969;129:305.

28. Roseman JM, Tench D, Bryant LR. The safe use of cisplatin in hyperthermic isolated limb perfusion systems. Cancer 1985;56:742–744.

29. Hahn GM. Potential for therapy of drugs and hyperthermia. Cancer Res 1979;39:2264–2268.

30. Song CW, Kang MS, Rhee JG, Levitt SH. The effect of hyperthermia on vascular function, PH, and cell-survivalval. Radiology 1980;137:795–803.

31. Alberts DS, Peng YM, Chen HSG, Moon TE, Cetas TC, Hoeschele JD. Therapeutic synergism of hyperthermia-Cis-platinum in A mouse-tumor model. J Natl Cancer Inst 1980;65:455–461.

32. Herman TS. Temperature-dependence of adriamycin, cis-diamminedichloroplatinum, bleomycin, and 1,3-bis(2-chloroethyl)-1-nitrosourea cyto-toxicity in vitro. Cancer Res 1983;43:517–520.

33. Meyn RE, Corry PM, Fletcher SE, Demetriades M. Thermal Enhancement of DNA damage in mammalian-cells treated with cis-diamminedichloroplatinum(Ii). Cancer Res 1980;40:1136–1139.

34. Herman TS, Teicher BA, Chan V, Collins LS, Abrams MJ. Effect of heat on the cyto-toxicity and interaction with DNA of a series of platinum complexes. Int J Radiat Oncol Biol Phys 1989;16:443–449.
35. Wallner KE, Degregorio MW, Li GC. Hyperthermic potentiation of cis-diamminedichloroplatinum(Ii) cytotoxicity in chinese-hamster ovary cells resistant to the drug. Cancer Res 1986;46:6242–6245.
36. Cavalier R, Ciocatto EC, Giovanel BC, et al. Selective heat sensitivity of cancer cells—biochemical and clinical studies. Cancer 1967;20:1351.
37. Kase K, Hahn GM. Differential heat response of normal and transformed human cells in tissue-culture. Nature 1975;255:228–230.

3

Isolated Limb and Organ Perfusion Laboratory Models

Timo L. M. ten Hagen, PhD and
Alexander M. M. Eggermont, MD, PhD

CONTENTS

INTRODUCTION
REGIONAL CANCER THERAPY
INTRATUMORAL INJECTION, REGIONAL PERFUSION AND INFUSION
    MODELS
PERFUSION AND INFUSION MODELS
RESULTS WITH REGIONAL THERAPY
CONCLUSIONS
REFERENCES

SUMMARY

When treating patients with solid tumors one is faced with a plethora of factors that may influence clinical outcome. Drugs tested with success on tumor cells in vitro do not always turn out to be that promising when used in humans. It is clear that although a drug may have strong activity on tumor cells in vitro, the usefulness of this drug also depends (for instance) on its availability when injected in the body. Factors such as pharmacokinetics, toxicity profile, intratumoral distribution, and activity in hypoxic or acidic regions are likely to be of even greater importance than the cytotoxic potential of a drug. To allow better prediction of the activity of a drug in the clinical setting, the use of clinically relevant animal models is imperative. Here we describe the use of animal models for solid tumor therapy and in particular regional treatment application.

Key Words: Animal models; regional therapy; perfusion; infusion; tumor; cancer.

1. INTRODUCTION

Solid tumors account for at least 85% of cancer-related mortality, and cancer is one of the leading causes of death in developed countries. Solid tumor therapy is therefore an important research area in the medical field. To study tumor therapeutic treatment modalities, whether from a clinical, preclinical, or fundamental point of view, the use of clinically relevant animal models is indispensable. Particularly when the treatment comprises

From: *Cancer Drug Discovery and Development: Regional Cancer Therapy*
Edited by: P. M. Schlag and U. S. Stein © Humana Press Inc., Totowa, NJ

a multitargeted approach (e.g., both tumor cells and stromal compartments such as endothelial cells are targeted), in vitro data will be of limited value. Also, for studies related to the development of regional cancer therapies, the use of animal models is essential to obtain insight into the pharmacokinetics, drug distribution, and tumor response. Well-chosen animal models will provide conclusive data on the activity of the drug in the complex in vivo setting. In this chapter animal models are discussed that are useful for the evaluation of regional cancer therapies.

2. REGIONAL CANCER THERAPY

Treatment of solid tumors is dramatically impaired by typical characteristics, which work against drug delivery to the tumor cells. Generally solid tumors have a highly disorganized tumor vasculature, with chaotic and immature vessels that are tortuous and curved *(1)*. Together with the presence of shunts and uncontrolled branching, this results in irregular or even absent blood flow. These features contribute to a heterogeneous blood flow in solid tumors, resulting in an inadequate delivery of active components. In addition, tumors tend to exhibit an elevated interstitial fluid pressure (IFP) *(2,3)*, which works against the accumulation of drugs. Moreover, lymphatic vessels may be compressed, impairing the flow of lymph *(4,5)*. Next to these hurdles in drug delivery to solid tumors, treatment is compromised by toxicity of the applied agents. Most anticancer drugs express toxicity toward tumor cells as well as to normal cells, and therefore the drug dose of is limited by normal tissue tolerance. Inadequate drug delivery could lead to regrowth of tumors and possible development of resistant tumor cells. Last, the blood volume of solid tumors is rather low compared with the total blood volume, meaning that relatively little of the blood-borne therapeutic agent is flowing through the tumor at a given time point. Moreover, after the drug enters the bloodstream, massive dilution occurs.

As it is quite difficult to achieve adequate concentrations of anticancer agents at the tumor site, methods have been developed to deal with some of these drawbacks in solid tumor therapy. One such method is regional application of the therapeutic agent. First, by limiting the area of distribution, higher local drug levels can be reached. Depending on the type of local therapy, for instance, isolated perfusion or single-pass infusion, augmented drug concentrations can be prolonged or initially reached. Second, inhibition of distribution of the chemotherapeutic agent throughout the body not only impairs clearance and dilution of the applied agent but also minimizes systemic toxicity, therefore allowing higher dosages to be applied.

The major aim of course of regional cancer therapy is to improve tumor response and clinical outcome. To develop new treatment modalities, understand mechanisms related to this approach, and provide insight into pharmacokinetics, animal models are key.

3. INTRATUMORAL INJECTION, REGIONAL PERFUSION, AND INFUSION MODELS

Several approaches can be used to treat solid tumors more or less regionally. First, intratumoral injections allow specific delivery of drugs in the center of a tumor. However, this method has met with several complications such as drainage of the injected agents from the tumor to the system, limited spread of the injected drug (typical needle track distribution). and difficulty in locating the tumors (Fig. 1). Tumors can also be treated by regional intraarterial infusion, making use of a so-called first-pass effect. In this setting an important fraction of the drug passes the tumor site relatively undiluted, resulting in an increased exposure of the tumor to the blood-borne agent. However, right after that the drug enters the circulation, with obvious disadvantages. A setting that most effectively limits systemic exposure is isolated perfusion. Several isolated perfusion modalities will be discussed.

4. PERFUSION AND INFUSION MODELS

4.1. Animals

The choice of animal greatly depends on the type of study. Although mice seem quite attractive owing to the availability of a great number of genetically modified strains, their size limits the reproducible application of a perfusion, or at least makes it an exercise that will test your technical skills and patience. Although infusion of a limb or organ may be rather simple, performing an isolated perfusion is complex. Thus most surgical procedures including an infusion or perfusion are performed on rats, but rabbits or larger animals are used also. To test the applicability of the (newly developed) method in a clinical setting, or to obtain pharmacokinetic profiles that allow translation to the human setting, the use of pigs is preferred. Application of the different animal species is discussed below.

4.2. Methodologies

A selection of possible regional therapy methods will be described in detail, with an emphasis on isolated perfusion. Typically isolated perfusion allows recirculation of the perfusate, resulting in continuous high local drug levels, while leakage to the system is kept to a minimum. This in contrast to an infusion, in which the (venous) effluent is not collected and the entire agent disappears into the body. This method creates the possibility of enhanced local exposure through a so-called first-pass effect. As an alternative, perfusate may be collected at the venous side and discarded. The single-pass system provides initial high local concentration, as is obtained with the infusion method, but is not accompanied by systemic exposure.

4.2.1. ISOLATED LIMB PERFUSION

Creech and coworkers pioneered the technique of isolated limb perfusion (ILP) in 1958 *(6)*, which we and others adapted for rats *(7–9)*. An important improvement of this technique is that regional concentrations of chemotherapeutic agents 15 to 25 times higher than those reached after systemic administration can be achieved in the tumor-bearing extremity without systemic side effects. Isolation of the blood circuit of a limb is achieved by clamping and canulation of the major artery and vein, connection to an oxygenated extracorporeal circuit, ligation of collateral vessels, and application of a tourniquet. Once isolation is secured, drugs can be injected into the perfusion circuit. In rats a similar setup can be accomplished allowing fast and reliable screening of antitumor agents alone or combined (Fig. 2).

In the rat model an ILP is performed as follows. Generally small fragments (3–5 mm) of an appropriate tumor (for instance, we use the rapidly growing and metastasizing BN-175 soft tissue sarcoma) are implanted subcutaneously into the right hindlimb.

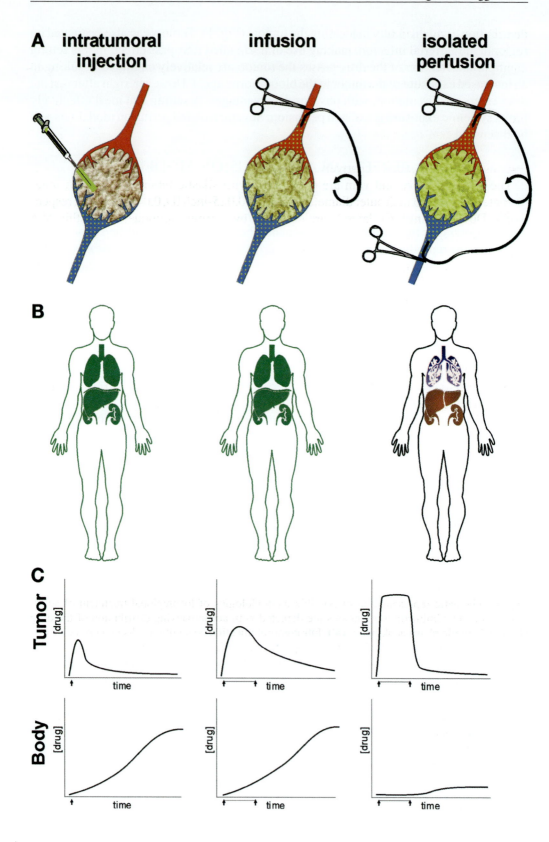

Perfusion is performed at a tumor diameter of 12 to 15 mm; however, this may depend on scientific question as well as the tumor type under study. Animals are anesthetized with inhalation anesthetics (isoflurane oxygen mixture), and 50 IU of heparin are injected intravenously to prevent coagulation. The hindlimb is kept at a constant temperature by a warm water mattress. The temperature of the tumor is measured with a temperature probe, which is fixed on the skin covering the tumor and is normally set on mild hyperthermia (38–39°C). We previously evaluated other temperature settings, i.e., room temperature (24–26°C) and true hyperthermia (42–43°C), but these appeared to affect tumor response or local toxicity negatively.

The femoral artery and vein are cannulated with silastic tubing (0.012-inch inner diameter [ID], 0.025 inch outer diameter [OD] and 0.025-inch ID, 0.047-inch OD, respectively; Dow Corning). Collaterals are occluded by a groin tourniquet, consisting of a rubber band applied high around the leg and fixed in such way that the vessels in the inside of the limb are easy accessible. Isolation time starts when the tourniquet is tightened. An oxygenation reservoir, consisting of a small tube that is constantly oxygenated with a mixture of O_2/CO_2 (95%:5%), and a roller pump are included in the circuit. The perfusion solution is 5 mL Haemaccel (Behring Pharma, Amsterdam, The Netherlands) and the hemoglobin (Hb) content of the perfusate in this rat model is 0.9 mmol/L. Generally the agents, for instance, melphalan and tumor necrosis factor (TNF), are added as boluses to the oxygenation reservoir. A roller pump (Watson Marlow, Falmouth, UK; type 505 U) recirculates the perfusate at a flow rate of 2.4 mL/min. A washout with 5 mL oxygenated Haemaccel is performed at the end of the perfusion. Subsequent tumor growth after perfusion is recorded daily by caliper measurement. Although other methods can be used, we calculate the tumor volume using the formula $0.4(A^2B)$, where A is the minimal tumor diameter and B the diameter perpendicular to A.

4.2.1.1. Assessment of Surgery-Related Complications

To assess the quality of the ILP limb function was clinically observed in which the rat's ability to walk and stand on the perfused limb was scored 5 d after ILP. On this scale a severe impaired function (grade 0) means that the rat drags its hindlimb without any function; a slightly impaired function (grade 1) means the rat does not use its hindlimb in a usual manner, but stands on it when rising; an intact function of the hindlimb (grade 2) means a normal walking pattern.

Fig. 1. Schematic representation of possible methodologies of locoregional treatment of solid tumors. In (**A**) administration methods are depicted with accompanying distribution of the drug (**B**) and theoretic pharmacokinetics (**C**). Intratumoral injection generally results in a limited distribution of the injected agent in the tumor, with a characteristic localization around the needle track. Infusion and isolated perfusion results in a more widespread distribution of the drug in the tumor, although in especially necrotic parts no or limited drug levels are reached. Because of the recirculation properties of the isolated perfusion, higher end local drug levels can eventually be reached. Bodily exposure to the drug is maximal in both the intratumoral injection and infusion methods, in which all organs experience certain levels of the drug administered. With the aid of an isolated perfusion, this can be abrogated or kept to a minimum. Therefore intratumoral injection and infusion results in only short and low local drug levels, whereas perfusion may result in much higher drug concentrations in the tumor. Here theoretic examples of tumor and systemic drug levels are presented, which of course depend strongly on the typical pharmacokinetic behavior of the drug administered. The drug used as an example preferentially stays in the blood during the chosen monitoring period. Arrow, injection time point; between arrows, time of infusion or perfusion.

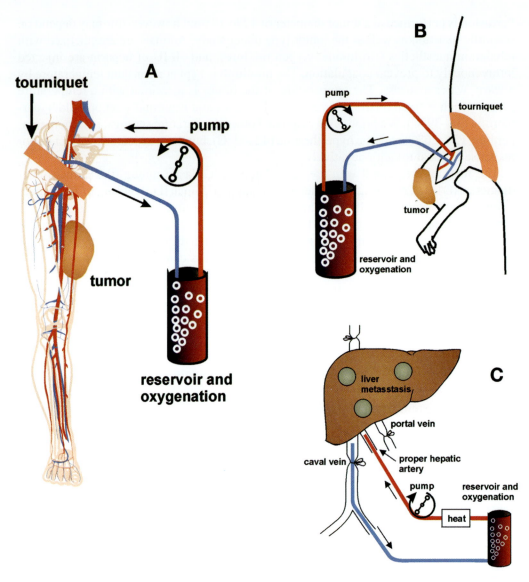

Fig. 2. Isolated perfusion of the extremity, e.g., isolated limb perfusion (ILP), seems an obvious approach for the locoregional treatment of solid tumors confined to arms or legs. This setting, depicted in (**A**), proved beneficial for the treatment of advanced sarcoma or bulky and multiple in transit melanoma. The success of the ILP initiated the development of a preclinical testing model in the rat (**B**), with features, such as the perfusion method but also tumor response and drug pharmacokinetics, closely resembling the clinical setting. This model allowed thorough testing of the method and evaluation of optimal prerequisites. Moreover, with the aid of the rat model, the mechanism of action of, for instance, tumor necrosis factor-α (TNF) could be unraveled. New, and possibly better, drugs could be identified and tested with success with the data acquired. The advantages of ILP led to testing of the perfusion method for organs such as the liver (**C**), with likewise superior pharmacokinetics and efficacy. The schematic illustration clearly shows the importance of well-developed and representative animal models.

4.2.2. ISOLATED LIVER OR HEPATIC PERFUSION

The isolated hepatic perfusion (IHP) procedure is a modification of the technique described by de Brauw et al. *(10,11)*. Small viable tumor fragments of 1 to 2 mm are implanted under the liver capsule in the left and central liver lobe with a 19-gage Luer lock needle in a standardized manner, under anesthetia. IHP is performed at a diameter of approximately 6 mm, which for the BN-175 soft tissue sarcoma is 6 d after implantation. During follow-up, tumor diameters are assessed under anesthetia through a small midline incision by caliper measurement. We evaluated the effect of this surgical procedure on tumor growth by checking end-point volumes of tumors, from rats that were operated on and controls, and found no effect. Evaluation of tumor progression in rats by MRI confirmed these findings. Tumor volume is calculated as described in the ILP method. Animals are sacrificed when tumor diameter exceeds 20 mm or when abdominal adhesions prohibit further assessment of tumor size.

Two types of perfusion can be used. In one, the perfusion comprises both arterial and portal inflow, and in the other, only an arterial inflow is applied. We found the latter to be accompanied by less liver-related toxicity, certainly when TNF was used. The perfusion circuit further consists of a venous outflow limb and a collection reservoir/oxygenator. The circuit is primed with 30 mL Haemaccel containing 50 IU heparin. The perfusate is oxygenized in the reservoir with a mixture of O_2/CO_2 (95%:5%) and kept at 38 to 39°C by means of a heat exchanger connected to a warm water bath. A temperature probe is positioned in the lumen of the portal catheter 5 cm from the catheter tip. Arterial and portal flow is maintained with two low-flow roller pumps (Watson Marlow, type 505 U) and kept at 2.5 mL/min and 10 mL/min, respectively. Rats are perfused for 10 min with Haemaccel and dissolved agents, after which a washout of agents is performed with oxygenized Haemaccel for 2 min.

Anesthesia is induced and maintained with inhalation anesthetics (isoflurane/oxygen). During the surgical procedure, which on average takes 60 to 80 min, rats are kept at constant temperature with a warmed mattress. A midline laparotomy is performed and the hepatic ligament exposed. In the dual-inflow setting the pyloric side branch of the portal vein and the gastroduodenal side branch of the common hepatic artery are cannulated, positioning the tips of the Silastic cannulas (0.025-inch OD, 0.012 inch ID; Dow Corning) in the hepatic artery and portal vein. In the single-inflow setting, only the gastroduodenal side branch of the common hepatic artery is cannulated. Through an inguinal incision the femoral vein is exposed.

To collect hepatic venous outflow, a silicon cannule (0.025-inch ID and 0.047-inch OD; Dow Corning) is femorally introduced and retrogradely inserted in the caval vein with the tip positioned at the level of the hepatic veins. Isolation of the hepatic vascular bed is obtained by clamping the hepatic artery and the portal vein. The venous outflow limb is isolated by clamping the suprahepatic caval vein and by applying a temporary ligature around the infrahepatic caval vein containing the cannule, cranial to the right adrenal vein. During isolation the mesenteric artery is clamped to reduce splanchnic blood pressure and the risk for translocation of intestinal bacteria. After the IHP procedure, clamps on the caval vein, portal vein, hepatic artery and mesenteric artery are released. The gastroduodenal artery, pyloric vein, and femoral vein are ligated, and the gastroduodenal and pyloric cannules are removed.

4.2.3. Isolated Lung or Pulmonary Perfusion

Lung perfusions are not performed in our department and therefore we discuss here a method for rats as described originally by Weksler et al. *(12)* and modified as described by Wang et al. *(13)*. The lung is retracted from the thoracic cavity and the pulmonary vessels dissected. The pulmonary artery and vein are clamped and the artery is cannulated with a PE-10 catheter (0.26-mm ID, 0.61 OD; Becton Dickinson). A suction catheter collects the effluent through a pulmonary venotomy. After perfusion, the catheteres are removed and the artery closed with a 9–0 suture; the venotomy is not repaired. To facilitate reexpansion of the lung a 16-gage catheter connected to a 5-mL syringe is introduced in the left chest cavity.

Dr. P. van Schil's group describes a modification to this technique, which allows better access of the pulmonary artery *(14)*. Rats are anesthetized with inhalation anesthetia (isoflurane oxygen mixture). Instead of posterior luxation, retractor and lung are positioned anteriorly, and the hilus is dissected free from the posterior side. After the pulmonary artery and vein are clamped with curved microclips, a 16-gage angiocath is placed through the chest wall. The PE-10 perfusion catheter (Becton-Dickinson) is introduced into the chest through this angiocath and secured by a 4–0 silk tie after insertion into the pulmonary artery. After perfusion, both catheter and angiocath are removed, and the procedure is finished as described by Wang et al. *(13)*.The animal is then supplied with room air until it begins to breath spontaneously, after which the pleural drain and endotracheal tube are removed.

4.2.4. Isolated Kidney Perfusion

Perfusion of the kidney is performed by us in a manner resembling ILP *(15)* and is described and used also by others *(16,17)*. Anesthesia is induced and maintained with inhalation anesthetics (isoflurane/oxygen). During the surgical procedure, which on average takes 90 and 120 min, rats are kept at constant temperature with a warmed mattress. Through a median laparotomy, the left kidney and vessels are exposed in the retroperitoneum by sharp and blunt dissection. Branches of the renal artery and vein (adrenal and spermatic) are dissected when needed and temporarily occluded with ligatures. A tobacco-pouch ligature is placed in the vein with nylon 9-0 (SSC, B Braun). A bolus of 50 IU heparin (Heparin Leo, Weesp, The Netherlands) is injected intravenously. Isolation of the renal artery and vein is carried out by means of microvessel clamps. Via a venotomy and arteriotomy, the vessels are cannulated with Silastic tubing (0.025-inch ID, 0.047 inch OD and 0.012-inch ID, 0.025-inch OD, respectively; Dow Corning). Another bolus of 50 IE heparin is added to the perfusion circuit.

Perfusion is carried out for 15 min. Flow through the kidney is regulated by a nonpulsatile roller pump (Watson-Marlow, 505U). Perfusion pressure is recorded on a Datex AS/3 monitor and kept between 100 and 120 mmHg, adjusting the flow generated by the roller pump accordingly. Perfusion fluid is warmed to approximately 37°C by countercurrent (Polyscience 210, Merck, Amsterdam, The Netherlands) and temperature is recorded constantly (Thermodig KJ-11, Mera, Benelux). Flow through the kidney is approximately 1 mL/min. The perfusion reservoir is oxygenated with a mixture of O_2/ CO_2 (95%/5%), to keep the oxygen pressure of the perfusate at 350 to 400 mm Hg and the saturation at 99.5%. Drugs are added to the perfusion circuit as bolus. A washout is carried out with 6 mL perfusion fluid (about four times the intravascular rat kidney volume). At the end of the perfusion period, the venotomy is closed by tightening the tobacco-pouch ligature. The arteriotomy is closed with nylon 10-0 (SSC, B Braun). The laparotomy is closed with silk 2-0 (B Braun) in one layer in a running way. During the recovery period, the animal is kept warm with a heating lamp or warm water mattress.

4.2.5. Cardiac Perfusion

Isolated cardiac perfusion has been explored for the treatment of cardiovascular diseases, rather than treatment of solid tumors. In these cases gene therapy is performed in animal models. Cardiac perfusion is not performed by our department but is described for rats by Hajjar et al. *(18)* and for piglets by Davidson et al. *(19)*. Rats are anesthetized and the chest is opened on the left side at the third intercostal space. Through the pericardium a 7-0 suture is placed at the apex of the left ventricle. A 22-gage catheter is advanced from the apex of the left ventricle to the aortic root. The aorta and pulmonary arteries are clamped distally from the catheter, and the solution with agents under study is injected. The clamp is maintained for 10 s while the heart pumps against a closed system (isovolumically). This procedure allows the injected solution to circulate through the coronary arteries and perfuse the heart without direct manipulation of the coronaries. After 10 s, the clamp on the aorta and pulmonary artery is released. After removal of air and blood, the chest is closed, and animals are extubated and transferred to their cages.

On larger animals cardiac perfusion can be performed as follows. One-week-old piglets (3 kg) are anesthetized, and a median sternotomy is performed. After systemic heparinization, a cardiopulmonary bypass (CPB) is established via an aortic and a right atrial cannula. The CPB circuit consists of a reservoir, a hollow fiber oxygenator/heat exchanger, and a roller pump. After stabilization, the aorta is cross-clamped and the heart arrested by infusion of cold (4°C) hyperkalemic cardioplegia solution (30 mL/kg) into the aortic root. Immediately after cardioplegic arrest, agents can be injected into the aortic root and maintained in the myocardium. After 30 min of cardiac arrest, the cross-clamp is removed and the heart reperfused. The animals are weaned off CPB and allowed to recover.

4.2.6. Pelvic and Abdominal Perfusion: A Balloon Catheter Approach

The success obtained with locoregional approaches for treatment of solid tumors or organ-selective delivery of (viral) vectors in gene therapy initiated endeavors in more demanding settings. Moving from limb to liver as a target for isolated perfusion was obvious and appeared workable although demanding on the technical skills of the surgeons *(20)*. Therefore the application of balloon catheters was thought of and applied with success in pigs *(21,22)*. In this method liver isolation is obtained by using single and double balloon catheters, reducing the surgical procedure. Whereas in the pigs isolation was quite good, with minimal leakage to the system, in the human setting applications of this technique appeared troublesome. Massive leakage through an extensive collateral network was observed, making it impossible to use this highly toxic agent *(23,24)*.

For the treatment of malignancies such as pelvic recurrences of colorectal carcinoma, advanced primary gastric and pancreatic carcinomas, and locally extensive ovarian malignancies, perfusion of the abdominal or pelvic area is explored *(25,26)*. It is quite difficult to obtain a leakage-free area in such a setting. However, the initial high dose, together with the advantage of a single-pass effect, may be the key to a better response rate. This was tested in pigs. The perfusion circuit of 220 mL, consisting of an aorta occlusion balloon catheter, a caval vein occlusion balloon catheter (12F, balloon capacity

25 mL), and a tubing set (PfM, Cologne, Germany), included a roller pump and a bubble trap. Drugs are infused through a side-line into the perfusion circuit. Pigs are anesthetized, an arterial line is introduced into a carotid artery, and a double-lumen central venous catheter is placed in an external jugular vein on either side. After a midline laparotomy is performed, the pyloric vein is cannulated. Pigs are subsequently heparinized with 2 mg/kg heparin. After surgical exposure of the femoral vessels, arteriotomy and venotomy are performed, and the aorta-occlusion catheter and the caval vein occlusion catheter are introduced into the common femoral vessels and retrogradely moved up into the aorta and caval vein.

For abdominal perfusion, balloons are positioned at the level of the diaphragm, above the hepatic veins. When a pelvic perfusion is undertaken, balloons are positioned just above the bifurcations of the major abdominal vessels. Temporary relative isolation of the abdominal vascular bed is achieved by inflating the balloons and placing pneumatic tourniquets around both upper thighs of the hind extremities. To compensate for the decrease in cardiac preload, the aorta occlusion balloon is inflated prior to inflating the caval balloon. After the catheters are connected to the perfusion system, primed with 220 mL Haemaccel, the perfusate is circulated by means of a roller pump with a constant flow of 200 mL/min. Stable perfusion is assessed by monitoring the blood level in the bubble trap. Then, drugs are rapidly administered as a bolus infusion into the perfusate during approximately half a minute. After 20 min of perfusion, isolation is terminated by subsequently deflating the caval and aortic balloons.

4.2.7. OTHER PERFUSION OR INFUSION POSSIBILITIES

In addition to the perfusion modalities just described, still other organs or body sites can be treated locally by perfusion or infusion, i.e., isolated splenic perfusion *(27)*, which will be not be described here.

4.3. Important Factors To Be Considered When Performing Animal Studies

Several factors, which can be controlled before, or during, and after treatment, contribute to the success of local therapy and will add to the quality of the experiment. The weight and condition of the animal at the beginning of the experiment is crucial. One should check the microbiological status of every new animal and demand that suppliers adhere closely to standard regulations such as those of the Federation of European Laboratory Animal Science Association (FELASA). In particular, when a liver perfusion is conducted, rats should not be too light in weight and should be in perfect condition. When rats weigh less than 250 g, it is difficult to perform this demanding technique, and animals tend to have less resistance. Monitoring of animal weights is mandatory, especially when one is working with TNF or other toxic substances. Weight loss is typically associated with TNF-related toxicity and is a sensitive parameter for systemic toxicity. Unusual animal behavior (lethargy), erection of hair, and diarrhea are indications of possible TNF-related discomfort. We found that oxygenation of the perfusion or infusion fluid diminished local toxicity and improved animal survival. Moreover, the type of perfusion fluid (e.g., Haemaccel) and the temperature (38–39°C) are important. Especially for kidney perfusion, but also for IHP, pressure applied during the procedure strongly influences damage to the organ and should therefore be kept low.

During perfusion the animal is anesthetized. To prevent body temperature changes, the animal is kept at a constant temperature with a warm water mattress. Especially for

IHP, which demands longer and more intensive surgery, this is of crucial importance. Second, in the IHP setting the rats are anesthetized with inhalation anesthetics. We found that it is necessary to manipulate the anesthesia as directly as possible in this setting. During recovery animal temperature should be monitored and controlled, with heating lamps, for instance. A surgical microscope is indispensable for perfusion experiments, in particular for isolated organ perfusions. Although complete sterility is difficult to obtain, working in a setting that is as clean as possible will contribute to success. Also, the speed with which the procedure is performed may have a strong impact on the end result.

An important parameter in performing local cancer therapy is tumor volume. Tumors can be generated by injection of a cell suspension but also by transplantation of small tumor fragments from a donor animal. We routinely transplant tumors, as we found this to result in highly reproducible outgrowth of the tumor. The small standard deviation allows a reduction in the number of animals to be used in experiments. Moreover, in the liver setting, with this technique single nicely defined tumors can be grown, whereas injection of cells often results in spillage and subsequent tumor growth around the wound and in the cavities.

4.4. Assessment of Tumor Response in ILP and IHP

In the ILP setting tumor growth can easily be recorded daily after perfusion by caliper measurement. Tumor volume is calculated with the formula $0.4(A^2B)$, where A is the minimal tumor diameter and B the diameter perpendicular to A. Rats are sacrificed when tumors reach a size of 25 mm in diameter or animals show obvious signs of discomfort. Recording of the size of liver tumors is more difficult. Normally after IHP, tumor size is measured with a standardized caliper, via a small midline laparotomy every fourth day, and tumor volume is calculated as described above.

Classification of tumor response is as follows: progressive disease (PD) = increase of tumor volume (>25%) within 5 d; no change (NC) = tumor volume equal to volume during perfusion (in a range of –25% and + 25%); partial remission (PR) = decrease in tumor volume (–25% and –90%); complete remission (CR) = tumor volume 0 to 10% of volume during perfusion or skin necrosis.

5. RESULTS WITH REGIONAL THERAPY

5.a. Animal models as key tools in cancer therapy studies.

ILP is probably one of the most favorable examples of regional cancer therapy. Both the ease of the technique and superior control over drug distribution contribute to success in the treatment of locally advanced sarcoma and multiple or bulky melanoma of the extremity. With ILP, local concentrations can be increased 15 to 25 times while exposure of the rest of the body is kept to a minimum. We and others have demonstrated that application of melphalan together with the highly toxic agent TNF rendered inoperable tumors resectable (sarcoma or bulky melanoma). An 80 to 100% limb salvage rate can be obtained with this approach *(28–32)*. Acknowledging the possible importance of understanding the underlying mechanisms involved in melphalan/TNF-based ILP, we developed several animal models. Rat models in particular, and to a lesser extent mouse models, are instrumental in elucidating mechanisms and studing new combinations.

Larger animals, such as pigs, have been used to practice new techniques and gain insight into pharmacokinetics.

5.1. Advances in Local Cancer Therapy With Animal ILP Models

Using the rat ILP model we fine-tuned certain aspects that could not be explored in humans, such as:

1. Interferon-γ only marginally adds to the tumor response *(33)*.
2. Actinomycin D drastically enhances local toxicity of TNF *(34)*.
3. Nitric oxide (NO) inhibition further improves TNF-based ILP with melphalan *(35)*.
4. The TNF dose can be lowered fivefold *(9)*.
5. The optimal temperature is 38 to 39°C.
6. Hypoxia does not improve response *(9)*.
7. Application of the TNF mutant SAM2 results in comparable synergistic tumor response *(36)*.
8. Whereas TNF was thought to affect the tumor-associated vasculature directly, animal models showed that the presence of endothelial monocyte-activating polypetide II (EMAP-II) made tumors more susceptible to TNF *(37,38)*.

More importantly, we demonstrated that ILP with TNF alone has no or marginal effect on tumor progression *(7–9)*. However, TNF changes the pathophysiology of the tumor, resulting in augmented accumulation of the coadministered drug melphalan or doxorubicin *(39,40)*. This was also observed in the IHP and systemic setting, in which lower local levels of TNF are reached *(11,41–43)*. TNF increases the permeability of the endothelial lining, facilitating better leakage of melphalan or doxorubicin from more vessels (manuscript in preparation). This initiated the search for agents that could mimic the permeability-enhancing effect of TNF while lacking the typical TNF-related toxicity. We found that both histamine and interleukin-2 (IL-2) were good candidates and showed strong synergy between these agents and melphalan for the treatment of soft tissue sarcoma in ILP *(44,45)*. Both agents augmented tumor drug accumulation but lacked the toxicity of TNF.

We also showed the potential power of a useful animal model when testing the applicability of liposomal formulated doxorubicin in ILP. Although melphalan is the drug of choice in ILP, some groups use doxorubicin instead, with good results *(46,47)*. However, effective use of this drug is accompanied by increased local toxicity. One way to lower the toxicity of doxorubicin is encapsulation in liposomes. Indeed, the stealth liposomal formulation of doxorubicin (Doxil) has a tendency to accumulate better in solid tumors, and toxicity to the heart is lessened *(48–50)*. We tested the usefulness of Doxil in ILP in combination with TNF and found reduced efficacy compared with free doxorubicin, which is important for the outcome of clinical trials *(51)*.

In addition to chemotherapy studies, gene therapy studies have also demonstrated the usefulness of local delivery. Although intratumoral injection of an adenoviral construct coding for IL-3β in a soft tissue sarcoma had no effect on tumor growth, transendothelial delivery by ILP resulted in a pronounced tumor response *(52)*. We observed that the latter delivery resulted in impressive transfection of tumor cells in the well-perfused regions of the tumor, whereas intratumoral injection resulted in a typical needle-track transfection of tumor cells *(53)*. ILP results in a more homogeneous distribution of the viral vector, which is also true for delivery of chemotherapeutics. We hypothesize that, in addition to enhanced delivery of the chemotherapeutic or vector, the more homogeneous distribution in vital areas of the tumor resulting from the isolated perfusion procedure is crucial in obtaining a better response.

5.3. Translating ILP Research to Organ Perfusion

The success obtained with ILP initiated the translation of this approach to the liver. Not only is the liver more difficult to isolate from the body than an extremity but it is also more likely to respond to (toxic) agents. It is therefore imperative to provide conclusive data on the feasibility, toxicity, and efficacy of this approach before application in the human setting is warranted. We used IHP in the rat to study the interaction between melphalan and TNF in liver-confined primary tumors. The first objective was to establish the feasibility of the approach with emphasis on (local) toxicity and to test our hypothesis that, as in ILP, a synergistic antitumor activity can be obtained when one is using melphalan and TNF in IHP. Although we needed to lower the TNF dose in IHP, an effective concentration can be used, with minimal leakage into the system *(11)*. Moreover, we demonstrated synergy between TNF and melphalan with dramatic tumor response. The model allowed us to pinpoint a high vascular density of the liver tumor as an important prerequisite for effective application of TNF *(41)*, which could very well explain the discrepancy in tumor response observed by Alexander et al. *(54)*.

In pigs the surgical procedure and pharmacokinetic profile of chemotherapeutics in IHP was evaluated *(20)*. In this setting also, balloon catheter-based IHP was tested with success *(22)*. However, in patients this approach was accompanied by extensive collateral leakage, clearly demonstrating the limitations of animal models and the necessary precautions when translation is made to patients.

5.4. Isolated Kidney Perfusion

Like perfusion of the liver, local treatment of the kidney is complicated by the response of this organ to the procedure and agents administered. We found, for instance, that only low concentration of TNF can be tolerated *(15)*.

5.5. Isolated Lung Perfusion

In animal isolated lung perfusion (ILuP), the efficacy of a number of agents and agent combinations has been tested (reviewed in ref. *14*). ILuPs are performed in a number of different animals such as rats, dogs, rabbits, pigs, and sheep. In these models the efficacy of several agents (e.g., doxorubicin, melphalan, and cisplatin) toward sarcoma and melanoma has been shown. Moreover, in this setting the combination of melphalan with TNF was also tested but did not exhibit the same synergistic response as observed in ILP *(55)*. This might correlate with our conclusion that a high vascular density is needed for TNF to have an effect *(41)*. Carcinomas, as used in the ILuP, tend to have a lower vascular density compared wih sarcomas.

6. CONCLUSIONS

Although in vitro data may provide useful information on the direct cytotoxicty of agents toward tumor cells, efficacy in vivo may be hard to predict. The complexity of the in vivo setting is such that although an agent is highly potent in vitro, its usefulness in patients may be absent. Not only does the sensitivity of the tumor cells predict outcome but also the pharmacokinetic behavior of the agent, in addition to specificity, effect on organs and healthy tissues, binding to blood-borne elements, and, most importantly, the exact target. In vitro, the activity of an agent is generally tested using a single tumor cell line at one time. In vivo a tumor comprises a number of different cell types; tumor cells are present as well as leukocytes, fibroblasts, endothelial cells, and other cells, which may make up 50% of the tumor mass. TNF is an excellent example. Whereas TNF is only toxic toward 30% of the tumor cell lines tested, it is highly potent in an ILP setting. We demonstrated that TNF exhibited antitumoral activity irrespective of the sensitivity of the tumor cell line used. Thus, based on in vitro testing, TNF would have been dismissed. However, TNF mainly targets the tumor-associated vasculature, in particular the endothelial cell, such that increased permeability of the endothelial lining facilitates an augmented accumulation of the coadministered melphalan. This example, like many others, clearly proves the enormous power of a translational, well-chosen, and validated animal model.

REFERENCES

1. Jain RK. Normalization of tumor vasculature: an emerging concept in antiangiogenic therapy. Science 2005;307:58–62.
2. Kristensen CA, Nozue M, Boucher Y, Jain RK. Reduction of interstitial fluid pressure after TNF-alpha treatment of three human melanoma xenografts. Br J Cancer 1996;74:533–536.
3. Jain RK. Transport of molecules in the tumor interstitium: a review. Cancer Res 1987;47:3039–3051.
4. Jain RK, Munn LL, Fukumura D. Dissecting tumour pathophysiology using intravital microscopy. Nat Rev Cancer 2002;2:266–276.
5. Jain RK, Fenton BT. Intratumoral lymphatic vessels: a case of mistaken identity or malfunction? J Natl Cancer Inst 2002;94:417–421.
6. Creech OJ, Krementz ET, Ryan RF, Winblad JN. Chemotherapy of cancer: regional perfusion utilizing an extracorporeal circuit. Ann Surg 1958;148:616–632.
7. Manusama ER, Nooijen PTGA, Stavast J, Durante NMC, Marquet RL, Eggermont AMM. Synergistic antitumour effect of recombinant human tumour necrosis factor alpha with melphalan in isolated limb perfusion in the rat. Br J Surg 1996;83:551–555.
8. Manusama ER, Stavast J, Durante NMC, Marquet RL, Eggermont AMM. Isolated limb perfusion with TNF alpha and melphalan in a rat osteosarcoma model: a new anti-tumour approach. Eur J Surg Oncol 1996;22:152–157.
9. de Wilt JHW, Manusama ER, van Tiel ST, Van Ijken MGA, ten Hagen TLM, Eggermont AMM. Prerequisites for effective isolated limb perfusion using tumour necrosis factor alpha and melphalan in rats. Br J Cancer 1999;80:161–166.
10. de Brauw LM, van de Velde CJ, Tjaden UR, et al. In vivo isolated liver perfusion technique in a rat hepatic metastasis model: 5-fluorouracil concentrations in tumor tissue. J Surg Res 1988;44:137–145.
11. Van IJken MG, van Etten B, de Wilt JH, van Tiel ST, ten Hagen TL, Eggermont AM. Tumor necrosis factor-alpha augments tumor effects in isolated hepatic perfusion with melphalan in a rat sarcoma model. J Immunother 2000;23:449–455.
12. Weksler B, Schneider A, Ng B, Burt M. Isolated single lung perfusion in the rat: an experimental model. J Appl Physiol 1993;74:2736–2739.
13. Wang HY, Port JL, Hochwald SN, Burt ME. Revised technique of isolated lung perfusion in the rat. Ann Thorac Surg 1995;60:211–212.
14. Van Putte BP, Hendriks JM, Romijn S, Van Schil PE. Isolated lung perfusion for the treatment of pulmonary metastases current mini-review of work in progress. Surg Oncol 2003;12:187–193.
15. Van Der Veen AH, Seynhaeve ALB, Breurs J, Nooijen PTGA, Marquet RL, Eggermont AMM. In vivo isolated kidney perfusion with TNF-alpha in tumour bearing rats. Br J Cancer 1999;79:433–439.
16. Asbach HW, Bersch W. The effect of in situ isolated perfusion of experimental renal tumors with cytotoxic agents in high concentration. Urol Int 1980;35:112–124.
17. Walther MM, Jennings SB, Choyke PL, et al. Isolated perfusion of the kidney with tumor necrosis factor for localized renal-cell carcinoma. World J Urol 1996;14(Suppl 1):S2–7.

18. Hajjar RJ, Schmidt U, Matsui T, et al. Modulation of ventricular function through gene transfer in vivo. Proc Natl Acad Sci U S A 1998;95:5251–5256.

19. Davidson MJ, Jones JM, Emani SM, et al. Cardiac gene delivery with cardiopulmonary bypass. Circulation 2001;104:131–133.

20. de Vries MR, Rinkes IH, van de Velde CJ, et al. Isolated hepatic perfusion with tumor necrosis factor alpha and melphalan: experimental studies in pigs and phase I data from humans. Recent Results Cancer Res 1998;147:107–119.

21. Eggermont AM, Van Ijken MG, van Etten B, et al. Isolated hypoxic hepatic perfusion (IHHP) using balloon catheter techniques: from laboratory to the clinic toward a percutaneous procedure. Hepatogastroenterology 2000;47:776–781.

22. Van IJken MGA, de Bruijn EA, de Boeck G, ten Hagen TLM, van der Sijp JRM, Eggermont AMM. Isolated hypoxic hepatic perfusion with tumor necrosis factor-alpha, melphalan and mitomycin C using balloon catheter techniques: a pharmacokinetic study in pigs. Ann Surg 1998;228:763–770.

23. Van IJken MG, van Etten B, Brunstein F, et al. Bio-chemotherapeutic strategies and the (dis) utility of hypoxic perfusion of liver, abdomen and pelvis using balloon catheter techniques. Eur J Surg Oncol 2005;31:807–816.

24. van Etten B, Brunstein F, Van IJken MG, et al. Isolated hypoxic hepatic perfusion with orthograde or retrograde flow in patients with irresectable liver metastases using percutaneous balloon catheter techniques: a phase I and II study. Ann Surg Oncol 2004;11:598–605.

25. Van IJken MG, de Bruijn EA, ten Hagen TL, de Boeck G, van Eijck CH, Eggermont AM. Balloon catheter hypoxic abdominal and pelvic perfusion with tumour necrosis factor-alpha, melphalan and mitomycin C: a pharmacokinetic study in pigs. Eur J Surg Oncol 2004;30:699–707.

26. Van IJken MG, van Etten B, Guetens G, et al. Balloon catheter hypoxic abdominal perfusion with mitomycin C and melphalan for locally advanced pancreatic cancer: a phase I-II trial. Eur J Surg Oncol 2004;30:671–680.

27. Parpala-Sparman T, Liakka A, Kortteinen P, Lukkarinen O. Surgical organ perfusion method for gene transfer into cells of the perifollicular area of the spleen: an experimental trial on farm pigs. Scand J Clin Lab Invest 2001;61:293–299.

28. Eggermont AMM, Schraffordt Koops H, Klausner JM, et al. Isolated limb perfusion with tumor necrosis factor and melphalan for limb salvage in 186 patients with locally advanced soft tissue extremity sarcomas. The cumulative multicenter European experience. Ann Surg 1996;224:756–764;discussion 764–765.

29. Eggermont AMM, de Wilt JH, ten Hagen TL. Current uses of isolated limb perfusion in the clinic and a model system for new strategies. Lancet Oncol 2003;4:429–437.

30. Eggermont AMM, ten Hagen TL. Isolated limb perfusion for extremity soft-tissue sarcomas, in-transit metastases, and other unresectable tumors: credits, debits, and future perspectives. Curr Oncol Rep 2001;3:359–367.

31. Eggermont AMM, Schraffordt Koops H, Lienard D, et al. Isolated limb perfusion with high-dose tumor necrosis factor-alpha in combination with interferon-gamma and melphalan for nonresectable extremity soft tissue sarcomas: a multicenter trial. J Clin Oncol 1996;14:2653–2665.

32. ten Hagen TLM, Eggermont AMM, Lejeune FJ. TNF is here to stay—revisited. Trends Immunol 2001;22:127–129.

33. Manusama ER, de Wilt JHW, ten Hagen TLM, Marquet RL, Eggermont AMM. Toxicity and anti-tumor activity of interferon gamma alone and in combination with TNF alpha and melphalan in isolated limb perfusion in the BN175 sarcoma tumor model in rats. Oncol Rep 1999;6:173–177.

34. Seynhaeve ALB, de Wilt JHW, van Tiel ST, Eggermont AMM, ten Hagen TLM. Isolated limb perfusion with actinomycin D and TNF-alpha results in improved tumour response in soft-tissue sarcoma-bearing rats but is accompanied by severe local toxicity. Br J Cancer 2002;86:1174–1179.

35. de Wilt JHW, Manusama ER, van Etten B, et al. Nitric oxide synthase inhibition results in synergistic anti-tumour activity with melphalan and tumour necrosis factor alpha-based isolated limb perfusions. Br J Cancer 2000;83:1176–1182.

36. de Wilt JH, Soma G, ten Hagen TL, et al. Synergistic antitumour effect of TNF-SAM2 with melphalan and doxorubicin in isolated limb perfusion in rats. Anticancer Res 2000;20:3491–3496.

37. Lans TE, ten Hagen TL, van Horssen R, et al. Improved antitumor response to isolated limb perfusion with tumor necrosis factor after upregulation of endothelial monocyte-activating polypeptide II in soft tissue sarcoma. Ann Surg Oncol 2002;9:812–819.

38. Lans TE, van Horssen R, Eggermont AM, ten Hagen TL. Involvement of endothelial monocyte activating polypeptide II in tumor necrosis factor-alpha-based anti-cancer therapy. Anticancer Res 2004;24:2243–2248.

39. de Wilt JHW, ten Hagen TLM, de Boeck G, van Tiel ST, de Bruijn EA, Eggermont AMM. Tumour necrosis factor alpha increases melphalan concentration in tumour tissue after isolated limb perfusion. Br J Cancer 2000;82:1000–1003.

40. Van Der Veen AH, de Wilt JHW, Eggermont AMM, van Tiel ST, Seynhaeve ALB, ten Hagen TLM. TNF-alpha augments intratumoural concentrations of doxorubicin in TNF-alpha-based isolated limb perfusion in rat sarcoma models and enhances anti-tumour effects. Br J Cancer 2000;82:973–980.

41. van Etten B, de Vries MR, Van Ijken MGA, et al. Degree of tumour vascularity correlates with drug accumulation and tumour response upon TNF-alpha-based isolated hepatic perfusion. Br J Cancer 2003;88:314–319.

42. ten Hagen TLM, Van Der Veen AH, Nooijen PTGA, van Tiel ST, Seynhaeve ALB, Eggermont AMM. Low-dose tumor necrosis factor-alpha augments antitumor activity of stealth liposomal doxorubicin (DOXIL) in soft tissue sarcoma-bearing rats. Int J Cancer 2000;87:829–837.

43. Brouckaert P, Takahashi N, van Tiel ST, et al. Tumor necrosis factor-alpha augmented tumor response in B16BL6 melanoma-bearing mice treated with stealth liposomal doxorubicin (Doxil) correlates with altered Doxil pharmacokinetics. Int J Cancer 2004;109:442–448.

44. Brunstein F, Hoving S, Seynhaeve AL, et al. Synergistic antitumor activity of histamine plus melphalan in isolated limb perfusion: preclinical studies. J Natl Cancer Inst 2004;96:1603–1610.

45. Hoving S, Brunstein F, aan de Wiel-Ambagtshear G, et al. Synergistic antitumor response of interleukin 2 with melphalan in isolated limb perfusion in soft tissue sarcoma-bearing rats. Cancer Res 2005;65:4300–4308.

46. Rossi CR, Foletto M, Di Filippo F, et al. Soft tissue limb sarcomas: Italian clinical trials with hyperthermic antiblastic perfusion. Cancer 1999;86:1742–1749.

47. Di Filippo F, Giannarelli D, Botti C, et al. Hyperthermic antiblastic perfusion for the treatment of soft tissue limb sarcoma. Ann Oncol 1992;3(Suppl 2):S71–S74.

48. Coukell AJ, Spencer CM. Polyethylene glycol-liposomal doxorubicin. A review of its pharmacodynamic and pharmacokinetic properties, and therapeutic efficacy in the management of AIDS-related Kaposi's sarcoma. (Review). Drugs 1997;53:520–538.

49. Gabizon A, Shiota R, Papahadjopoulos D. Pharmacokinetics and tissue distribution of doxorubicin encapsulated in stable liposomes with long circulation times. J Natl Cancer Inst 1989;81:1484–1488.

50. Gabizon A, Meshorer A, Barenholz Y. Comparative long-term study of the toxicities of free and liposome-associated doxorubicin in mice after intravenous administration. J Natl Cancer Inst 1986;77:459–469.

51. ten Hagen TL, Hoving S, Ambagtsheer G, van Tiel ST, Eggermont AM. Lack of efficacy of Doxil in TNF-alpha-based isolated limb perfusion in sarcoma-bearing rats. Br J Cancer 2004;90:1830–1832.

52. de Wilt JH, Bout A, Eggermont AM, et al. Adenovirus-mediated interleukin 3 beta gene transfer by isolated limb perfusion inhibits growth of limb sarcoma in rats. Hum Gene Ther 2001;12:489–502.

53. de Roos WK, de Wilt JH, van Der K, Manusama ER, et al. Isolated limb perfusion for local gene delivery: efficient and targeted adenovirus-mediated gene transfer into soft tissue sarcomas. Ann Surg 2000;232:814–821.

54. Alexander HR, Brown CK, Bartlett DL, et al. Augmented capillary leak during isolated hepatic perfusion (IHP) occurs via tumor necrosis factor-independent mechanisms. Clin Cancer Res 1998;4:2357–2362.

55. Hendriks JM, Van Schil PE, de Boeck G, et al. Isolated lung perfusion with melphalan and tumor necrosis factor for metastatic pulmonary adenocarcinoma. Ann Thorac Surg 1998;66:1719–1725.

II TECHNIQUES AND PREREQUISITES FOR REGIONAL THERAPY

4 Interventional Radiotherapy

Enrique Lopez Hänninen, MD
and Timm Denecke, MD

SUMMARY

Brachytherapy is an established technique in radiation oncology. The radiation source is placed into the tissue, next to or directly into the tumor. In contrast to percutaneous implantation of applicators into superficial tumors or insertion of applicators into body cavities, interventional minimally invasive application of brachytherapy addresses the internal organs, particularly the liver, which is a common site of metastatic and primary tumor manifestations. For interventional application of radiation treatment agents to hepatic malignomas, two methods are currently used: the percutaneous approach using cross-sectional imaging, usually computed tomography, for guidance of applicator positioning and radiation therapy planning purposes, and the transarterial approach, using angiographic as well as scintigraphy techniques for targeting and dosimetry. Percutaneous afterloading has been shown to be suitable for treatment of lung malignomas as well. This chapter reviews the indications, methodology, and clinical outcome of both interventional modalities, percutaneous interstitial brachytherapy and transarterial radioembolization, in hepatic malignomas.

Key Words: Interstitial radiation, brachytherapy; transarterial radioembolization; microspheres; afterloading; liver malignancy; radiation oncology; local ablative therapy; interventional radiology.

1. INTRODUCTION

Radiation oncology represents one important pillar of cancer treatment. Radiation treatment is usually applied percutaneously by external beam radiation. However, there are a few indications for which the radiation source is brought next to the tumor, such as endobronchial or endovaginal irradiation of lung and cervical cancer, or interstitial

From: *Cancer Drug Discovery and Development: Regional Cancer Therapy*
Edited by: P. M. Schlag and U. S. Stein © Humana Press Inc., Totowa, NJ

irradiation of superficial tumors (e.g., breast cancer, head and neck cancer). This approach is called brachytherapy and is usually realized in an afterloading technique, whereby a radiation source, e.g., Iridium-192, is inserted into prepositioned applicators, which offers the opportunity for high dose rate irradiation ([HDR] >12 Gy/h) with minimal exposure of neighboring tissues. The sites accessible for traditional noninvasive brachytherapy are limited, as body cavities like the trachea or the vagina are needed to insert the afterloading catheter, or else invasive implantation of catheters is required.

Tumor localizations like the liver are more difficult to reach, since invasive procedures are required to introduce the radiation source into the tumor region. Intraoperative radiation therapy has been successfully used in the past to treat internal organs. However, since most of the indications are palliative approaches, minimally invasive procedures with a low risk of morbidity and mortality are warranted. This can be achieved by employing radiological interventional procedures, which are mainly based on image guidance. In the liver, the interventional approach is either percutaneously in an afterloading technique or transarterially. The latter is called transarterial radioembolization (RE), as radioactive (Yttrium-90) microspheres are injected into the hepatic artery and embolize semi-selectively into the peripheral capillaries of the metastases. The semiselectivity of transarterial RE is given by the dominant arterial supply of hepatic malignomas as opposed to the normal liver parenchyma, which is predominantly supplied by the portal vein. For patients with irresectable metastatic disease or primary hepatic malignomas confined to the liver, interstitial therapy is an interesting option. The aim is the complete ablation of all hepatic lesions or at least the achievement of local tumor control. Specifically, radiofrequency ablation (RFA) has gained increasing interest since it is easy to use and can also be used as an outpatient procedure in selected patients (1). Laser-induced thermotherapy (LITT) offers the opportunity of real-time therapy monitoring by magnetic resonance thermometry, which is thought to be advantageous to other locally ablative procedures (e.g., RFA) (2,3). However, these procedures have limitations concerning the number, localization, size, and shape of tumor lesions.

More recently, there hs been growing interest in applying radiotherapy to hepatic metastases of colorectal cancer. However, since the tolerance dose of liver parenchyma is lower than that of most tumor tissues, the therapeutic efficacy of percutaneous irradiation interferes with the mandatory maintenance of sufficient liver function. The main problems are the breathing excursion of the liver and the flat dose shoulder surrounding the target volume, resulting in a relatively high radiation exposure of the normal hepatic parenchyma. Even though innovations exist like triggered irradiation, stereotactic irradiation, or tomotherapy devices, these problems have not generally been solved to date (4).

The drawbacks of external beam radiotherapy can be overcome when irradiation is combined with locally ablative treatment. Inserting a radiation source into the tumor in an afterloading technique via percutaneous transhepatic catheters placed under computed tomography (CT) guidance is largely independent of breathing motion and offers a steep dose reduction to the periphery for optimally focused dosing of the tumor lesion. This technique is invasive, thus requires a short radiation time, and is therefore applied as single-fraction HDR brachytherapy (5).

For multiple hepatic tumor lesions or diffuse hepatic spread, local ablation is not suitable. Here, in addition to the established and evolving systemic chemotherapeutic concepts, alternative approaches such as transarterial application of therapeutic agents (chemoembolization, infusion chemotherapy, or tumor perfusion) can be used as pallia-tive strategies to achieve a regional coverage of the hepatic tumor burden (6). Another promising approach for regional treatment of hepatic malignancies is the transarterial implantation of radioactive microspheres (7). This regional concept is mainly based on the characteristically different blood supply of the normal liver and hepatic malignomas. It has been shown that hepatic metastases from colorectal cancer have a dominantly arterial blood supply, whereas the liver parenchyma is supplied to a great extent (approxi-mately 80–85%) by the portal vein (8). Flooding the liver with an embolizing agent via the hepatic arteries will thus affect the metastases predominantly. This semiselectivity allows targeting of tumors inside the liver, even if the lesions are multiple and diffusely distributed.

In the following discussion, aspects of interstitial brachytherapy with percutaneous afterloading and transarterial RE will be explored including patient selection, treatment planning, procedures, technical considerations, adverse effects, and clinical outcome.

2. PERCUTANEOUS AFTERLOADING

2.1. Background

Intraoperative radiotherapy in a high single dose has been used to treat unresectable liver metastases. Safety and efficacy have been shown in previous studies. The typical doses applied range between 15 and 30 Gy, with reference to the tumor margin and accepting dose inhomogeneity in the target volume depending on the particular radiation technique (9–11). Thomas et al. (11) reported on 22 patients with irresectable liver metastases who underwent laparotomy and interstitial HDR brachytherapy with Iridium-192 with doses in the tumor periphery ranging from 20 to 30 Gy (11). No acute or chronic radiation toxicity was observed at a median follow-up of 11 mo. Median actuarial local control at irradiated sites was 8 mo, with 26% actuarial local control at 26 mo by CT or magnetic resonance imaging (MRI). This phase I/II trial demonstrates the feasibility of single-fraction HDR brachytherapy in the treatment of liver metastases. However, since most of these procedures are palliative, a minimally invasive approach without the risk of laparotomy and the opportunity of imaging guidance by MRI or CT is favorable. This may be achieved by an image-guided procedure, e.g., CT-guided percutaneous puncture of the hepatic tumor and catheter placement for subsequent afterloading, as described by Ricke et al. (5). This interventional radiological approach has been successfully em-ployed for treatment of several secondary and primary hepatic malignomas, and also in malignomas of the lung and other sites (5,12).

2.2. Patient Evaluation

Locally ablative treatment should be preserved for patients with solitary tumor mani-festations, regionally confined disease, or symptomatic lesions. Local overtreatment with an unnecessary risk should be avoided. Whether a patient might profit from locally ablative treatment depends in general on the tumor entity, tumor spread, and overall clinical condition. The indication has to be made individually after thorough examination and careful assessment of alternative treatment options. Clinical and paraclinical param-eters such as comorbidity, liver function, or blood coagulation have to be taken into consideration, as well as the patients's decision.

Theoretically, minimally invasive interstitial afterloading is applicable to many potential tumor localizations. It has already been successfully applied for treatment of pulmonary and hepatic malignomas, but also in the mediastinum, in the retroperitoneum, or in bone. The limitation is primarily the technical feasibility of catheter placement, as a minimal risk of the procedure has to be ensured. A secondary limitation is the possibility of placing surrounding tissues at risk for adverse effects of irradiation, such as the bowel, stomach, spinal canal, skin, neuronal tissue, and so on. The size and number of lesions to treat is of course an issue. However, the procedure can be adapted to achieve a sufficient dose coverage in target volumes larger than those suitable for thermal ablation techniques *(13)*. Additionally, it has been shown that CT-guided interstitial brachytherapy is independent of the cooling effects of large vessels or bile ducts in the ablation zone, which have been identified as potential causes of inadequate heating and local recurrent tumor growth in thermal ablation techniques *(13)*. As the widest experience has been had with hepatic malignomas, the following will mainly focus on interstitial HDR brachytherapy via percutaneous transhepatic afterloading. However, these technical aspects of locally ablative treatment apply not only to hepatic malignomas but also to other organs involved by tumor, such as the lung, where patients may benefit of interstitial therapy, predominantly in a palliative scenario *(12)*.

2.3. Therapy Application

For therapy planning, cross-sectional imaging, CT or MRI is needed. The chosen imaging modality has to be capable of outlining the tumor precisely against the surrounding tissue. A gross planning of catheter positions is done using the axial slices, as this is the orientation of the fluoroscopic CT monitoring of the intervention. In addition to the puncture direction, dose coverage of the clinical target volume and sparing of surrounding tissues at risk have to be taken into account during catheter placement. It is useful to place the needle such that a bridge of normal liver parenchyma lies between the liver capsule and the tumor border. This buffer provides a hold for the catheter and prevents bleeding of commonly hypervascularized tumors and potential spilling of tumor cells into the abdominal cavity. The puncture is performed under aseptic conditions and CT (or MRI) guidance after intravenous sedation and anesthesia as well as local anesthesia at the cutaneous puncture site. A guide wire is inserted through the needle, and the needle is replaced by a flexible catheter sheath (opaque on X-ray). After removal of the guide wire, an afterloading catheter is placed into the catheter sheath. The system is stitched to the skin for fixation. Upon completion of catheter placement, a contrast-enhanced scan is acquired for documentation of the exact catheter location in relation to the tumor. These data are the basis for 3D reconstructions and radiation therapy planning on a dedicated workstation by outlining the clinical target volume (CTV), the catheters, and the surrounding risk tissues (e.g., bowel, stomach wall, gall bladder, kidney, spinal canal, skin). This technique, with retrospective registration of the catheter positions, is highly accurate and less complex compared with prospectively arranged catheter positions with templates or intraoperative raster placement *(14,42)*.

With a selected minimal CTV dose, usually 15 to 25 Gy, an afterloading plan is generated giving stop locations and dwell times for the Iridium-192 source (half-life, 78.8 d; decay, beta [672 keV] and gamma [<469 keV]) inside the afterloading catheters. This plan needs to be controlled and may be manually adjusted if necessary. Although the number of catheters is theoretically unlimited, it is recommended not to exceed six to eight catheters, depending on the tumor size and shape. Because of the stress situation, the radiation time should be limited to 1 h depending on the patient's condition. Using this plan, the afterloading procedure is performed and subsequently the catheters are slowly removed, sealing the puncture channels with tissue glue or other thrombogenic material to prevent bleeding.

2.4. Adverse Events

Adverse events can be subdivided into acute complications occurring during or imme-diately after treatment and late inadvertent effects. The acute adverse events are mainly owing to mechanical alterations caused by the puncture and catheter placement. These are bleeding, or perforation of the bowel, stomach, or gall bladder. These and other supradiaphragmatic organs may be traumatized with the needle, which, however, occurs very rarely since CT-guided puncture is a safe way to avoid severe injuries of nontarget tissues. Major bleeding from the liver is a very rare complication and can be prevented by sufficient sealing of the puncture channel during retraction of the catheter sheaths. Other acute effects are pain, emesis, and shivers, which should be treated medically.

Late effects besides infectious complications are mainly related to radiation exposure of nontarget tissues. When one is treating hepatic malignomas, exposure of surrounding healthy liver tissue to a relevant radiation dose cannot be avoided. This consecutive safety margin is generally advantageous and desired. However, a sufficient hepatic reserve has to be ensured before one treats hepatic malignomas, particularly in patients with large and/or multiple lesions, preexisting liver disease (e.g., hepatocellular carcinoma in cir-rhosis), previously irradiated liver (dose accumulation), or otherwise impaired liver func-tion reserve owing to prior chemotherapy. The tolerance dose of the liver ranges from 30 Gy to the whole organ to 50 Gy to approximately one-third of the liver volume. For external radiotherapy, the clinical end points are liver failure and severe hepatitis. If the irradiated volume of normal liver tissue is reduced down to approximately 100 mL or less, the tolerated doses are much higher—in principle, without any upper limit with respect to the clinical end points mentioned. Additionally, the different radiobiologic effects of a single high-dose fraction to the tissue compared with fractionized strategies has to be considered. It is well known that healthy tissue tolerates larger doses applied in multiple fractions. The options for the irradiated liver tissue are either destruction or recovery to normal liver function. Additionally, compensating mechanisms of the remaining nonirradiated liver parenchyma have to be taken into account. In a study by Ricke et al. (13), it was shown that in interstitial brachytherapy with iridium-192 and an afterloading technique, the tolerance dose causing an early functional loss of hepatocytes, as deter-mined by MRI with hepatotrope contrast material 6 wk after irradiation, was 9.9 Gy (±2.3 SD). This and the careful assessment of the hepatic reserve has to be taken into consid-eration when one is planning the treatment, to avoid posttherapeutic hepatic failure.

Other tissues at risk are the bile ducts, gallbladder, gastrointestinal tract, skin, kidney, and spinal cord. Previously described complications have included strictures of the com-mon bile duct or gastric ulcers (5,15). Concerning gastric complications, a threshold dose of of 15.5 Gy/mL tissue for the clinical end point ulceration of gastric mucosa has been estimated (15). This in vivo assessment is in accordance with tolerance data by Emami et al. (16). Regarding the small and large bowel, dose thresholds have not been estimated yet, but it has been hypothesized that they are similar to those described for the gastric wall. Overall, however, these complications and late effects are rare (5,17). Concerning gastric exposure, proton pump inhibitor therapy is being recommended as ulcer prophy-laxis. In all cases, a careful evaluation of the risk/benefit ratio has to be performed before treatment initiation and during radiation planning.

2.4. Clinical Outcome

Image-guided local tumor ablation has been established as a valuable adjunct in onco-logical treatment concepts. Most locally ablative procedures are performed by applying thermal ablation, such as radiofrequency or laser. However, in view of the limitations of thermal ablations regarding tumor size, shape, and location, or adjacent risk structures, novel techniques combining brachytherapy with modern interventional techniques have demonstrated favorable outcomes. In contrast to thermal ablation therapies, CT-guided brachytherapy is independent of complex geometric configurations of the lesions, as dwell times and dwell locations of the source within the applicators can be adjusted to fit the outlines of the tumor (18). Furthermore, adjacent ducts and vessels do not influence the ablation zone, as brachytherapy is not prone to disturb cooling effects. In contrast to external beam radiation, breathing motions are not an issue, because the catheters move with the tumor (13).

Initial data suggest that with minimal dose levels of 12 to 20 Gy, local tumor control may be as high as 87% after 6 mo (5). An analysis of treatment of 200 colorectal liver metastases between 1 and 11 cm (median 4 cm) in a phase III study revealed a local tumor control rate of 96% after 12 mo with 25 Gy, and 67% with 20 Gy as the minimal tumor dose. Major adverse events were hemorrhage in three patients (2%), which ceased after blood transfusion (19).

CT-guided brachytherapy of lung malignancies has also demonstrated favorable results with respect to side effects and local tumor control. In a phase I trial, 15 patients with 28 lung metastases and non-small cell lung cancer in two patients were treated with a single fraction of 20 Gy minimal tumor dose. No major adverse events were recorded. Minor events included radiographically visible local hemorrhage in two patients (12). In contrast to thermal ablation techniques, air cavities in the lung were not seen. Radiobiologically, the cytotoxic effect after single-fraction HDR irradiation shows within weeks to months, with only moderate acute injury and, in particular, no mechanical alterations (20).

3. TRANSARTERIAL RADIOEMBOLIZATION

RE is a one-time procedure and is usually not repeated. The therapeutic agent consists of microspheres, 20 to 40 nm in diameter, which contain radionuclide emitting beta-radiation (e.g., Yttrium-90) (21–24). The effective path length of Yttrium-90 is only 5.3 mm, meaning that 90% of the energy is deposited within a 5.3-mm radius of the microsphere. Yttrium-90-microspheres, both resin and glass, were recently approved by the U.S. Food and Drug Administration (FDA) for transarterial treatment of hepatic malignancies (7). The microspheres are delivered into the hepatic artery and embolize the microvessels and capillaries of tissues. The dominance of arterial supply of hepatic malignancies in contrast to the normal liver is used for a semiselectivity of drug delivery (8). The typical vascular architecture of liver metastases leads to a predominant seeding of the microspheres into the outer regions of the tumors, which are hypervascularized and thus hyperoxygenated, making radiation in these areas more effective (22). In addition to colorectal cancer metastases, promising data exist from controlled phase I to III trials for the use of RE in hepatocellular carcinoma (7). Benefits from RE application in other secondary hepatic malignomas, such as breast cancer metastases, have been reported occasionally (25).

3.1. Patient Evaluation

The planning of transarterial RE requires certain imaging procedures. Proper patient selection and treatment rationale, taking disease status and cancer entity into account, are important. Tumor staging to exclude extrahepatic progression is mandatory. This should be done at least by CT imaging of the thorax and abdomen, to gain information about lesion dynamics. In this context, it should be thoroughly discussed whether or not a patient might benefit from RE. This is unlikely when progressive extrahepatic disease is present or when a hepatic failure is preexistent. For preinterventional staging of patients with colorectal liver metastases, we recommend the performance of additional FDG-PET scans or combined FDG-PET-CT scans, since it has been shown that patient selection before invasive focused treatment like surgery or thermal ablation can be improved (26,27). Additionally, MRI of the liver can be helpful in individual cases to define the topography of the hepatic tumor burden and to discuss technical options of alternative locally ablative procedures. Since the approach is dependent on the vascular situation, it is desirable to perform helical CT scanning with multirow detector CT including arterial and portal venous phase imaging. This is important to rule out arterial or portolvenous occlusions and to visualize anatomic variants of hepatic arteries and can be helpful in planning digital subtraction angiography (DSA) (28).

Aside from tumor and vascular status, other clinical and paraclinical parameters, such as signs of liver failure or diminished hepatic synthesis, are important. Since relevant radiation exposure of hepatic parenchyma cannot be avoided, careful risk stratifications have to be made concerning the maintenance of sufficient liver function. This is why studies on risk stratification are mainly focused on hepatic parameters. In a study with 121 hepatocellular carcinoma patients, Goin et al. (29) identified the high risk factors (i.e., infiltrative disease, large tumor burden [>70% of the liver], reduced albumin levels, elevated bilirubin levels, or estimated lung dose >30 Gy) that have resulted in significantly worse clinical outcome compared with low risk patients (median survival at low-risk, 466 d; at high risk, 108 d). A total of 12 patients died from complications considered to be therapy related (n = 6, liver failure; n = 2, pneumonitis; and n = 1, gastric ulceration; three patients were not specified). Pulmonary and gastrointestinal therapy-related complications are predominantly caused by nontarget seeding of microspheres into nonhepatic arteries or through arteriovenous intrahepatic shunts. Therefore, therapy planning with DSA and scintigraphy is needed to rule out predisposing risk factors such as relevant shunt volumes or aberrant nonhepatic arteries within the area of microsphere release (29).

3.2. Treatment Planning and Dosimetry

DSA is routinely performed before RE for two reasons. One is the visualization of hepatic arteries and their anatomic variants to find the optimal localization for releasing the microspheres. The other purpose of DSA is the identification of nontarget vessels arising in the area of agent release, supplying organs other than the liver. Avoidance of extrahepatic implantation of microspheres, potentially causing gastritis, ulcers, pancreatitis, and other gastrointestinal morbidities, is decisive (7). Therefore, sufficient and careful planning of the procedure is mandatory. Even though coil embolization of the right gastric artery and the gastroduodenal artery is recommended before RE, there may exist small collateral or accessory vessels, supplying gastrointestinal structures from the hepatic arteries after coiling. Intervention planning should include selective arterial catheterization with application of ^{99m}Tc-macroaggregated albumin (MAA) and subsequent planar scintigraphy to define the distribution of microspheres, which are subsequently released at the same intraarterial location, with respect to shunting to the lung and gastrointestinal accumulations (7).

DSA is performed via transfemoral arterial access including selective mesentericoportography, which is used to visualize the vascular anatomy of the liver and to explore technical options to determine the optimal location for microsphere release. Technical considerations have been extensively reviewed elsewhere by Liu et al. (30).

The desired position of the catheter tip is the proper hepatic artery, distally from origins of arterial branches supplying organs other than the liver. With the high number of anatomic variants of the arteries supplying the liver and other organs in the upper abdomen, there are a few nontarget arteries, which are potentially included in the perfusion territory. The cystic artery usually arises from the right hepatic artery (71%) (31). This implies the risk of therapy-related cholecystitis. If the gallbladder has not been resected previously, intraarterial drug delivery should be performed distally from the origin of the cystic artery. The right gastric artery is a minor contributor to the gastric blood supply. Variation of the right gastric artery is common. It may arise from the proper hepatic artery (51%), the left (23%) or right (3%) hepatic artery, the origin of the gastroduodenal artery (GDA) (3%), or the common hepatic artery (9%) (32). The identification of this vessel is imperative for regional treatment, as inflammation with gastric necrosis, mucosal ulceration, and perforation are potential complications of inadvertent delivery of RE, as in intraarterial infusion chemotherapy (33). Here, with insufficient coiling of the right gastric artery during minimally invasive port implantation, the incidence of endoscopically confirmed mucosal lesions is 36%, compared with 3% in cases with sufficient coiling (34). Thus, it is important to exclude insufficient coiling with vessel recanalization (4% of cases; 34), subsequent opening collateral vessels of the right gastric artery before application of therapeutic agents proximally to its origin. The GDA and its branches may be responsible for duodenal ulceration or pancreatitis during regional therapy, when coiled insufficiently or subsequently opening collaterals were initially not visible during coiling and MAA test injection (30).

The location of drug release depends on the anatomy of the hepatic arteries. Injection into the proper artery in case of regular arterial anatomy allows treatment of the entire liver in a single therapy session. It is also possible to divide the amount of MAA, and subsequently of therapeutic agent, into two or more portions and to administer them over an angiographic catheter selectively into the supplying arteries of the liver or single liver lobes in more than one location. This is advantageous, not only because this technique is independent from anatomic variants with separate hepatic arteries but also for fractionation of the therapy into two single-lobe treatment sessions, in order to preserve a hepatic reserve.

Nonetheless, knowledge of accessory arteries and aberrant origins of arteries is important to ensure regional coverage of the entire tumor bearing liver, as it has been shown that ignored minor feeders may cause accumulation deficits in the liver (35). An aberrant

or accessory right hepatic artery occurs in 10 to 31% of cases, with 96% of these originating from the superior mesenteric artery *(30)*. An accessory or replaced left hepatic
artery is present in 12 to 21% of cases. It usually arises from the left gastric artery and thus
communicates with the gastric and esophageal bed. Other relevant variants are double
hepatic arteries with separate origins from the aorta or an accessory middle hepatic artery
(30). Alternatively to fractionation of drug delivery to address separately originating
hepatic arteries, especially if one of the arteries is difficult to catheterize or drug application is insecure owing to near nontarget vessels, a central coil embolization of the
smaller vessels can be performed to induce an intrahepatic arterial collateralization from
the dominant artery. This strategy has the advantage of maintaining a single location for
drug release in the dominant artery. However, the collateralization is often not fully
compensatory, resulting in the dependent liver parenchyma being poorly supplied with
microspheres.

After angiographic assessment of arterial anatomy and MAA injection at the desired
location, scintigraphy is performed including planar anterior and posterior scans covering the thorax and abdomen, as well as single-photon emission computed tomography
(SPECT) scans of the upper abdomen. It has been shown that performing the SPECT scan
with SPECT-CT hybrid systems for anatomic mapping of scintigraphic findings is advantageous *(35)*. Based on this examination, extrahepatic inadvertent MAA accumulations can be accurately detected or excluded, the intrahepatic perfusion pattern can be
assessed, and arteriovenous shunting to the lung can be quantified by comparing the
count rate over the lung with that of the liver. Whereas the presence of nontarget MAA
seeding makes a repeated DSA necessary to occlude the responsible vessel or to modify
the location of drug release, the shunt quantification accounts for the dosimetry. A high
shunt volume predisposes for a radiation-induced pneumonitis and fibrosis; thus, the
delivered dose of microspheres has to be diminished according to the shunt volume. The
dose of Yttrium-90-microspheres, approximately 1 to 3 GBq, is related to the body
surface, the shunt volume, and the hepatic tumor burden. Other models of dosimetry are
adapted to the tumor and liver volume.

3.3. Therapy Application

For the drug application procedure, radiation protection is mandatory. Therefore,
specific devices have been developed, to prevent direct and prolonged contact of the
radiologist with the therapeutic agent. Again, DSA is performed with selective intraarterial catheterization with line placement similarly to the test injection of MAA. Then
yttrium-90-microspheres are infused alternating with small bolus injections of contrast
agent for maintenance of the correct catheter position and to check for retrograde flow.
Afterward another scintigraphy on the basis of bremsstrahlung emission is performed as
described above for documentation of microsphere distribution.

3.4. Adverse Events

As aforementioned, the adverse treatment-related events can be subdivided into hepatic and nonhepatic. The nonhepatic complications are mainly owing to nontarget seeding of microspheres into the gastrointestinal tract and lung. For the latter, consecutive
pneumonitis and fibrosis have been described in rare cases. This was significantly related
to high shunt volumes and high estimated doses delivered to the lungs (>30 Gy) *(29)*.

Gastrointestinal seeding may result in mucositis, ulceration, perforation, or pancreatitis, depending on the location and the amount of microsphere implantation. This is why the pretherapeutic test injection of ^{99m}Tc-MAA with assessment of shunting and nontarget implantation is so important.

Hepatic toxicity is of course an issue, as relevant radiation doses reach the nonmalignant portion of the liver. This is particularly the case in hepatocellular carcinoma (HCC) patients in whom liver function is commonly impaired owing to viral hepatitis and cirrhosis. In a retrospective study with 88 HCC low-risk patients, it was shown that radiation dose (up to 150 Gy) and pretreatment bilirubin levels elevations correlated with the occurence of posttherapeutic liver toxicity. Portal vein occlusion and ascitis was not significantly related to therapy-related liver toxicity (36).

3.5. Clinical Outcome

The arterial administration of Yttrium-90 loaded glass and resin microspheres to the liver for treatment of hepatic malignancies is currently approved by the FDA for specific indications, the stand-alone or presurgical or pretransplant radiation therapy of irresectable hepatocellular carcinoma (glass device, approved in 2000) and the treatment of irresectable colorectal metastases in combination with intraarterial fluorodeoxyuridine (FUDR) (resin device, approved in 2002). The widest experiences have been with colorectal liver metastases and hepatocellular carcinoma, and there is evidence that both devices are suitable for the treatment of HCC and colorectal metastases alike (7). However, RE of other tumor entities in the liver (e.g., breast cancer, gallbladder cancer, thyroid cancer, non-small cell lung cancer) has also shown encouraging results in regards to local control and may prove beneficial in the future (25,37).

In HCC, a phase II trial has shown improved mean survival in those patients receiving higher doses of Yttrium-90 glass microspheres (>104 Gy, 635 d; <104 Gy, 323 d) (38). Comparable survival benefits were observed in patients receiving higher doses of Yttrium-90 resin microspheres (39). Data from another trial, summarizing 80 patients with hepatocellular carcinoma treated at different disease stages and doses of 47 to 270 Gy showed similar survival times as those reported for transarterial chemoembolization. The response rate in a trial including 71 patients was 27%; in 4 of these patients resection was allowed by therapy-related shrinkage of the tumors.

Concerning colorectal cancer metastases, the most relevant (randomized phase III) trial so far has included 71 patients who had received intraarterially either FUDR alone or FUDR in combination with Yttrium-90 resin microspheres. A significant difference was observed in the mean time to disease progression in both groups, which was favorable for those patients who were treated with RE (9.7 vs 15.9 months, $p = 0.001$) (24). Similar survival benefits were demonstrated in other trials for RE plus chemotherapy vs chemotherapy alone, with a mean survival time of 29.4 vs 12.8 mo (40). Studies employing the glass microsphere device also achieved encouraging results, with stable disease or partial response in more than 50% of patients (41).

4. CONCLUSIONS

Employing features of established therapies, such as the efficacy of brachytherapy, the safety of CT-guided organ puncture, principles of afterloading technique, and minimal invasiveness of superselective arterial catheterization, a novel therapeutic approach in radiation oncology has been developed by means of interventional radiation therapy. Transarterial RE and percutaneous afterloading of hepatic malignomas are therapeutic instruments enabling effective treatment even in those patients who are not suitable for surgical or thermal ablations because of tumor size or location. Results are promising for the treatment of HCC and colorectal liver metastases as well, and further studies are upcoming. This and the increasing interest in interventional radiotherapy will help to establish these procedures and to define their roll in modern concepts of cancer treatment.

REFERENCES

1. Meyers MO, Sasson AR, Sigurdson ER. Locoregional strategies for colorectal hepatic metastases. Clin Colorectal Cancer 2003;3:34–44.
2. Nolsoe CP, Torp-Pedersen S, Burcharth F, et al. Interstitial hyperthermia of colorectal liver metastases with a US-guided Nd-YAG laser with a diffuser tip: a pilot clinical study. Radiology 1993;187:333–337.
3. Vogl TJ, Müller PK, Hammerstingl R, et al. Malignant liver tumors treated with MR imaging-guided laserinduced thermotherapy: technique and prospective results. Radiology 1995;196:257–265.
4. Herfarth KK, Debus J, Wannenmacher M. Stereotactic radiation therapy of liver metastases: update of the initial phase-I/II trial. Front Radiat Ther Oncol 2004;38:100–105.
5. Ricke J, Wust P, Stohlmann A, et al. CT-guided interstitial brachytherapy of liver malignancies alone or in combination with thermal ablation: phase I-II results of a novel technique. Int J Radiat Oncol Biol Phys 2004;58:1496–1505.
6. Meyer L, Hildebrandt B, Riess H. 5-Fluorouracil, folinic acid and oxaliplatin administered via hepatic arterial infusion as regional second-line therapy for advanced colorectal cancer. Oncology 2003;64:473–474.
7. Murthy R, Nunez R, Szklaruk J, et al. Yttrium-90 microsphere therapy for hepatic malignancy: devices, indications, technical considerations, and potential complications. Radiographics 2005;25(Suppl 1):S41–S55.
8. Breedis C, Young G. The blood supply of neoplasms in the liver. Am J Pathol 1954;30:969–797.
9. Nauta RJ, Heres EK, Thomas DS, et al. Intraoperative single-dose radiotherapy. Observations on staging and interstitial treatment of unresectable liver metastases. Arch Surg 1987;122:1392–1395.
10. Dritschilo A, Harter KW, Thomas D, Nauta R, Holt R, Lee TC, Rustgi S, Rodgers J. Intraoperative radiation therapy of hepatic metastases: technical aspects and report of a pilot study. Int J Radiat Oncol Biol Phys 1988;14:1007–1011.
11. Thomas DS, Nauta RJ, Rodgers JE, et al. Intraoperative high-dose rate interstitial irradiation of hepatic metastases from colorectal carcinoma. Results of a phase I-II trial. Cancer 1993;71:1977–1981.
12. Ricke J, Wust P, Wieners G, et al. CT-guided interstitial single-fraction brachytherapy of lung tumors: phase I results of a novel technique. Chest 2005;127:2237–2242.
13. Ricke J, Wust P, Wieners G, et al. Liver malignancies: CT-guided interstitial brachytherapy in patients with unfavorable lesions for thermal ablation. J Vasc Interv Radiol 2004;15:1279–1286.
14. Tonus C, Debertshauser D, Strassmann G, et al. CT-based navigation systems for intraoperative radiotherapy using the afterloading-flab technique. Dig Surg 2001;18:470–474.
15. Streitparth F, Pech M, Bohmig M, et al. In-vivo assessment of the gastric mucosal tolerance dose after single fraction, small volume irradiation of liver malignancies by computed tomography-guided high-dose-rate brachytherapy. Int J Radiat Biol Oncol Phys 2006;65(5):1479–1486.
16. Emami B, Lyman J, Brown A, et al. Tolerance of normal tissue to therapeutic irradiation. Int J Radiat Oncol Biol Phys 1991;21(1):109–122.
17. Ricke J, Seidensticker M, Ludemann L, et al. In vivo assessment of the tolerance dose of small liver volumes after single-fraction HDR irradiation. Int J Radiat Oncol Biol Phys 2005;62:776–784.
18. Rühl R, Ricke J. Image-guided microtherapy for tumor ablation: from thermal coagulation to advanced irradiation techniques. Onkologie 2006;29:210–224.
19. Ricke J, Mohnike K, Pech M, Wieners G, Wust P, Felix R. CT-guided interstitial HDR-brachytherapy of liver malignancies: results of a prospective phase III trial in colorectal liver metastasis. Radiology 2005;230:164.

20. Manning MA, Zwicker RD, Arthur DW, Arnfield M. Biologic treatment planning for high-dose-rate brachytherapy. Int J Radiat Oncol Biol Phys 2001;49:839–845.
21. Arie IM. Treatment of inoperable primary pancreatic and liver cancer by the intra-arterial administration of radioactive isotopes (Y90 radiating microspheres). Ann Surg 1965;162:267–278.
22. Campbell AM, Bailey IH, Burton MA. Tumor dosimetry in human liver following hepatic yttrium-90 microsphere therapy. Phys Med Biol 2001;46:487–498.
23. Gray B, Van Hazel G, Hope M, et al. Randomised trial of SIR-spheres plus chemotherapy vs. chemotherapy alone for treating patients with liver metastases from primary large bowel cancer. Ann Oncol 2001;12:1711–1720.
24. Rubin D, Nutting C, Jones B. Metastatic breast cancer in a 54-year-old woman: integrative treatment with yttrium-90 radioembolization. Integr Cancer Ther. 2004;3:262–267.
25. Fernandez FG, Drebin JA, Linehan DC, Dehdashti F, Siegel BA, Strasberg SM. Five-year survival after resection of hepatic metastases from colorectal cancer in patients screened by positron emission tomography with F-18 fluorodeoxyglucose (FDG-PET). Ann Surg 2004;240:438–447.
26. Amthauer H, Denecke T, Hildebrandt B, et al. Evaluation of patients with liver metastases from colorectal cancer for locally ablative treatment with laser induced thermotherapy. Impact of PET with 18F-fluorodeoxyglucose on therapeutic decisions. Nuklearmedizin 2006;45(4):177–184.
27. Lehmkuhl L, Denecke T, Warschewske G, et al. Multislice computed tomography angiography for pre-interventional planning of port placement for intra-arterial hepatic infusion chemotherapy. J Comput Assist Tomogr 2006, in press.
28. Goin JE, Salem R, Carr BI, et al. Treatment of unresectable hepatocellular carcinoma with intrahepatic yttrium 90 microspheres: a risk-stratification analysis. J Vasc Interv Radiol 2005;16:195–203.
29. Liu DM, Salem R, Bui JT, Courtney A, Barakat O, Sergie Z, Atassi B, Barrett K, Gowland P, Oman B, Lewandowski RJ, Gates VL, Thurston KG, Wong CY. Angiographic considerations in patients undergoing liver-directed therapy. J Vasc Interv Radiol 2005;16:911–935.
30. Arora R, Soulen MC, Haskal ZJ. Cutaneous complications of hepatic chemoembolization via extra-hepatic collaterals. J Vasc Interv Radiol 1999;10:1351–1356.
31. Yamagami T, Nakamura T, Iida S, et al. Hepatic encephalopathy secondary to intrahepatic portosystemic venous shunt: balloon-occluded retrograde transvenous embolization with n-butyl cyanoacrylate and microcoils. Cardiovasc Intervent Radiol 2002;25:219–221.
32. Nakamura H, Hashimoto T, Oi H, Sawada S, Furui S. Prevention of gastric complications in hepatic arterial chemoembolization. Balloon catheter occlusion technique. Acta Radiol 1991;32:81–82.
33. Inaba Y, Arai Y, Matsueda K, Takeuchi Y, Aramaki T. Right gastric artery embolization to prevent acute gastric mucosal lesions in patients undergoing repeat hepatic arterial infusion chemotherapy. J Vasc Interv Radiol 2001;12:957–963.
34. Denecke T, Hildebrandt B, Lehmkuhl L, et al. Fusion imaging using a hybrid SPECT-CT camera improves port perfusion scintigraphy for control of hepatic arterial infusion of chemotherapy in colorectal cancer patients. Eur J Nucl Med Mol Imaging 2005;32:1003–1010.
35. Goin JE, Salem R, Carr BI, et al. Treatment of unresectable hepatocellular carcinoma with intrahepatic yttrium 90 microspheres: factors associated with liver toxicities. J Vasc Interv Radiol 2005;16: 205–213.
36. Wong CY, Qing F, Savin M, et al. Reduction of metastatic load to liver after intraarterial hepatic yttrium-90 radioembolization as evaluated by [18F]fluorodeoxyglucose positron emission tomographic imaging. J Vasc Interv Radiol 2005;16(8):1101–1106.
37. Dancey JE, Shepherd FA, Paul K, et al. Treatment of nonresectable hepatocellular carcinoma with intrahepatic 90Y-microspheres. J Nucl Med 2000;41:1673–1681.
38. Lau WY, Leung WT, Ho S, et al. Treatment of inoperable hepatocellular carcinoma with intrahepatic arterial yttrium-90 microspheres: a phase I and II study. Br J Cancer 1994;70(5):994–999.
39. van Hazel G, Blackwell A, Anderson J, et al. Randomised phase 2 trial of SIR-Spheres plus fluorouracil/leucovorin chemotherapy alone in advanced colorectal cancer. J. Surg Oncol 2004;88:78–85.
40. Andrews JC, Walker SC, Ackermann RJ, et al. Hepatic radioembolization with yttrium-90 containing glass microspheres: preliminary results and clinical follow-up. J Nucl Med 1994;35(10):1637–1644.
41. Kolotas C, Roddiger S, Strassmann G, et al. Palliative interstitial HDR brachytherapy for recurrent rectal cancer. Implantation techniques and results. Strahlenther Onkol 2003;179:458–463.

5 Surgical Strategies

Sandra Grünberg, MD and
Peter M. Schlag, MD, PhD

CONTENTS

SUMMARY

In this chapter regional cancer treatment of tumors/metastases of the peritoneum, liver, lung, pleura, and the limbs is summarized and, especially, surgical technical principles and prerequisites of regional chemotherapy are described.

Regional chemotherapy can be applied via vascular or cavital access. Prior to regional therapy extra-regional tumor spread has to be excluded and the individual anatomy of the region to be treated must be clarified. Intraoperatively, a skillfull management and postoperatively a thoughtful monitoring of the patient is mandatory. Therefore, a close collaboration between different medical specialities is necessary.

Key Words: Pre-, peri- and postoperative prerequisites/management; surgical techniques; cavital access; vascular access; perfusion; infusion.

1. INTRODUCTION

Regional therapy is an important option in the treatment of unresectable or metastatic tumors. The aims of regional therapy are to increase the exposure of regional confined cancers to drugs and to decrease their systemic levels. Regional therapy is used as a rescue therapy for tumors that have not responded to systemic chemotherapy or as an alternative to reduce systemic side effects of high-dose chemotherapy. Two main routes for access are available: vascular or intracavital (Table 1). In this chapter the technical principles and prerequisites for regional therapy, the periinterventional management, and the special risks of the different strategies are summarized. The reader will find further specific information in the corresponding chapters of this book.

From: *Cancer Drug Discovery and Development: Regional Cancer Therapy*
Edited by: P. M. Schlag and U. S. Stein © Humana Press Inc., Totowa, NJ

Table 1
The Most Relevant Techniques and
Procedures in Regional Chemotherapy

Vascular access
Intravascular infusion
Liver
Head-neck
Pancreas
Breast
Perfusion
Liver
Limb
Lung
Stop-flow procedures
Pelvis
Pancreas

Cavital access
Cavital infusion
Peritoneum
Pleura
Bladder
Cavital perfusion
Peritoneum

2. PREOPERATIVE DIAGNOSTICS AND PREREQUISITES

Prior to therapy, the benefit of regional chemotherapy in comparison with systemic chemotherapy must be evaluated. Regional therapy requires a close collaboration between different medical specialists (Fig. 1). To exclude extraregional tumor spread, contrast-enhanced computed tomography (CT) or magnetic resonance tomography (MRT) are essential. Additionally, positron emission tomography and CT (PET/CT) have become valuable diagnostic tools to rule out extraregional tumor spread. Diagnostic laparoscopy/thoracoscopy is recommended when other imaging procedures are not conclusive. Because of the side effects of regional therapy, the operability of patients should be evaluated by standard cardiopulmonary examinations (electrocardiogram, pulmonary function tests), complete blood count, and liver and kidney function tests. The use of contrast media that require good renal function must be restricted when nephrotoxic substances will be used for regional therapy. Furthermore, specific diagnostic tests such as echocardiograms, extended lung function tests, or stress electrocardiograms should be performed when cardio- or pulmotoxic (especially prior to extracorporal perfusion) procedures will be used or when extended surgery is planned in combination with regional therapy. Preoperative evaluation of tumor markers should be done to establish an early trend parameter for tumor response. Ulcerated or infected tumors should be recognized as a septic risk.

2.1. Vascular Access

The vascular approach requires reliable access to the tumor, supplying the vascular system with homogenous distribution of the drug in the target (1).

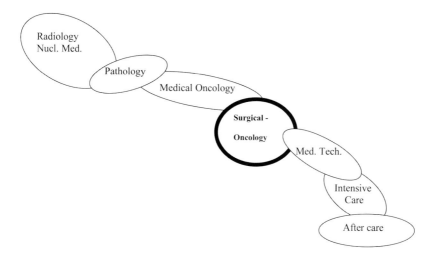

Fig. 1. Medical specialities and expertise needed for regional therapy.

The vascular supply of the target organ needs to be known in detail. Therefore, angiography or multislice contrast-enhanced CT must be performed prior to surgery to identify vascular anomalies, collaterals, or occluded vessels. To prevent systemic side effects, aberrant vessels might be occluded preoperatively by the radiologist or might be ligated/clamped intraoperatively by the surgeon. In cases of additional supply vessels, the placement of a double-lumen catheter for infusion therapy might be an alternative to vascular ligature. Additionally, the venous or portal vein system should be examined by ultrasound Doppler to exclude thrombosis. Patients with severe lymph edema are unsuitable candidates for regional therapy. Finally, the neurological status of the patient should be carefully recorded. The limb volume, body surface, and body weight must be measured to calculate the drug dosage *(2)*.

2.2. Cavital Access

In case of peritoneal carcinomatosis, the peritoneal cancer index needs to be evaluated. This index is a quantitative prognostic indicator of carcinomatosis *(3)*. Generally, prior to cavital chemotherapy tumor debulking should be done as extensively as possible. In cases of captured lung owing to pleural carcinomatosis, decortication has to be performed prior to regional therapy.

3. PRE-, PERI-, AND POSTOPERATIVE MANAGEMENT

In association with hyperthermic chemotherapy, body temperature must be monitored by means of temperature probes placed, e.g., into the esophagus and the bladder. The temperature of the target organ must also be controlled during hyperthermic regional therapy. Before applying nephrotoxic substances, at least 3 L of isotone saline solution must be infused. If there is a risk of a crush kidney owing to myoglobinemia (e.g., after isolated limb perfusion [ILP] or the aortic stop flow technique), the urine pH should be controlled regularly. If the pH of the urine drops below 7.0, $NaHCO_3$ (50 mL) should be given. To prevent a crush kidney, diuresis should be higher than 200 mL/h. Because of the risk of renal failure, the equipment and experience for hemodialysis must be available. Leakage of cytostatic drugs into the systemic circuit must be controlled continuously. Patients need to be intubated with a double-lumen endotracheal tube prior to isolated lung or pleural perfusion. Extended cardiac monitoring should be available. During ILP and stop flow procedures, catheters should be used, which allow the interpretation of the left heart function. For the early postoperative phase a well-equipped intensive care unit should be readily available.

To prevent clotting of surgically placed catheters a mixture of about 5 mL saline solution and heparin (5000 IE heparin [1 mL heparin]/4 mL NaCl) should be injected into the chamber of the port after the catheter is connected to the port or directly into the catheter.

3.1. Vascular Access: Infusion Chemotherapy

3.1.1. HEPATIC ARTERIAL INFUSION (HAI) THERAPY

The following drugs are mainly used for HAI: 5-fluorouracil (5-FU), 5-fluoro-2-deoxyuridine (FUDR), cisplatin, and Adriamycin (8).

Several techniques are used for the delivery of HAI chemotherapy, including:

1. A **catheter** connected to an external **infusion** pump.
2. Arterial access **port systems**.
3. Surgically placed implantable vascular **pump systems**.

The vascular anatomy of the liver must be known in detail. About 15 to 30% of the patients have anomalies in hepatic vascular supply. The different anomalies in liver perfusion are depicted in Table 2 (4). The catheter should be inserted so that infusion with the chemotherapeutic agent results in complete hepatic perfusion. Arterial branches distal to the catheter and proximal to the liver should be ligated to prevent extrahepatic perfusion. A cholecystectomy is recommended to prevent drug-induced cholecystitis (7). Homogenous liver perfusion and correct catheter placement is confirmed intraoperatively by injection of patent blue or fluoroscein and visualization with a Wood lamp (6). For arterial catheter placement, the distance between the end of the gastroduodenal artery and the bifurcation of the common hepatic artery is important. If the distance is less than 1 cm, the gastroduodenal artery goes directly into the right liver artery, and homogenous distribution of the chemotherapeutic agent is uncertain.

Currently, there are no studies comparing the feasibility of silicon or polyurethane catheters for long-term use. Most catheters have an open tip, but some have a vent at their tip. If shortening of the catheter is necessary, it should not be cut with scissors (4). Cutting the catheter causes roughness at the tip, which may result in thrombosis. Nonabsorbable sutures should be used to fix the catheter at the vessel. For direct implantation of the catheter in the mainstream off an artery, the use of a Holter catheter is recommended (4).

3.1.1.1. Percutanously Placed Catheter Connected to an External Pump.
Early studies with percutaneously placed hepatic artery catheters showed considerable success. However, the risk of catheter clotting, bleeding, and infection led physicians to use this method less frequently (5). Nevertheless, it can be valuable to check the patient's response to a chemotherapeutic agent prior to treatment via a permanent regional vascular access system.

Table 2
Anomalies in Hepatic Arteries

Type	Anomaly
I	Right, middle, and left liver arteries resolve from the A. hepatica communis
II	Right and middle liver arteries resolve from the A. hepatica communis; left liver artery resolves from the A. gastrica sinistra (10%)
III	Left and middle liver arteries resolve from the A. hepatica communis; right liver artery resolves from the A. mesenterica superior (11%)
IV	Only the middle liver artery resolves from the A. hepatica communis; right artery resolves from the A. mesenterica superior and the left from the A. gastrica sinistra (1%)
V	Right, middle, and left liver arteries resolve from the A. hepatica communis; one small left liver artery, relatively accessory liver artery, resolves from the A. gastrica sinistra (8%)
VI	Right, middle, and left liver arteries resolve from the A. hepatica communis; one small right, relatively accessory liver artery, resolves from the A. mesenterica superior (7%)
VII	Right, middle, and left liver arteries resolve from the A. hepatica communis; but with small or normal diameter, additional accessory right liver artery resolves from the A. mesenterica superior and an accessory liver artery resolves from the A. gastrica sinistra (1%)
VIII	Combinations: (1) atypical origin of the A. hepatica dextra and accessory left artery or (2) accessory right liver artery and atypical origin of the A. hepatica sinistra (2%)
IX	Absence of the A. hepatica communis; whole arterial blood supply by A. mesenterica superior (2.5%)
X	Absence of the A. hepatica communis; whole arterial blood supply by the A. gastrica sinistra (0.5%)

a According to Michels *(4)*.

3.1.1.2 Arteria Hepatica Port Catheter. To place a permanent arteria hepatica port catheter, either a laparoscopy or a laparatomy must be performed. After the ligation of the peripancreatic part of the gastroduodenal artery, the catheter is placed and fixed in the hepatic part of the artery.

The tip of the catheter has to be placed tangential to the blood flow of the A. hepatica propria. Before connecting the catheter to the port, the port and the catheter must be filled with saline solution (heparin block). The port is implanted in a subcutaneous pocket on top of the distal rib cage. The port is accessed with strict sterile technique, using a Huber needle.

3.1.1.3. Surgically Placed Implantable Pumps. In principle, the implantation of a drug delivery pump does not differ from the implantation of the catheter port system. The pump is placed in a subcutaneous pocket in the right abdominal area. The pro and cons of the pump system are discussed in Chapter 13 of this book, about regional chemotherapy of liver tumors. The major disadvantage of the implantable pump is the small drug reservoir, which does not allow the use of drugs other than FUDR.

3.2. Vascular Access: Perfusion Chemotherapy

3.2.1. ISOLATED LIVER PERFUSION

Isolated liver perfusion techniques with several technical variations have been used with 5-FU, mitomycin C, cisplatin, and melphalan with or without tumor necrosis factor-alpha (TNF-alpha) *(1)*.

Prior to perfusion, all the retroperitoneal venous tributaries of the vena cava, including the adrenal vein and the suprahepatic phrenic veins must be clamped. A segment of the gastroduodenal artery is dissected to serve as the arterial cannulation site for the isolated hepatic perfusion. A veno-venous bypass circuit is set up with the inferior vena cava, and portal blood flow is incorporated into this circuit. After this procedure, the inferior vena cava can be occluded and shunted to the axillary vein *(6)*. A venous return cannula is positioned in the retrohepatic portion of the inferior vena cava just below the hepatic veins to collect the venous effluent from the liver. This cannula is connected to the venous outflow line of the extracorporal bypass circuit for isolated perfusion. The arterial inflow catheter is introduced into the gastroduodenal artery and positioned at the confluence of the common hepatic artery and the gastroduodenal artery. Supra- and infrahepatic caval cross-clamps are applied, and the perfusion is initiated using a roller pump, a heat exchanger, and a bubble oxygenator. The hepatic temperature is monitored to ensure adequate hyperthermia and uniform delivery of the perfusate to both hepatic lobes *(6)*. After perfusion is completed, the liver is flushed to remove residual chemotherapy or biological agents. After the flush the vessels are decannulated, and vascular repairs are made.

3.2.2 ISOLATED LUNG PERFUSION

Human isolated lung perfusion studies from 1958 to 2004 have used mitomycin C, doxorubicin, TNF-α, cisplatin, and melphalan for the treatment of lung metastases *(7)*.

In cases of advanced metastases, perfusion may be performed before surgical resection *(7)*. Perfusion of lung tumors depends on the tumor entity. Experience has been gained mainly with regional chemotherapy along the bronchial-arterial system *(4)*. Chemotherapeutic agents such as doxorubicin, cisplatin, and melphalan with or without hyperthermia have proved useful in particular for the treatment of recurrent or unresectable lung metastases in sarcoma patients *(12,14)*.

Single-lung perfusion can be accomplished by cannulation of the pulmonary artery. Total lung perfusion requires a systemic and a pulmonary circuit. For the systemic circuit, a standard cardiopulmonary bypass is used, with arterial cannulation of the ascending aorta and a venous cannula placed in the right arterial appendage. The pulmonary circuit consists of a pulmonary artery cannula and a venous cannula in the left arterial appendage *(8)*. The main pulmonary artery and both pulmonary veins have to be isolated. The pericardium needs to be opened in order to clamp the pulmonary artery and veins centrally. The pulmonary artery and veins are cannulated by standard techniques. The main bronchus must be snared in order to occlude bronchial artery blood flow. The perfusion circuit contains a heat exchanger, a centrifugal pump, and special extracorporal circuit tubing primed with a mixture of 6% hydroxyethyl starch and 2% heparin *(7)*. The remaining volume of the perfusion circuit is contributed by the blood volume of the isolated lung.

Perfusion of the collapsed lung is carried out for 20 to 30 min at a rate of 300 to 500 mL/min at ambient temperatures *(9)*. Intraoperatively, malperfusion can be identified by the use of dye injection (patent blue, methylene blue). At the end of the perfusion, the chemotherapeutic agent must be washed out of the lung and the pulmonary vein effluent must be discharged

3.2.3. ISOLATED LIMB PERFUSION

The main indications for ILP are intrinsic metastases of malignant melanoma or advanced musculoskeletal tumors. Treatment of skeletal tumors is described in detail in the corresponding chapter of this book.

Melphalan is the standard cytotoxic drug for ILP. Actinomycin D, darcabacin, cisplatin, mitomycin, adriamycin, mioxantrone, and thiopenta are also used. TNF-alpha was first introduced to ILP by F. Lejeune and D. Lienard in 1988. The drugs must be placed into the arterial line of the perfusion circuit. Hyperthermia may intensify the effect of ILP. In case of cisplatin perfusion, tissue temperature should not increase above 40.5°C.

The limbs are isolated from the central circulation by dissecting the vessel. Depending on the tumor localization and spread, this can be done at three levels: in the region of the iliacal femoral vessels and in the femoropopliteal axis. All side branches and potential collaterals must be ligated or occluded during the time of perfusion. A tourniquet is applied above the cannulated vessels to compress the small vessels perfusing the muscle, the subcutaneous tissue, and the skin. Then the isolated extremity is provided with artificial circulation by means of an oxygenated extracorporeal circuit containing a heart-lung machine and an oxygenator. The temperature of the perfusate and the limb and parameters such as blood oxygen concentration, hematocrit, and pH of the perfusate are continuously monitored. Leakage monitoring is performed by using a precordial scintillation probe to detect leakage of radiolabeled albumin or erythrocyte suspension. Adjustment of the flow rate and tourniquet may be required to ensure that leakage from the perfusion circuit to the systemic circulation is stable and does not exceed 10%. In particular, TNF-α should only be administered if leakage is less than 3 to 5% per 60 min.

ILP consists of a 90-min-long perfusion at mild hyperthermia. At the end of the perfusion, washout fluid (albumin or hydroxyethyl-starch fluid) should be injected. The systemic reperfusion is followed by decannulation and suturing of the vessels.

3.2.4. AORTIC STOP FLOW PROCEDURES

Aortic stop flow procedures have been described for the treatment of advanced pancreatic and pelvic cancer (e.g., rectal cancer, gynecological cancers, and bladder cancer).

The cytostatic agents mitomycin C, doxorubicin, epirubicin, and cisplatin can be used as chemotherapeutic agents *(10,11)*.

Using the aortic stop flow technique, an isolated compartment is created including the whole abdominal cavity below the diaphragm, the retroperitoneal space, and the pelvis. Perfusion of this compartment is achieved by connecting the balloon catheters to the perfusion system. *(10)*. The stop-flow balloon catheter is placed via transfemoral arterial and venous access within the vena cava inferior and the abdominal aorta near the diaphragm. In the periphery, distal to the pelvis, cessation of blood flow can be achieved by means of pneumatic blockade of both thighs. Angiography can be used to check correct and tight placement of the balloon catheters and to exclude leakage *(11)*. Because of the complexity of blood perfusion, normally homogenous perfusion cannot be reached.

3.3. Cavital Access: Infusion Chemotherapy

For initial tumor debulking, see also Chapters 15 and 16 about peritoneal carcinomatosis and peritoneal mesothelioma.

Any tumor adherent to vital structures that cannot be resected may be cytoreduced with the cavitronic ultrasonic surgical aspirator device or electrocautery.

3.3.1. INTRAPLEURAL CHEMOTHERAPY USING AN IMPLANTABLE ACCESS SYSTEM

Hyperthermic intrapleural chemotherapy in pleural malignancies is described in detail in Chapter 24.

The implantable access system consists of a catheter and a port site. The silicon rubber catheter has multiple perforations along the proximal end. The catheter of the implantable access system is placed in the pleural space by video-assisted thoracoscopic surgery (VATS). The port is positioned in a subcutaneous pocket in the hypochondrium. The port and the catheter are connected via a subcutaneous tunnel *(12)*. The position of the catheter needs to be controlled by intraoperative X-ray. The portal is accessed transcutaneously using a Huber needle. It is important to avoid sharp bends in the catheter.

3.3.2. INTRAVESICAL THERAPY

Regional therapy of bladder tumors is described in Chapter 20.

3.3.3. INTRAPERITONEAL CHEMOTHERAPY

Intraperitoneal chemotherapy can be indicated for peritoneal carcinomatosis of the ovary or the gastrointestinal tract or pseudomyxoma peritonei.

Usually, cisplatin, mitomycin C, and doxurubicin are used for intraperitoneal (hyperthermic) perfusion *(13,14)*. For intraperitoneal chemotherapy using implantable systems, 5-FU and mitomycin C has been mainly used *(15)*.

3.3.3.1. Intraperitoneal Chemotherapy Using Implantable Catheters or Port Systems. Most experience with intraperitoneal chemotherapy has been obtained with the Tenckhoff-type catheter *(16)*. The device consists of an implantable catheter of 42 cm with perfusion holes in the distal part. There are two dacron cuffs, one placed adjacent to the fascia and the other in midposition within a subcutaneous tunnel. Separate peritoneal entry and skin exit sites via a s.c. tunnel serve to reduce peritoneal infection rates. Removal following completion of the therapy usually requires a minilaparotomy with adhesiolysis. The peritoneal Port-a-Cath system is an implantable version of the Tenckhoff system. Insertion can be carried out either at the time of laparotomy or as a separate limited procedure, utilizing two small incisions: one over the lower anterior rib cage, slightly above the costal margin, and another lateral to the umbilicus *(17)*. In case insertion takes place during laparotomy, the ports may be placed just above the costal margin over the lower anterior right and left rib cage. The incision over the anterior rib cage is carried down to the fascia, and a pocket large enough to house the port is created bluntly within the s.c. space. The port is sutured to the fascia with permanent sutures. Finally, the tunnelled Tenckhoff catheter is attached to the port *(17)*. The portal is accessed transcutaneously using a Huber needle. Before the first treatment cycle is started, an evaluation of the intraperitoneal distribution using radioisotopes should be performed (distribution scintigraphy).

3.4. Cavital access: Perfusion Chemotherapy

3.4.1. HYPERTHERMIC INTRAPERITONEAL CHEMOPERFUSION (HIPEC)

Intraperitoneal hyperthermic chemoperfusion can be performed simultaneously with tumor debulking or 5–7 d after cytoreductive surgery to prevent anastomotic leakage. However, because of adhesions, HIPEC should not be initiated later than 8 d after primary surgery. HIPEC can be performed by either an open or a closed technique. The open abdominal cavity technique involves covering the abdomen with a plastic sheet during circulation of hyperthermic chemotherapeutic agents (18). After the completion of cytoreductive surgery, peritoneal perfusion catheters are placed during surgery using small separate incisions (3). Two inflow catheters are placed in the left and right hemidiaphragma. Then another two catheters are placed. One catheter is placed in the deep pelvis and one in the superficial pelvis (19). Drainage bulbs are attached to the end of the outflow catheters. The abdominal skin incision is temporarily closed with a running suture to prevent leakage of peritoneal perfusate during the closed technique. A perfusion circuit is typically established with 3 L of crystalloid solution. Flow rates of approximately 300–1000 mL/min are maintained by using a roller pump managed by a perfusionist. The pelvic catheters drain to a standard cardiotomy reservoir containing a coarse filter to catch debris and reduce foaming. The circuit continues through a single roller pump and heat-exchanger to the patient. Heated water is pumped to the heat exchanger device heating/cooling blanket reservoir. The temperature of the fluid in the patient-return and patient-directed tubing is monitored with stainless steel couplers with temperature probe connectors and needle probes at the tips of one inflow and outflow cannula. The abdomen is gently massaged throughout the perfusion to improve drug distribution to all peritoneal surfaces. Constant temperature monitoring is performed at all temperature probes. Once outflow temperatures exceed 39°C, the antineoplastic drugs are added to the perfusate. A maximum inflow temperature of 42.5°C is tolerated during the perfusion. The target outflow temperature is 40°C. The total perfusion time after initial addition of the chemotherapeutic agent varies from 60 to 120 min in the literature. After the perfusion, the peritoneum is washed out with 2 to 5 L of lactated Ringer's solution. The skin is opened, and the cannulas are removed under direct vision. The abdomen is inspected, and the required anastomoses are created. The fascia and the skin are then closed in a standard fashion (3).

4. RISKS OF VASCULAR AND CAVITAL ACCESS

The main risks of regional cancer therapy using different access systems are catheter sepsis or catheter dislocation or leak, and surgical infection. Abscesses and fistulas (vascular-enteric, entero-cutan, porto-venous, pleuro-pulmonary, etc.) are common risks. Even in inexperienced hands the implanted systems can only be used in average for a less than 12–18 mo owing to local catheter or port or vessel complications (20). Leakage of cytostatic drugs into the systemic circulation or malperfusion result in the specific systemic side effects of the cytostatic drugs.

Hematological, gastrointestinal, pulmonary, and cardiological side effects have been seen. The risk of systemic toxicity rises when the dose of a cytostatic agent is higher for regional therapy than for systemic therapy (21).

A risk of thrombosis exists owing to catheter occlusion or dissection of vessels. Skin and muscle necrosis can occur in case of leakage.

Table 3
Complications With Hepatic Infusion Chemotherapy[a]

Complications	%
Gastric and duodenal ulcers	15
Biliary sclerosis (with FUDR)	6–35
Catheter occlusion/dislocation	5–30
Occlusion of liver artery	
By use of port systems	30
By use of implantable pumps	5
Hematoma/seroma	6
Catheter infection	1

[a] From ref. 4.

4.1. Vascular Access- Infusion Therapy

Systemic side effects may occur if the blood flow to aberrant vessels or to structures that should not be reached by regional chemotherapy has not been interrupted. Rare lethal complications, mainly because of pulmonary embolism, are described.

4.1.1. HEPATIC ARTERIAL INFUSION THERAPY (HAI)

Table 3 summarizes the complications with liver infusion therapy (4).

4.1.1.1. Method-Related Specific Risks. Early postinterventional complications include arterial injury leading to hepatic artery thrombosis; incomplete perfusion of the liver caused by the lack of recognition of an accessory hepatic artery; malperfusion to the stomach, duodenum, or pancreas; and pump/port pocket hematoma and infection (22). Five to 10% of patients have gastric or duodenal ulcers caused by malperfusion. Late complications tend to be more common and include pump/pocket infections, catheter thrombosis, and gastric or duodenal ulcer.

Pump failure, catheter breakage, thrombosis, and serious infections occurred in less than 10% in different clinical trials (23). The malpositioning of catheters may cause thrombosis. The catheter must be of the appropriate length. If the catheter is too short, there is a risk of disconnection between the port and the catheter, and owing to thoracic movements the catheter might rub on the ribs. Bowel strangulation in case of an intraabdominal catheter is possible.

4.1.1.2. Systemic Toxicity. Myelosuppression, stomatitis, nausea, vomiting, and diarrhea have been described (23).

4.1.1.3. Regional Toxicity. Chemical hepatitis refers to an elevation of liver enzymes or bilirubin and is the most common toxicity, occuring in 42% of patients in the different trials (5). When managed appropriately, most cases of hepatic toxicity resolve. In some patients, particularly those treated with FUDR, a progressive biliary sclerosis has been observed (5,23).

Table 4
Grade 3/4 Toxicities After Intraarterial Isolated Hepatic Perfusion *(5)*

	No. of Grade 3/4 Toxicities	
Toxicity	TNF + melphalan (n = 32)	Melphalan + HAI (n = 19)
Hypotension	1	0
Weight gain	4	1
Cardiac	0	1
Decrease in platelets	3	1
Increase in:		
Bilirubin	22	9
Transaminase	16	9
Alkaline Phosphatase	2	0

[a] With melphalan and tumor necrosis factor (TNF) or with melphalan followed by hepatic artrial infusion (HAI) in 51 patients with metastatic colorectal cancer.

4.2. Vascular Access Perfusion Therapy

4.2.1. ISOLATED LIVER PERFUSION

4.2.1.1. Method Related Special Risks and Systemic Toxicity. The perioperative morbidity includes liver failure, bleeding, pulmonary edema, and acute respiratory distress syndrome (ARDS). Table 4 summarizes the grade 3/4 toxicities after isolated hepatic perfusion with melphalan with or without TNF in 51 patients *(6)*.

4.2.2. ISOLATED LUNG PERFUSION

Experience with isolated lung perfusion is limited, and risk evaluation remains to be clarified.

4.2.2.1. Method-Related Special Risks. In a study including the perfusion of melphalan described by Hendriks et al., there was no operative or postoperative mortalitiy. One patient with bleeding required reintervention *(6)*. Interstitial or alveolar oedema as a result of contusion syndrome has been described *(8)*.

4.2.2.2. Local Toxicity. Lung edema and radiographic changes resembling a chemical pneumonitis of the whole perfused lung have been described. Owing to necrosis after treatment with TNF, 1 patient in 16 had an abscess *(8)*.

4.2.2.3. Systemic Toxicity. Cardiopulmonary toxicity was graded by a system devised by Burt et al. *(12)*. Two of seven patients showed grade 2 pulmonary toxicity, meaning a decrease of more than 20% in ventilation or perfusion of the treated lung, and dyspnea on exertion or rest. In a study by Ratto et al. with six patients there were no systemic toxicities *(8)*.

4.2.3. Isolated Limb Perfusion

4.2.3.1. Method-Related Special Risks. Mild disturbance of limb function was described in a study performed between 1991 and 2003 in 4 of 53 cases *(24)*.

4.2.3.2. Systemic Toxicity. Because of myoglobinemia, after perfusion there is always the risk of a crush kidney. Systemic toxicity was absent or mild: only 1 of 217 patients had a mild fever above 40° for more than 24 h *(24)*.

4.2.3.3. Local Toxicity. Acute local toxicity of the ILP procedure can be classified according to Wieberdink et al. *(18)*: grade I, no reaction; grade II, slight erythema or edema; grade III, considerable erythema or edema with some blistering, slightly disturbed motility permissible; grade IV, extensive epidermolysis or obvious damage to the deep tissues, causing definite functional disturbance and threatening or manifest compartmental syndrome; and grade V, reaction that may necessitate amputation. Late morbidity of the ILP led to lymphoedema in 28%, muscle atrophy in 12%, neuropathies in 3%, recurrent erysipelas in 3%, and motor deficiency in 20%. In 217 patients treated with ILP, local toxicity was mild (grade 1–2) to moderate (grade 3).

4.2.4. Stop Flow Technique

4.2.4.1. Method-related risks. There is a risk of rhabdomyolysis and a crush kidney. Intrainterventional problems and complications such as problems with the balloon catheter placement and disturbance of the blood circulation have been observed *(25)*. Duodenal ulcers causing gastrointestinal bleedings and paralytic ileus with subsequent development of peritonitis and severe enterocolitis have been described as well *(25)*. De Santis et al. described deaths owing to pulmonary embolism in 2 of 10 patients. In 1 of 10 patients the balloon ruptured intraarterally, and one hospitalization 10 d after perfusion was required owing to inguinal hematoma *(11)*.

4.2.4.2. Systemic side effects. Hematological abnormalities, in particular decrease in white blood cell and platelet counts, and gastrointestinal problems such as nausea, vomiting, diarrhea, and stomatitis of grade III/IV (WHO grading) have been described *(25)*. Chemotherapy-induced side effects could not be discriminated exactly from complications of the hypoxia induced by the abdominal perfusion *(10)*.

4.3. Cavital Access: Infusion Therapy

4.3.1. Intrapleural Chemotherapy

The special risks of intrapleural chemotherapy are described in Chapter 24. A hemothorax is rarely described *(12)*.

4.3.2. Intraperitoneal Chemotherapy

4.3.2.1. Method-Related Risks. In a study of 91 patients, the total number of complications was nine (7.63%), seen during catheter evacuation (eight bowel incisions and one hernia of the linea alba). In the same study 10 patients required cessation of chemotherapy prior to its expected completion for the following reasons: two fistulas of the catheter to the vagina, two fistulas to the bowel, four cases in which the intraperitoneal catheter spontaneously fell out owing to abscess (two after cytostatic flow under the skin and two without a clear reason, probably because of improper fixation), one abscess in the peritoneal cavity, and problems with cytostatic inflow, one because of a subileus *(26)*.

4.4. Cavital Access: Perfusion Therapy

4.4.1. Intraperitoneal Chemotherapy

For more detailed information see Chapter 16.

4.4.1.1. Method-Related Special Risks. Because of the extent of surgery necessary to obtain optimal cytoreduction, the morbidity and mortality of the procedures are significant *(3)*. Current morbidity rates range between 27 and 56%. The most common complications include abscess, bowel fistula, prolonged ileus, pneumonia, and hematological toxicity *(3)*. Other risks that need to be considered are chemical or infectious peritonitis, pancreatitis, and abdominal adhesions with (sub)ileus. Perforations may also occur in a delayed or late time frame, from weeks to many months after i.p. chemotherapy. Nausea and vomiting can be caused by local complications but also by systemic side effects of the chemotherapy and need supportive therapy. The risk of an anastomotic dehiscence is increased.

4.1.1.2. Systemic Side Effects. A risk of renal failure exists because of the use of cisplatin. The literature has noted that side effects for chemotherapy of mitomycin C and cisplatin are common. In a retrospective study by Pilati et al. of 34 patients treated for peritoneal carcinomatosis from colon adenocarcinoma, hematological toxicity (grade I or II anemia, according to the WHO classification) occurred in 4 patients *(27)*.

5. CONCLUSIONS

This overview shows that locoregional therapy is in its beginning. Its potential awaits further evaluation in clinical trials. The outcome of different treatment options must be evaluated in further thoroughly planned phase III studies with adequate control groups. For these trials a tight cooperation among surgical and medical oncologists, diagnostic and interventional radiologists, and medical technologists is essential.

REFERENCES

1. Schlag P, Hohenberger P. The rationale of intraarterial chemotherapy of liver cancer, in Domellöf L ESO Monographs: Drug Delivery in Cancer Treatment II, 1st ed., vol. 2. (Veronesi U, ed.), Berlin: Springer-Verlag, 1987:44–53.
2. Wieberdink J, Benckhuysen C, Braat RP, et al. Dosimetry in isolation perfusion of the limbs by assessment of perfused tissue volume and grading of toxic tissue reaction. Eur Cancer Clin Oncol 1982;18:905–910.
3. Stewart JH, Perry S, Levine EA. Intraperitoneal hyperthermic chemotherapy for peritoneal surface malignancy: current status and future directions. Ann Surg Oncol 2005;12:765–778.
4. Boese-Landgraf J. Spezielle chirurgische Kathetertechniken, in Regionale Tumortherapie, 1st ed. (Boese-Landgraf J, Gallkowski U, Layer G, Schallhorn A, eds.), Berlin: Springer Verlag, 2003:35–46.
5. Cohen AD, Kemeny NE. An update on hepatic arterial infusion chemotherapy for colorectal cancer. Oncologist 2003;8:553–566.
6. Grover AC, Richard HA. The past decade of experience with isolated hepatic perfusion. Oncologist 2004;9:653–664.
7. Hendriks J, Grootenboers M, Schramel FM, et al. Isolated lung perfusion with melphalan for resectable lung metastases: phase I clinical trial. J. Thoracsur 2004;78:1919–1927.
8. Liu D, Burt M, Ginsberg RJ. Lung perfusion of treatment of metastatic sarcoma of the lungs, in Regional Chemotherapy: Clinical Research and Practice, 1st ed. (Markmann M, ed.), Totowa, NJ: Humana, 2000:87–100.
9. Burt M, Liu D, Abolhoda A, et al. Isolated lung perfusion for patients with unresectable metastases from sarcoma a phase I trial. Ann Thorac Surg 2000;69:1542–1549.

10. Meyer F, Gebauer T, Grote R, et al. Pharmacokinetics of the antineoplastic drug mitomycin C in regional chemotherapy using the aortic stop flow technique in advanced pancreatic carcinoma, Chemotherapy 2005;51:1–8.

11. De Santis M, Arioso P, Calo GF, et al. Antineoplastic perfusion with percutanous stop-flow control in the treatment of advanced pelvic malignant neoplasms. Radiol Med 2000;100:56–61.

12. Shoji T, Tanaka F, Yanagihara K, et al. Phase II study of repeated intrapleural chemotherapy using implantable access system for management of malignant pleural effusion. Chest 2002;121:821–824.

13. Sugarbaker PH, Mora JT, Carmignani P, et al. Update on chemotherapeutic agents utilized for perioperative intraperitoneal chemotherapy. Oncologist 2005;10:112–122.

14. Sugarbaker PH. Peritoneal surface oncology: review of a personal experience with colorectal and appendical malignancy. Tech Coloproctol 2005;9:95–103.

15. Culliford AT, Brooks AD, Sharma S, et al. Surgical debulking and intraperitoneal chemotherapy for established peritoneal metastases from colon and appendix cancer. Ann Surg Oncol 2001;8:787–795.

16. Tenkhoff H. Manual for Chronic Peritoneal Dialysis. Seattle: University of Washington School of Medicine, 1974.

17. Wiper DW, Kennedy AW. Surgical considerations in intraperitoneal chemotherapy, in Regional Chemotherapy: Clinical Research and Practice, 1st ed. (Markmann M, ed.), Totowa, NJ: Humana, 2000:151–177.

18. Sugarbaker PH. Succesful management of microscopic residual disease in large bowel cancer. Cancer Chemother Pharmacol 1999;4:15–25.

19. Kuhn A, McLoughlin JM, Harris DC, et al. Intraperitoneal hyperthermic chemotherapy: experience at Baylor University Medical Center. Proc Bayl Univ Med Cent 2002;15:359–362.

20. Jakob AR, Kühl M, Jauch KW, et al. Complications using implantable port-systems for regional chemotherapy of liver metastases. Reg Cancer Treat 1996;9:33–36.

21. Schallhorn A. Allgemeine Pharmakologie, in Regionale Tumortherapie, 1st ed. (Boese-Landgraf J, Gallkowski U, Layer G, Schallhorn A, ed.), Berlin: Springer Verlag, 2003:5–10.

22. Kemeny NE, Atiq OT. Intrahepatic chemotherapy for metastatic colorectal cancer, in Regional Chemotherapy: Clinical Research and Practice, 1st ed. (Markmann M, ed.), Totowa, NJ: Humana, 2000: 5–20.

23. Pelley RJ, Regional hepatic arterial infusion chemotherapy for hepatic colorectal metastases, in Regional Chemotherapy: Clinical Research and Practice, 1st ed. (Markmann M, ed.), Totowa, NJ: Humana, 2000:21–32.

24. Grünhagen DJ, Brunstein F, Graveland WJ, et al. Isolated limb perfusion with tumor necrosis factor and melphalan prevents amputation in patients with multiple sarcomas in arm or leg. Ann Surg Oncol 2005;12:473–479.

25. Meyer F, Ridwelski K, Gebauer T. Pharmacokinetics of the antineoplastic drug mitomycin C in regional chemotherapy using the aortic stop flow technique in advanced pancreatic cancer. Chemotherapy 2005;51:1–8.

26. Milczek T, Emrich J, Klasa-Mazurkiewicz D. Surgical complications connected with intraperitoneal chemotherapy in ovarian cancer. Ginekol Pol 2003;74:817–823.

27. Pilati P, Mocellin S, Rossi CR, et al. Cytoreductive surgery combined with hyperthermic intraperitoneal intraoperative chemotherapy for peritoneal carcinomatosis arising from colon adenocarcinoma. Ann Surg Oncol 2003;10:508–513.

6 Regional Thermotherapy

Peter Wust, MD *and Johanna Gellermann,* MD

CONTENTS

SUMMARY

A broad range of temperatures is useful in oncology. Thermoablation (heat alone) requires temperatures of >45 to 50°C and is only clinically possible in circumscribed lesions. High-intensity focused ultrasound (HIFU) and nanotherapy are suitable methods. The largest volume heated is the whole body, using whole-body hyperthermia (WBHT); 42°C is the highest temperature permitted. Clinical experience and some positive studies suggest, however, that higher temperatures (e.g., 43°C) are required at least in certain specific (e.g., hypoxic) parts of the tumors to increase local control in conjunction with radiotherapy and/or chemotherapy and to be beneficial for patients. Dedicated multiantenna applicators operating in the radiofrequency range (60–200 MHz) must be designed for each indication accounting for the anatomical region. Magnetic resonance monitoring is the first candidate for noninvasive control.

The technical problems have been solved to integrate such applicators into an MR-tomograph. Although commercially available systems (for *regional hyperthermia*) are adequate for pelvic and extremity tumors, adaption/optimization is still desired for abdominally disseminated disease. Here, the term *part-body hyperthermia* has been created, for which a large number of clinical indications (gastrointestinal tumors) exist.

Key Words: Thermotherapy; thermoablation; nanotherapy; regional hyperthermia; part body hyperthermia; MR monitoring; thermography.

1. THERMAL DOSE AND DOSE-EFFECT RELATIONSHIP

Heat has a reproducible and predictable effect on cells *(1)*: the effect is quantified according to the thermal dose concept, taking the sum over a weighted product of temperature and exposure time. From the dependence of chemical reactions on temperature (the Arrhenius equation), we derive that above 42 to 43°C (the so-called breaking point)

From: *Cancer Drug Discovery and Development: Regional Cancer Therapy*
Edited by: P. M. Schlag and U. S. Stein © Humana Press Inc., Totowa, NJ

a temperature increase of 1°C shortens the treatment time by a factor of 2 to achieve an isoeffective thermal dose, e.g., 60 min at 43°C is equivalent to 30 min at 44°C. However, below the breaking point, a further decrease of temperature by 1°C enforces a fourfold treatment time for the same effect, i.e., 4 h at 40°C instead of 1 h at 41°C. We conclude that at temperatures < 43°C effective heat treatments are increasingly difficult.

From typical survival curves it follows that 60 min at 43°C can reduce the cell number by a factor of 10 (1). However, to control a macroscopic tumor, we need to eradicate 10^9 cells or more, resulting theoretically in a required time of 10 h (at 43°C) or approximately 10 min at 50°C. We conclude that for thermal ablation (destruction of tumors with heat alone), temperatures >45°C, or better, 50°C, are required (depending on the exposure time). This is only realistic under clinical conditions for small volumes (<4–5 cm; *see* Subheading 2.). Excessive treatment times at lower temperatures (e.g., for hours) or a higher number of fractions are also problematic because of the phenomenon of *thermotolerance*.

For locally advanced tumors and large regions, we must employ the sensitizing effect of heat that has been found in conjunction with radiation and/or certain cytotoxic drugs. Here, the thermal enhancement ratio (TER) has been introduced. The TER describes the factor by which the dose might be reduced to get the same effect. Typical values of TER ≅ 1.2 to 1.5 for 41 to 42°C (60 min) are known from laboratory studies. Therefore, lower temperatures in the range of 40 to 41°C might also be effective for a combination of heat with radiation (or chemotherapy). However, a precise estimation becomes more difficult, because of the high number of variables including physiological parameters (tumor environment) and the timing between both modalities. Note that a true simultaneous application of radiotherapy and heat has not been realized, for technical reasons.

Other temperature-dependent effects are also known, such as various immunological trigger points, intracellular processes, and physiological changes (especially perfusion changes). The clinical impact of these mechanisms is not yet clear until now. In addition, the required temperature is not precisely fixed, even though for certain immunological effects in particular (T-cell activation), a so-called danger signal (cell necrosis at temperatures ≥43°C) is postulated. In addition to the well-known enhancement of radiation and cytostatic drugs, other agents has been found that can be modulated by a temperature increase. Among them are thermosensitive liposomes (2) and heat control of gene expression (3).

All in all, the actual required temperatures for a certain therapeutic objective are not well defined. Therefore, a reasonable strategy is the attempt to get a temperature as high as possible. In fact, in a number of clinical studies, higher thermal parameters are statistically correlated with clinical end points describing local efficacy (*see* Subheading 3.).

From in vitro and in vivo studies there is a sound rationale to apply heat in cancer treatment. The problem in patients is technical realization of the heating itself and the appropriate temperatures under clinical conditions.

2. BASIC UNDERSTANDING OF THERMODYNAMICS IN BIOLOGICAL TISSUES

Temperature increase in any material requires deposition of energy and is characterized by a material constant called *heat capacity* in kJ/kg (kilojoule per kilogram) required to increase the temperature of 1 kg of this material by 1°C. For instance, for *water*, the heat capacity is 4.2 kJ/kg/°C (at 20°C), and this value is a good approximation for human tissue.

We note that 1000 Ws = 1 kJ, which implies that 1 W/kg over 4200 s (roughly 1 hr) results in a temperature increase of 1°C in a closed system (i.e., no energy is transferred out of the specimen). Because the basal metabolic rate in humans is 1 W/kg, thermal isolation would lead to a core temperature of approx 42°C in 3 to 4 h (considering that the metabolic rate increases with temperature). This appears to be the easiest way to ensure a temperature of 42°C in tumors, and for metastatic diseases it is the only option to achieve a therapeutic temperature in all tumor lesions. The speed of heating (warm-up period) can be enhanced (down to 90–120 min) by external (infrared) radiation, which deposits several hundred watts in the body *(4)*.

However, for whole-body hyperthermia (WBHT), 42°C is the absolute limit of systemic temperature (and consequently in the tumor also) and includes various risks for complications. The dose-effect estimations of Subheading 2. suggest that 42°C might be the lower threshold of temperatures that must be exceeded for beneficial effects in tumors. In fact, clinical studies evaluating WBHT in conjunction with chemotherapy have revealed only slight additional efficacy together with some toxicity and nonneglectable burden for most patients *(5)*. On the other hand, a systemic temperature increase above 39 to 40°C is only tolerated by patients in deep sedation or even general anesthesia, contributing to further patient stress *(6)*.

In consequence, other local or regional heating techniques are required that potentially achieve temperatures >42°C in tumors (for higher efficacy), at least in selected parts, without relevant systemic heating (for better tolerance). For that purpose, any method should be considered that can be used to apply a certain amount of power in a target volume, given in W/kg. This power density is termed the specific absorption rate (SAR) and can be deduced from the gradient of temperature rise or fall-off (after switching on or switching off of power) by a simple formula:

$$\text{SAR [W/kg]} = 66.7 \times \Delta T/\text{time [°C/min]} \tag{1}$$

Therefore, a low temperature increase (ΔT) of 0.1°C per minute is caused by a power density of approx 7 W/kg, i.e., seven times the basal metabolic rate. For a higher temperature increase of 1°C/min, a SAR $\cong$ 70 W/kg is needed, which is difficult to achieve with available systems (*see* Subheading 3.).

If the material is unperfused, e.g., in a static phantom or in necrotic areas of a tumor, and the exposed volume is high enough, the temperature increase becomes strictly linear. In biological tissues, perfusion w (in mL/100 g/min) and (thermal) conduction λ (in W/°C) will finally limit the temperature increase and result in a steady-state temperature distribution (plateau), mathematically described by the stationary bioheat-transfer equation. This partial differential equation can be numerically solved *(7,8)*, and the solution will depend on the perfusion, the SAR (as a source term), the thermal conductivity λ, and their spatial distribution, including the boundary conditions describing the heat transfer to the surroundings.

For sufficiently large volumes with constant perfusion *w*, SAR, and λ the temperature elevation ΔT in the steady state is given by another simple formula:

$$\Delta T \text{ [°C]} = 1.4 \times \text{SAR [W/kg]}/w \text{ [mL/100 g/min]} \tag{2}$$

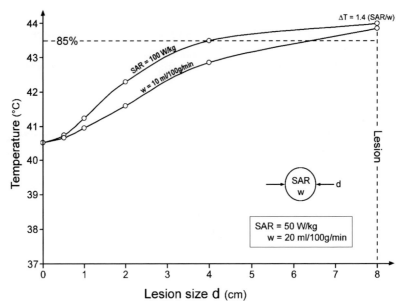

Fig. 1. Illustration of Eq. 2. The accuracy depends on the diameter of a lesion if either the perfusion w is lowered or the SAR is increased inside d. The background temperature is 40.6°C (50 W/kg in tissue perfused with 20 mL/100 g/min.)

Therefore, in a tumor with a mean perfusion of 10 mL/100 g/min, we need a SAR of 30 to 40 W/kg to achieve (42°C (ΔT = 4–6°C). The validity of this formula depends on the size of the lesion and is illustrated in Fig. 1. We will discuss two cases:

1. If we lower the perfusion in a circumscribed volume of diameter d, the temperature increases if a constant SAR everywhere is assumed. For $d \rightarrow$, the formula is exact. However, for small d = 1.5 cm, only 20% of this temperature increase is achieved, and for d = 3.5 cm, 60% is achieved. Nevertheless, a necrotic region in a well-perfused tumor (w = 20 mL/100 g/min) exposed to 50 W/kg will rise 0.2°C for d = 5 mm (40.8°C vs 40.6°C), 0.7°C for d = 10 mm (41.3°C vs 40.6°C), 1.4°C for d = 15 mm (42.0°C vs 40.6°C), and 2.4°C for d = 20 mm (43.0°C vs 40.6°C) in comparison with the well-perfused part of the tumor. We conclude that a thermotherapy technique achieving only 40.6°C in well-perfused parts of a tumor (SAR = 50 W/kg, w = 20 mL/100 g/min) will *achieve 43°C in every necrosis of 2 cm extension or more.* Therefore, this external technique (e.g., radiofrequency hyperthermia) might be more effective than WBHT. Even a single necrosis of 5 mm extension achieves a few tenths of °C higher temperature. Of course, an accumulation of necrotic areas will further enhance this effect, even if they are small and distributed.

2. If we deposit a constant SAR in a circumscribed lesion (with less SAR outside), again a relevant temperature increase is only achieved for diameters of a few centimeters, similar to case 1. The increase of ΔT with d is steeper and shifted about 1 cm to smaller diameters (Fig. 1). For d = 2 cm, 50% of the theoretical ΔT is achieved, and for d = 4 cm, 85%. In conclusion, isolated SAR elevations of <5 up to 10 mm extension must be excessively high (hundreds of W/kg) to induce a relevant temperature elevation. If the diameter is <1 mm, we are unable to raise the temperature to some °C for realistic SAR. This means in particular, that an isolated intracellular heating (cell diameter of about 10 μm) is impossible for physical reasons.

Achievable SAR and the temperature elevation induced strongly depend on the volume. We can roughly classify thermotherapy methods into thermoablative techniques (often interstitial) and locoregional techniques (mostly external). Very large SARs of 2500 W/kg are applied with high-intensity focused ultrasound (HIFU), but only in a focus of ≅1 to 3 mL *(9)*, which corresponds to temperature increases of 10°C per minute (see Eq. 1). For larger volumes (of 100 mL or more), we have to scan along the target. Considering the cooling time between every sonification, the total treatment time can be considerable. HIFU is presently under consideration for uterine myoma, breast cancer, prostate cancer, and liver malignoma. Similar power densities are deposited in limited volumes by laser-induced thermotherapy (LITT) or radiofrequency ablation (RFA) (up to 4 cm extension).

Nanotherapy is an interstitial treatment with SAR of some 100 W/kg that is theoretically and practically achieved *(10)* in a volume of up to 50 to 100 mL at maximum (*see* Subheading 3. for further details).

Much less SAR is achieved by use of locoregional thermotherapy. For local applications *(11)*, we achieve a mean SAR of 100 W/kg depending on the tissue depth.

In regional hyperthermia for pelvic tumors we have measured SARs of 30 to 50 W/kg *(12,13)*. This is a strong limitation to achieve >42°C reliably in human tumors, and further technical improvement is required (*see* Subheading 3.).

3. THERMOTHERAPY METHODS

3.1. Nanofluids and Other Interstitial Methods

Generally, interstitial methods are employed to heat circumscribed tumor lesions; they can be used as a single treatment in localized tumors or as an enhancing procedure during systemic treatment in resistant areas. Thermoablation (e.g., achieving ≥60°C in the target volume for some minutes) is achieved by laser fibers (LITT), radiofrequency electrodes or antennas (RFA or high-frequency induced thermotherapy [HITT]), and currents (bipolar electrodes). These devices have a given power deposition pattern around their tip and are aiming to coagulate a certain range of the surrounding tissue with therapeutic ranges up to 2 cm (typically less). Therefore, the greatest lesion diameter for a single-application use is about 4 to 5 cm.

Recently, an interstitial technique has been introduced based on a fluid with nanoparticles *(14)*. This fluid can be instilled and distributed in a tissue by thin needles; it absorbs power from an external alternating magnetic field in a controlled manner, as described elsewhere *(15)*. Thus the quality of the pattern (and therefore the effectivity) depends on the intervention, which is an advantage (flexibility) and a disadvantage (user dependency) at the same time.

The physical characteristics (the power absorption in particular, and consequently the heat generation) per nanoparticle in a magnetic alternating field are known for the magnetic fluid MFL AS 082A *(14)*. For example, a moderate power density of 50 W/kg is achieved if 1 mL of nanofluid is distributed in 10 mL of tumor tissue, and a 100-kHz magnetic field of 5 kA/m field strength (continuous wave, peak value) is applied.

This calibration allows an estimation of the power density (SAR) for employing any volume v[mL] of nanofluid homogeneously distributed in a target volume V[mL] in a magnetic field H [kA/m] of frequency f [100 kHz]:

$$\text{SAR [W/kg]} = (10 \, v/V) \, (H/5)^2 \, f^2 \, 50 \text{ W/kg} \qquad (3)$$

We can create from this formula a broad range of SARs covering moderate levels of 50 W/kg (typical for locoregional hyperthermia), up to several thousand W/kg with higher concentrations (e.g., $v = V$) and/or higher fields (e.g., $H = 10–15$ kA/m). Such high levels are usable for thermoablation.

The distribution of the nanoparticles in the target volume can be quantitatively determined via computed tomography (CT) utilizing the known relationship between Hounsfield unit (HU)-elevation above the HU of the tissue of interest and the iron (Fe) concentration (according to Gneveckow et al. *[14]*).

In short, an undiluted instillation of $v = 1$ mL nanofluid in $V = 1$ mL target volume (i.e., 75 mg Fe in 1 mL) results in an HU elevation of 600, decreasing to 60 for a dilution of 1:10 (i.e., 7.5 mg Fe in 1 mL tissue). The lowest measurable concentration is 1:50, 0.02 mL nanofluid in 1 mL tissue, resulting in an HU elevation of 20. Considering both characteristics of nanofluids together (the potential for calculating the absolute SAR in every point for given parameters $v/V, H, f$, and the ability to scan the amount of nanofluid), makes this approach very attractive for controlled interstitial treatment.

For clinical use we have exclusion criteria, in particular, metallic implants <30 cm distant from the treatment area. For lesions in the head and neck region, amalgam fillings or gold crowns must be replaced by ceramics. Metallic clips or seeds of some millimeter length and less than 1 mm diameter are not a contraindication, because we have found a power absorption of only a few mW per seed in a magnetic field of $H = 10$ kA/m.

The first clinical experiences are available with various nonresectable and recurrent (i.e., pretreated) solitary lesions (most of them preirradiated), which were treated in a phase I study *(10)*. Two different methods of nanofluid application were evaluated.

3.1.1. Prospective Planning

According to the *first strategy, prospective planning* of nanofluid distribution on a three-dimensional CT data set is performed by selecting a 2.5-mm slice distance in the treatment position. In a planning system, a segmentation module is included to define regions of different extension and shape with a given constant SAR (in W/kg) in and around the target volume. This target volume is contoured by the oncologist beforehand. Every SAR region is targeted with a specific amount of nanofluid v in mL, which can be calculated from Eq. 3. For this preplan, an assumption about the achieved magnetic field H [kA/m] is made. Then, for a given tumor perfusion [mL/100 g/min], the temperature distribution is calculated by solving the bioheat-transfer equation on a tetrahedral grid generated by utilizing the finite-element method.

For realization of this plan, the number of nanofluid depots is limited for practical reasons. If the depots are injected under CT control, the direction and positions of the puncture tracks are also preplanned to guide the radiologist. The total amount of nanofluid, the amount per depot, and their positions are optimized to achieve a given minimum temperature (e.g., 42°C) enclosing the target volume and to give a certain homogeneity, i.e., to limit the maximum temperature. The predicted temperature value critically depends on the assumed perfusion, which is only approximately known.

The nanofluid depots are shaped like either spheres (i.e., injection in a defined point) or cylinders (i.e., gradual injection by retracting the canule along the puncture track). The tracks and positions of the depots are selected according to anatomical considerations (sparing of critical structures), if possible in standardized settings (e.g., transverse planes). Then the number and distribution of the depots are manually modified until the 42°C isotemperature line (or any other defined temperature) is covering the target volume.

The preplanned tracks and coordinates are targeted by the interventional radiologist under CT fluoroscopy. The standardized technique is described by Ricke et al. *(16)*. It is advisable to leave a catheter in (<1 mm diameter) for a direct temperature measurement in the tumor after implantation. Permanent seed implantation with 125-I seeds is based on a standardized procedure to place the seeds with millimeter precision under transrectal ultrasound and X-fluoroscopy *(17)*. For the special indication of recurrent prostate cancer (after definitive external radiotherapy), the nanofluid is distributed along the needle tracks on the same template as that used for seed implantation in the same session.

3.1.2. INTRAOPERATIVE IMPLANTATION

The *second strategy* is an intraoperative implantation of the nanofluid *intraoperatively* under visual control. Here a prospective plan is not possible, because after tumor debulking, an individual (nonresectable) tumor rest or risky area (R1/R2 situation) must be infiltrated. The quality and coverage of the nanofluid distribution depends on the ability of the surgeon and his/her knowledge of the location and extension of the tumor-involved area. The surgeon is also advised to leave a catheter in for temperature measurement *in situ*. Cervical cancer recurrences at the pelvic wall (after primary treatment) are typical clinical examples. The nanofluid concentration in the target area should be as high as possible. In these patients retrospective planning based on a postoperative CT data set is performed.

We treated 20 patients with recurrent lesions by the three methods described, i.e., using either CT guidance, transrectal ultrasound (TRUS)-guidance for the prostate, or during operation under visual control. Different amounts of nanofluid (1.5–10 mL) were applied. The tolerated magnetic field strength ranged from 3 to 8 kA/m, with the typical value in the pelvis being 4.5 kA/m. Discomfort in skin folds is a limiting factor. In the upper thorax and neck the tolerance is higher (6–8 kA/m). Postimplantation analysis via CT revealed a high mean SAR of 190 W/kg after CT-guided implantation and 50 to 70 W/kg for the prostate and R1/R2 regions. These values are higher than those achieved with external locoregional systems. Therefore, the mean maximum temperatures are estimated in the lesions as 44.5°C after CT-guided implantation and 42 to 42.5°C for the other implantation methods, which is again superior to regional hyperthermia *(13)*. Dependency on the skill of the therapist is a shortcoming. Therefore, standardization and refinement of application modes are needed for further improvement.

A particularly effective method to increase the SAR further (and the temperature) is the use of higher magnetic fields, because SAR is proportional to the square of H. Adjusting H to 10 kA/m, i.e., doubling of H, would increase the SAR up to $\geq$200 W/kg. Technical solutions are under way.

3.2. Locoregional Hyperthermia

Antennas radiating electromagnetic waves are suitable to generate SAR distributions of a given shape and extension, if they are positioned outside the patient and near the target volume. Suitable frequencies lie in the radiofrequency (RF) range between 70 and 200 MHz. Theoretical considerations have shown that the best frequency depends on the

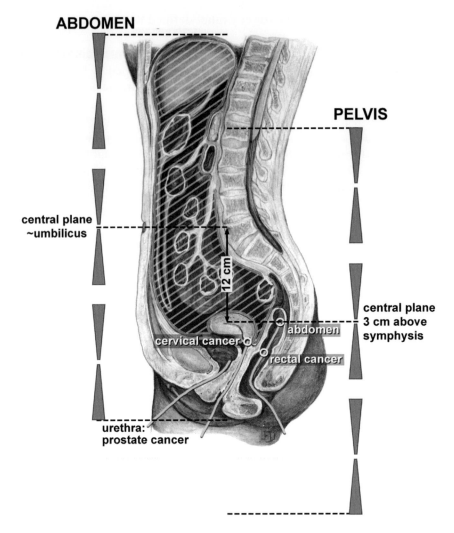

ABDOMEN

PELVIS

central plane
~umbilicus

12 cm

central plane
3 cm above
symphysis

abdomen

cervical cancer

rectal cancer

urethra:
prostate cancer

Fig. 2. Schematic arrangement of small-dipole antennas around the body either to heat a pelvic tumor or to expose the whole abdomen (called part-body hyperthermia). This applicator is called the Sigma-Eye applicator.

special problem (location of the target) *(18)*. Because the penetration of electromagnetic waves with lower frequencies increases, the frequencies (e.g., 70 MHz) are better suited for deeply located and largely extended volumes.

The optimal arrangement of RF antenna arrays must be formulated as a general problem, which is shown in Fig. 2. Antennas are radiating structures fed by an amplifier, which have a certain radiation profile at a given frequency. The matching to this frequency must be ensured by a transforming network between the amplifier and antenna feed point. The near-field range of such antennas is typically not suitable to generate a clinically useful power deposition pattern in patients.

Recently we have investigated attributes of antennas to design better dedicated applications. Among these attributes are form, thickness, coating, and special environment (dielectric structures) of the antennas. We have found possibilities to reduce the near-field range. Outside the near-field range the field pattern is easier to control. A water load (presently used as a water bolus) is required to direct the radiation to the patient. However, this bolus probably does not need direct pressure/contact to the patients' surface in an advanced hyperthermia system. This would contribute to a much easier and more comfortable application of RF hyperthermia.

Another feature of antenna arrays are the coupling conditions, which depend on both the network and the particular position of the antennas (field coupling). It has been found that flexibility (control) and efficiency of antenna arrays are inversely correlated. If the antennas of an array approach each other, they are automatically coupled for physical reasons. Then, the technical possibilities for decreasing the coupling are limited. The antenna arrays generate so-called resonance modes. In or near such a resonance mode the power (efficiency), which is deposited in the patient, is quite high. Adjustments far away from those resonance modes are difficult to realize and have certain disadvantages (see next paragraph).

Planning systems are now available for calculating and optimizing the SAR distribution (and consequently the temperature distribution) generated by these antenna arrays *(12,20)*. The solution in the patient is quite reliable, if the antenna models are correct. However, the antenna models and the transforming networks are probably too simple. Recently, improved algorithms have been developed that take into account special antennas and networks. These algorithms are the basis for the improved design of applications *(8)*. The most important parameters for controlling SAR patterns are the phases in the feed points of the antennas. Theoretically, using simplified antenna models we can calculate complicated SAR patterns with sometimes atypical and erratic phase values. In doing this we overestimate the flexibility of SAR control. However, if we want to adjust these phases under practical conditions, we measure increasing phase errors from ±10° (near the resonance modes) up to ±20 to 30° (far away from the resonance modes). Furthermore, high reactive power is then deposited for these adjustments for off-resonance in the water bolus or network. Of course, this high reactive power results in ohmic losses in reality, which further decreases the efficiency of the power deposition. As a consequence, we have found technical limitations (amplifier power) to achieve the desired temperatures (e.g., >42°C). We conclude that these "optimized" patterns are not as useful for practical applications, and we have developed other strategies to improve the temperature distribution in tumors.

3.2.1. SWITCHING BETWEEN STANDARD PATTERNS CREATING HOT SPOTS AT DIFFERENT LOCATIONS

In the pelvis, total power is mostly limited by a single hot spot, which might be either at the symphysis or at the dorsal sacral bone (Fig. 3A). Switching between both SAR patterns (by changing the phases) at time intervals of 1 to 8 min results in temperature-time curves (Fig. 3B) that still successfully heat the tumor up to 43°C (solid gray line), but distribute the thermal dose between both hot spot regions (fluctuating lines). The shorter the switching time, the smoother the curves, but there are technical/practical limitations. Increasing the number of patterns with different hot spots further improves the heating possibilities. Note that for this strategy we use standard patterns (with only slight phase delays of maximally 30°), which minimizes aberrant power losses.

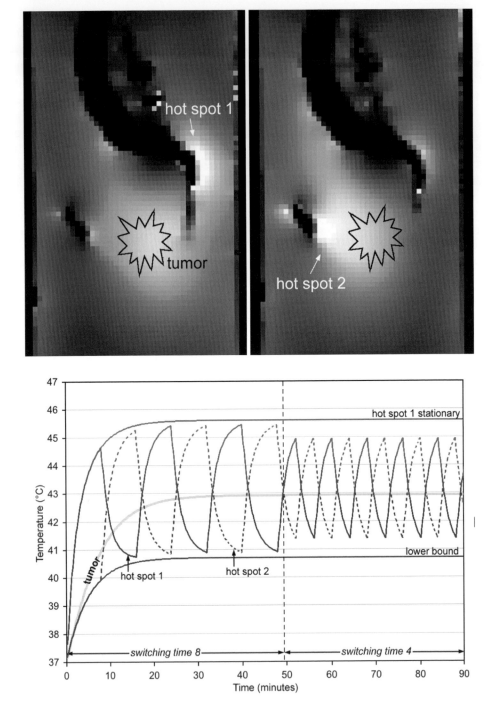

Fig. 3. Strategy to increase the intratumoral SAR in the pelvis: (1) for two SAR distributions, the power density is approximately equal in the tumor, but hot spots occur at different locations (at the sacral bone, left; at the symphysis, right); (2) switching between both adjustments allows a temperature of 43°C in the tumor, and a tolerable temperature at the hot spots. Decreasing the switching time from 8 to 4 min results in better tolerance. Switching times of 1 min would nearly avoid the peak temperatures in hot spots.

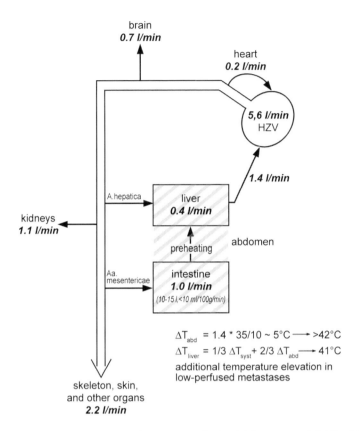

Fig. 4. Concept of part-body hyperthermia with a realistic (fairly constant) SAR of 35 W/kg in the abdomen. With a mean perfusion of <10 mL/100 g/min, we achieve 42 to 43°C in the peritoneum, and we consider the preheating effect in the liver as well as effective temperatures in liver metastases.

3.2.2. PART-BODY HYPERTHERMIA

With a special applicator, a reasonably homogeneous SAR in the abdomen (with a typical volume of 15–20 L), including the liver, should be possible. The Sigma-Eye applicator (Fig. 2) positioned with the central plane at the umbilicus is a possible solution, if phase delay is adjusted at the outer rings.

However, better applicator concepts exist. For a SAR distribution to be as homogeneous as possible, lower frequencies are better (e.g., 70 MHz instead of 100 MHz for the Sigma-Eye applicator). Then, a large aperture angle, a small near-field range, and a good match (with a minimum of transforming network components) are desirable. It is evident that small antennas (as in Fig. 2) are not optimal for this special task.

The objective of such an applicator is the generation of a constant SAR in the whole abdomen according to the hatched region shown in Fig. 4. A SAR of 35 W/kg in 15 L (525 W) results in a temperature elevation of 1.4×35 W/kg/10 mL/100 g/min, i.e., approx 5°C, corresponding to >42°C. This conforms to common heat treatments with regional hyperthermia, but a well-adapted applicator would be a precondition. We note that 15 L fits in a sphere of 30-cm diameter (which corresponds to the volume, in which a constant SAR should be generated by the array to be designed). This concept is consistent with the observation that perfusion through the abdomen (and entering the liver via the portal vein) is not increased during part-body hyperthermia.

3.2.3. LOCAL APPLICATORS

In principle, every additional clinical application needs special arrangements of antennas or applicators. For malignant lymph nodes in the neck, we used single applicators *(11,21)*. Dedicated equipment (dual-applicator operation) has been developed by the Rotterdam group for recurrent breast cancer of the chest wall *(22)*. The group at Duke has developed applicators for primary breast carcinoma *(23)*.

Locoregional hyperthermia is feasible, but improved understanding and manufacture of applicators will be indispensable, if we want to optimize the heating conditions for different indications. Dedicated applicators are needed for the abdomen (part-body hyperthermia), the neck region (including the primary tumor), the chest wall (including advanced and extended recurrences), and other areas.

For the pelvic region and lower extremities, the available applicators are already appropriate (*see* the Sigma-Eye applicator in Fig. 2), but nevertheless they must be controlled with sufficient certainty.

3.3. Thermotherapy and Monitoring

We clearly need a measuring parameter to classify our thermotherapy as effective (or not) and to detect potentially risky constellations, e.g., temperatures that are too high in normal tissues. When hyperthermia began, an intratumoral temperature measurement was demanded *(24)*. This measurement has been justified by various correlations between the local efficacy of the treatment (clinically described by response according to the World Health Organization [WHO] or a similar parameter) and thermal parameters, e.g., the thermal dose achieved in 90% of the measurement points *(25,26)*. To increase the acceptance, tolerance, and practicality of heat treatments *(27,28)*, endoluminal reference points were introduced as substitutes in pelvic tumors, as indicated in Fig. 3 *(29)*. These points can be arrived at with catheters by using minimally invasive procedures.

Endoluminal SAR measurements (see Eq. 1) do not differ from intratumoral SAR measurements, if interpreted properly *(12,13)*. Therefore, endoluminal data are useful for a check of the SAR distribution. Not unexpectedly, endoluminal temperature measurements display characteristic differences in comparison with intratumoral measurements, as described in Wust and colleagues in 1998 *(12)*. Nevertheless, the same correlations were found as in intratumoral measurements, as documented for rectal carcinomas *(30)*, prostate carcinomas *(31)*, and cervical carcinomas *(32)*. For standard situations in the pelvis, including bladder cancer, an endoluminal temperature measurement for control is equivalent.

For regional hyperthermia in the abdomen, especially part-body hyperthermia (Figs. 3 and 4), reference points are not available under patient-friendly conditions. This is the first reason to integrate antenna arrays (applicators) into a magnetic-resonance (MR) tomograph in order to establish a *noninvasive* monitoring capability. Second, by this technique a full three-dimensional data set is acquired comprising much more information than any direct thermometry. Third, online monitoring of thermotherapy can account for online corrections or improvements in heating and provide the basis for optimization of the adjustments.

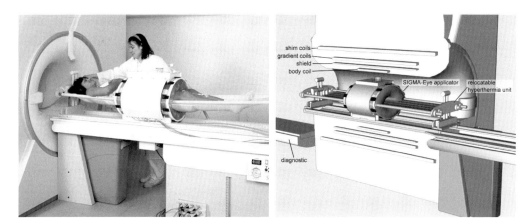

Fig. 5. In the hybrid system at the Berlin group, a multiantenna applicator (here the Sigma-Eye applicator) is moved together with the patient into the gantry of a tunnel MR tomograph (here the Magnetom Symphony, Siemens). On the right, we see more details of the components, which partially interact.

Basically, the hybridization of both systems is electrotechnically realized by separating the signal paths, filtering out the heating frequency (e.g., 100 MHz) in the receiving path of the MR, and filtering out the resonance frequency (64 MHz at 1.5 Tesla) in the power path to the antennas *(33)*. The mechanical integration is shown in Fig. 5; the patient and the applicator are moved together from the back into the gantry *(34)*. At the front, the diagnostic table is held ready, and a change between heating under MR monitoring or MR examination for diagnostic purposes is accomplished in a few minutes.

Magnetic resonance imaging (MRI) has been used for monitoring of thermoablative interventions for more than a decade. While researchers were evaluating MRI approaches for this indication, it became clear that the MR signals are influenced by a mixture of tissue-effects (e.g., coagulation) in addition to temperature changes *(35)*. As a result, more recent studies attempted to separate the temperature out as an observable factor in laser-induced thermotherapy *(36,37)* and focused ultrasound *(38,39)* and to elucidate the reliability and limitations of MR-guided thermography. Basically, three methods are available for MR thermography and are discussed in the literature. They are based on the temperature dependency of the relaxation time T1 *(40)*, the diffusion (apparent diffusion coefficient [ADC-value]) *(41,42)*, or the proton resonance frequency shift (PRFS) *(43,44)*. As T1-weighted sequences are particularly dependent on the type and status of the tissue *(45,46)*, they are mainly recommended in low-field systems because of their higher contrast. On the other hand, diffusion methods still suffer from technical and methodical limitations in clinical practice *(47)*. Therefore, for magnetic fields ≥1 Tesla, PRFS-based methods are preferred by most investigators today *(48–50)*.

However, temperature accuracies of MR-based thermography used for ablation techniques are still in the range ±3 to 4.5°C even under favorable in vitro conditions with liver specimens *(36,37,51)*. This is because *in vivo* MR thermography is hampered not only by motion but also by various (treatment-induced) tissue alterations, which are reversible or irreversible and depend on the temperature level, heating time, and tissue type. Therefore, MR thermography of larger target volumes, e.g., during regional hyperthermia, appears to be even more challenging, especially as the expected temperature differences in the course of a treatment (37–43°C) are near the uncertain values referenced for high-temperature applications.

In a small series, Carter et al. *(52)* employed a self-developed cylindrical phased-array hyperthermia applicator (25-cm diameter) to treat sarcomas of the lower leg in a 1.5-Tesla MR scanner (Signa General Electric, Milwaukee, WI). The investigators acquired phase images during regional hyperthermia and demonstrated a satisfactory correlation with measured temperatures (standard error ±1°C) at moderate power levels of about 150 W. Peller et al. *(53)* described a hybrid system consisting of a Sigma-Eye applicator (BSD Medical, Salt Lake City, UT) integrated into a low-field system (0.2 Tesla, Magnetom Open Viva, Siemens, Erlangen, Germany). With T1 imaging, they claimed to control the heat of treatments (hot spot detection) and presented selected cases (lower extremity) with good correlation of T1 and directly measured temperatures *(54)*.

A hybrid system installed by Wust et al. 2004 *(34)* has been validated with the PRSF method in an anthropomorphic phantom *(33)*. Special acquisition and postprocessing methods have been developed. We note that for rectal recurrences after abdominoperineal resection, an endoluminal reference point is difficult to specify or does not exist, and therefore the introduction of noninvasive MR thermography represents real progress with respect to tolerance and safety. For rectal recurrences and soft tissue sarcomas, an analogue correlation between response and mean MR temperature in the tumor has been found *(55)*.

In the abdomen, the present standard method for noninvasive thermometry (PRFS) cannot be applied because of motion (breath-dependent) and strong susceptibility gradients leading to severe artifacts (especially because of air conglomerations in the intestine). Navigated acquisition techniques might compensate for motion in the liver and allow the PRFS method. The most stable monitoring technique is gained by perfusion (contrast media dynamics), which is not dependent on susceptibility discontinuities and is less vulnerable to motion. With the known SAR distribution (at least from a computer plan), the temperature distribution can be estimated.

4. CLINICAL RESULTS AND INDICATIONS

A series of randomized studies have demonstrated the enhancing effect of heat in addition to radiotherapy, as summarized by Wust et al. *(56)* or Falk and Issels *(57)*, and Issels et al. *(58)*. The most convincing study employed the standard system for regional hyperthermia (RHT) (BSD 2000) for pelvic tumors and found a survival benefit in the study arm (radiotherapy plus hyperthermia) for cervical cancer ≥ IIB *(59)*. Recently, radiochemotherapy has become the new standard for this patient group, and the role of regional hyperthermia will be defined in a running study comparing radiochemotherapy with hyperthermic radiochemotherapy *(60)*. Other prospective randomized studies evaluating chemotherapy (±RHT) in soft tissue sarcomas *(58)* or radiochemotherapy (±RHT) in rectal cancer *(61)* are not yet completed.

Further randomized studies have succeeded in demonstrating the enhancing effect for superficial tumors of different histologies *(62–64)*, with increased local control and/or response in the hyperthermia arm. Recently, considerably improved local control (recurrence-free survival) was found in the hyperthermia (plus intravesical mitomycin C) arm for patients with bladder cancer by Colombo et al. *(65)*.

There are various problems with these studies related to the clinical use of hyperthermia:

1. There are not many clinical data, and they are not sufficient to give unequivocal answers.
2. For oncological reasons, a survival benefit was found only in the study of Van der Zee *(59)*. The improved local control found in other studies might be informative for the users, but is not accepted as a clinical end point constituting an imperative indication.
3. Further clinical studies would be strongly desirable. However, these studies are demanding and difficult to perform, because only a few centers are involved, which prolongs the recruiting time.
4. Technological developments are still in progress (*see* Subheadings 2 and 3), which might be crucial for achievement of effective temperatures.

Existing commercial systems are suitable for heating pelvic tumors (prostate, cervix, rectum, bladder) and tumors of the lower extremity (soft tissue sarcoma).

Abdominal and liver metastases are frequently seen. Primary tumors are gastrointestinal (colorectal, pancreas, stomach) and ovarian cancers. Part-body hyperthermia might be helpful to enhance the chemotherapy effect (± innovative substances in addition). We found that WBHT is not ideal for that indication, because of high burden and temperature limits (42°C). Better applications have been described (part-body hyperthermia), which heat only the abdomen to (ideally) >42°C, and do not greatly affect the systemic temperature. The adaption of present technology (Fig. 2) for this indication is under way, and clinical studies are in preparation. The objective of these studies must be survival improvement in patients receiving systemic standard chemotherapy.

Other oncological indications exist, when standard radiochemotherapy will not lead to a fully satisfactory outcome, e.g., inoperable head and neck carcinoma (with a present long-term survival of at best 30–40%, *see*, e.g., ref. 66) or malignant brain tumors (with present curative rates near zero) *(67)*.

Dedicated applicators and treatment strategies are required for these indications, but they are not yet available. Planning tools and technical know-how are evolving to make the design of such applicators possible (e.g., antenna arrays) for every specific location— and to integrate these applicators into an MR gantry for noninvasive monitoring. In conclusion, suitable and effective applicators must be designed for every specific oncological indication (when they are needed by clinical reasons), and the general rules for constructing them must be understood.

REFERENCES

1. Hildebrandt B, Wust P, Ahlers O, et al. The cellular and molecular basis of hyperthermia. Crit Rev Oncol Hematol 2002;43:33–56.
2. Lindner LH, Eichhorn ME, Eibl H, Teichert N, Schmitt-Sody M, Issels RD. Novel temperature-sensitive liposomes with prolonged circulation time. Clin Cancer Res 2004;10:2168–2178.
3. Li CY, Dewhirst MW. Hyperthermia-regulated immunogene therapy. Int J Hyperthermia 2002;18: 586–596.
4. Wust P, Riess H, Hildebrandt B, et al. Feasibility and analysis of thermal parameters for the whole body hyperthermia system IRATHERM-2000. Int J Hyperthermia 2002;16:325–339.
5. Hildebrandt B, Dräger J, Kerner T, et al. Whole-body hyperthermia in the scope of von Ardenne's systemic cancer multistep therapy (sCMT) combined with chemotherapy in patients with metastatic colorectal cancer: a phase I/II study. Int J Hyperthermia 2004;20:317–333.
6. Kerner T, Hildebrandt B, Ahlers O , et al. Anesthesiological experiences with whole body hyperthermia. Int J Hyperthermia 2003;19:1–12.

7. Wust P, Nadobny J, Felix R, Deuflhard P, John W, Louis A. Numerical approaches to treatment planning in deep RF-hyperthermia. Strahlenth Onkol 1989;165(10)751–757

8. Nadobny J, Wlodarczyk W, Westhoff L, Gellermann J, Felix R, Wust P. A clinical water-coated antenna applicator for MR-controlled deep-body hyperthermia: a comparison of calculated and measured 3-D temperature data sets. IEEE Trans Biomed Eng 2005;52:505–519.

9. Hengst SA, Ehrenstein T, Herzog H, et al. Magnetic resonance tomography guided focused ultrasound surgery (MRgFUS) in tumor therapy—a new noninvasive therapy option. Radiologe 2004;44: 339–346.

10. Wust P, Gneveckow U, Ricke J, et al. Nanofluids for interstitial thermotherapy—feasibility, tolerance, achieved temperatures. Int J Hyperthermia, 2006, in press.

11. Wust P, Stahl H, Dieckmann K, et al. Local hyperthermia of N2/N3 cervical lymphnode metastases: correlation of technical/ thermal parameters and response. Int J Radiat Oncol Biol Phys 1996;34: 635–646.

12. Wust P, Gellermann J, Harder C, et al. Rationale for using invasive thermometry for regional hyperthermia of pelvic tumors. Int J Radiat Oncol Biol Phys 1998;41:1129–1137.

13. Tilly W, Wust P, Rau B, et al. Temperature data and specific absorption rates in pelvic tumours: predictive factors and correlations. Int J Hyperthermia 2001;17:172–188.

14. Gneveckow U, Jordan A, Scholz R, et al. Description and characterization of the novel hyperthermia- and thermoablation-system MFH300F for clinical magnetic fluid hyperthermia. Med Phys 2004;31:1444–1451.

15. Jordan A, Wust P, Fähling H, John W, Hinz A, Felix R. Inductive heating of ferrimagnetic particles and magnetic fluids: physical evaluation of their potential for hyperthermia. Int J Hyperthermia 1993;9:51–68.

16. Ricke J, Wust P, Stohlmann, A, et al. CT-guided interstitial brachytherapy of liver malignancies alone or in combination with thermal ablation: phase I-II results of a novel technique. Int J Radiat Oncol Biol Phys 2004;58:1496–1505.

17. Wust P, Wischka von Borczyskowksi D, Henkel T, et al. Clinical and physical determinants for toxicity of 125-I seed prostate brachytherapy. Radiother Oncol 2004;73:39–48.

18. Seebass M, Beck R, Gellermann J, Nadobny J, Wust P. Electromagnetic phased arrays for regional hyperthermia—optimal frequency and antenna arrangement. Int J Hyperthermia 2001;17:321–336.

19. Gellermann J, Wust P, Stalling D, et al. Clinical evaluation and verification of the hyperthermia treatment planning system HyperPlan. Int J Radiat Oncol Biol Phys 2000;47:1145–1156.

20. Sreenivasa G, Gellermann J, Rau B, et al. Clinical application of the hyperthermia treatment planning system HyperPlan—comparison of algorithms and clinical observables. Int J Radiat Oncol Biol Phys 2003;55:407–419.

21. Valdagni R, Amichetti M, Pani V. Radical radiation alone versus radical radiation plus microwave hyperthermia for N3 (TNM-UICC) neck nodes: a prospective randomized clinical trial. Int J Radiat Oncol Biol Phys 1998;15:13–24.

22. Van der Zee J, van der Holt B, Rietveld PJ, et al. Reirradiation combined with hyperthermia in recurrent breast cancer results in a worthwile local palliation. Br J Cancer 1999;79:483–490.

23. Jones EL, Prosnitz LR, Dewhirst MW, et al. Thermochemoradiotherapy improves oxygenation in locally advanced breast cancer. Clin Cancer Res 2004;10:4287–4293.

24. Sapozink MD, Corry PM, Kapp DS, et al. RTOG quality assurance guidelines for clinical trials using hyperthermia for deep-seated malignancy. Int J Radiat Oncol Biol Phys 1991;20:1109–1115.

25. Leopold KA, Dewhirst MW, Samulski TV, et al. Cumulative minutes with T90 greater than TempIndex is predictive of response of superficial malignancies to hyperthermia and radiation. Int J Radiat Oncol Biol Phys 1993;25:841–847.

26. Issels R, Prenninger SW, Nagele A, et al. Ifosfamide plus etoposide combined with regional hyperthermia in patients with locally advanced sarcoms: a phase II study. J Clin Oncol 1990;8:1818–1829.

27. van der Zee J, Per-Valstar JN, Rietveld PJ, de Graaf-Strukowska L, van Rhoon GC. Practical limitations of interstitial thermometry during deep hyperthermia. Int J Radiat Oncol Biol Phys 1998;40:1205–1212.

28. Wust P, Gellermann J, Harder C, et al. Rationale for using invasive thermometry for regional hyperthermia of pelvic tumors. Int J Radiat Oncol Biol Phys 1998;41:1129–1137.

29. Lagendijk J, van Rhoon G, Hornsleth S, et al. ESHO quality assurance guidelines for regional hyperthermia. Int. J. Hyperthermia 1998;14:125–133.

30. Rau B, Wust P, Tilly W, et al. Preoperative radio-chemotherapy in locally advanced recurrent rectal cancer: regional radiofrequency hyperthermia correlates with clinical parameters. Int J Radiat Oncol Biol Phys 2000;48:381–391.

31. Tilly W, Gellermann J, Graf R, et al. Regional hyperthermia in conjunction with definitive radio-therapy against recurrent or locally advanced prostate cancer T3 pN0 M0. Strahlenther Onkol 2005;181:35–41.

32. Sreenivasa G, Hildebrandt B, Kümmel S, et al. Preoperative hyperthermic radiochemotherapy in non-resectable cervical carcinoma (FIGO IIB-IVA)—a pilot phase II study. 2005; submitted.

33. Gellermann J, Wlodarczyk W, Ganter H, et al. A practical approach to perform the thermography in a hyperthermia/MR hybrid system—validation in an anthropomorphous phantom. Int J Radiat Oncol Biol Phys 2005;61:267–277.

34. Wust P, Gellermann J, Seebass M, et al. [Partt-body hyperthermia with a radiofrequency multiantenna applicator under online control in a 1.5 T MR-tomograph] Fortschr Röntgenstr 2004;176:363–374.

35. McDannold N, Hynynen K, Jolesz F. MRI monitoring of the thermal ablation of tissues: effects of long exposure times. J Magn Reson Imaging 2001;13:421–427.

36. Bär NK, Schulz T, Puccini S, Schirmer T, Kahn T, Busse H. MRT-gestützte laserinduzierte Thermoablation bei Lebertumoren—Klinische Aspekte und Konzept eines Überwachungssystems. Z Med Phys 2003;13:209–213.

37. Heisterkamp J, Matheijssen NAA, van Hillegersberg R, et al. Accuracy of MR phase mapping for temperature monitoring during interstitial laser coagulation (ILC) in the liver at rest and simulated respiration. Magn Reson Med 1999;41:919–925.

38. Hynynen K, Pomeroy O, Smith DN, et al. MR imaging-guided ultrasound surgery of fibroadenomas in the breast: a feasibility study. Radiology 2001;219:176–185.

39. McDannold N, Hynynen K, Wolf D, Wolf G, Jolesz F. MRI evaluation of thermal ablation of tumors with focused ultrasound. J Magn Reson Imaging 1998;8:91–100.

40. Parker DL, Smith V, Sheldon P, Crooks LE, Fussell L. Temperature distribution measurements in two-dimension NMR imaging. Med Phys 1983;10:321–325.

41. Delannoy J, Chen CN, Turner R, Levin RL, Le Bihan D. Noninvasive temperature imaging using diffusion MRI. Magn Reson Med 1991;19:333–339.

42. Samulski TV, MacFall J, Zhang Y, Grant W, Charles C. Non-invasive thermometry using magnetic resonance diffusion imaging: potential for application in hyperthermic oncology. Int J Hyperthermia 1992;8:819–829.

43. De Poorter J, De Wagter C, De Deene Y, Thomsen C, Stahlberg F, Achten E. Noninvasive MRI thermometry with the proton resonance frequency (PRF) method: in vivo results in human muscle. Magn Reson Med 1995;33:74–81.

44. Kuroda K, Oshio K, Chung AH, Hynynen K, Jolesz FA. Temperature mapping using the proton chemical shift: a chemical shift selective phase mapping method. Magn Reson Med 1997;38:845–851.

45. Fried MP, Morrison PR, Hushek SG, Kernahan GA, Jolesz FA. Dynamic T1-weighted magnetic resonance imaging of interstitial laser photocoagulation in the liver: observations on in vivo temperature sensitivity. Lasers Surg Med 1996;18:410–419.

46. Young IR, Hand JW, Oatridge A, Prior MV. Modeling and observation of temperature changes in vivo using MRI. Magn Reson Med 1994;32:358–369.

47. Gellermann J, Wlodarczyk W, Feussner A, et al. Methods and potentials of magnetic resonance imaging for monitoring radiofrequency hyperthermia in a hybrid system. Int J Hyperthermia 2005;21:497–513.

48. De Poorter J, De Wagter C, De Deene Y. The proton-resonance-frequency-shift method compared with molecular diffusion for quantitative measurement of two-dimensional time-dependent temperature distribution in a phantom. J Magn Reson 1994;B103:234–241.

49. Quesson B, de Zwart JA, Moonen CTW: Magnetic resonance temperature imaging for guidance of thermotherapy. J Magn Reson Imaging 2000;12:525–533.

50. Wlodarczyk W, Hentschel M, Wust P, et al. Comparison of magnetic resonance methods for mapping of small temperature changes. Phys Med Biol 1999;44:607–624.

51. Vogl TJ. Weinhold N, Mack MG, et al. [Verification of MR thermometry by means of an in vivo intralesion, fluoroptic temperature measurement for laser-induced thermotherapy of liver metastases]. RoFo Fortschr Geb Rontgenstr Neuen Bildgeb Verf 1998;169:182–188.

52. Carter DL, MacFall JR, Clegg ST, et al. Magnetic resonance thermometry during hyperthermia for human high-grade sarcoma. Int J Radiat Oncol Biol Phys 1998;40:815–822.

53. Peller M Löffler R, Baur A, et al. MRT-gesteuerte regionale Tiefenhyperthermie. [MRI-controlled regional hyperthermia]. Radiologe 1999;39:756–763.

54. Peller M, Reinl HM, Weigel A, Meininger M, Issels RD, Reiser M. T1 relaxation time at 0.2 Tesla for monitoring regional hyperthermia: feasibility study in muscle and adipose tissue. Magn Reson Med 2002;47:1194–1201.

55. Gellermann J, Wlodarczyk W, Hildebrandt B, et al. Non-invasive magnetic resonance thermography of recurrent rectal carcinoma in a 1.5 Tesla hybrid system. Cancer Research 2005;65:1–9.

56. Wust P, Hildebrandt B, Sreenivasa G, et al. Hyperthermia in a combined treatment of cancer. Lancet Oncology 2002;3:487–497.

57. Falk MH, Issels RD. Hyperthermia in oncology. Int J Hyperthermia 2001;17:1–18.

58. Issels RD, Abdel-Rahman S, Sendtner C, et al. Neoadjuvant chemotherapy combined with regional hyperthermia (RHT) for locally advanced primary or recurrent high-risk adult soft-tissue sarcomas (STS) of adults: Long-term results of a phase II study. Eur J Cancer 2002;31:1599–1608.

59. Van der Zee J, Gonzalez Gonzalez D, van Rhoon GC, van Dijk JD, van Putten WL, Hart AA. Comparison of radiotherapy alone with radiotherapy plus hyperthermia in locally advanced pelvic tumours: a prospective, randomised, multicentre trial. Dutch Deep Hyperthermia Group. Lancet. 2000;355:1119–1125.

60. Prosnitz L. A new phase III trial for treatment of carcinoma of the cervix. Int J Hyperthermia 2002:18:31–32.

61. Rau B, Wust P, Hohenberger P, et al. Preoperative hyperthermia combined with radiochemotherapy in locally advanced rectal cancer. A phase II clinical trial. Annals Surg 1998;227:380–389.

62. Overgaard J, Gonzalez Gonzalez D, Hulshof MC, et al. Randomised trial of hyperthermia as adjuvant to radiotherapy for recurrent or metastatic malignant melanoma. Lancet 1995;345:540–543.

63. Vernon CC, Hand JW, Field SB, et al. Radiotherapy withz or without hyperthermia in the treatment of superficial localized breast cancer: results from five randomized controlled trials. International Collaborative Hyperthermia Group. Int J Radiat Oncol Biol Phys 1996;35:731–744.

64. Jones E, Oleson JR, Prosnitz LR, et al. Randomized trial of hyperthermia and radiation for superficial tumors. J Clin Oncol 1995:23:3079–3085.

65. Colombo R, Da Pozzo LF, Salonia A, et al. Multicentric study comparing intravesical chemotherapy alone and with local microwave hyperthermia for prophylaxis of recurrence of superficial transitional cell carcinoma. J Clin Oncol 2003;23:4270–4276.

66. Budach V, Stuschke M, Budach W, et al. Hyperfractionated accelerated chemoradiation with concurrent fluorouracil-mitomycin is more effective than dose-escalated hyperfractionated accelerated radiation therapy alone in locally advanced head and neck cancer: final results of the Radiotherapy Cooperative Clinical Trials Group of the German Cancer Society 95–06 Prospective Randomized Trial. J Clin Oncol 2005;23:1125–1135.

67. Graf R, Hildebrandt B, Tilly W, et al. Dose-escalated conformal radiotherapy of glioblastomas— results of a retrospective comparison applying radiation doses of 60 and 70 Gy. Onkologie 2005; 28:325–330.

7 Radiofrequency Thermal Ablation

Eren Berber, MD and Allan E. Siperstein, MD

CONTENTS

INTRODUCTION
INDICATIONS
TECHNIQUE
RESULTS
DISCUSSION
REFERENCES

SUMMARY

Over the last decade, radiofrequency thermal ablation (RFA) has become an accepted treatment modality for unresectable primary and metastatic liver tumors. It can be performed either percutaneously, laparoscopically, or via an open approach. With experience, indications and selection criteria have been determined for each tumor type. RFA has become the first-line therapy for unresectable HCC before chemotherapy or chemoembolization. It is also used as a bridge to transplantation. The purpose of RFA for unresectable colorectal liver metastasis is to debulk the liver in these patients who are predicted to die of liver failure owing to tumor progression. Neuroendocrine liver metastases benefit from debulking with RFA because of the frequent presence of debilitating symptoms from hormonal oversecretion. A selected group of patients with non-HCC, nonneuroendocrine, and noncolorectal liver metastases and without evidence of extrahepatic disease on imaging studies may benefit from debulking of the liver involvement with RFA and when other conventional modalities have failed. RFA provides effective local tumor control with minimal morbidity and short hospital stay. Recent studies also suggest a survival advantage of RFA for colorectal liver metastases and HCC.

Key Words: Radiofrequency thermal ablation; primary liver cancer; metastatic liver cancer; laparoscopic.

1. INTRODUCTION

Hepatocellular carcinoma (HCC) is the most common primary malignancy of the liver and one of the world's most common malignancies, causing almost one million deaths annually. Metastasis to the liver is also a significant problem, for which the management

From: *Cancer Drug Discovery and Development: Regional Cancer Therapy*
Edited by: P. M. Schlag and U. S. Stein © Humana Press Inc., Totowa, NJ

is challenging. Colorectal cancer is responsible for up to 75% of liver metastases that undergo surgical treatment. Of 160,000 new cases of colorectal carcinoma in the United States each year, liver metastases will develop in approx 40,000. Liver metastases develop in 5 to 90% of patients with neuroendocrine tumors that, in contrast to most metastatic adenocarcinomas, have an indolent course, which may be dominated by symptoms related to hormonal activity *(1–3)*.

Although surgery is the gold standard for treating liver tumors, most of these patients are unfortunately excluded from resectional therapy either because of bilobar or multifocal disease within the liver or because of the presence of extrahepatic disease. Chemotherapy has a limited benefit, although studies are under way using newer chemotherapeutic agents. Radiofrequency thermal ablation (RFA) is gaining increased acceptance for the management of patients with unresectable primary and metastatic tumors of the liver. It causes local tissue destruction by delivering electrical energy at a frequency of 400 kHz into the tissues. This creates resistive heating as a result of the movement of electrons within the tissues. Once cells are heated above 50°C, their cell membranes melt and fuse, and protein denaturation and irreversible cell death occurs *(4,5)*.

Initial human trials focused on percutaneous RFA of liver tumors *(6,7)*. With the percutaneous approach, the lesions in the periphery of the liver are more difficult to target and there is a risk of injury to other organs adjacent to the liver. Although the open approach overcomes these limitations and also allows for abdominal staging, it carries the morbidity of a laparotomy. The laparoscopic approach, on the other hand, is minimally invasive. Tumor targeting is facilitated by the upward movement of the diaphragm, and laparoscopic ultrasonography allows for highly sensitive staging of the liver. Our group has shown that in 20% of the patients undergoing RFA of liver tumors, laparoscopic ultrasound shows at least one additional tumor compared with preoperative tri-phasic CT scans *(8)*.

2. INDICATIONS

The current selection criteria include (1) unresectable primary or metastatic liver tumors, (2) either no or limited amounts of extrahepatic disease, and (3) enlarging liver lesions, worsening of symptoms, and/or failure to respond to other treatment modalities.

2.1. Hepatocellular Carcinoma

Patients with primary liver tumors usually present with a small number of liver lesions. Nevertheless, their surgical risks are high because of accompanying cirrhosis and other medical problems. As a well-tolerated procedure with good local tumor control, RFA has been accepted in many centers as a first-line treatment before chemoembolization or chemotherapy. RFA is also being used as a bridge to liver transplantation. Child's A or B cirrhotic patients generally tolerate the procedure well; however, the risk of complications, including liver failure, may be increased for Child's C patients.

2.2. Metastatic Adenocarcinoma

The purpose of RFA for unresectable colorectal liver metastasis is to debulk the liver in these patients, who are predicted to die of liver failure owing to tumor progression. Our current selection criteria for RFA in these patients are: (1) no more than eight liver lesions, (2) less than 20% of total liver volume replaced with tumor, (3) largest lesion smaller than 8 cm in diameter, and (4) normal biliary ductal diameters. Generally, RFA is performed after the patients have failed chemotherapy. On the other hand, synchronous ablation with bowel resection may be performed in selective cases when liver metastases are detected at the time of surgery for primary disease and when concomitant liver resection may be too risky or not indicated *(9)*.

2.3. Neuroendocrine Metastases

Although neuroendocrine liver metastases are often multifocal, they benefit from debulking owing to the frequent presence of debilitating symptoms from hormonal oversecretion. In addition to dominant tumors, at surgery these patients are often found to have multiple subcentimeter lesions. Our practice has been to ablate those metastases greater than 1 cm. Symptomatic improvement is noted immediately after surgery, and the degree of improvement is related to the extent of cytoreduction achieved.

2.4. Nonneuroendocrine, Noncolorectal Liver Metastases

Although there are abundant data in the literature about the use of RFA for the tumor types discussed above, little is known about the outcome of patients with nonneuroendocrine, noncolorectal liver metastases. The rationale for treating patients with liver metastases from sarcoma, breast cancer, pancreatic adenocarcinoma, and other tumor types is less clear-cut. These patients are predicted to succumb from diffusely disseminated disease; therefore, for most of them, it is not predicted that treating liver metastasis would prolong survival. On the other hand, a selected group of patients with atypical tumors and without evidence of extrahepatic disease on imaging studies may benefit from debulking of the liver involvement with RFA when other conventional modalities have failed.

3. TECHNIQUE

Laparoscopic RFA is performed under general endotracheal anesthesia. We use 1 g of cefazolin for surgical prophylaxis. The patients are positioned supine on the operating table. We use two 11-mm trocars beneath the right costal margin, one for the laparoscope and one for the laparoscopic ultrasound transducer (Fig. 1). We prefer to enter the abdominal cavity under direct view using an optical access trocar, as many of these patients have had prior abdominal surgeries. The falciform, triangular, or coronary ligaments do not need to be mobilized; however, anterior perihepatic adhesions from prior abdominal surgeries are divided using scissors or the ultrasonic scalpel to allow for sonographic evaluation of the liver. It is important to identify any adherent viscera that may be close to the zone of ablation and to dissect them away from the liver if necessary. For lesions encroaching on the gallbladder fossa, the gallbladder should also be removed prior to ablation, so as to avoid thermal injury to the wall of the gallbladder with delayed bile leakage.

Diagnostic laparoscopy is first performed to inspect the diaphragm, abdominal wall, omentum, viscera, and pelvic cavity for the presence of metastases not evident on preoperative imaging studies. For most tumor types, the finding of limited amounts of extrahepatic disease is not a contraindication to proceed with ablation, but widespread disease is.

Next, laparoscopic ultrasonography of the liver is performed using a high-frequency laparoscopic transducer. We use a 10-mm rigid, linear, side-viewing transducer. The

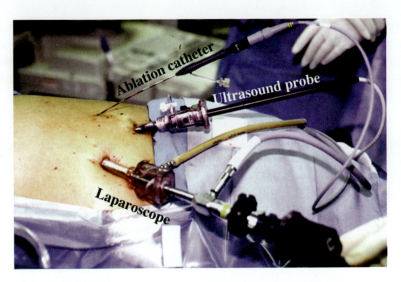

Fig. 1. Placement of subcostal trocars for the laparoscope and laparoscopic ultrasound transducer. The radiofrequency ablation catheter is placed through a separate percutaneous puncture.

liver parenchyma is scanned by moving the transducer linearly from the cephalad to caudad aspects of the liver, and the lesions are mapped out. The use of a picture-in-picture box to superimpose a quarter-sized laparoscopic image over the full-sized ultrasound image is helpful to coordinate the movement of the laparoscopic ultrasound transducer with the laparoscopic image (Fig. 2). Once the lesions are identified, core biopsies of representative lesions are obtained with an 18-gage spring-loaded biopsy gun with an echogenic needle tip using the free-hand technique. Frozen section is obtained. It is most useful to insert the biopsy needle in parallel and within the plane of the ultrasound transducer, so that the entire path of the needle can be imaged as it traverses the liver parenchyma. Tumor vascularity is assessed using Doppler color flow.

There are different RFA devices available, which work on the same principles but have variations in probe and generator designs. The ablation catheter, which is either a straight-tip electrode or composed of a needle with deployable prongs with or without thermocouples, is targeted into the center of the tumor through a skin puncture without using an additional trocar. Then the generator delivers radiofrequency energy to the tissue to create heat. This is performed using different algorithms based on the type of RFA device used. If a catheter with thermocouples is used, once the programmed ablation time is over, the power is turned off to determine the tissue temperature with continued monitoring of the thermocouples. In the first 10 to 20 s, the temperature of the metal prongs decreases rapidly by 20–30°C to equilibrate with the surrounding tissue. This decrease in temperature then proceeds at a slower rate as heat is dissipated from the zone of ablation. Thermocouple temperatures in the 60 to 70°C range 1 min after the ablation process has ceased indicates that a successful ablation has been performed. Another way of assessing the ablation is by the observation of outgassing of dissolved nitrogen into the heating tissues. As the tissues are heated, the solubility of dissolved nitrogen decreases, resulting in microbubble formation within the tissue. This appears as an echogenic blush that enlarges to encompass the zone of ablation (Fig. 3). In those tumors that demonstrate tumor flow

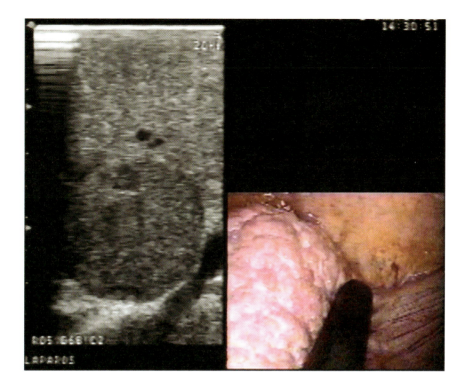

Fig. 2. A picture-in-picture box is useful, providing the laparoscopic and ultrasound images on the same screen. This intraoperative capture shows a hepatocellular cancer lesion in the liver seen with laparoscopic ultrasound.

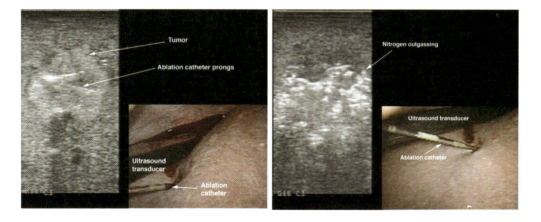

Fig. 3. This intraoperative capture demonstrates (**A**) deployment of the ablation catheter inside the tumor under laparoscopic ultrasound guidance. Then ablation is started, and nitrogen outgassing is seen within the tumor (**B**). This hypoechoic image thus obtained can be used to assess the ablation margins around the tumor.

before ablation, color flow Doppler is repeated after ablation to demonstrate the absence of blood flow within the ablated zones.

Bleeding from the needle track is rarely a problem on withdrawal of the needle. Nevertheless, the needle tract may be coagulated with 20 to 30 W of power during withdrawal of the needle.

Patients require only routine care in the postoperative period without any requirement for narcotics in most. Those patients not undergoing a concomitant surgical procedure are discharged within 24 h. In our series, laparoscopic thermal ablation was performed on all identified lesions, and this treatment did not preclude any subsequent chemotherapy or other treatment modalities. In a number of patients who developed new or recurrent liver disease in follow-up, laparoscopic RFA was applied repeatedly to maintain local tumor control in the liver.

Laboratory studies consist of CBC, renal panel, liver function panel, serum albumin, prothrombin time (PT), partial thromboplastin time (PTT), and tumor markers obtained before, 1 d, and 1 wk after operation. Quality of life is assessed using the SF-36 questionnaire. Radiologic studies include plain chest films and triphasic (noncontrast, arterial, and portal-venous) computed tomography (CT) scans obtained 1 wk before and 1 wk after the thermal ablation procedure. The patients are followed up by repeating the quality of life questionnaire and the laboratory and radiologic studies every 3 mo.

4. RESULTS

Between January 1996 and August 2005, a total of 521 ablations were performed in 428 patients with primary and secondary liver tumors. Three hundred and forty-six patients underwent a single ablation and 82 repeat ablations. The pathology was metastatic adenocarcinoma in 269 (52%), hepatocellular cancer in 106 (20%), metastatic neuroendocrine cancer in 77 (15%), and other tumors in 69 (13%). A total of 1636 lesions (mean 3.1 per patient, range 1–16) were ablated. The mean ±SD tumor size was 2.7 ±1.6 cm (range 0.3–11.5 cm). All cases were completed laparoscopically. The 30-d mortality was 0.4 % ($n = 2$), and morbidity was 3.8 % ($n = 20$), self-limited conditions delaying discharge/requiring readmissions in 6 patients, including liver abscess in four patients, intraabdominal hemorrhage in two patients, trocar injury in two patients, and flank abscess, arrhythmia, pneumonia, wound infection, pestop hypotension and esophageal variceal bleeding in one patient each. The average length of stay was 1.0 d.

In the CT scan obtained 1 wk after RFA, the ablated lesion looks larger than the original lesion in the preop CT scan because of ablation of a rim of normal tissue around the tumor. The lesion shows a progressive decline in size in the absence of a local recurrence (Fig. 4). In our initial evaluation of local recurrence, the local recurrence rate was 12%, with larger adenocarcinomas and sarcomas being at greatest risk. Local recurrence of tumor occurred early in follow-up, with most occurring by 6 mo. Predictors of failure included lack of increased lesion size at 1 wk , adenocarcinoma or sarcoma, larger tumors, and vascular invasion on laparoscopic ultrasound (10).

In our analysis of 67 consecutive patients with HCC undergoing laparoscopic RFA, the median Kaplan-Meier survival was 25.3 mo after RFA treatment (Fig. 5). Patients with an AFP < 400 ng/mL had improved survival compared with those with an α-fetoprotein (AFP) > 400 (25.2 vs 6.7 mo, $p < 0.05$). Patients with a bilirubin of < 2 mg/dL had a survival of 25.2 mo (vs 5.9 mo for those with > 2 mg/dL, $p < 0.05$). Patients with

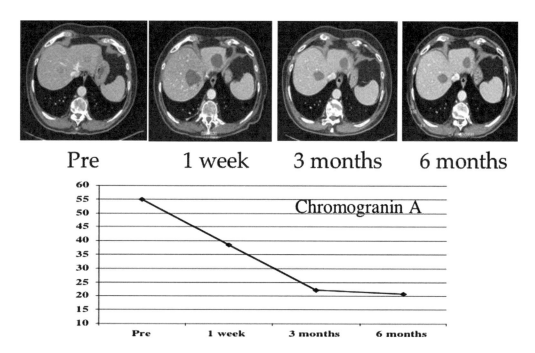

Fig. 4. CT and tumor marker response of a 72-yr-old man with two carcinoid liver metastases. CT scans demonstrate ablated areas larger than the original tumors in the postoperative 1-wk scan owing to ablation of a rim of normal tissue around the tumors. In serial follow-up scans, the lesions show a reduction in tumor size and volume, accompanied by a dramatic decrease in serum chromogranin A levels.

no ascites had a median survival of 29 mo vs 10.1 mo for mild ascites and 4.7 mo for moderate/severe ascites ($p < 0.001$). Patients in Child A classification had a median survival of 29 mo compared with 14.7 mo in Child B and 10.1 mo in Child C classifications ($p < 0.001$). There was no survival advantage based on age, gender, time interval between the diagnosis of liver metastases and RFA, tumor size and number, serum albumin, and PT. Seven patients underwent RFA as a bridge to liver transplantation *(11)*.

We previously reported our results for colorectal liver metastases in 135 consecutive patients . These patients were not candidates for resection, and 80% had tumor progression despite chemotherapy. The median Kaplan-Meier survival for all patients was 28.9 mo after RFA treatment (Fig. 6). Patients with a carcinoembryonic antigen (CEA) < 200 ng/mL had improved survival compared with those with a CEA > 200 (34 vs 16 mo, $p = 0.01$). Those patients with a time from diagnosis of liver metastases to RFA of less than 1 yr had a survival time of 34 mo compared with patients diagnosed more than 1 yr previously (21 mo, $p = 0.01$). Patients whose dominant lesion was < 3 cm in diameter had a median survival of 38 mo vs 34 mo for lesions 3 to 5 cm and 21 mo for lesions > 5 cm ($p = 0.03$). Survival approached significance for patients with one to three tumors vs more than three tumors (29 vs 22 mo, $p = 0.09$). There was no survival advantage based on sex, age, colon vs rectal primary, nodal status at time of diagnosis, metachronous vs synchronous disease, bilobar vs unilobar disease, pretreatment chemotherapy, or documented extrahepatic disease at the time of treatment. Risk of death by the Cox proportional

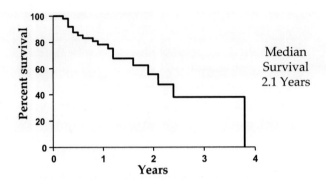

Fig. 5. Overall Kaplan-Meier survival of patients with unresectable hepatocellular cancer undergoing laparoscopic RFA. The median survival was 2.1 yr after radiofrequency thermal ablation treatment.

hazard model was 2.4 for patients with CEA > 200, 2.2 for > 1 yr from diagnosis to RFA, and 1.7 for patients with the largest lesion > 5 cm ($p < 0.05$) *(12)*.

In neuroendocrine patients, amelioration of symptoms was obtained in 95%, with significant or complete symptom control in 80%, for a mean of 10+ mo (range 6–24 mo). Mean ± SEM survival times after diagnosis of primary disease, detection of liver metastases, and performance of RFA were 5.5 ± 0.8 yr, 3.0 ± 0.3 yr, and 1.6 ± 0.2 yr, respectively. Sixty-five per cent of the patients demonstrated a partial or significant decrease in their tumor markers at follow-up *(13)*.

An analysis of 53 patients with noncolorectal, nonneuroendocrine liver metastases undergoing ablation of 192 lesions revealed a local recurrence rate of 17% over a mean follow-up of 24 mo. The overall median survival was 33 mo for the whole series, with > 51 mo for breast cancer and 25 mo for sarcoma *(14)*. This was a highly selected group of patients without evidence of extrahepatic disease.

In 69 cases (13%), RFA was combined with another general surgical procedure including laparoscopic cholecystectomy, colon and small bowel resections, open liver resections, ventral hernia repairs, and various oncologic minor procedures. The morbidity was not increased in these procedures, and recovery was determined by convalescence from the concomitant procedure. Although patients undergoing laparoscopic RFA in combination with a clean-contaminated procedure could be at high risk for secondary infection of ablated foci, this was not observed *(9)*.

5. DISCUSSION

Laparoscopic RFA is a promising safe and effective treatment modality for patients with primary and metastatic liver malignancies. It provides excellent local tumor control with overnight hospitalization and low morbidity for otherwise untreatable lesions. Laparoscopic ultrasonography is a critical part of the procedure, as it allows identification and targeting of the lesions, as well as monitorizing of the ablation process. Technically, it is the most challenging part of the procedure. With the development of larger ablation catheters and more powerful RF generators, it has been possible to ablate large sizes of tumors with a decreased need for overlapping ablations, theoretically decreasing the risk of local recurrence. Still, the general principles of RFA should be followed, and

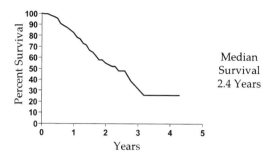

Fig. 6. Overall Kaplan Meier survival of patients with unresectable colorectal liver metastases undergoing RFA. Survival is from the time of the RFA treatment, not from the time of diagnosis of liver metastases.

lesions near the major bile ducts in the porta hepatis should be approached with caution to avoid a possible bile duct injury. Serial triphasic CT scans are essential for documenting objective tumor responses and for identifying recurrent tumor in the liver or elsewhere that may benefit from additional therapy.

It is very important that RFA be performed with minimal morbidity in these advanced-stage cancer patients with already depressed immune systems. In this regard, laparoscopic surgery, is superior to open surgery as it is associated with a lesser degree of immune suppression *(15)*, shorter hospital stay, and faster recovery. Compared with percutaneous RFA, the laparoscopic approach allows imaging of the entire liver, more precise targeting, abdominal staging, and treatment of peripheral tumors. Local recurrence has been the highest in series of patients treated percutaneously, despite smaller and fewer lesions being treated in this group.

RFA technology is evolving rapidly. The initial survival results of our group for HCC, colorectal, neuroendocrine, and other metastases are encouraging compared with historical controls undergoing chemotherapy alone. Our results suggest the use of RFA as the first line of treatment for HCC not amenable to resection. An analysis of colorectal patients suggested a survival advantage in addition to a high local control rate as well. Application of RFA to neuroendocrine liver metastases with a debulking intent is important for palliation of symptoms. Finally, our results also suggest that RFA can play a role in the treatment algorithm of selected patients with noncolorectal, nonneuroendocrine liver metastases who have liver-only disease.

The determining of long-term survival and the performance of randomized clinical studies will better establish the role of RFA in the treatment of liver tumors. In our experience, application of laparoscopic RFA with a debulking intent in a large number of patients resulted in significant palliation of symptoms, especially in neuroendoocrine liver metastases, and also rendered the other types of metastases more susceptible to other treatment modalities such as systemic chemotherapy. These results underscore the concept of "palliative liver ablation" for patients with liver metastases who are not candidates for surgical resection. Our patient population and results also support RFA of liver tumors as a palliative liver surgery model. Another important advantage of laparoscopic RFA is that it can be applied multiple times during the disease course, analogous to chemotherapy, to obtain local tumor control without increasing the morbidity of the procedure.

REFERENCES

1. Berber E. Liver cancer and resection, in *The Cleveland Clinic Guide to Surgical Patient Management* (Ponsky J, ed.), Mosby, St. Louis, MO, 2001, pp. 151–158.
2. Siperstein AE, Berber E. Cryoablation, percutaneous alcohol injection, and radiofrequency ablation for treatment of neuroendocrine liver metastases. World J Surg 2001;25:693–696.
3. Silverberg E, Boring CC, Squires TS. Cancer statistics, 1990 [see comments]. CA Cancer J Clin 1990;40:9–26.
4. Lounsberry W, Goldschmidt V, Linke C. The early histologic changes following electrocoagulation. J Urol 1961;86:291–297.
5. McGahan JP, Brock JM, Tesluk H, et al. Hepatic ablation with use of radiofrequency electrocautery in the animal model. J Vasc Interv Radiol 1992;3:291–297.
6. Rossi S, Fornari F, Buscarini L. Percutaneous ultrasound guided radiofrequency electrocautery for the treatment of small hepatocellular carcinoma. J Interv Radiol 1993;8:97–103.
7. McGahan J, Schneider P, Brock J. Treatment of liver tumors by percutaneous RF electrocautery. Sem Interv Radiol 1993;10:143–149.
8. Foroutani A, Garland AM, Berber E, et al. Laparoscopic ultrasound vs triphasic computed tomography for detecting liver tumors. Arch Surg 2000;135:933–938.
9. Berber E, Senagore A, Remzi F, et al. Laparoscopic radiofrequency ablation of liver tumors combined with colorectal procedures. Surg Laparosc Endosc Percutan Tech 2004;14:186–190.
10. Siperstein A, Garland A, Engle K, et al. Local recurrence after laparoscopic radiofrequency thermal ablation of hepatic tumors. Ann Surg Oncol 2000;7:106–113.
11. Berber E, Rogers S, Siperstein A. Predictors of survival after laparoscopic radiofrequency thermal ablation of hepatocellular cancer: a prospective study. Surg Endosc 2005;19:710–714.
12. Berber E, Pelley R, Siperstein AE. Predictors of survival after radiofrequency thermal ablation of colorectal cancer metastases to the liver: a prospective study. J Clin Oncol 2005;23:1358–1364.
13. Berber E, Flesher N, Siperstein AE. Laparoscopic radiofrequency ablation of neuroendocrine liver metastases. World J Surg 2002;26:985–990.
14. Berber E, Ari E, Herceg N, Siperstein A. Laparoscopic radiofrequency ablation for unusual hepatic tumors: operative indications and outcome. Surg Endosc 2005;19:1613–1617.
15. Vittimberga FJ Jr, Foley DP, Meyers WC, Callery MP. Laparoscopic surgery and the systemic immune response. Ann Surg 1998;227:326–334.

8 Cryoablation for Primary and Secondary Liver Tumors

Tristan D. Yan, BSc, MBBS,
Faruque Riffat, BSc, MBBS, and
David L. Morris, MD, PhD

CONTENTS

INTRODUCTION
TECHNIQUES AND PREREQUISITES
RESULTS
CONCLUSIONS
REFERENCES

SUMMARY

Primary and secondary liver tumors are common. Without a definitive treatment, most patients will succumb to their disease usually within 12 months. As to date, neither regional nor systemic chemotherapy alone has made any significant impact on long-term survival, whereas liver resection or ablation can prolong overall survival in selected patients. However, only a small proportion of patients are suitable for liver resection. Cryoablation alone or in conjunction with resection and intra-arterial chemotherapy is another important tool, which considerably increases the scope of patients who can be treated with a curative intent. This review presented current data on cryoablation therapy for primary and secondary liver tumors.

Key Words: Cryoablation; cryotherapy; hepatic neoplasms; hepatocellular carcinomas; colorectal liver metastases.

1. INTRODUCTION

Primary and secondary liver malignancies are common, and their prognosis is poor without surgical interventions. Hepatocellular carcinoma (HCC) alone leads to more than one million annual deaths worldwide [1,2]. It is common in Asia, where hepatitis B and hepatitis C are more prevalent. Without treatment, patients would succumb to their disease within 12 mo, but in carefully selected patients, liver resection, ablation, or liver transplant can achieve a 5-yr survival rate of 35% [3–8].

From: *Cancer Drug Discovery and Development: Regional Cancer Therapy*
Edited by: P. M. Schlag and U. S. Stein © Humana Press Inc., Totowa, NJ

Colorectal adenocarcinoma is the most common cause of metastatic cancer to the liver and is the second leading cause of cancer-related deaths in the United States. Fifteen to 25% of patients are found to have liver metastases simultaneously with a colorectal primary. Another 30% of patients will develop a metachronous liver secondary *(9,10)*. Over the past decade, surgeons have become more radical in treating colorectal liver metastases. Many ablative techniques, such as cryotherapy, laser therapy, and, more recently, radiofrequency ablation (RFA), have been used in patients who are not candidates for resection. However, controversy still exists as to the extent to which surgery can offer a better survival outcome compared with medical treatment. To date, neither regional nor systemic chemotherapy alone has made any significant impact on long-term survival.

Neuroendocrine cancers have substantially better survival even with multiple liver metastases. Cytoreductive liver surgery is known to offer long-term palliation in this group of patients *(11–13)*.

The only curative treatment for primary and secondary liver tumors to date is resection, yielding a 5-yr survival rate of 50% *(14-19)*. However, this depends on strict patient selection, and, as a result, only a few patients are suitable for surgery *(20–26)*. Cryoablation alone or in conjunction with resection and intraarterial chemotherapy is another important tool; it considerably increases the scope of patients who can be treated with a curative intent. The theoretical basis for this combined treatment modality is to use cryotherapy with or without resection to remove the macroscopically visible tumor with a zone of clearance, followed by regional chemotherapy infusion to eradicate the potentially remaining microscopic tumor cells.

The effects of cryotherapy are several, including vascular injury, disruption of intracellular organelles and the cell membrane, cellular dehydration, and changes in intracellular pH and osmolarity. Rapid cooling, slow thawing, and repetition of freeze-thaw cycles achieve the ablative end point by intra- and extracellular ice crystal formation, coalition of ice crystals, and vascular injury *(27–30)*. The effect of thawing is most marked when it is done slowly and completely. Repetition of freeze-thaw cycles produces more extensive and more certain tissue damage because cells are subjected to additional deleterious physicochemical changes in passing again through damaging thermal conditions. Disruption of cellular elements and cell membranes during a previous freeze-thaw cycle leads to increased thermal conductivity and results in faster cooling and rapid enlargement of the volume of frozen tissue.

2. TECHNIQUES AND PREREQUISITES

2.1. Patient Selection

We do not use this treatment modality as an alternative to resection, but it is certainly our intention to offer a greater proportion of patients a potentially curative treatment option. Some surgeons recommend cryotherapy as an alternative to resection, but it is not yet well supported because of less certain long-term results. However, in general, cryoablation should be considered in patients with multiple bilobar tumors beyond the reach of multiple subsegmental resections to achieve total clearance, whereas cryotherapy allows focal destruction of liver tumors and preservation of functional liver tissue. Percutaneous treatment can also be considered in patients with poor performance status.

2.2. Preoperative Management

All patients should undergo an extensive preoperative workup, which consists of the following:

1. Imaging.
   a. Contrast-enhanced abdominal computed tomography (CT): with intravenous and oral contrast.
   b. Dynamic CT arterial portography: more sensitive and less specific than conventional CT and requires more invasive angiography.
   c. Chest and pelvic CT scans and whole-body bone scan: to exclude extrahepatic lesions.
   d. Positron emission tomography (PET): for the diagnosis of extrahepatic disease. Strasberg et al. reported a 3-yr survival and 3-yr disease-free survival rate of 40% in patients evaluated with a PET scan prior to liver resection *(31)*.

2. Tumor markers.
   a. α-Fetoprotein (AFP) for hepatocellular carcinoma.
   b. Carcinoembryonic antigen (CEA) for colorectal liver metastases.

3. Biopsy: biopsy of tumors is not advised because of the risk of peritoneal seeding.
4. Performance status: general tests for fitness for anesthesia *(32)*.

2.3. Operative Techniques

The initial laparotomy is performed via a right subcostal incision to exclude extrahepatic malignancy and recurrent local disease. Any suspicious lymph nodes or peritoneal nodules are submitted for frozen section histology. A thorough examination of the liver is performed by both palpation and intraoperative ultrasonography (IOUS) to confirm the number, size, and location (especially in relation to hepatic and portal veins). When surgery is feasible, the incision is extended to a bilateral subcostal or triradiate incision. The liver is mobilized after retracting the costal margins by strong retractors attached to a horizontal bar fixed to the operating table. When synchronous resection of colon and liver metastases is planned, a long midline incision is used.

The cryoprobe is placed under IOUS guidance, using stereotacic technique, so that the tip of the probe lies in the center of the lesion *(33)*. In superficial lesions probe is inserted under direct vision. For deeper lesions, the probe insertion can be done using a spinal needle, as a guide, to determine the depth and direction of the lesion, or else with the Seldinger technique. In this technique, an 18-gage needle is followed by a 60-cm stiff mandrill, a 0.964-mm J guide wire, and a subsequent dilator with a 3-, 5-, or 8-mm sheath depending on the probe size to be used (Onik Percutaneous Access Kit, Cook, Spencer, IN). The sheath remains in place while the wire and dilator are exchanged for the selected cryoprobe under continuous IOUS monitoring in two planes. Once the probe is confirmed to be in the lesion, the sheath is pulled out for 5 cm to expose the freezing portion of the cryoprobe. Before commencement of freezing, all tubing and joints of the system are checked and tightened and at the beginning of the operation the probe is run under water to detect gas leaks. Inlet and exhaust tubes are supported by a hand-held gage sling. The skin and viscera of the patient are protected to prevent inadvertent thermal injury to the surrounding structures.

The probe should be kept supported during freezing. Real-time monitoring of the ice ball is done by IOUS from multiple directions, including from the back of the liver. Freezing is continued until the ice ball is seen to exceed the tumor by a margin of at least

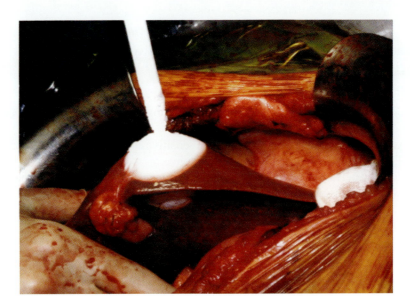

Fig. 1. Cryoablation of a hepatic tumor.

1 cm in all planes. (Fig. 1) When the liver tumor is close to a major portal sheath or hepatic vein, the Pringle maneuver is performed during the cryotherapy to avoid the "heat sink" effect. The average time for a 5-cm ice ball using a single probe is roughly 30 min. For lesions greater than 3 cm in the largest diameter, two or more cryoprobes are usually used simultaneously to ensure total clearance and reduce the time. In patients who have had cryotherapy and liver resection, resection is used preferentially for large tumors, because of the relationship of the cryovolume to the cryoshock phenomenon *(34)*, and the remaining smaller metastases in the contralateral lobe were treated with cryoablation (Fig. 2).

After complete freezing, the edge of the ice ball is allowed to thaw for 1 cm (partial thaw) before refreezing is commenced. The second freeze is allowed to extend at least to the edge of the first ice ball. The first partial thaw is done passively. The final thaw is done actively using heated nitrogen gas. In most patients, we perform this partial double freeze-thaw cycle, whereby thawing of the outer rim of the ice ball by approx 1 cm prior to refreezing increases the lethality of freezing. Complete thawing and refreezing can be time consuming, and, more importantly, it is associated causally with the cryoshock phenomenon. Movement of the probe indicates that thawing has occurred around it, and the probe is removed. Precut fingers of oxidized cellulose foam are packed in the probe track to prevent bleeding. After complete thawing, hemostasis is done and the abdomen is closed in layers after placing two suction drains. Ice-ball cracks may require suture after thawing to control bleeding.

A hepatic arterial catheter is routinely inserted in cryotherapy patients; details of the technique are described elsewhere *(35)*.

2.4. Postoperative Management

We routinely monitor our patients in either the intensive care unit or the high dependency unit for the first 24 h after surgery. Deep venous thrombosis prophylaxis and chest physiotherapy are imperative.

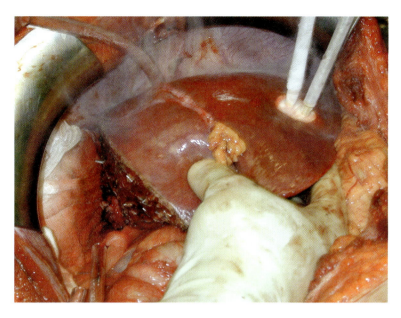

Fig. 2. Resection of the larger hepatic lesion, followed by cryoablation of the smaller contralobar lesion.

Patients are followed at monthly intervals for the first 3 mo and at 3-mo intervals thereafter, unless they become symptomatic. Follow-up includes clinical examination and measurement of tumor markers. Any rise in tumor markers is investigated by CT to identify recurrent disease.

3. RESULTS

3.1. Morbidity and Mortality (Table 1)

1. Cryoshock: this is a syndrome of multiorgan failure characterized by severe coagulopathy, disseminated intravascular coagulation (DIC), acute adult respiratory distress syndrome (ARDS), renal failure, liver failure, profound hypotension, and shock. It is found in 1% of patients undergoing hepatic cryoablation and has a 30% mortality. The exact etiopathogenesis is not known, but it is associated with activation of cytokines and increased production of acute phase proteins, e.g., interleukin-6 (IL-6) and tumor necrosis factor-α (TNF-α). We have, however, never seen full cryoshock, and have not lost any patients from this syndrome, because we use a partial double free-thaw cycle, which produces less cytokine release.

2. Cracking of the ice ball: cracks in the liver may develop when the ice ball is allowed to extend to the liver capsule they are caused by thermal stress occurring during the rapid freezing and thawing process. They can lead to intraoperative and postoperative hemorrhage and are more common in cryoablation of large lesions. Pressure, packing with hemostatic material, application of fibrin glue, or argon plasma coagulation controls bleeding in most cases, but we frequently use liver suturing.

3. Thrombocytopenia: depending on the volume of tissue frozen, the level of serum transaminases rises and the thrombocyte count falls postoperatively *(36)*. The enzyme levels normalize within 1 wk and the platelet count usually reaches its nadir on the third

Table 1
Published Series of Morbidity and Mortality Following Hepatic Cryoablation[a]

Reference	Year	No. of patients	Mortality	Cracking of ice ball	Bleeding	Nephropathy	Chest infection	Pleural effusion	Biloma/ fistula	Abscess
Zhou et al. (57)	1993	113	0	—	0	—	—	—	0	0
Zhou et al. (58)	1995	145	0	—	0	—	—	—	0	0
Ravikumar et al. (59)	1991	32	0	—	0	—	—	—	0	1 (3)
Kane (60)	1993	64	0	5 (8)	2 (3)	—	—	—	2 (3)	2 (3)
Onik et al. (61)	1993	86	3 (3)	1 (1)	1 (1)	3 (3)	—	—	1 (1)	1 (1)
Weaver et al. (62)	1995	140	6 (4)	—	10 (7)	3 (2)	—	7 (5)	6 (4)	2 (1)
Morris et al. (63)	1996	110	2 (2)	—	10 (9)	1 (1)	28 (25)	4 (4)	9 (8)	2 (2)
Gueuthar et al. (64)	1994	100	1 (1)	—	3 (3)	—	—	—	—	—
Saranton et al. (65)	1997	155	1 (1)	39 (25)	—	1 (1)	—	—	1 (1)	—
Korpan et al. (66)	1997	63	0	—	0	—	3 (5)	—	0	0
Seifert et al. (67)	1998	116	1 (1)	—	4 (4)	5 (4)	8 (7)	4 (3)	4 (3)	5 (4)

[a]Numbers in parentheses are percents.

Table 2
Published series of Survival Data of Cryoablation for Hepatocellular Carcinoma (HCC)

References	Year	No. of Patients	Survival (%)		
			1-year	3-year	5-year
Zhou et al. *(68)*	1988	60	52	21	11
Zhou et al. *(69)*	1992	87	61	32	20
Zhou et al. *(57)*	1993	107	—	—	22
Zhou et al. *(58)*	1995	145	69	49	35
Zhou et al. *(70)*	1998	245	78	54	40
Weaver et al. *(71)*	1998	136	85	40	20

postoperative day. These changes are more profound with the double freeze-thaw cycle, probably owing to more extensive hepatocytic damage. Platelet transfusion is rarely indicated.

4. Aseptic pyrexia: aseptic pyrexia (up to 39°C) is very common in the postoperative period and resolves by the end of the first week on its own. It might be caused by tumor cell and hepatocyte lysis.
5. Cardiac arrhythmia: transient hyperkalemia produced by cell lysis can cause cardiac arrhythmias, but it is very rare and is sometimes associated with vena caval freezing.
6. Subphrenic and intrahepatic abscesses: as cryoablation leaves necrotic tissues *in situ*, such tissue is prone to infection, especially if cryoablation of secondary liver cancer and resection of primary colorectal cancer are done simultaneously. It is very rarely seen in the absence of synchronous colorectal surgery. This can be managed by percutaneous pigtail drainage under CT or ultrasound guidance.
7. Biloma and biliary fistula: this can occur when freezing is done near a major biliary structure; however, biliary structures within the liver appear to be well protected by blood flow in the portal sheaths.
8. Pleural effusion, atelectasis, lung collapse and chest infection: pulmonary complications are common after cryoablation of liver tumors, as they are after other types of upper abdominal surgery.

3.2. Survival Results of Hepatocellular Carcinoma (Table 2)

The literature on the cryoablative treatment of HCC is limited. The common use of multimodal therapy for HCC makes it difficult to comment on cryotherapy alone as treatment for HCC.

Zhou's group in China is credited with the largest volume of cryoablation experience in HCC in the world. They have published many series; one of the largest included 167 patients with survival rates at 1, 3, and 5 yr of 74, 48, and 32%, respectively *(37)*. Tumors of less than 5 cm had a better prognosis compared with tumors larger than 5 cm, with 5-yr survival rates of 48 and 25%, respectively.

We have earlier reported a median survival of 640 d for patients with unresectable HCC undergoing cryoablation *(38)*. Pearson et al. achieved complete tumor necrosis assessed by avascularity on post-treatment imaging in 60 to 85% of tumors treated with cyrotherapy *(39)*. However, incomplete tumor eradication can occur owing to large tumor size or close proximity to a large vessel.

Crews et al. *(40)* treated eight HCC patients with intraoperative cryoablation. They saw no tumor progression after 18 mo. In a recent series, Adam et al. *(41)* compared cryotherapy and RFA in 36 patients (18 in each group). They found no significant differences between the two groups in tumor progression. Once again, their results supported a superiority of cryotherapy for HCC compared with other metastases.

One of the major advantages of cryoablation in the treatment of HCC is the fact that patients with HCC often have concurrent cirrhosis, for which cryoablation has a safety advantage over liver resection. The perioperative mortality in cirrhotic patients is about three times higher than in patients without cirrhosis. Such patients with impairment of liver function (Child's B or C) would generally do better with nonresectional therapy for HCC. As long as the tumor is small enough for safe freezing (less than 6 cm), then cryotherapy is a reasonable option for unresectable HCC. Helling et al. *(42)* performed cryoablation in two patients with HCC and cirrhosis with Child's B liver dysfunction and achieved good results. No controlled trial of cryotherapy or RFA has been reported for these patients.

3.3. Survival Results of Colorectal Metastases (Table 3)

Many high-volume series on cryoablation of metastatic liver disease from colorectal adenocarcinoma have been reported world wide, with encouraging results *(43)*. Ravikumar et al. *(44)* have reported on a series of 24 patients who underwent cryotherapy of liver metastases under IOUS guidance between 1985 and 1990. At median follow-up of 24 mo, 29% of patients were disease free, 34% were alive with disease, 35% had recurrence in the liver, and 37% of patients had died. Onik et al. *(45)* also reported similar data: 22% disease-free survival with a median follow-up of 29 mo.

We have recently reported the long-term results of 224 patients who underwent cryotherapy and hepatic arterial chemotherapy with or without resection for unresectable colorectal liver metastases in the last 14 yr *(46)*. The overall median survival was 31 mo (range 1–130 mo), with a 5-yr survival rate of 23%. The median survival for the 200 patients with complete tumor eradication was 36 mo (range 3–130 mo), with a 5-yr survival rate of 26%. In the same study, four factors were independently associated with a favorable outcome: cryotherapy with resection, complete tumor eradication, low preoperative CEA level ($\leq$5 ng/mL), and low postoperative CEA level ($\leq$5 ng/mL).

3.4. Survival Results of Edge Cryotherapy

Numerous studies have shown that a surgical margin of less than 1 cm after liver resection is associated with poor survival. We have also been using cryotherapy to provide an area of tumor eradication up to another 1 cm on involved or close hepatic resection margins (edge cryotherapy). The results are very promising. One hundred and twenty patients with colorectal liver metastases had suboptimal surgical margins following liver resection, and they received edge cryotherapy *(47)*. The overall median survival was 39 mo (range 1–139 mo), with 5-yr survival rate of 36%.

3.5. Survival Results of Neuroendocrine Liver Metastases (NET) (Table 4)

Malignant neuroendocrine tumors are a heterogeneous group of tumors that are generally slow growing; patients have the potential for long-term survival. Even in the setting of advanced disease, a mean survival of up to 8 yr from symptom onset to death has been reported *(48)*. Rapid liver dysfunction and failure is rarely a complication of hepatic NET metastasis despite tremendous tumor bulk *(49)*. Liver metastases from these tumors often present with disabling symptoms owing to syndromes of hormonal excess.

We have earlier reported on a series of 13 patients with metastatic neuroendocrine tumors of the liver who were cryoablated *(11)*. Seven of them were symptomatic, and five had elevated hormonal tumor markers. Twelve patients were alive and asymptomatic at a median follow-up of 14 mo. All patients had complete radiological and marker responses postoperatively. Two patients (15%) had postoperative bleeding owing to coagulopathy requiring reexploration. Cryoablation offers a useful treatment option for this group of patients by alleviating symptoms and probably has impact on survival. Cozzi et al. *(12)* reported similar results earlier.

Goering et al. *(50)* reported on a series of 48 hepatic tumor ablations in 42 patients; 13 of them underwent treatment for neuroendocrine tumors. They achieved a 91% 3-yr survival rate and 32% 3-yr recurrence-free survival rate for NET treated with resection and cryotherapy or cryotherapy alone. Nine of 13 patients required cryotherapy to achieve complete tumor clearance. These results for cryotherapy are comparable to those of other groups, which achieved actuarial survival rates of 73% at 4 yr *(51)*. However, the advantage of cryoablation of application to a broader range of patients including those with unresectable disease means that such a survival benefit can be obtained even in those who would not be candidates for curative resections. In resectable patients, the addition of cryoablation may not only improve survival but would also provide more effective palliation in those patients than by surgery alone.

3.6. Recurrence Rates

Recurrence is not uncommon after cryoablation, as we are treating a biologically different group of patients from those undergoing resection. The most common sites for tumor recurrence are the liver, lung, and lymph nodes. Adam et al. *(52)* previously demonstrated that 35% of the patients had cryosite recurrence in the cryoablation with resection group and 80% in the cryoablation alone group. Johnson et al. *(53)* also had similar results, showing cryosite recurrence rates of 29 and 71% in the cryoablation with resection group and cryoablation group, respectively. Between 1990 and 2003, at our institution, 135 patients had complete macroscopic tumor eradication at the end of the cryooperation. Overall, 115 patients (85%) developed tumor recurrence. Sites of recurrence were the cryosite (44%), the remaining liver (62%), and extrahepatic sites (71%). Univariate analysis demonstrated that an elevated serum CEA level (>5 ng/mL) was a significant prognostic factor for shorter overall and extrahepatic disease-free intervals. Cox regression analysis demonstrated that with the use of resection and cryotherapy, rather than cryotherapy alone, fewer colorectal liver metastases and <3 cm of the largest cryotreated lesions were independent significant prognostic variables for a longer disease-free interval at the cryosite. Our results are comparable to others reported in the literature (Table 3).

The hypothesis that cryotherapy leads to more tumor cell dissemination and tumor recurrence is still controversial. Cuschieri et al. *(54)* carried out an experimental study designed to investigate the risk of tumor dissemination cused by hepatic cryotherapy and to determine the final subzero temperature required for effective hepatic tumor cryoablation in rats. Complete ablation with no residual viable tumor was obtained only at $-38°C$ or below, and hepatic cryotherapy was not found to enhance tumor dissemination. In our opinion, a 1-cm margin of normal liver tissue should be frozen beyond the tumor margin to ensure effective local control. Allen et al. *(55)*, in an experimental study, found that cryoablation of HCC does not accelerate residual tumor growth in rats.

Table 3
Published Series on Survival and Recurrence After Cryoablation for Colorectal Liver Metastases

Reference	Year	No. of patients	Median follow-up [mo (range)]	DFS rate (%)	Recurrence rate [no (%)]					
					Overall	Liver	Cryosite	Remaining liver	Extra-hepatic	Lung
Ravikumar et al. (59)	1991	18	24 (5–60)	39	11/18 (61)	—	—	—	—	—
Weaver et al. (71)	1995	47	26 (24–57)	11 / 23	17/22[b] (77)	12/22[b] (55)	—	—	13/22[b] (59)	8/22[b] (36)
Yeh et al. (72)	1997	21	19	43	10/21 (48)	4/21 (19)	1/21 (5)	—	8/21 (38)	—
Adam et al. (73)	1997	25	16[c] (2–27)	20	20/25 (80)	15/25 (60)	11/25 (44)	—	10/25 (40)	—
Crews et al. (74)	1997	27	15 (1–31)	15	23/27 (85)	—	2/27 (7)	19/27 (70)	7/27 (26)	—
Johnson et al. (75)	1997	7[d]	14 (1–21)	29	5/7 (71)	5/7 (71)	5/7 (71)	2/7 (29)	2/7 (29)	—
Johnson et al. (75)	1997	7[e]	6 (3–17)	71	2/7	2/7	2/7	1/7	1/7	1/7

Reference	Year	n			(29)	(29)	(29)	(14)	(14)	(14)
Weaver et al. (76)	1998	136	—	21	107/136 (79)	88/136 (65)	—	—	70/136 (51)	—
Seifert et al. (77)	1999	85	22 (0–64)	22	66/85 (78)	40/85 (47)	21/85 (25)	36/85 (42)	33/85 (39)	19/85 (22)
Wallace et al. (78)	1999	106	14 (1–60)	38	66/106 (62)	52/106 (49)	—	—	45/106 (42)	—
Ruers et al. (79)	2001	30	26 (9–73)	7[f]	25/30 (83)	18/30 (60)	6/30 (20)	—	14/30 (47)	6/30 (20)
Rivoire et al. (80)	2002	24	48	24[g]	19/24 (79)	18/24 (75)	—	—	17/24 (71)	11/24 (46)
Our results	2003	135	24 (0–98)	15	115/135 (85)	92/135 (68)	60/135 (44%)	84/135 (62)	96/135 (71)	60/135 (44)

[a] Patients with complete treatment of colorectal liver metastases.
[b] Patients alive.
[c] Mean.
[d] Cryotherapy only.
[e] Cryotherapy + Liver resection.
[f] 2-year disease-free survival.
[g] 4-year disease-free survival.

Table 4
Published Series of Cryoablation for Neuroendocrine Liver Metastases

Reference	Year	No. of patients	Median follow-up [mo (range)]	Symptomatic response [no. (%)]	Marker response [no. (%)]	Survival (%)
Cozzi et al. *(81)*	1995	6	24 (6–72)	7/7 (100)	3/3 (100)	100
Bilchik et al. *(82)*	1997	19	17 (3–49)	19/19 (100)	17/18 (94)	72
Shapiro et al. *(83)*	1998	5	30	5/5 (100)	4/4 (100)	20
Seifert et al. *(84)*	1998	13	13.5	5/7 (71)	3/3 (100)	92

However, in our previous animal work, we have shown that cryotherapy stimulates the systemic release of the proinflammatory cytokines IL-6 and TNF-α, which is directly proportional to the size of the cryoablations *(34)*. It is known that increasing cytokine levels will upregulate the cellular expression of adhesion molecule, which might facilitate tumor cell implantation in distant organs. We have recently demonstrated that hepatic cryoablation is related to the incidence of pulmonary metastases in patients with secondary colorectal liver cancer *(56)*.

4. CONCLUSIONS

Hepatic cryotherapy is a relatively safe procedure. To optimize its efficacy, the authors recommend the following: (1) the concurrent use of IOUS to monitor the extension of a cryo ice ball of at least 1 cm beyond the tumor in all planes to ensure complete tumor eradication; (2) resecting the larger hepatic lesions to avoid the cryoshock phenomenon, which might improve the long-term survival results; (3) applying the Pringle maneuver when a cryoprobe is deployed close to a major vessel to avoid the "heat sink" effect and maximize its killing power; (4) to avoid the cryoshock phenomenon feared by many surgeons, using a partial double freeze-thaw cycle, with thawing of the outer rim of the ice ball by approximately 1 cm prior to refreezing, but not complete thawing and refreezing. The complete double freeze-thaw cycle might produce more cytokine release, which is thought to be causally associated with the cryoshock phenomenon. With this partial double freeze-thaw technique, we have not experienced a single case of cryoshock phenomenon in the 371 cases of cryotherapy that we have performed for primary and secondary hepatic tumors.

REFERENCES

1. London WT. Primary hepatocellular carcinoma: etiology, pathogenesis, and prevention. Hum Pathol 1981;12:1085–1097.
2. Zhao J, Dwerryhouse SJ, Ross WB, Morris DL. Cryotherapy for hepatocellular carcinoma. Asian J Surg 1997;20:140–145.
3. Nagasue N, Yukaya H, Hamada T, Hirose S, Kanashima R, Inokuchi K. The natural history of hepatocellular carcinoma. A study of 100 untreated cases. Cancer 1984;54:1461–1465.
4. Falkson G, Cnaan A, Schutt AJ, Ryan LM, Falkson HC. Prognostic factors for survival in hepatocellular carcinoma. Cancer Res 1988;48:7314–7318.
5. Bismuth H, Chiche L. Comparison of hepatic resection and transplantation in the treatment of liver cancer. Semin Surg Oncol 1993;9:341–345.

6. Farmer DG, Rososve MH, Shaked A. Current treatment modalities for hepatocellular carcinoma. Ann Surg 1994;219:59–71.

7. Onodera H, Ukai K, Minami Y. Hepatocellular carcinoma cases with five-year survival and prognostic factors affecting the survival time. Tohoku J Exp Med 1995;176:203–211.

8. Stuart KE, Anand AJ, Jenkins RL. Hepatocellular carcinoma in the United States. Prognostic features, treatment outcome, and survival. Cancer 1996;77:2217–2222.

9. Bengmark S, Hafstrom L, Jeppsson B, Jonsson PE, Ryden S, Sundqvist K. Metastatic disease in the liver from colorectal cancer: an appraisal of liver surgery. World J Surg 1982;6:61–65.

10. Adson MA, van Heerden JA, Adson MH, Wagner JS, Ilstrup DM. Resection of hepatic metastases from colorectal cancer. Arch Surg 1984;119:647–651.

11. Seifert JK, Cozzi PJ, Morris DL. Cryotherapy for neuroendocrine liver metastases. Semin Surg Oncol 1998;14:175–183.

12. Cozzi PJ, Englund R, Morris DL. Cryotherapy treatment of patients with hepatic metastases from neuroendocrine tumors. Cancer 1995;76:501–509.

13. Bilchik AJ, Sarantou T, Foshag LJ, Giuliano AE, Ramming KP. Cryosurgical palliation of metastatic neuroendocrine tumors resistant to conventional therapy. Surgery 1997;122:1040–1047; discussion 1047–1048.

14. Seifert JK, Morris DL. Prognostic factors after cryotherapy for hepatic metastases from colorectal cancer. Ann Surg 1998;228:201–208.

15. Ballantyne GH, Quin J. Surgical treatment of liver metastases in patients with colorectal cancer. Cancer 1993;71(12 Suppl):4252–4266.

16. Hughes KS. Resection of the liver for colorectal carcinoma metastases: a multi-institutional study of indications for resection. Registry of Hepatic Metastases. Surgery 1988;103:278–288.

17. Scheele J, Stang R, Altendorf-Hofmann A, Paul M. Resection of colorectal liver metastases. World J Surg 1995;19:59–71.

18. Seifert JK, Junginger T. Resection of liver metastases of colorectal tumors. A uni- and multivariate analysis of prognostic factors. Langenbecks Arch Chir 1996;381:187–200.

19. Nordlinger B, Guiguet M, Vaillant JC, et al. Surgical resection of colorectal carcinoma metastases to the liver. A prognostic scoring system to improve case selection, based on 1568 patients. Association Française de Chirurgie. Cancer 1996;77:1254–1262.

20. Morris DL. Shiv K Ganandha. Cryoablation of liver tumors. Chapter 14. "Malignant liver tumors: Current and emerging therapies" 2nd ed., 2004.

21. Adam R, Lucidi V, Bismuth H. Hepatic colorectal metastases: methods of improving resectability. Surg Clin North Am 2004;84:659–671.

22. Doci R, Gennari L, Bignami P, Montalto F, Morabito A, Bozzetti F. One hundred patients with hepatic metastases from colorectal cancer treated by resection: analysis of prognostic determinants. Br J Surg 1991;78:797–801.

23. Rees M, Plant G, Bygrave S. Late results justify resection for multiple hepatic metastases from colorectal cancer. Br J Surg 1997;84:1136–1140.

24. Adam R, Avisar E, Ariche A, et al. Five-year survival following hepatic resection after neoadjuvant therapy for nonresectable colorectal. Ann Surg Oncol 2001;8:347–353.

25. Littrup PJ, Lee FT Jr, Rajan D, Meetze K, Weaver D. Hepatic cryotherapy (state-of-the-art techniques and future developments). Ultrasound Q 1998;14:171–188.

26. Elias D, de Baere T, Sideris L, Ducreux M. Regional chemotherapeutic techniques for liver tumors: current knowledge and future directions. Surg Clin North Am 2004;84:607–625.

27. Gage AA, Baust J. Mechanisms of tissue injury in cryosurgery. Cryobiology 1998;37:171–186.

28. Hill AG. Initiators and propagators of the metabolic response to injury. World J Surg 2000;24:624–629.

29. Xin-Da Z, Zhao-You Y, Ye-Qin U. Cryosurgery for liver tumors, in Novel Regional Therapies for Liver Tumors, 1995.

30. Kariappa SM, Links M, Morris DL. Non-surgical treatment options in Hepatocellular carcinoma. Cancer reviews: Asia-Pacific 2003;1:245–279.

31. Strasberg SM, Dehdashti F, Siegel BA, Drebin JA, Linehan D. Survival of patients evaluated by FDG-PET before hepatic resection for metastatic colorectal carcinoma: a prospective database study. Ann Surg 2001;233:293–299.

32. Schneider PD. Preoperative assessment of liver function. Surg Clin North Am 2004;84:355–373.

33. Lee FT Jr, Mahvi DM, Chosy SG, et al. Hepatic cryosurgery with intraoperative US guidance. Radiology 1997;202:624–632.

34. Seifert JK, France MP, Zhao J, et al. Large volume hepatic freezing: association with significant release of the cytokines interleukin-6 and tumor necrosis factor α in a rat model. World J Surg 2002;26:1333–1341.

35. McCall JL, Jorgensen JO, Morris DL. Hepatic artery chemotherapy for colorectal liver metastases. {Review.] Aust N Z J Surg 1995;65:383–389. Review.

36. Cozzi PJ, Stewart GJ, Morris DL. Thrombocytopenia after hepatic cryotherapy for colorectal metastases: correlates with hepatocellular injury. World J Surg 1994;18:774–776; discussion 777.

37. Zhou XD, Tang ZY, Yu YQ. Ablative approach for primary liver cancer: Shanghai experience. Surg Oncol Clin N Am 1996;5:379–390.

38. Zhao J, Dwerryhouse SJ, Ross WB, Morris DL. Cryotherapy for hepatocellular carcinoma. Asian J Surg 1997;20:140–145.

39. Pearson AS, Izzo F, Fleming R, et al. Intraoperative radiofrequency ablation or cyroablation for hepatic malignancies. Am J Surg 1999;178:599–603

40. Crews K, Kuhn J, McCarty T, et al. Cryosurgical ablation of hepatic tumors. Am J Surg 1997;174:614–617

41. Adam R, Hagopian E, Linhares M, et al. A comparison of percutaneous cryosurgery and percutaneous radiofrequency for unresectable hepatic malignancies. Arch Surg 2002;137:1332–1339

42. Helling T. Realistic expectations for cryoablation of liver tumor. J Hepatobiliary Pancreat Surg 2000;7:510–515

43. Morris DL, Ross WB, Iqbal J, McCall JL, King J, Clingan PR. Cryoablation of hepatic malignancy: An evaluation of tumor marker data and survival in 110 patients. GI Cancer 1996;1:247–251.

44. Ravikumar TS, Kane R, Cady B, Jenkins R, Clouse M, Steele G Jr. A 5-year study of cryosurgery in the treatment of liver tumors. Arch Surg 1991;126:1520–1523; discussion 1523–1524.

45. Onik G, Rubinsky B, Zemel R, et al. Ultrasound-guided hepatic cryosurgery in the treatment of metastatic colon carcinoma. Preliminary results. Cancer 1991;67:901–907.

46. Yan TD, Padang R, Morris DL. Long-term results and prognostic indicators after cryotherapy and hepatic arterial chemotherapy with or without resection for colorectal liver metastases in 224 patients long-term survival can be achieved in patients with multiple bilteral liver metastases. J Am Coll Surg 2006;202:100–111.

47. Yan TD, Padang R, Xia H, Zhao J, Li J, Morris DL. Management of involved or close resection margins in 120 patients with colorectal liver metastases: edge cryotherapy can achieve long-term survival. Am J Surg 2006;191:735–742.

48. Moertel C. Karnofsky Memorial Lecture: an odyssey in the land of small tumors. J Clin Oncol 1987;5:1503–1522

49. Chamberlain R, Canes D, Brown K, et al. Hepatic neuroendocrine metastasis does intervention alter outcome. J Am Coll Surg 2000;190:432–445

50. Goering J, Mahvi D, Neiderhuber, et al. Cyroablation and liver resection for noncolorectal liver metastasis. Am J Surg 2002;183:384–389

51. Que F, Nagorney D, Batts K, et al. Hepatic resection for metastatic neuroendocrine carcinomas. Am J Surg 1995;174:610–613

52. Adam R, Akpinar E, Johann M, Kunstlinger F, Majno P, Bismuth H. Place of cryosurgery in the treatment of malignant liver tumors. Ann Surg 1997;225:39–38; discussion 48–50.

53. Johnson LB, Krebs TL, Van Echo D, et al. Cytoablative therapy with combined resection and cryosurgery for limited bilobar hepatic colorectal metastases. Am J Surg 1997;174:610–613.

54. El-Shakhs SA, Shimi SA, Cuschieri A. Effective hepatic cryoablation: does it enhance tumor dissemination? World J Surg 1999;23:306–310.

55. Allen PJ, D'Angelica M, Hodyl C, Lee J, You YJ, Fong Y. The effects of hepatic cryosurgery on tumor growth in the liver. J Surg Res 1998;77:132–136.

56. Yan TD, Chiang G, Zhao J, Chan D, Morris DL. Lung metastases after liver resection and cryotherapy—is there a difference? HPB, in press.

57. Zhou X-D, Tang Z-Y, Yu Y-Q, et al. The role of cryosurgery in the treatment of hepatic cancer: a report of 113 cases. J Cancer Res Clin Oncol 1993;120:100–102.

58. Zhou X-D, Tang Z-Y, Yu Y-Q. Cryosurgery for liver tumors, in Novel Regional Therapies for Liver Tumors, 1995.

59. Ravikumar TS, Kane R, Cady B, Jenkins R, Clouse M, Steele G Jr. A 5-year study of cryosurgery in the treatment of liver tumors. Arch Surg 1991;126:1520–1523; discussion 1523–1524.

60. Kane RA. Ultrasound guided hepatic cryosurgery for tumor ablation. Sem Interv Radiol 1993;10: 132–142.

61. Onik GM, Atkinson D, Zemel R, Weaver ML. Cryosurgery of liver cancer. Semin Surg Oncol 1993;9:309–317.

62. Weaver ML, Atkinson D, Zemel R. Hepatic cryosurgery in the treatment of unresectable metastases. Surg Oncol 1995;4:231–236.

63. Morris DL, Ross WB, Iqbal J, McCall JL, King J, Clingan PR. Cryoablation of hepatic malignancy: an evaluation of tumor marker data and survival in 110 patients. GI Cancer 1996;1:247–251.

64. Guenther D, Kirgan R, Klein L, Foshag L, Ramming K. Coagulopathy associated with cryosurgery for hepatic metastases of colorectal cancer. Proc ASCO 1994;13:A213.

65. Sarantou T, Bilchik A, Ramming K. Cryoablation of primary and metastatic liver cancer unresponsive to conventional therapy. Proc ASCO 1997;16:304A.

66. Korpan NN. Hepatic cryosurgery for liver metastases. Long-term follow-up. Ann Surg 1997;225: 193–201.

67. Seifert JK, Morris DL. Prognostic factors after cryotherapy for hepatic metastases from colorectal cancer. Ann Surg 1998;228:201–208

68. Zhou XD, Tang ZY, Yu YQ, Ma ZC. Clinical evaluation of cryosurgery in the treatment of primary liver cancer. Report of 60 cases. Cancer 1988;61:1889–1892.

69. Zhou XD, Yu Yq, Tang ZY et al. An 18-year study of cryosurgery in the treatment of primary liver cancer. Asian J Surg 1992;15:43–47.

70. Zhou XD, Tang ZY. Cryotherapy for primary liver cancer. Semin Surg Oncol 1998;14:171–174.

71. Weaver ML, Atkinson D, Zemel R. Hepatic cryosurgery in treating colorectal metastases. Cancer. 1995;76:210–214.

72. Yeh KA, Fortunato L, Hoffman JP, Eisenberg BL. Cryosurgical ablation of hepatic metastases from colorectal carcinomas. Am Surg 1997;63:63–68.

73. Adam R, Akpinar E, Johann M, Kunstlinger F, Majno P, Bismuth H. Place of cryosurgery in the treatment of malignant liver tumors. Ann Surg 1997;225:39–38; discussion 48–50.

74. Crews KA, Kuhn JA, McCarty TM, Fisher TL, Goldstein RM, Preskitt JT. Cryosurgical ablation of hepatic tumors. Am J Surg 1997;174:614–617; discussion 617–618.

75. Johnson LB, Krebs TL, Van Echo D, et al. Cytoablative therapy with combined resection and cryosurgery for limited bilobar hepatic colorectal metastases. Am J Surg 1997;174:610–613.

76. Weaver ML, Ashton JG, Zemel R. Treatment of colorectal liver metastases by cryotherapy. Semin Surg Oncol 1998;14:163–170.

77. Seifert JK, Morris DL. Indicators of recurrence following cryotherapy for hepatic metastases from colorectal cancer. Br J Surg 1999;86:234–240.

78. Wallace JR, Christians KK, Pitt HA, Quebbeman EJ. Cryotherapy extends the indications for treatment of colorectal liver metastases. Surgery 1999;126:766–772; discussion 772–774.

79. Ruers TJ, Joosten J, Jager GJ, Wobbes T. Long-term results of treating hepatic colorectal metastases with cryosurgery. Br J Surg 2001;88:844–849.

80. Rivoire M, De Cian F, Meeus P, Negrier S, Sebban H, Kaemmerlen P. Combination of neoadjuvant chemotherapy with cryotherapy and surgical resection for the treatment of unresectable liver metastases from colorectal carcinoma. Cancer 2002;95:2283–2292.

81. Cozzi PJ, Englund R, Morris DL. Cryotherapy treatment of patients with hepatic metastases from neuroendocrine tumors. Cancer 1995;76:501–509.

82. Bilchik AJ, Sarantou T, Foshag LJ, Giuliano AE, Ramming KP. Cryosurgical palliation of metastatic neuroendocrine tumors resistant to conventional therapy. Surgery 1997;122:1040–1047; discussion 1047–1048.

83. Shapiro RS, Shafir M, Sung M, Warner R, Glajchen N. Cryotherapy of metastatic carcinoid tumors. Abdom Imaging 1998;23:314–317.

84. Seifert JK, Cozzi PJ, Morris DL. Cryotherapy for neuroendocrine liver metastases. Semin Surg Oncol 1998;14:175–183.

9 A Personal History of Photodynamic Therapy

Thomas J. Dougherty, PhD

CONTENTS

SUMMARY

Photodynamic therapy (PDT), which utilizes a photoactivated drug (photosensitizer) to destroy malignant or certain other undesirable tissue, is approved by health agencies worldwide, mainly for the treatment of early- and late-stage lung cancer and premalignant and obstructive esophageal cancer. The clinical and scientific development of PDT began in the early 1970s at Roswell Park Cancer Institute in Buffalo, NY. This paper presents the history of this process at Roswell Park.

Key Words: Photodynamic therapy; PDT; development.

1. PHOTODYNAMIC THERAPY

Photodynamic therapy (PDT) involves the use of photoactivated drugs to destroy or modify certain undesirable tissues and/or tissue components. PDT is approved by health agencies in the United States, Europe, Canada, and Japan mainly for treatment (palliation) of obstructive esophageal cancer and endobronchial cancers and for curative intent for early-stage lung and esophageal cancer. Mechanistically, PDT requires a photosensitizer, light to match the absorption of the sensitizer (usually in the red range), and singlet oxygen formed by energy transfer from the excited sensitizer to endogenous oxygen. Vascular effects, direct cellular effects, and immunological effects accompany PDT. Since there are numerous excellent reviews of both the clinical use and basic mechanisms involved (e.g., refs. *1* and *2*), it is my intention to provide here my personal experience in helping develop PDT.

From: *Cancer Drug Discovery and Development: Regional Cancer Therapy*
Edited by: P. M. Schlag and U. S, Stein © Humana Press Inc., Totowa, NJ

2. THE BEGINNING

In February 1970, I joined a biology research group at Roswell Park Cancer Institute, basically as a postdoctoral graduate student. I was supported by a National Institute of Health research grant and asked to use nuclear magnetic resonance to study gramacidin transport into cells. I had been recommended to Roswell by Professor George S. Hammond, the Chairman of Chemistry at Cal Tech, whom I had met and had many discussions with in his role as consultant for DuPont (where I spent the first 10 years after receiving my PhD in physical-organic chemistry from Ohio State University). I had worked on a photochemical problem at DuPont, and George Hammond was the foremost photochemist in the world. This was my introduction to photochemistry, with which I became fascinated.

While I was doing the research required on the gramacidin project at Roswell, there was plenty of time to browse in the library. I was particularly interested in finding problems with current cancer treatment and if there was any way I could use my background to address any of them. In looking at radiation therapy, I found considerable information on the so-called oxygen effect, i.e., hypoxic tumors tend to be considerably more resistant to radiation damage than fully oxygenated tumors. (This is largely because the oxygen radicals generated by radiation attack the tumor and assist in destroying it.) I reasoned that if a drug could be found that would release oxygen upon radiation, it might help reverse this resistance.

Looking through the chemical literature, I came upon a class of compounds called endoperoxides, which I evaluated for this application. Irradiation indeed caused release of oxygen (in what form was unknown) and regeneration of the parent compound. Also, in cell culture (melanoma cells), a combination of the endoperoxide and irradiation appeared to be more toxic to the cells than radiation or the drug alone. However, by this time I was beginning to realize that the in vivo situation would be very different—the peroxides would likely be toxic, not survive detoxification in vivo, and so on. I had been using fluorescein diacetate to measure viability of the melanoma cells in vitro. (The nonfluorescent diacetate is enzymatically cleaved to fluorescent fluorescein only in viable cells.) The technician who was helping me warned me to be careful to shield the labeled cells from light or they would die. Naturally, I tried this (exposed the labeled cells to sunlight through the window), and sure enough the cells died. I repeated this several times to be sure it was true (it was) and then went to the literature, where of course I "discovered" the photodynamic effect, going all the way back to Raab in 1900 (3).

The next step was to try light exposure against tumors in mice. (Again I relied on numerous scientists and technicians at Roswell to teach me the relevant techniques—they were wonderfully responsive.) We obtained a mammary tumor and implanted it into mice; when it was about 4 to 5 mm in diameter, we injected fluorescein and then used a filtered lamp (approx 500 nm) to illuminate the tumors. The tumor growth slowed compared with untreated controls, but this was not exactly what I was looking for. However, we published these results in the *Journal of the National Cancer Institute* in 1974 (4). I had realized by then that if there was any hope of this working in vivo I needed a nontoxic compound that absorbed in the red spectrum (for deeper tissue penetration) and that did not clear as quickly as did fluorescein. About this time I was talking to a pharmacologist from the State University at Buffalo who mentioned a material called hematoporphyrin derivative (Hpd) being used at the Mayo Clinic for detecting cancers by virtue of its red fluorescence. I went to the literature and found that several groups were actually doing this in the 1960s. They were finding that virtually all kinds of cancers took up Hpd and that they could be located by virtue of Hpd fluorescence. I also realized that porphyrins were excellent generators of singlet oxygen, the same cytotoxic agent produced by fluorescein (albeit in very low yields)—and the porphyrins had an absorption in the red. Thus began my quest with Hpd, which really laid the foundation for modern-day PDT using Photofrin (a purified form of Hpd).

When I read the Mayo Clinic papers and others, it was not very clear what the structure of Hpd was nor how to make it, except that it came from hematoporphyrin (Hp) and was formed when the Hp was treated with acetic acid. Nonetheless, I set out to prepare Hpd, and after a few failures, finally got something that I thought was similar to the Hpd reported in the literature. We (by this time I was joined by colleagues Donn Boyle and Ken Weishaupt, both of whom I had met at DuPont) continued modifying the synthesis until it was reproducible as tested in vivo in a mouse breast tumor model. After playing around with Hpd doses, time intervals, and light doses, we actually were able to destroy the entire tumor and "cure" some of the mice, which we reported in the *Journal of the National Cancer Institute* in 1975 *(5)*. I recall that one of the reviewers objected to my use of the term "cure." It seemed appropriate to me at the time since in some of the mice the tumor never recurred. By 1974 we had treated literally hundreds of mice and rats, honing in on the optimum PDT conditions for "control" of the tumors.

2.1. First PDT Clinical Protocol

At this point, it seemed appropriate to me that we should consider beginning a phase I clinical trial of this "new" treatment. The road we took, which is described below, should not be taken as a model for beginning a clinical trial with an experimental drug—but in those days we actually thought we were proceeding appropriately.

We prepared several bottles of Hpd in our lab according to our optimized synthetic methods, and then Arnold Mittelman, a senior surgeon here, and I wrote a clinical protocol that was submitted to our Institutional Review Board (IRB) for approval to begin a phase I clinical trial (technically to test toxicity, but PDT also requires light treatment and therefore measurement of tumor response). This was readily approved by our IRB. (It was easy in those days.) The protocol called for treatment of any solid tumor involving the skin, metastatic cancers of the breast, colon, and so on. This was before we used lasers. The light source was a xenon arc lamp filtered to emit light in the red region of the spectrum. In 1974 we treated our first patient—a woman with a metastatic colon tumor protruding through the abdominal wall. Note that there is no mention of the FDA here! We reasoned that the Food and Drug Administration (FDA) has jurisdiction only over interstate activity, and we were operating strictly intrastate (or so we thought—see below).

We learned in the very first patient that a human is not a mouse! We used treatment conditions in this patient similar to that we had found optimal in mice. She was severely overtreated, with necrosis to the entire treatment field including apparently normal skin. She was in considerable pain. I felt terrible that we had done this to her. I remember returning to the hospital late at night to be with her. She was magnificent—she tried to console me. Obviously we reduced the Hpd and light dose in subsequent patients and attempted to determine the optimum conditions (Hpd dose, time interval, light dose) for obtaining selective treatment. We eventually found what appeared to be optimum conditions and reported in 1978 on a series of 25 patients with a total of 113 lesions treated by Hpd-PDT *(6)*. In 1976, Kelly and Snell *(7)* had actually reported on the treatment of a patient with superficial bladder cancer, although no further clinical data were subsequently reported by them. Also, I eventually found that Richard Lipson of the Mayo Clinic, who had initiated the use of Hpd for cancer detection *(8)*, had also recognized the therapeutic potential of Hpd as a photosensitizer and had treated a patient with metastatic breast cancer (skin) with Hpd-PDT. This report was only published in an abstract from a meeting in Japan in 1966 *(9)*; I obtained it from Denis Cortese of the Mayo Clinic several years after we started our study. The studies published from Roswell Park *(6,10)* still represent the first clinical trial of PDT.

Okay, what's wrong with this picture? In 1979, following the presentation of some of our clinical results at a meeting of the American Society for Photobiology in Washington, D.C., I received a phone call from someone at the FDA who apparently had heard my presentation. He wanted to know why we had not filed for an Investigational New Drug Exemption (IND) with the FDA before initiating patient treatment. I confidently explained that all the patients were from within New York state, that the Hpd was prepared in New York State, and so on and so forth, and that the FDA therefore did not have jurisdiction over this study. The next question he asked me was "Where do you buy the bottles for the Hpd?" Oops! The message was loud and clear. We were in fact subject to the FDA regulations and were told to stop the study. We agreed to file an IND. However, this created a dilemma. We had several patients in the pipeline ready for treatment. The FDA agreed to allow us to continue on a case-by-case basis. We had to make the case to the FDA as to why a particular patient had to be treated and they would consider our argument and determine if we could proceed. This was a clumsy process, but at least it kept things going while we prepared and filed the IND. As I recall, they in fact agreed to treatment for all patients we requested. We filed all the necessary paperwork, including the data on all the patients we had treated up to that time, and obtained the IND in 1979. Now we were legitimate (at least bureaucratically!).

Over the next few years we continued our clinical trials on Hpd-PDT, published results *(6,10)*, and gave presentations at meetings and various hospitals and universities. A few investigators became interested in using PDT in their institutions. Among these were Jim McCaughan (surgeon at Grant Laser Center in Columbus, OH), Jim Kennedy (medical oncologist at the Royal Military College of Canada in Kingston, ON), and Yosihiro Hayata (head of Thoracic Surgery at the Tokyo Medical College). They picked up on PDT and confirmed what we had been reporting. However, they were able to expand the clinical use beyond tumors on the skin. By this time we had all gotten laser systems equipped with fiberoptics, allowing for endoscopic use (e.g., esophagus, lung). Professor Hayata was the first to use PDT to treat lung cancer and the first to apply PDT endoscopically—with spectacular results *(11)*.

Jim McCaughan also treated many cancer types, with excellent results *(12)*. It was very exciting in those days to attend meetings at which clinical PDT work was presented—all for the first time. It became clear that PDT had potential for a broad range of applications in cancer.

In the early 1980s I encountred a typical situation showing how difficult it was to convince physicians that PDT was a viable treatment for certain patients. I received a letter from Ian Forbes (a medical oncologist in Adelaide, Australia), who had been using PDT for cutaneous metastatic breast cancer. He was receiving a lot of flack from the radiation therapists in Adelaide, who were treating this disease with radiation therapy

(XRT), which was the standard treatment. However, they objected to Ian using PDT to treat recurrences of the disease—after XRT! Their argument was that no one knew whether PDT could be applied to the skin after radiation therapy, in spite of the fact that we had been doing just that successfully at Roswell Park for several years. On the other hand, it was not a totally unreasonable concern, so our group at Roswell carried out experiments in mice combining PDT with radiation, and using the PDT both before and after radiation. What we found was that there was no synergism between the damage incurred by PDT and radiation. The effects were additive. We put together the data with numerous pathological slides and sent them to Ian, who discussed the data with his radiation therapists. They still were not convinced, and for all practical purposes, they shut down Ian's clinical PDT program. It should be noted that in patients who have experienced heavy doses of XRT to the chest wall (e.g., >60 gy), especially when combined with chemotherapy, one does have to be cautious with the PDT dose. For these patients we generally use 0.75 mg/kg Photofrin and light doses of 175 J/cm^2, 48 hours after injection.

In the late 1970s we began a collaboration with a local veterinarian, Richard Thoma. We began to treat primary cancers in cats and dogs. These were not experimental animals. They were pets, many of which would not have been treated at all. However, they were excellent models for treatment of humans. These results were initially reported in *Cancer Research (13)* and subsequently in various veterinarian journals. By the time of our last publication, we had treated over 100 animals. An interesting incident occurred with Dick Thoma. When we began this study, we treated his animals here at Roswell—after hours. Our laser was installed in one of the X-ray rooms used for patient treatment (both XRT and PDT). One day I met Dick at the back entrance bringing in his Labrador retriever for treatment. As we entered the elevator, lo and behold there was the Institute director, whom we assumed would not look favorably on bringing a dog into a patient treatment area. Dick, who happened to be wearing sunglasses, reacted quickly. He took up the leash very short and stared straight ahead, pretending that he was blind! It worked. The director never asked where we were going with that dog!

2.2. Mechanistic Studies

In addition to the clinical studies being reported by several physicians, papers began to appear papers dealing with in vitro mechanisms of PDT. Many of these came from the laboratory of Johan Moan at the Norwegian Radium Hospital and represented one of the first attempts to understand the underlying mechanisms of PDT *(14,15)*. David Kessel of Wayne State University (Detroit) began research in PDT at about the same time *(16)*. It was David who first suggested that the "tumor-localizing" component of Hpd was likely a high-molecular-weight material. (He was correct!).

In 1981 Barbara Henderson joined our group. Barbara is among those responsible for converting PDT from an anecdotal clinical technique to a legitimate scientific therapy. Barbara demonstrated conclusively that PDT (at least with Hpd) produces a direct vascular effect and mainly sublethal damage to cells, which ultimately die due to loss of oxygen and nutrients *(17,18)*.

It was becoming increasingly clear that Hpd was a mixture of porphyrins, probably consisting of inactive as well as active material. I had tried unsuccessfully to separate the material on various columns. One day in the summer of 1981, returning from a meeting in California, I was sitting with Kendric Smith (Stanford) in the airport discussing this dilemma and he suggested trying a size exclusion column. (Luckily Hpd is water soluble.)

I had not considered this, but as soon as I got back into the lab I ordered the materials and tried to separate Hpd this way. To my amazement, as soon as I applied the Hpd to the column, it began to separate into two distinct bands—one brown (rapid moving) and one red (slow moving). It was one of those Eureka moments—thanks Kendric! Ultimately we determined that the red band was inactive (consisting of monomers of hematoporphyrin, the vinyl hematoporphyrin derivatives, and protoporphyrin). All the PDT activity resided in the brown band. It was clear that it was a large molecule, likely at least a dimer or larger. (It later turned out to be a mixture of porphyrin oligomers ranging from 2 to 8 *[19]*.) Luckily this provided the basis for a patent (Hpd was not patentable since it had been in the literature for years). The critical importance of a patent is described below.

3. PATENTS, COMPANIES, AND PROTOCOLS

Why was the patent important? We realized that if PDT was ever to become widely available to patients, it had to be approved by the FDA and other health agencies. The only way this could be accomplished was to be able to license Photofrin (the purified active material of Hpd) to a pharmaceutical company capable of spending hundreds of millions of dollars on its development and clinical testing. Without a patent (for exclusivity), no company would touch it. Therefore, granting of the first PDT patent in 1985 was a crucial step in bringing PDT to the general public. This is where Ken Weishaupt (a longtime colleague) of mine and his company (Oncology Research and Development [ORD]) became important. It should be noted that Roswell Park, through its agent (Research Corp.), declined to patent the Photofrin (after looking at it for 11 months—after 12 months patents are no longer granted in the United States). Therefore, Ken, some others, and myself found our own patent attorney and filed the patent, which was eventually issued in 1985. Interestingly, Roswell Park claimed that they were still the rightful owners of the patent since I was employed there. Luckily this turned out well since ORD wanted to work with Roswell Park and gave them the patents, which were then licensed back to ORD. I became a consultant to the company, which eventually had about seven or eight people total.

This fledgling little company (in the beginning Ken was CEO and chief bottle washer) was soon investigated by the FDA. Thus began the "fun." Every time they investigated, we got a long list of "deficiencies." Most involved buying more equipment and hiring more people. The problem with this was that we had no money! We had managed to get a $60,000 loan from a local bank, but that was it. When we tried to skimp at one point they threatened to lock the doors and put Ken in jail! The company provided Hpd (and later the purified Photofrin) to investigators carrying out clinical studies of PDT. At one point there were 25 to 30 investigators both in the United States and abroad. Naturally the income (we charged $10 for shipping) did not come anywhere near the expenses. We had brought in two people with business and fund-raising experience. Some money was raised from the laser companies that kept us alive temporarily.

Shortly thereafter (about 1983), after I presented some of our clinical results at a meeting in Santa Barbara, I was approached by a woman who introduced herself as working on acquisitions for Johnson & Johnson. She was interested in PDT. I suggested that she should talk to our business people, who were attending the meeting. The upshot was that we began a long series of negotiations with Johnson & Johnson to acquire ORD.

(This is where the existence of a functioning company became important, i.e., ORD had gone through the regulatory morass and was able to provide Hpd and later Photofrin to investigators—and there "appeared" to be a market for the drug.) There were numerous meetings over an entire year. Finally, on December 26, 1984, Johnson & Johnson acquired ORD and made an Agreement with Roswell Park. I won't go into details, but the upfront money was modest. A reasonable royalty to Roswell Park was agreed on in the event PDT actually got FDA approval for commercialization (which happened first in 1995, as described later). Royalties were to be shared with the inventors listed on the PDT patents.

When Johnson & Johnson acquired the rights to Photofrin, they set up a lab near Roswell Park to continue Photofrin studies (i.e., testing each batch for activity against a mammary tumor in mice, since this became a release criteria, seeking alternate testing, carrying out pharmacokinetic studies, and so on). They declined to set up at Roswell Park, since they were afraid that the "trade secrets" would leak out too easily—and they were probably right. Ken Weishaupt became lab director. He hired a chemist, Ravi Pandey, PhD, who had been recommended to me by Kevin Smith, whom I considered to be the foremost porphyrin chemist in the United States. He said Ravi was the best chemist he had ever worked with. (Ravi has proved to be outstanding.) He also hired two biologists Dave Bellnier, an excellent biologist and experimentalist (one of my former PhD students who was largely responsible for establishing the pharmacokinetic data on Photofrin, an essential part of the FDA approval process), and Kwan Ho, a PhD in biology from the State University at Buffalo, and two or three lab techs. Since my group at Roswell met regularly with the people at this Johnson & Johnson lab, the question of leaking of proprietary information became moot.

In order to work toward FDA approval for Photofrin, Johnson & Johnson set up a free-standing company headed by an individual who had run one of their large divisions. He was a very capable and considerate person, which was not true of some others we encountered at Johnson & Johnson. The company was called Photofrin Medical (later changed to Photomedica). We were concerned that our people at ORD would lose their jobs after Johnson & Johnson acquired the company. They told us that this would not happen as they did not want to change anything that was already in place and FDA approved (sort of). Within a few weeks, people from Johnson & Johnson visited the ORD facility and declared that it was "not up to their standards." They announced their intention of moving the Photofrin manufacturing to their plant in Raritan, NJ. Of all the ORD personnel (about eight or nine by now), they would keep only Ken Weishaupt.

In the 4 to 5 years that ORD had operated, Photofrin had always passed sterility and pyrogenicity testing (at least 40 to 50 different batches). When Johnson & Johnson manufactured their first batch of the drug, not only did the bottles break when frozen owing to overfilling, the drug failed sterility testing. As did the next, and the next. Our investigators (to whom ORD had been supplying Photofrin) were furious, as they could not obtain the material for their patients. Jim McCaughan went so far as to have one of his patients call the President of Johnson & Johnson and ask why they could not make the drug. Finally, Johnson & Johnson discovered that the room where they were preparing the Photofrin was contaminated. They moved to a different facility and solved the problem. They were, in fact, correct in saying that the ORD facility "was not up to their standards"—ours was clean! The intention was to begin Phase III clinical trials immediately for FDA approval. Two trials were started: bladder (superficial cancer, carcinoma *in situ*) and lung (advanced), since there were published papers indicating the best

On September 12, 1994, I attended this Advisory Board meeting along with Bill Potter (the physicist in our PDT group) and several members of Photomedica. The FDA was considering PDT approval for palliation of obstructive esophageal cancer. It was one of the most excruciating experiences of my life. The meeting began benignly enough with brief presentations from QLT on pharmacology (partly David Bellnier's data) by Julia Levy, who is a founder of QLT and was CEO during most of its critical growth. Then Charles Lightdale, gastroenterologist from Columbia Presbyterian Medical Center and one of the clinical trial investigators, presented the clinical data on PDT vs Nd-YAG laser for palliation of obstructive esophageal cancer. The data basically showed that at 1 wk after treatment, the two modalities were equivalent; however, at 1 month, PDT was superior in maintaining the open lumen and palliating the disease. Also, seven perforations (to the trachea) had resulted from the Nd-YAG laser and only one from the PDT treatment.

Following the presentations, the members of the Advisory Committee asked numerous questions, which went on for hours. Some were just technical—attempting to understand what was presented and the implications. Others were very pointed, indicating (at least so it appeared) a certain skepticism or antagonism on the part of the questioner. One factor that was jumped on by the panel was that the Photofrin formulation was changed in the middle of the trial—from an aqueous-based solution to a freeze-dried solid. The problem was that it appeared there were some differences, especially in increased toxicity associated with the freeze-dried formulation—and QLT could not explain why! (This was a very low point in the proceedings—I was convinced it was all over and Photofrin would not be approved. However, it got worse.)

A well-known medical oncologist who sits on many of the FDA Advisory Committees asked a question something like the following. A patient with an obstructive esophageal cancer comes into his office and he is going to explain PDT for treatment. He is going to tell the patient the following: (1) PDT has a 5% mortality rate; (2) there is a 30% chance you will have a life-threatening toxicity; (3) there is a 52% chance of a severe toxicity; (4) and there is only a 33% chance that you will have a benefit, and in any case it will only last 30 days. (This of course was a setup, since the YAG laser side effects were just as bad and included seven life-threatening complications.) This was really the lowest point in the entire meeting. Here was probably the most influential member of the Advisory panel expressing great skepticism about the safety and usefulness of PDT. The responses from QLT and Dr. Lightdale pointed out that many of the problems he brought up in relation to PDT treatment were, in fact, disease related and that the control arm (Nd-YAG) had most of the same toxicity profile. Finally, there was an open discussion among the Advisory Committee members, who brought up more questions, e.g., is it too toxic? What is the risk-to-benefit ratio? During this discussion one member suggested the risk vs benefit was too high for approval. However, his comments were somewhat countered by other members, who noted that PDT was much easier on the patient and physician than the ND-YAG laser and that some patients did, in fact, benefit from PDT more than from Nd-YAG (those with long tumors, angular tumors, and proximal and distal tumors).

In the end, 11 of 12 members (all except the statistician) voted to approve PDT for treatment of patients with completely or partially obstructing esophageal tumors that in the judgment of the physician cannot be satisfactorily treated by Nd-YAG laser. The last phrase was added because there actually were more toxicities for PDT than for Nd-

YAG—but by the same token there are certain patients (described above) for whom the Nd-YAG is quite dangerous but who can be satisfactorily treated by PDT.

Bill Potter and I were numb when it all ended. Stu Marcus, the Medical Director for Photofrin at Lederle at the time, was seated behind us. He poked me on the shoulder and said "It's okay—they approved it!" My emotions were still bouncing around, and it took me several hours before I realized that the first PDT drug (which came out of our lab and clinic at Roswell Park) had actually just been approved by the FDA—23 years (1995 was the final approval date) after we carried out the first PDT experiments in a tiny lab in the basement of the hospital. Other approvals followed for palliation of obstructive lung cancer, "cure" of early-stage lung cancer, and "cure" of high-grade dysplasia in Barrett's esophagus. Thus, the approval process itself has continued for 9 years and still continues. (Axcan plans to seek approval for treatment of cholangiocarcinoma, an invariably fatal cancer that has responded spectacularly to PDT.)

4. THE TRIP TO CHINA

Early in 1983 I received a call from Joseph Saunders of the Office of International Affairs, National Cancer Institute (NCI), which was involved in travel exchanges for various technical people between the United States and other countries. They offered to send me to China for a few weeks to teach them about PDT techniques. The arrangement was that the United Stateswould be responsible for the travel outside China and the Chinese would cover our expenses within the country. Ken Weishaupt, then President of ORD, agreed to go, as he would be able to supply Hpd or Photofrin to the Chinese if they wanted to get into PDT. (We found out later that the Chinese do not operate that way. They prepared their own Hpd and in addition built their own lasers.) I also wanted a clinician, so Jim McCaughan accompanied us. I don't recall exactly how it happened, but a local TV reporter for CBS (Rich Newberg) got wind of the trip and asked to join us, along with his wife and photographer Mike Mombray and his wife. He thought there might be a good story.

So a few months later, off we went: myself, Ken, Rich Newberg, his wife, Mike Mombray and his wife, and Jim McCaughan and what seemed like tons of equipment— cameras, film, and so on. We first spent a week in Japan, mainly with Hayata and Kato at Tokyo Medical College to film the PDT lung treatment there. Then on to China. We landed in Beijing about 10 p.m. and were met by several gentlemen, none of whom I knew. I was herded into a black limousine with two men in front. All the others were in other cars, and we proceeded to the hotel—the Beijing Hotel, formerly owned and oper-ated by the British. It had seen better days. One could still see traces of former grandeur, but the hotel was now worn down—and dirty! I was put into a large room with bath, and the others had somewhat smaller rooms. I found all the attention rather embarrassing. For breakfast we gathered in a restaurant on the first floor that was large enough for about 1000 people, but only about 20 people were there. Then, on to the hospitals. I gave a PDT lecture that was simultaneously translated into Chinese until the lights went off. Every-one, especially me, welcomed the break.

The hospitals were old and not the cleanest places, many patients were on gurneys in the hallways, and the rooms were lit by single hanging light bulbs. We watched the pharmacists mixing up the various Chinese medicines (herbs, and other substances) individualized for each patient. We also watched a patient being treated by acupuncture—

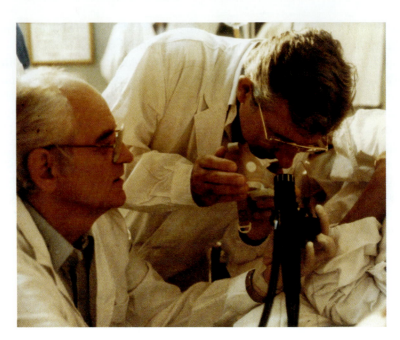

Fig. 1. Beijing, 1983. Dr. James McCaughan (left) of Grant Laser Center, Columbus, Ohio demonstrates to Chinese physicians the art of photodynamic therapy for treatment of esophageal cancer. Dr. Dougherty (right) is at the endoscope.

after the needles were inserted the punk on the other end was lighted. We also saw a high-tech version of acupuncture in which the needles were heated with an HeNe laser. Jim McCaughan wanted to take a picture, but this was not allowed. Jim examined several patients with esophageal cancer (Fig. 1) and described to the physicians how to carry out PDT.

This same routine was repeated in several other cities, e.g., Shanghai and Zhengzhou. At a banquet in Zhengzhou. Jim McCaughan was sitting next to the Mayor. Jim asked him how many children he had. (We had all noted the posters around the cities reminding couples that they were allowed only one child.) The Mayor replied that he had three. Jim being Jim, he asked the mayor why he could have three and the ordinary people only one. At this point I was kicking him under the table. However, the banquet continued without incident. On another occasion we finished early at one of the hospitals and they returned us to the hotel. Since the weather was good we decided to take a walk. As we began to walk we noted a pair of gentlemen on the opposite side of the street who were following us. (We were never left alone while there.) I asked them if they would please leave us alone, and they did—at least we could no longer see them!

While in Beijing, Rich Newberg met with the CBS correspondent. The meeting took place one morning during breakfast in the huge restaurant at the Beijing Hotel. Rich and the correspondent sat in the middle of the room, which was empty. The correspondent explained that they are being constantly spied upon, so he was taking no chances of being overheard. One day Rich returned to his room unexpectedly. When he entered he found six men in suits. They never explained what they were doing there, but it was clear that the room had been searched.

I had been corresponding with Ha Hsien-wen of the Cancer Institute at the Chinese Academy of Medical Sciences in Beijing. He had been using PDT on patients since 1981, primarily for esophageal cancer, which is endemic in Henan Province. He was relying on us to help to advance this program. I had expected to see quite a lot of him during our trip and had thought it curious that he was not among the welcoming party at the airport but thought no more of it. On the first day he did give us a tour of his hospital, but he was very circumspect in what he told us. He spoke perfect English, so that was not the problem. He indicated to me that he was limited in what he could show or tell us. The next day I gave a lecture to a large group of physicians and noted that Dr. Ha was not present, nor was he present at that evening's banquet. In fact, we saw no more of him during the entire trip, and he was not among those seeing us off at the airport. Some of the others indicated to us that he was in trouble with the authorities, although we got no details. We had been informed that among those who were always with us when we moved around was a member of the "party," apparently to keep the others in line.

When we arrived in the hotel in Zhengzhou, where we had gone by train, a necktie was hanging on the door of Jim McCaughan's room that he had left behind in Beijing. We could not figure out how the tie got to the hotel before we did. Apparently they actually did have flights between the cities, although we had been told they didn't. In fact, Mike Mombray's wife became homesick and wanted to return home earlier than planned. We were informed that there were no planes flying, so she could not leave. She had to stick it out to the end.

We were booked to fly from Shanghai to Hong Kong and then home. When we arrived at the airport in Shanghai, it was a mob scene. We could barely get in the door. Luckily our hosts must have had some clout, as they took us and all the extensive accompanying baggage to the front of the line and we were rushed through the boarding process. As we waited to board the plane, Jim McCaughan became convinced that they would not let us out of the country. There was a big sigh of relief when we actually took off (in an old DC-3 that began spewing vapor from the ceiling. We were told not to worry about it, it was just the ventilating system!). We landed a few hours later in Hong Kong—what a contrast! We were met at the airport in a chauffeured Mercedes Benz limousine and taken to a beautiful hotel with flowers and fresh fruit in each room. We dined in the hotel restaurant that evening—superb! (I was especially impressed when we arrived at our table, which I had reserved earlier, to find books of matches engraved with my name.) We had a great few days touring Hong Kong and eating great meals. Then the trip was over— to the relief of several of us.

5. A NEW PHOTOSENSITIZER

By 1995 things seemed to be going well and I was slowly getting back to PDT research at Roswell Park. Then, as now, I was involved not only in science but also in the PDT clinical program. Along with the clinical staff, then as now, I initiated many of the PDT protocols, dealt with our Scientific Review Committee (SRC), our IRB, and the FDA. Up until about 1995 most of the protocols involved Photofrin. In 1995 that changed. Ravi Pandey, the chemist we had originally hired to work in the Johnson & Johnson established lab and now the head of our chemistry group in the PDT Center here at Roswell Park, had synthesized a chlorin, which we called MPH (the methyl ester of pyropheophorbide-a hexyl ether) and which looked like a possible candidate for further development for PDT.

In 1990, after QLT had closed the lab that Johnson & Johnson had established in 1985, both Ravi Pandey and David Bellnier had joined our PDT Center at Roswell Park. Here we further evaluated MPH and discovered a problem. The serum esterases were cleaving the methyl esters and providing a mixture of acids and esters. We therefore decided to remove the esters chemically and deal only with the diacid, now known as HPPH. In our laboratory HPPH "appeared" to be equivalent to Photofrin in efficacy (at 1/15 the dose, since the red absorption at 665 nm was 15 times that of Photofrin at 630 nm). Further, HPPH was not retained in skin past a few days in mice (23,24).

We attempted to interest QLT in HPPH to no avail. No one else was interested either. Therefore, in 1994, just as we had done with Photofrin 21 years earlier (but now the correct way!) we obtained the necessary toxicological, pharmacological, and animal data (from David Bellnier, Barbara Henderson, and Bill Potter), prepared a clinical protocol to use HPPH-PDT to treat skin cancer, and filed for an IND with the FDA for initiation of a human clinical trial. Unfortunately, the FDA had just established a new division for dermatology. Prior to this time all applications for an IND for cancer (including skin cancer) went to the Oncology Division, whose staff was by this time well versed in Photofrin and PDT. Not so for the dermatologists at the FDA. They were not used to injecting a new drug into patients with a non-life-threatening disease. I guess I can't blame them. (Of course, by this time we and others had treated many such patients with Photofrin-PDT.)

At any rate, Allan Oseroff (Chief of Dermatology at Roswell Park) and I spent the next 5 years going back and forth (letters, conference calls, and so on) with the people in the Dermatology Division of the FDA. Seeing the long delay in getting approval for the dermatology study, in 1996 Hector Nava (GI surgeon at Roswell Park) and I put together a PDT-HPPH protocol for treatment of obstructing esophageal cancer, knowing that this IND application would go to the Oncology Division at the FDA. This IND was granted in late 1996, and we began our first clinical study of HPPH. It would be 4 more years before the dermatology IND would be granted. (You have to be persistent)!

When we treated the very first patient with HPPH (a woman with a long history of esophageal cancer), we told her that she could have Photofrin-PDT (an approved indication), but she wanted to take a vacation in the Caribbean and did not want to be photosensitive. Of course, we also had to inform her that we did not know for sure that HPPH would work for her as the protocol called for drug escalation starting at the lowest dose. Nonetheless, she opted for HPPH. It's always a bit unnerving to inject a brand new drug into a human for the first time, no matter what the animal toxicity studies told us (essentially nontoxic at doses considerably greater than those planned in our human protocols). The reaction of the tumor to the light treatment which was delivered 48 hours after injection, was excellent, to say the least. Although we had designed a dose escalation study and were starting at the lowest dose, we subsequently amended the protocol to a dose de-escalation study. Also, we had designed in our studies a test of cutaneous photosensitivity using a solar simulator and found that in this patient and all subsequent patients (about 80 as of this writing) usually no reaction was elicited past about 5 days, even at the highest dose of HPPH used (about 0.15 mg/kg). This has subsequently been verified in patients, most of whom have gone into sunlight at 5 to 7 days post injection without a problem. One patient did complain of a sunburn 3 weeks post injection, but he had spent several hours in the sun flying a model airplane, so we were not sure we could blame it on HPPH. Another had a slight sunburn at about 10 days post injection.

As previously noted, we had tried to interest QLT in licensing HPPH. After lengthy discussions with the company, they decided not to pursue a license. This was frustrating, since we were convinced that HPPH had very similar efficacy to Photofrin—but without the long-term cutaneous photosensitivity. Currently (2005) we are negotiating with another company to license HPPH, but as of this writing that agreement has run into a snag. (So, what else is new?) We have consistently found that negotiations for licensing Photofrin or HPPH take the better part of a year to come to fruition. This was true with the Johnson & Johnson, QLT (when QLT/Lederle picked up the Photofrin license agreement from Johnson & Johnson, they insisted on renegotiating and changing a substantial portion of the terms), and with Light Sciences Corporation (with whom we had only a short relationship). We are now going on 6 months and counting with the current HPPH negotiations. This is always a stressful situation. It seems each side sets out conditions that the other side views as unreasonable, often because of a misunderstanding between the parties. However, to get FDA approval such arrangements are generally necessary.

Currently it looks like HPPH will be licensed for development initially in Asia. We'll see how that goes. At least the beat goes on, albeit requiring a little life support from time to time.

REFERENCES

1. Henderson BW, Gollnick SO. Mechanistic principles of photodynamic therapy, in CRC Handbook of Organic Photochemistry and Photobiology (Horspool W, Lenci F, eds.), Boca Raton, FL: CRC Press, 2003:145-1–145-25.
2. Dougherty TJ, Gomer CJ, Henderson BW, et al. Photodynamic therapy. J Natl Cancer Inst 1998;90:889–905.
3. Raab O. Ueber die Wirkung fluoreszierender Stoffe auf Infusorien. Z Biol (Munich) 1900;39: 524–546.
4. Dougherty TJ. Activated dyes as anti-tumor agents. J Natl Cancer Inst 1974;51:1333–1336.
5. Dougherty TJ, Grindey GB, Fiel R, Weishaupt KR, Boyle DG. Photoradiation therapy. II. Cure of animal tumors with hematoporphyrin and light. J Natl Cancer Inst 1975;55:115–121.
6. Dougherty TJ, Kaufman JE, Goldfarb A, Weishaupt KR, Boyle D, Mittelman A. Photoradiation therapy for the treatment of malignant tumors. Cancer Res 1978;38:2628–2635.
7. Kelly JF, Snell ME. Hematoporphyrin derivative: a possible aid in the diagnosis and therapy of carcinoma of the bladder. J Urol 1976;115:150–151.
8. Lipson RL, Baldes EJ, Olsen AM. Hematoporphyrin derivative: a new aid for endoscopic detection of malignant disease. J Thorac Cardiovasc Surg 1962:623–629.
9. Lipson RL, Gray MJ, Baldes EJ. Hematoporphyrin derivative for detection and management of cancer, in Proceedings of the 9th International Cancer Congress, 1966.
10. Dougherty TJ, Lawrence G, Kaufman JH, Boyle D, Weishaupt KR, Goldfarb A. Photoradiation in the treatment of recurrent breast carcinoma. J Natl Cancer Inst 1979;62:231–237.
11. Hayata Y, Kato H, Konaka C, Ono J, Takizawa N. Hematoporphyrin derivative and laser photoradiation in the treatment of lung cancer. Chest 1982;81:269–277.
12. McCaughan JS. Overview of experiences with photodynamic therapy for malignancy in 192 patients. Photochem Photobiol 1987;46:903–909.
13. Thoma RE, Stein RM, Weishaupt KR, Dougherty TJ. Phototherapy: a promising cancer therapy. Vet Med/Small Anim Clinician 1989;33:1693–1699.
14. Christensen T, Moan J, Wibe E, Oftebro R. Photodynamic effect of haematoporphyrin throughout the cell cycle of the human cell line NHIK 3025 cultivated in vitro. Br J Cancer 1979;39:64–68.
15. Moan J, Pettersen EO, Christensen T. The mechanism of photodynamic inactivation of human cells in vitro in the presence of haematoporphyrin. Br J Cancer 1979:398–407.
16. Kessel D. Components of hematoporphyrin derivatives and their tumor-localizing capacity. Cancer Res 1982;42:1703–1706.

17. Henderson BW. The significance of vascular photosensitization in photodynamic therapy. Future Dir Applic Photodyn Ther 1990;156:153–166.
18. Henderson BW, Farrell G. Possible implications of vascular damage for tumor cell inactivation in *vivo*: comparison of different photosensitizers, in Photodynamic Therapy: Mechanisms (Dougherty TJ, ed.), Bellingham, WA: SPIE—The International Society for Optical Engineering, 1989:2–10.
19. Siegel MM, Tabei K, Tsao R, et al. Comparative mass spectrometric analyses of Photofrin oligomers by fast atom bombardment mass spectrometry, UV and IR matrix-assisted laser desorption/ionization mass spectrometry, electrospray ionization mass spectrometry and laser desorption/jet-cooling photoionization mass spectrometry. J Mass Spectrom 1999;34:661–669.
20. Lam S, Haussinger K, Leroy M, Sutedja T, Huber R. Photodynamic therapy (PDT) with Photofrin®, a treatment with curative potential for early stage superficial lung cancer. Proceedings of the 34th Annual Meeting of the American Society of Clinical Oncology, 1998.
21. Balchum OJ, Doiron DR. Photoradiation therapy of endobronchial lung cancer. Large obstructing tumors, nonobstructing tumors, and early-stage bronchial cancer lesions. Clin Chest Med 1985;6:255–275.
22. Balchum OJ, Doiron DR, Huth GC. HpD photodynamic therapy for obstructing lung cancer. Prog Clin Biol Res 1984;170:727–745.
23. Bellnier DA, Greco WR, Loewen GM, et al. Population pharmacokinetics of the photodynamic therapy agent 2-[-1-hexyloxyethyl]-2-devinyl pyropheophorbide-a in cancer patients. Cancer Res 2003;63:1806–1813.
24. Bellnier DA, Greco WR, Nava H, Loewen GM, Oseroff AR, Dougherty TJ. Mild skin photosensitivity in cancer patients following injection of Photochlor (2–1-[1-hexyloxyethyl]-2-devinylpyropheophorbide-a) for photodynamic therapy. Cancer Chemother Pharmacol 2006;57:40–45.

10   Ultrasound-Guided Therapy

Robert F. Wong, MD, Amanjit S. Gill, MD, and Manoop S. Bhutani, MD

CONTENTS

SUMMARY

Utilizing-high frequency sound waves to define internal structures, ultrasound (US) provides an opportunity not only to diagnose disease but also to target treatment to malignant tumors. US has several advantages over other radiology-assisted techniques that highlight its important role as a component of anticancer therapy. US provides an opportunity to administer therapy with real-time guidance. In other words, the physician can deliver treatment while synchronously visualizing the US images to ensure proper targeting.

By placing US transducers within gastrointestinal (GI) lumens, periluminal structures can be readily visualized with US. The concept has led to the development of rigid US probes that can provide high-quality images of perirectal organs, such as the prostate, and, in recent years, endoscopic ultrasound (EUS). The creation of these US-endoscopy hybrids permits placement of high-frequency US probes in close proximity to structures that can be difficult to image with percutaneous US. EUS is not only limited to abdominal viscera, but can also image thoracic organs as well and therefore provides the endoscopist with minimally invasive access to evaluate and potentially treat abdominal and thoracic malignancies. This chapter will discuss US-based delivery of regional cancer therapy, introducing the reader to the methods and requirements for successful treatment. Examples of therapy will be provided; however, an in-depth discussion of indications and results for specific cancers will be reserved for chapters focusing on specific regional therapies.

Key Words: Endoscopic ultrasound; ultrasound; cancer; therapy; endosonography.

From: *Cancer Drug Discovery and Development: Regional Cancer Therapy*
Edited by: P. M. Schlag and U. S. Stein © Humana Press Inc., Totowa, NJ

1. INTRODUCTION

Utilizing high-frequency sound waves to define internal structures, ultrasound (US) provides an opportunity not only to diagnose disease but also to target treatment to malignant tumors. US has several advantages over other radiology-assisted techniques that highlight its important role as a component of anticancer therapy. First, US avoids radiation exposure, distinguishing US from other modalities, such as fluoroscopy and computed tomography (CT). Radiation exposure becomes more significant when one considers the often multiple sessions necessary for effective therapy. Second, US is relatively inexpensive, portable, and commonly available. Third, US provides an opportunity to administer therapy with real-time guidance. In other words, the physician can deliver treatment while synchronously visualizing the US images to ensure proper targeting.

A disadvantage of US-guided therapy is the potential limited accessibility to different organs and structures. Because US relies on the transmission of sound energy through an acoustic medium, several structures, like bone and air-filled organs, are not penetrable with US. An air-filled lumen (such as the small intestine) or a bony structure that lies between the US transducer and the potential target often preclude US-guided therapy. This is important for several abdominal organs, like the retroperitoneal pancreas, that can lie underneath loops of small bowel or colon. Furthermore, depth of penetration and resolution share an inverse relationship that limits access to organs distant from the US transducer. Therefore, higher frequency (shorter wavelength) US waves provide better resolution of structures near the transducer at the expense of penetration depth *(1)*. Thus percutaneous US has been used as a delivery method for anticancer therapy, but mostly for tumors of superficial organs, such as the liver.

This major limitation of US has been addressed through the clever use of techniques to use US transducers to reach organs residing in deeper compartments of body cavities. By placing US transducers within gastrointestinal (GI) lumens, periluminal structures can be readily visualized with US. The concept has led to the development of rigid US probes that can provide high-quality images of perirectal organs, such as the prostate, and, in recent years, endoscopic ultrasound (EUS). The creation of these US-endoscopy hybrids has permitted placement of high-frequency US probes in close proximity to structures that can be difficult to image with percutaneous US. Based on the position of the transducer within the GI lumen, EUS provides high-resolution, real-time images of important organs, including the pancreas, lymph nodes, and major vascular structures. EUS is not limited to abdominal viscera but can also be used for thoracic organs and therefore allows the endoscopist (with minimally invasive access) to evaluate and potentially treat abdominal and thoracic malignancies.

This chapter discusses US-based delivery of regional cancer therapy, introducing the reader to the methods and requirements for successful treatment. Examples of therapy will be provided; however, an in-depth discussion of indications and results for specific cancers will be found in chapters focusing on specific regional therapies.

2. PERCUTANEOUS ULTRASOUND-GUIDED THERAPY

2.1. Introduction

Percutaneous US-guided therapy has been a natural evolution from the ability to target tumors with needles for tissue diagnosis. This division of interventional oncology has

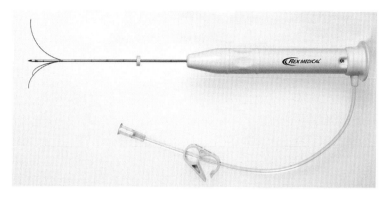

Fig. 1. Tip of the Quadra-Fuse* (Rex Medical) needle showing dispersion of injected material, with four holes along the distal aspect of each of the three deployable tines. .

exploded for many reasons. A large majority of the tumors treated percutaneously are unresectable, conventional surgical procedures are associated with considerable morbidity and mortality, and systemic chemotherapy has been largely ineffective.

A team approach to treatment planning is in the patient's best interest and should involve active consultation by a team consisting of a hepatologist, oncologist, surgeon, and interventional radiologist.

2.2. Techniques

Multiple techniques are now available for local tumor ablation; they can be subdivided into chemical and thermal techniques.

2.2.1. CHEMICAL ABLATION

Percutaneous chemical ablation is the most established local therapy; it acts by causing protein denaturation and small vessel thrombosis *(2,3)*. It has the advantage of being readily available, inexpensive, and rapid. Various agents used for this purpose include ethanol, acetic acid, and hot saline.

2.2.1.1. Ethanol. Percutaneous ethanol ablation (PEI) is most effective for single small hepatocellular carcinomas (HCCs) and has been shown to have an equivalent survival to surgery, with a 3-yr survival of 79% for resection and 71% for PEI *(4,5)*. PEI can be used to treat 3 or fewer lesions smaller than 3 cm in size. PEI is, however, relatively ineffective in the treatment of hepatic metastases *(6)*.

Different needles used to optimize diffusion of ethanol through the lesion are available. Examples are a multiside hole conical tip needle (Bernardino, Cook, Bloomington, IN), with good tip echogenicity and linear tracking, and Quadra-Fuse (Medical Device Technologies, Gainesville, FL), a multipronged injection needle (Figs. 1 and 2).

The volume of ethanol required to treat a tumor is calculated by the formula $(4/3)\pi$ $(d/2 + 0.5)^3$, where d is the average tumor diameter. Aliquots of 0.2 to 0.4 mL of absolute ethanol are injected into the tumor, with a total of 5 to 10 mL per session. The treatment is performed in multiple sessions, up to two to three times per week.

Ethanol injection is fairly safe, with an incidence of major complications ranging from 1.3 to 13.4% *(7–9)*. Hemorrhagic complications such as a self-limiting hemoperitoneum (less than 5% of patients) and subcapsular and parietal hematomas may be seen. Other

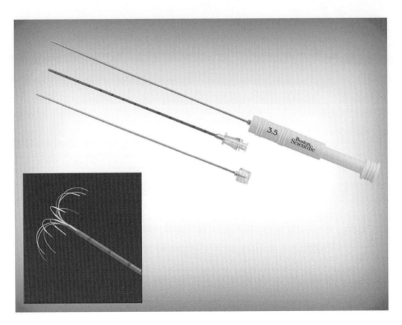

Fig. 2. A view of the entire Quadra-Fuse* needle.Quadra-Fuse* is a trademark of Rex Medical. Distributed by Inter•V®.

complications include vessel thrombosis, biloma formation, hemobilia, acute cholangitis, hepatic infarction, tumor seeding, liver abscess, and pleural complications such as pneumothorax and pleural effusion.

It is postulated that central ablation by PEI or radiofrequency ablation can have a synergistic effect with peripheral tumor therapy by chemoembolization. Devascularization by PEI may also facilitate thermal ablation, by reducing the heat sink effect, a phenomenon described in detail later.

2.2.1.2. Acetic Acid. Acetic acid has better diffusion characteristics than ethanol; it can diffuse through tumor septae, and this translates into a larger coagulation area and thus fewer treatment sessions. Maximum therapeutic effect is achieved at 50% concentration (approx 8 mol/L).

It is associated with the same risks and complications as ethanol, with isolated cases of liver capsule perforation and renal failure reported *(10,11)*.

Not enough literature is available at present to prove superiority of acetic acid over ethanol or a similar safety profile, in the clinical setting.

2.2.2. THERMAL ABLATION

Thermal ablation includes techniques that rely on temperature modification, either heat or cold, to achieve ablation.

2.2.2.1. Radiofrequency. Radiofrequency ablation (RFA) has found application in a wide variety of disease processes and organs. Tumors of the liver, kidney, lung, bone, adrenal gland, and breast have been ablated with this technology. It has also been used for neurolysis, for different pain syndromes. RFA produces 90% necrosis in HCCs measuring less than 3 cm in diameter, in comparison with 80% by PEI, but it is less successful in larger tumors *(12,13)*. Larger HCCs, up to 5 cm (especially if encapsulated)

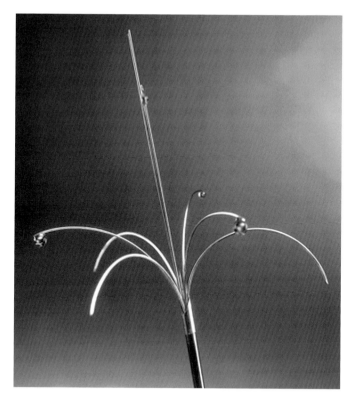

Fig. 3. Coaxial multitined expandable electrode (LeVeen, Boston Scientific) with insulated coaxial needle (in blue). Note the deployed tines (in inset), which are contained within the needle marked 3.5, and deployed once the tip of the needle is within the lesion.

or metastases up to 3 to 4 cm can be treated. Contraindications to performing the procedure include uncorrectable coagulopathy, Child's class C liver disease, central location, and proximity to bowel. However, the latter two are relative, and procedural modifications can be employed to perform the procedure safely in this subset of patients.

Most current systems available are monopolar in design, with a single active electrode, and they depend on a grounding pad to complete the circuit. Newer bipolar systems are now available, with two active electrodes in proximity; coagulation is created between the electrodes, eliminating the need for grounding pads. The electrodes are available in multitined expandable, internally cooled, and perfusion forms. The multitined expandable electrode consists of a cannula with contained deployable tines, of varying geometries, depending on the manufacturer (Fig. 3). The corresponding ablation zone varies according to the geometry and should be a consideration during planning. All multitined electrodes can be deployed partially to create a smaller ablation zone.

The internally cooled electrodes use a perfusate (water or saline) through an internal lumen, which thus has no contact with the tissue. A high temperature around the electrode may cause charring, with resultant high impedance to current, and a limited zone of ablation. The perfusate helps prevent charring around the electrode by reducing the temperature and thus promotes greater conduction of heat into the surrounding tissue and

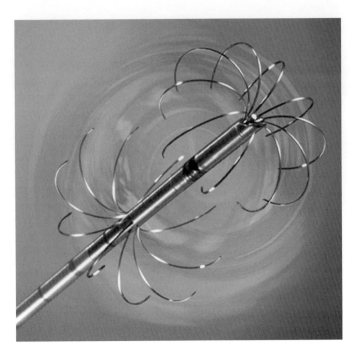

Fig. 4. A view of the tip of the Xli enhanced needle (RITA) with perfusion electrodes showing saline droplets at their tips.

a larger ablation zone. The internally cooled electrodes can either be single or a cluster of three or more, spaced less than 1 cm apart.

Perfusion electrodes (Fig. 4) have an aperture at the active tip to infuse sterile normal or hypertonic saline into the tissues. The three major manufacturers in the United States are RITA Medical Systems (Fremont, CA), Boston Scientific/Radiotherapeutics (Natick, MA), and Radionics/Valleylab (Boulder, CO).

RITA Medical Systems supplies monopolar multitined expandable electrodes with or without perfusion in sizes ranging from 16.5 to 13 gage, with an ability to create ablation zones up to 7 cm. The tines deploy in a Christmas-tree-like configuration, creating a teardrop-shaped ablation zone. Electrodes are also available in semiflexible and flexible designs to facilitate use in the CT and magnetic resonance imaging (MRI) gantry. MRI-compatible probes are available. Thermocouples on the electrodes provide real-time temperature feedback during the ablation. The generator operates at 460 kHz at a maximum power output of 250 W.

The Boston Scientific/Radiotherapeutics generator has an impedance-based feedback system and generates a maximum power of 200 W. Their monopolar electrodes are available in diameters of 2 to 5 cm, are 14 to 17 gage, have umbrella-like tines, and thus create a disc-shaped ablation zone. A new bipolar dual-umbrella electrode (Figs. 5 and 6) has been introduced capable of producing an ablation zone of 4 by 5.5 cm.

Radionics/Valleylab manufactures a 200-W generator, with an impedance-based feedback, and a 17-gage straight internally cooled electrode, capable of creating a 4- to 5-cm oval area of ablation.

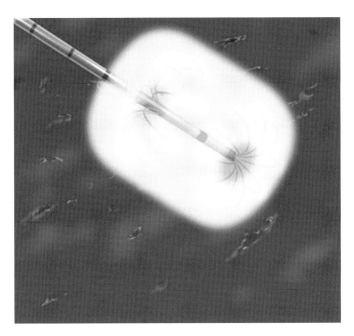

Fig. 5. The new bipolar electrode (Concerto, Boston Scientific) with a dual-umbrella configuration.

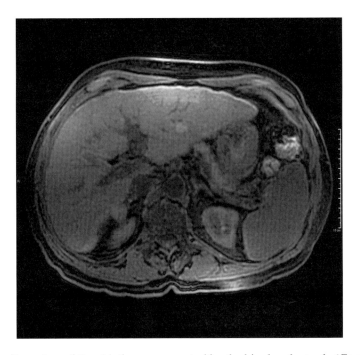

Fig. 6. The configuration of the ablation zone created by the bipolar electrode (Concerto, Boston Scientific).

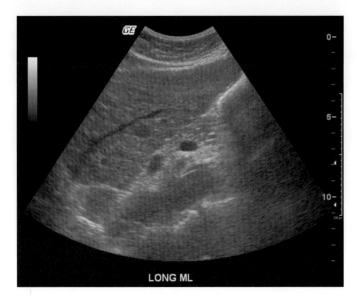

Fig. 7. MR image of a 72-yr-old man with hepatitis B and a biopsy-proven 1 cm hepatocellular carcinoma in segment II (left lobe of the liver).

In its monopolar multitined expandable form, the radiofrequency procedure uses a 14.5 to 17.5 G electrode, with an insulated shaft and a noninsulated deployable tip. Grounding pads are placed on the back or the thighs to complete the electrical circuit. Alternating current in the radiofrequency (RF) wave range (375–500 kHz) is applied to the electrode by an RF generator *(14)*. The passage of alternating electrical current through the electrode causes ionic agitation in the surrounding tissues with frictional heating. At temperatures above 60°C, cell proteins denature and coagulate, causing cell death by coagulation necrosis.

The preprocedure evaluation consists of an adequate mix of imaging, such as US, biphasic CT, MR (Figs. 7 and 8), positron emission tomography (PET), and chest X-ray, to delineate the extent of local disease and to rule out distant metastatic disease. Laboratory investigations that must be obtained include prothrombin time, partial thromboplastin time, chemistry screen, liver function tests, tumor markers (α-fetoprotein, carcinoembryonic antigen), complete blood count, hepatitis panel, electrocardiogram, and type and cross-match of packed RBCs.

Administration of preprocedure antibiotics is controversial, and the practice varies among institutions. A combination of ampicillin and gentamicin, or ciprofloxacin and metronidazole, can be administered before and for a week after the procedure. Patients with large or central liver lesions or those with ascites may benefit, as may those with renal tumors in contact with the collecting system. There is an increased risk for liver abscess formation in patients after hepatic artery embolization, biliary enteric anastomosis, sphincterotomy, or with focal biliary dilatation.

The patient is instructed to stop intake of solids 8 h before the procedure, and can ingest clear liquids up to 2 h before. Aggressive pre- and postprocedure hydration is believed to prevent renal toxicity or the development of acute tubular necrosis (related to tumor lysis) and to decrease the severity of the postembolization syndrome.

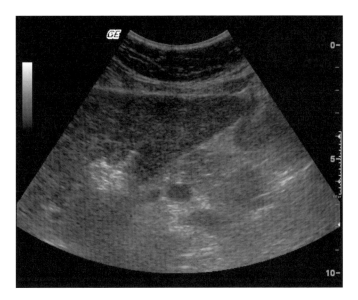

Fig. 8. Longitudinal ultrasound of the left lobe of the liver during the radiofrequency ablation procedure of the hepatocellular carcinoma of the patient in Fig. 7.

The procedure can be performed with local anesthesia and conscious sedation (midazolam and fentanyl). However, deep sedation (propofol, remifentanyl) or general anesthesia may be required for capsular, diaphragmatic, or large liver tumors, or with a history of prior surgery, owing to the greater amount of pain in these settings. It is prudent to bolus sedation prior to applying current, and the grounding pads should be removed before the sedation wears off.

The RF generator and the US machine should be attached to different electrical circuits to avoid artifacts during imaging.

In addition to US, imaging guidance with CT or MRI might be required in some cases. MRI has the potential to provide feedback about extent of ablation by the technique of thermography. US contrast agents are being used with varying degrees of success, to assess the early therapeutic effect of ablation on HCC.

The needle is advanced into the distal portion of the lesion under imaging guidance. During ablation, an echogenic area (Fig. 9) is seen around the active electrode and is thought to represent microbubbles owing to vaporization. This echogenic area has a poor correlation with actual lesion size on histology *(15)*, and images obtained 2 to 5 min after ablation (Fig. 10) may be more accurate at assessing the ablated volume. However, operators should depend more on the knowledge of actual needle placements in relation to the tumor for complete coverage. Ablation of a margin of 5 to 10 mm of normal parenchyma around the tumor is desired.

A single zone of ablation is created in 10 to 30 min. Multiple overlapping spheres will need to be created to cover a lesion larger than the size of the electrode. The needle tract should be cauterized (Fig. 11) with a lower energy setting during withdrawal of the electrode to prevent bleeding or tumor seeding (Fig. 12).

A *heat sink effect* has been well described; it is caused by the cooling effect of blood flow in major vessels, limiting coagulation necrosis in their vicinity. Strategies to limit

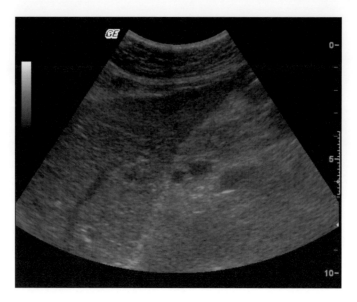

Fig. 9. During radiofrequency ablation of the lesion in Figs. 7 and 8. Note the intense echogenicity within the lesion, and some along the path of the needle.

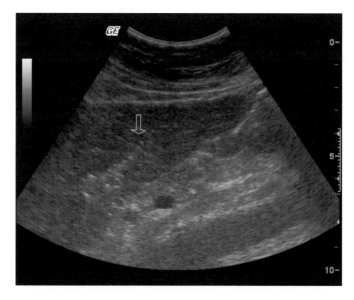

Fig. 10. Note the clearing of the echogenicity from the treated area, revealing the actual zone of ablation, seen as a hypoechoic area with some surrounding echogenicity.

the heat sink effect include pharmacological reduction of blood flow *(16)*, temporary balloon occlusion of a combination of the hepatic artery, the hepatic vein, and/or the portal vein *(17)*, intra-arterial embolization or chemoembolization *(18–20)*, or the Pringle maneuver (temporary occlusion of the hepatic artery and portal vein at the hepatic hilum) *(21,22)*. A beneficial *oven effect* has also been described, whereby the cirrhotic liver acts as a thermal insulator, potentiating and limiting the ablation to the tumor *(12)*.

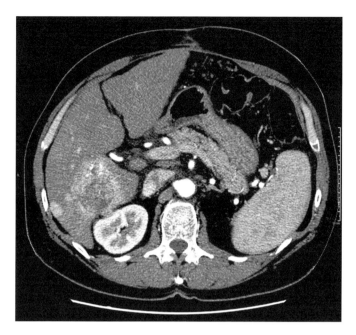

Fig. 11. Echogenicity along the needle track (solid arrow) represents cauterization of the needle tract during needle removal, to prevent hemorrhage, and tract seeding.

Tumors in certain locations require special consideration and techniques. A safety margin may not be possible in subcapsular tumors, and the capsule should be ablated if it is involved by the tumor. Subcapsular tumors located between the anterior and posterior capsule along the inferior edge of the liver can be approached with a straight internally cooled electrode, avoiding the risk of capsule perforation by one of the tines of the multitined electrode. The deeper portion of an exophytic subcapsular tumor should be ablated first, to decrease the blood supply to the more superficial portion. Alternatively, PEIn can be performed.

Central lesions, in close vicinity to large vessels, are difficult to ablate and require special techniques, as described in the above paragraph on the heat sink effect. When with expandable multitined electrode is used, the procedure can be performed with partial deployment of the array, with multiple overlapping ablations. The straight internally cooled electrode has the advantage of a lesser risk of blood vessel penetration and the potential creation of a large ablation zone, owing to reduced charring around the electrode. Alternatively, ablation can be performed during laparotomy or laparoscopy, with the Pringle maneuver, which can be safely applied to the normal liver for 1 h. (The safe duration for a cirrhotic liver is unknown.) These procedures do carry a higher risk of penetration of a large vessel with the electrode (causing bleeding, pseudoaneurysm formation, or damage to the biliary structures) and should be approached with caution.

The complication rate is low, with major complications seen in less than 2% and minor complications in up to 8% *(23)*. Abscess formation after ablation is difficult to differentiate from postablation changes by imaging. They must be treated aggressively by percutaneous drainage. Blockage of the biliary ducts secondary to the procedure should also

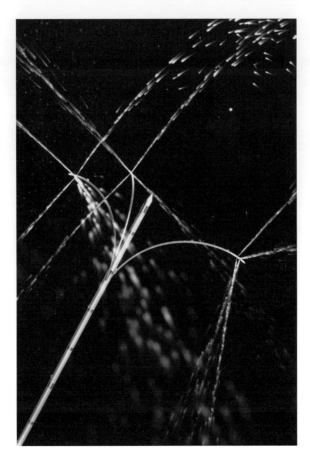

Fig. 12. An example of tumor seeding along the needle track. Note the small, well-defined hyperdense lesion in a subcapsular location, along the known needle track used to ablate the adjacent large lesion in the inferior aspect of the right lobe of the liver. The right lobe lesion itself has residual disease represented by the irregular enhancement around the well-defined hypodense central lesion.

be treated adequately by drainage. Pleural effusion or hemorrhage into the pleural or peritoneal cavities may occur *(12)*.

The major avoidable complication is injury to adjacent vital structures, and many strategies have been suggested, including injection of carbon dioxide and D5 to create thermal insulation barriers. The use of saline is not recommended, as it conducts thermal energy, owing to the presence of ions.

Ketorolac tromethamine is effective for postprocedure pain control but should be limited to one to two doses to avoid renal toxicity. A low-grade fever and a mild post-RFA pain are to be expected after the procedure. However, this is typically much less severe than the postembolization or tumor lysis syndrome. Any fever above 101°F must be investigated and treated. Depending on the complexity or extent of the procedure, the patient can be discharged on the same day or observed overnight.

The patient should be provided with detailed discharge instructions including a 24-h contact number. Warning signs include a fever above 101°F; no urine output for 4 h;

dizziness; difficulty breathing or chest pain; bleeding, swelling, redness, discharge, or tenderness at the probe insertion site; vomiting or coughing blood; or chills and back pain, with cloudy or foul-smelling urine.

Follow-up imaging for assessment of treatment response includes dynamic MRI, mutlislice CT, or PET. Postprocedure CT and MRI findings have a good correlation (within 2 mm) to the actual ablated zone by histology *(24,25)*. US, using microbubble contrast agents, has a sensitivity of only 50%, with a specificity of 100% *(26)*. Further improvements in US imaging and contrast agents are necessary before it can be considered a reliable follow-up imaging modality.

Same-day imaging can be performed to look for complications and to evaluate treatment. Thereafter, imaging can be performed at variable intervals, depending on many factors, including the size, histology, and expected rate of growth of the lesion, and confidence in adequate treatment. Early postprocedure imaging seeks to differentiate between the inflammatory granulation rind and residual or recurrent tumor. Benign periablational enhancement, consisting of reactive hyperemia, followed in time by fibrosis and giant cell reaction, can be seen for up to 6 mo, and is concentric, with smooth inner margins, usually 1 to 2 mm in thickness (up to 5 mm). Irregular peripheral enhancement in a scattered, nodular, eccentric pattern, in the portal venous or delayed (3 min) phases, is suggestive of residual tumor (Fig. 12). Failures of treatment are discernible within 3 to 6 mo.

The zone of ablation (tumor necrosis) is marked in vascular organs such as the liver and kidney by areas of low attenuation and absent perfusion (complete lack of enhancement during both the arterial and portal venous phases) in the parenchyma *(27–33)*. In the low-density surrounding tissues such as perinephric fat *(34,35)*, and in the lung *(36)*, the zone of ablation is marked by increased attenuation. The natural course of the ablated lesion is slow involution of coagulation, with a variable residual scar, lasting from months to years.

On MRI, treated lesions are hypointense on all sequences, with a hyperintense rim. The best tumor-to-treated thermal lesion contrast is brought out by T2-weighted sequences *(37,38)*.

Similar results to PEI have been achieved with RFA for HCC, with higher necrosis rates, fewer sessions (1.2 vs 4.8), and similar complication rates *(23)*. It is also safer compared with cryotherapy, when both are performed percutaneously. Complete local response can be expected in 70 to 75% of tumors between 3 and 5 cm, but response falls precipitously to 25% when lesion size exceeds 5 cm. With successful ablation, 5-yr survival rates of 40 to 50% are achieved, with new intrahepatic and extrahepatic disease seen in 25 to 50% of patients *(39,40)*.

RFA can be combined with PEI and chemoembolization to increase efficacy, albeit with a greater risk for complications. RFA has many other applications including management of arrythmias and ablation of nerve ganglia for treatment of trigeminal neuralgia, celiac ganglion pain, cluster headaches, chronic segmental thoracic pain, cervicobrachialgia, and plantar fascitis.

2.2.2.2. Microwave. Microwave ablation is a hyperthermic technique; like REI, it relies on the conversion of energy to heat, thus destroying tumors. Microwave needles can produce lesions of 3 to 6 cm in diameter, with larger lesions being created by using multiple needles and by selectively blocking the blood flow to the liver *(41,42)*. The lesions become hypoechoic on US immediately following treatment, providing an accurate and early assessment of the zone of ablation *(43)*. It provides a more uniform heating and shape, and is less dependent on thermal conduction than RFA. It is also questionably less prone to the heat sink effect and is faster than RFA, producing a lesion within 3 min. Complication rates of 14% for HCC and 20% for metastases have been reported following microwave ablation *(44)*. The local recurrence rate following microwave ablation varies from 0 to 10% *(45–47)*

2.2.2.3. Cryoablation. The principle of cryoablation is destruction of tumor by means of ice crystal formation *(48)*. Patients with a limited hepatic reserve and four or fewer lesions in different lobes are candidates for this procedure. Cryoablation has more commonly been performed at open surgery, with percutaneous ablation becoming more feasible, owing to the availability of smaller probe sizes (13–14 gage).

A vacuumiinsulated cryoprobe is placed into the tumor by US guidance, with large tumors requiring placement of multiple probes. The probe is anchored in place by rapidly lowering its temperature to –100°C *(49)*. Treatment is then begun by circulating liquid nitrogen at –196°C through the cryoprobe for one to three cycles lasting 15 minu each. Lethal temperatures of –20°C are achieved within the treated tissue. The probe is withdrawn, with Gelfoam embolization of the track *(50)*. The anterior margin of the ice ball is visualized on US as an area of increased echogenicity, with posterior acoustic shadowing. On MRI, the ice ball appears as a sharply marginated teardrop or ellipsoid area of signal void on all sequences *(51)*. Lesions near the portal vein or other major blood vessels can be treated (when a surgical margin may not be possible), as an ice ball can even form immediately adjacent to the portal vein, with very little risk of thrombosis.

Cryoablation, when compared with RFA, has a more marked inflammatory response, greater blood loss, and more complications; it is technically difficult owing to the larger probe size. The complications include hemorrhage, abscess formation, pleural effusion, splitting of the liver capsule, platelet consumption, small vessel ischemia, biliary strictures or perforation, myoglobinuria, and arteriovenous malformation formation *(52)*. The treated tissue appears on postprocedure CT as a low-density area mimicking an infarct or an abscess *(53)*, and as a signal void on MRI. Cryoablation appears to have similar recurrence rates as RFA for tumors less than 3 cm, and superior to RFA for large (>3 cm) liver lesions, with one study revealing a 38% recurrence rate for RFA-treated patients compared with 17% for cryoablation-treated patients *(54)*. A review article noted a survival rate of 46 to 89% for primary and secondary tumors, with a follow-up of 20 mo or more *(49)*.

2.3. Clinical Applications

This section provides pertinent details specific to the different tumors that can be treated with the modalities described earlier.

2.3.1. LIVER TUMORS

2.3.1.1. Primary. Approximately 90% of liver tumors are unresectable owing to underlying poor liver function or tumor multifocality *(55)*.

When the tumors are resectable, large series of surgical treatment of HCC report 3- and 5-yr survival rates of 38 to 65% and 33 to 44%, respectively *(56–60)*. This has to be balanced against the major morbidity and mortality of a major hepatic resection. Recurrence is common, even with a curative resection. Liver transplantation is a viable option for an unresectable small tumor burden (single tumor less than 5 cm, or three tumors less than 3 cm), with an 83% recurrence-free 4-yr survival rate, and a 6% perioperative mortality *(61)*.

The histological structure of primary liver tumors allows ethanol and the RFA-generated heat to be well distributed within the tumor, owing to the surrounding cirrhotic tumor, especially if the tumor is encapsulated. This is in contrast to the secondary tumors, as described next.

2.3.1.2. Secondary. Two-thirds of patients with colorectal cancer (CRC) have liver metastases by the time of their death *(62)*. Survival depends on the number and extent of the metastases, with a median survival of 4.5 to 15 mo.

Only 5 to 10% of all patients with CRC metastases are deemed suitable for resection, with a survival improvement of 16 to 40% after resection, a 2.6 to 4.5% operative mortality, and a perioperative morbidity of 7 to 16% *(6,63,64)*.

Metastases are more infiltrative than in HCC, and they are surrounded by normal liver; thus they are less well treated with PEI and RFA.

2.3.2. KIDNEY TUMORS

Candidates for local therapy include patients with small renal masses who are not surgical candidates, patients with recurrent malignancy, and patients with the potential for the development of multiple tumors such as von Hippel-Lindau syndrome and hereditary renal cell carcinoma (RCC). In the latter two, it is not necessary to obtain an ablative margin of 5–10 mm; it is more essential to try to preserve as much parenchyma as possible.

The ideal tumor for treatment is a small, exophytic tumor. However, selected larger or central tumors can be treated, keeping the heat sink effect in mind, as well as the greater propensity for complications. Encapsulated RCCs will benefit from the oven effect. Complications include hemorrhage, urinoma, abscess, paresthesias, transient hematuria, pain, ureteral stricture, and fistula formation. Minimal enhancement (<20 HU) on postprocedural CT is consistent with adequately ablated tissue. The long-term results of local therapy are awaited, for comparison with surgical treatment (partial or total nephrectomy) for renal tumors.

2.3.3. SOFT TISSUE TUMORS

The conventional treatment for painful soft tissue tumors includes radiation and pharmacologic therapy. Pain relief and tumor debulking can be obtained with local ablation, without much emphasis on clean margins. The mechanism of action is believed to be neurodestruction, decreased interstitial pressure and pressure, on adjacent organs.

2.3.4. LUNG TUMORS

RFA can be used to treat primary or metastatic lung tumors. Air in the surrounding lung provides insulation, with retention of heat energy within the lesion. A 10 to 20% pneumothorax rate has been encountered, more commonly with general anesthesia. A chest tube tray should always be available in the procedure room. Other complications include bleeding (more common in central tumors and possibly requiring unilateral intubation), hempoptysis, fistula, subcutaneous emphysema, effusions, infection, fever, and pain. One periprocedural death has been reported secondary to bleeding, as well as one stroke owing to cerebral embolism. The latter is a real risk because of the removal of the normal lung-filtering mechanisms and direct passage of bubbles created during RFA into the pulmonary vein and hence the arterial system.

RFA of lung tumors can be combined with experimental adjunctive therapies, conventional chemotherapy, and radiation in inoperable patients. Initial reports of small series are encouraging *(65–68)* and provide some data regarding safety and efficacy, but long-term results are awaited.

2.3.5. BONE TUMORS

Osteoid osteoma is a benign tumor and is seen most commonly in the cortex of long bones in the pediatric age group. The surgical treatment consists of osteotomy, with resultant risks of anesthesia, and wound healing, in addition to incomplete removal. RFA has a high success rate (90%) in the treatment of painful osteoid osteoma. A bone-cutting biopsy needle is placed into the lesion under CT guidance, followed by RFA of the prostaglandin-producing cells. Postprocedure imaging reveals bone demineralization after 6 wk, with persistence of the thermocoagulation radiologic defect for up to 1 yr.

Painful bone metastases unresponsive to other therapy constitute another indication for RFA. It can also be used to control hemorrhage and for local tumor eradication. A large tumor can be treated by a combination of RFA and radiotherapy: the central, less vascular tumor can be ablated with RFA because radiotherapy is less effective here. An intact cortex between the lesion and the spinal canal is essential when one is treating metastases in the spine, to avoid spinal cord injury. The procedure can also be combined with vertebroplasty when significant bone loss has occurred.

2.3.6. ADRENAL TUMORS

RFA can be used to treat primary (adrenocortical carcinoma), metastatic, and hormonally active tumors (pheochromocytoma, aldosteronoma) of the adrenal gland. Most of these tumors have limited treatment options. A full endocrine evaluation is essential. Hypertensive crisis during the ablation is a real concern, even in tumors not producing catecholamines, and thus the procedure should be performed under general anesthesia with blood pressure control. A high short-term technical success has been achieved for adrenocortical carcinoma less than 5 cm *(69)*.

2.3.7. BREAST

Large prospective trials have shown equivalent survival rates for mastectomy and for lumpectomy with radiation therapy. This has provided the background for attempted local ablation of breast tumors. However, in order to be a viable treatment option, RFA of breast tumors has to approach the nearly perfect success rate of surgery. RFA can, however, provide a debulking role, in inoperable tumors, in combination with radiation therapy. More surgical excision data with analysis of the pathology of ablation margins are required to assess the role of RFA in breast tumors.

2.3.8. OTHER ORGANS

Other potential applications for local ablation include tumors of the pancreas, thyroid, parathyroid, spleen, prostate, pelvis, head and neck, brain, lymph nodes, bronchus, retroperitoneum, and renal collecting system. However, these should be approached with extreme caution, owing to a high possibility of damage to nerves, vessels, and ducts.

3. EUS-GUIDED THERAPY

3.1. Introduction

EUS emerged in the 1980s as a research tool but now has become an invaluable method to diagnose and stage tumors of the aerodigestive tract. In many centers, EUS has assumed a major role in the management of GI and pulmonary cancers. More recently, interest has also developed in designing strategies to treat and palliate malignant tumors. Because of the access to several abdominal organs, EUS is an attractive method to deliver regional cancer therapy and provides an alternative to traditional, percutaneous techniques.

The general indications for EUS pertaining to malignancy include the following:

1. Diagnosis and staging of GI cancers.
2. Staging lung cancer (non-small cell).
3. EUS-guided therapy/palliation.

By far, the first two indications have received the most attention in the literature to date. However, several investigators have reported experiences with EUS-guided therapy, attesting to this rapidly developing and exciting field. For diagnosis and staging, EUS provides high-resolution images of the GI tract wall along with periluminal structures such as lymph nodes and blood vessels. Therefore, additional and often more accurate information regarding tumor T-stage and N-stage are obtainable with EUS—as a complement to traditional cross-sectional imaging, like CT or MRI. An added benefit of EUS is the ability to perform real-time fine needle aspiration (FNA) of suspicious masses or lymph nodes. The same concept also allows for EUS-guided cancer therapy.

The endosonographer is usually a gastroenterologist or, less commonly, a surgeon with special expertise in EUS. To perform EUS, specialized echoendoscopes are necessary as well as dedicated processors for EUS imaging. The basic design of an echoendoscope incorporates the standard video components of regular endoscopes together with an ultrasound transducer situated at the tip of the instrument.

3.2. EUS Principles

The endosonographer utilizes two different echoendoscopes—radial and linear—depending on the indication for the exam and the need to perform FNA or to deliver therapy (Fig. 13). In addition, diagnostic US probes, called miniprobes, can be advanced through the accessory channel of a standard endoscope and serve as another tool for the endosonographer. Common indications for miniprobe use include evaluation of small subepithelial tumors in the GI tract wall, tight malignant strictures that prohibit traditional echoendoscope passage, and intraductal imaging (intraductal US), as in evaluation of the proximal bile ducts. Typical US frequencies in EUS range from 5 to 20 MHz, although a 30-MHz miniprobe is available to provide high-resolution images of the luminal wall *(70)*. Based on the principals of ultrasound, lower frequencies provide greater depth of penetration to allow imaging of organs and structures outside the GI tract wall as opposed to higher frequencies that allow better definition of the wall layers at the expense of depth. For example, lower frequencies, such as 7.5 MHz, can define five GI wall layers (Fig. 14) but can also image organs such as the pancreas (Fig. 15). In comparison, a 20-MHz transducer often cannot visualize extraluminal structures but can provide a high-resolution image of the GI wall, commonly defining seven or more wall layers. The choice of frequency, therefore, often depends on the clinical indication.

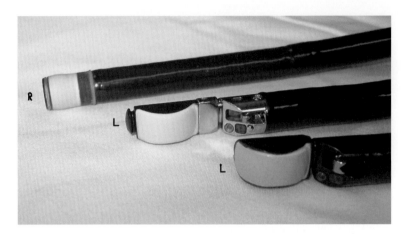

Fig. 13. Tips of radial (R) and linear (L) echoendoscopes used for endoscopic ultrasound procedures.

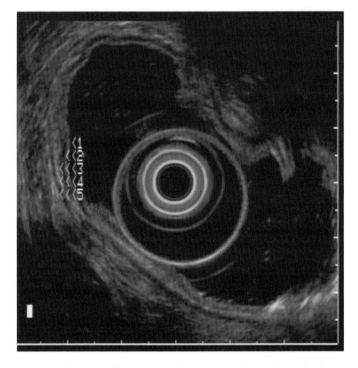

Fig. 14. Normal gastric wall seen with endoscopic ultrasound transducer in the stomach. 1: Superficial mucosa; 2: deep mucosa; 3: submucosa; 4: muscularis proproa; 5: serosa.

To provide acoustic coupling, a principle necessary for US transmission, water-filled balloons are attached to the tips of echoendoscopes. Another option is to fill the GI lumen with degassed water, although in some areas, such as the esophagus, this can be technically difficult and also presents an aspiration risk.

The radial echoendoscope enables the endosonographer to acquire images in a plane perpendicular to the long axis of the echoendoscope. Resulting EUS images can be a

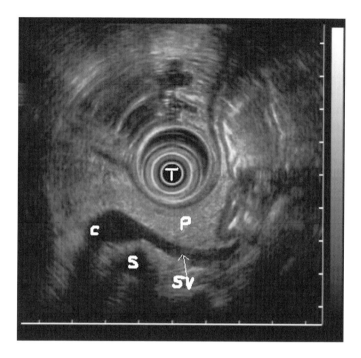

Fig. 15. Normal pancreatic body/tail and adjacent vasculature seen on EUS with the transducer (T) in the stomach. P, pancreas; C, confluence of splenic and portal vein; S, superior mesenteric artery; SV, splenic vein.

complete 360° or a partial 270°, depending on the echoendoscope manufacturer. Radial EUS is solely a diagnostic modality because its imaging characteristics do not allow for adequate and safe visualization of a needle advanced to perform FNA or therapeutic maneuvers. In contrast, linear echoendoscopes obtain a US image parallel to the long axis of the echoendoscope. They do not provide a circumferential view; however, with rotation and torque of the echoendoscope shaft, positioning and imaging of multiple longitudinal planes can be achieved. Linear EUS has the added advantage over radial EUS of permitting FNA and delivery of therapy through a small needle (usually 19 or 22 gage) advanced through the accessory channel of the echoendoscope. Therefore, real-time imaging can visualize the entire length of the needle with precise placement of the tip adjacent to vascular structures or into targeted lymph nodes or masses.

Echoendoscopes have an additional capability to perform simultaneous Doppler US to evaluate potential vascular structures. This tool is invaluable when one is defining anechoic structures of unknown etiology on EUS, to evaluate for malignant vascular invasion and to rule out intervening blood vessels in the projected path of an FNA needle.

3.3. Prerequisites for EUS-Guided Therapy

EUS is often an outpatient procedure and uses standard conscious sedation in the majority of cases. A complete history and physical exam are necessary to confirm the indications for the procedure, including a confirmation of the diagnosis, and to evaluate for contraindications. The contraindications for EUS are similar to those of standard GI endoscopy (i.e., uncooperative patient, unstable or unacceptable medical risk, suspected

GI perforation, and, for rectal EUS, fulminant colitis or diverticulitis) *(71)*. Potential limitations to EUS include altered GI tract abnormalities, for example, a gastrojejunostomy, which may make identification of relevant organs and structures more difficult or impossible. In addition, nontraversable malignant or benign strictures can limit the extent of the exam. For example, approx 30% of esophageal cancers result in high-grade strictures that do not allow echoendoscope passage *(72–74)*. Dilation of malignant esophageal strictures to allow echoendoscope passage is possible. The risk of perforation in this setting may be high *(73)*, although at least one study reported no perforations if dilation was less aggressive *(74)*. The endosonographer should review all prior cross-sectional imaging studies (CT or MRI) with a radiologist. This provides an opportunity to visualize the primary tumor, suspected invasion into adjacent structures, and lymphadenopathy that may alter the planned intervention.

Patients should have a complete blood cell count and standard coagulation studies prior to the procedure. Medications, including anticoagulants or antiplatelet drugs, should be held prior to interventional EUS per the recommendations of the American Society of Gastrointestinal Endoscopy *(75,76)*. Patients fast after midnight prior to the procedure as in standard GI endoscopy. Appropriate intravenous antibiotics should be available to administer at or near the time of the procedure if indicated (e.g., pancreatic cyst) *(77)*.

3.4. TECHNIQUE

After appropriate sedation with the patient in the left lateral decubitus position, the echoendosonographer advances the echoendoscope either orally or, for rectal EUS, by a transanal approach. Echoendoscopes provide either a traditional forward endoscopic view or oblique view depending on the type of echoendoscope (radial or linear) and the manufacturer. In the upper GI tract, the echoendoscope can generally be advanced to the distal segments of the duodenum, whereas in rectal EUS, the echoendoscope is often advanced proximally to 20 to 30 cm. Further advancement, although possible with rectal EUS, is generally not necessary. A colonoscope with EUS capabilities is available but is not commonly utilized or available because of a paucity of indications.

Both FNA- and EUS-guided therapy are readily performed with standard linear echoendoscopes (see ref. *78* for a technical review of EUS FNA). Through the accessory channel of the echoendoscope, a variety of needles and devices can be advanced to permit transluminal access to extraluminal structures or pathology. With FNA, typically a 22-gage needle can be directed into a lymph node or mass under real-time EUS guidance (Figs. 16 and 17). The FNA needle usually contains a stylet to decrease the amount of contaminating debris acquired as the needle traverses to its desired position. After removal of the stylet, the echoendosonographer uses short, smooth to-and-fro movements of the needle tip to obtain tissue. Sometimes a 10-mL syringe can be attached to the end of the needle to provide negative pressure and assist with tissue acquisition. After the needle is removed from the echoendoscope, technicians or nurses flush material from the needle tip for subsequent cytopathological review. In-room cytopathologists are helpful to provide immediate feedback with regard to adequate specimen retrieval and preliminary diagnostic results *(79–83)*. Depending on the adequacy of the sample, the endosonographer can repeat FNA with multiple needle passes if necessary to increase diagnostic yield. The procedure is similar when the goal is therapy as opposed to diagnosis. Potential therapeutic substances can be injected with the same needles used in FNA, a procedure called fine needle injection (FNI), or special

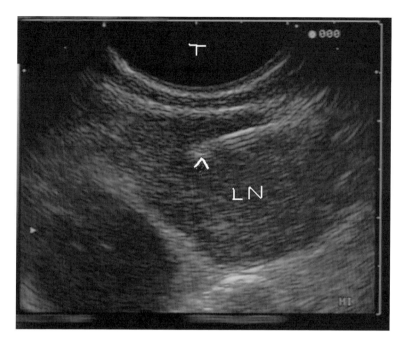

Fig. 16. Transesophageal endoscopic ultrasound guided fine needle aspiration of a large medias-tinal lymph node. LN, lymph node; T, transducer in the esophagus.

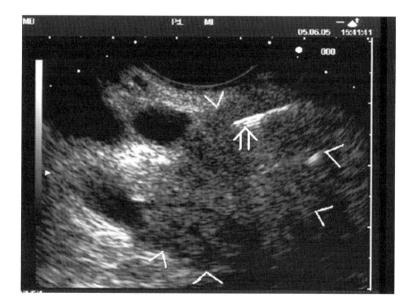

Fig. 17. Transduodenal endoscopic ultrasound-guided fine needle aspiration of a pancreatic head mass, outlined by arrowheads. Note the needle within the mass. The same technique can be used to perform transgastric or transduodenal fine needle aspiration of the pancreas or potentially to deliver targeted therapy via fine needle injection.

needles can be advanced through the accessory channel of the echoendoscope to deliver therapy, as in RFA.

3.5. Celiac Plexus Neurolysis

As a relatively new concept, published experience with therapeutic EUS is fairly limited. However, as more endosonographers are trained and new applications are discovered, delivery of therapy will potentially become a more common indication for EUS. The most clinical experience with therapeutic EUS is EUS-guided celiac plexus neurolysis (CPN). Similar to percutaneous CPN (84–86), EUS-guided CPN has also been used for palliation of pancreatic cancer-related pain, as first reported in 1996 (18). Whether percutaneous or EUS-guided, the concept of CPN is the same. Using radiographic guidance, a small-caliber needle can be placed in proximity to the celiac plexus and, subsequently, neurolytic agents can be injected. The main indication for CPN is palliation of pain resulting from intraabdominal cancers, particularly unresectable pancreatic cancer. Most patients with advanced pancreatic cancer experience significant pain associated with their disease (88). As opposed to a temporary celiac plexus block (CPB), commonly used for pain resulting from benign conditions, like chronic pancreatitis (89–91), CPN, in theory, destroys the celiac plexus and provides long-term, potentially lifelong palliation of pain. This is accomplished by injecting a neurolytic such as alcohol in lieu of a steroid (injected for a CPB).

EUS-guided CPN can be readily performed in experienced hands and requires minimal patient preparation (overnight fast and preprocedure coagulation studies/platelet counts) or equipment other than that required for traditional EUS and FNA. The procedure is often done on an outpatient basis with total procedural time usually less than 30 min. Because EUS can define the celiac axis and its origin from the aorta, EUS-guided CPN has a high technical success rate and an adequate safety and efficacy profile (87,90–92).

The procedure itself is fairly straightforward. After the linear echoendoscope is directed toward the posterior wall of the lesser curvature of the stomach, the abdominal aorta is identified in its longitudinal axis. The celiac axis can be imaged as the first vascular branch from the abdominal aorta (Fig. 18) below the diaphragm. With real-time EUS guidance, the endosonographer advances a 22-gage FNA needle through the accessory channel of the echoendoscope with placement of the needle tip just cephalad to the celiac axis takeoff. The needle is flushed with a small amount (3 mL) of saline to remove any debris and then aspirated to exclude inadvertent placement of the needle tip into a blood vessel. Subsequently, 3 to 6 mL of 0.25% bupivicaine and 10 mL dehydrated alcohol are injected, often creating an echogenic cloud visible by EUS imaging. Two methods of injection can be performed: either a single midline injection or two separate lateral injections. Altered anatomy secondary to the pancreatic tumor or lymphadenopathy may make bilateral injections difficult. At the end of the injection, the needle is injected with a small amount of either saline or bupivicaine (3 mL) as the needle is withdrawn.

EUS-guided CPN has been described for palliation of pain in the setting of pancreatic cancer. Initial experience with this technique was published by Wiersema and Wiersema in 1996, who included 30 patients treated with EUS-guided CPN (87). The same group published a larger prospective study that included the original patient group (92). In this series of 58 patients with unresectable pancreatic cancer, a reduction in pain was achieved in 78%, with a significant reduction in pain scores compared with baseline at 2 wk; this

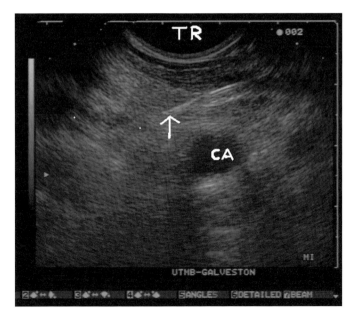

Fig. 18. Endoscopic ultrasound-guided celiac plexus neurolysis. The transducer (TR) is in the gastrointestinal lumen in the stomach near the gastroesophageal junction. A needle (arrow) is passed under real-time ultrasound guidance into the periceliac artery (CA) space to inject bupivacaine and alcohol.

remained significant for up to 8 wk. In addition, patients who received adjuvant chemotherapy alone or radiation and chemotherapy had an additional benefit with CPN that was durable to 24 wk. When the data were adjusted for opiate use and adjuvant therapy, CPN decreased pain scores by an average of 2.7 points at 2 wk. Beyond 2 wk, there was no further decrease in pain scores. Amounts of narcotic usage were no different before or after EUS-guided CPN.

In addition to potential complications associated with traditional endoscopy, endosonographers and patients should be aware of unique adverse events associated with EUS-guided CPN and prophylactic measures to decrease complications. Common side effects of CPN include postural hypotension (20%), transient diarrhea (15%) and transient exacerbation of abdominal pain (9%) *(92)*. Some advocate the prophylactic administration of half or a full liter of normal saline prior to the procedure to decrease the rates of postural hypotension *(91)*. Diarrhea generally can be managed with an anti-diarrhea agent such as loperamide as needed. An uncommon complication that has been noted with EUS-guided CPB, in which a steroid replaces the alcohol, is development of a peripancreatic abscess *(93)*. This complication has not been described for EUS-guided CPN with alcohol. In the case of CPB, some advocate administration of prophylactic antibiotics *(93)*. Reports of paraplegia after percutaneous or surgical CPN have been attributed to direct neurologic injury or spinal cord ischemia *(91,94–97)*, although no similar complication has been noted after EUS guidance. However, given the early experience with EUS-guidance, the authors generally include this theoretical risk in the informed consent process. Other uncommon complications of percutaneous CPN include visceral perforation and gastroparesis *(98,99)*.

3.6. EUS-Guided Fine Needle Injection

The relative ease with which needles can be accurately placing needles into targeted structures permits the endosonographer to inject therapeutic agents directly into tumors. The potential advantages of this site-specific therapy include delivery of a higher concentration of therapeutic agent to the tumor and avoidance of toxicity associated with systemic administration. During the same session, the endosonographer can make multiple injections at different sites within the tumor. In addition, because EUS is fairly well tolerated and minimally invasive, multiple sessions can readily be performed for tumor retreatment.

Despite the exciting and promising potential of EUS-guided FNI, only a few clinical studies have been reported. These include small trials designed to determine the feasibility, safety, and efficacy of intratumoral injection of various therapies, including biological agents. Cytoimplant is a collection of activated mononuclear cells created by incubating host and donor mononuclear cells. The incubation results in cytokine production and activation of immune effector cells. In the initial pilot study using Cytoimplant for unresectable pancreatic adenocarcinoma, Chang and colleagues used EUS-guided FNI to target injections into the main pancreatic tumor (100). In the initial study that included eight patients, either a partial or minor response was seen in slightly over a third of the patients. The results prompted a multicenter, randomized trial comparing conventional systemic gemcitabine with EUS-guided Cytoimplant. An interim analysis, however, disclosed favorable outcomes in the gemcitabine group, leading to cessation of the study.

Another biologic agent delivered with EUS-guided FNI was ONYX-015, a replication-sensitive adenovirus (101). The adenovirus has a deletion in the E1B-55kD gene— a p53 inhibitor—and selectively replicates and lyses tumor cells that are commonly p53 deficient. In the only trial with EUS-guided FNI of Onyx-015, 21 patients with pancreatic cancer underwent multiple injections over several separate sessions. Traditional gemcitabine was added at d 36. With Onyx-015 alone, no patient had an objective response. However, with combination therapy, 10% had a partial response and 38% had stable disease, with a median survival of 7.5 mo. Patients tolerated Onyx-015 well; however, there were procedural complications including infections and perforations. The future role of EUS-delivered Onyx-015 is doubtful based on the complications in conjunction with the multiple sessions necessary for treatment and the lack of clear benefit.

Most recently, Chang and colleagues reported clinical experience with a third biologic agent—TNFerade (102). The investigators injected TNFerade—a replication-deficient adenovirus expressing tumor necrosis factor-α (TNF-α) under the control of a radiation-inducible promoter—into the tumors of patients with unresectable pancreatic adenocarcinomas. Patients received weekly injections (both EUS-guided and percutaneous) with concomitant 5-FU and radiation. Although only published in abstract form, the results were promising. At 3 mo, 11% of patients had a partial response, 31% had a minor response, and 74% had tumor stabilization.

Other therapeutic agents for EUS-guided FNI include direct cytotoxins, such as alcohol or chemotherapeutic drugs. However, little clinical experience has been reported regarding either of these modalities. EUS-guided FNI of alcohol has been noted in case reports to treat successfully a GI stromal tumor (103) and a solid hepatic metastasis (104).

Additionally, in a pilot study, EUS-guided alcohol lavage showed some efficacy for the treatment of pancreatic cystic lesions *(105)*.

3.7. Other EUS-Guided Therapy

Investigators from Germany have reported their experience with EUS-guided radiation therapy for anal cancer *(106)*. After standard external beam radiation, patients undergo tumor restaging with endoanal US, and a 3D computer-generated model of the tumor is created. The investigators then implant afterloading needles with a transperineal approach using a specialized applicator that is permeable to ultrasound waves. Radiation is then delivered to the needles based on EUS-based dosimetry. In 42 such procedures in 18 patients, all subjects had complete response, and after a median follow-up of 24 mo, there were only two recurrences. Additional data from the same group in 36 patients again reported 100% complete response, with a recurrence rate of 13.9% after 44 mo *(107)*.

Other potential anticancer therapies delivered with EUS guidance are photodynamic therapy (PDT) and RFA. In feasibility studies using animal models, both PDT and RFA can be administered using EUS guidance. In the case of PDT, after systemic administration of a photosensitizer such as porfimer sodium, a small quartz optical fiber with a cylindrical diffuser can be advanced through the accessory channel of the echoendoscope into the desired location. With subsequent activation of the optical fiber, light results in the production of toxic singlet oxygen species in actively dividing cells that preferentially uptake the photosensitizer. RFA can be delivered through a special needle electrode, which can also be advanced through the accessory channel of the echoendoscope into a targeted lesion. In animal studies, both PDT and RFA can cause a well-circumscribed area of coagulative necrosis in various normal organs *(108,109)*. However, to date, there are no clinical data to support the use of either EUS-guided modality in the current treatment of cancer.

3.8. Post-EUS Care

After EUS, patients typically are observed in the endoscopy suite until they meet standard discharge criteria. The period of observation should be 2 h after CPN to ensure that postural hypotension does not develop that may require more intravenous fluids. Generally, there are no restrictions on oral intake or activity after EUS.

4. CONCLUSIONS

US guidance has proved to be an important method to deliver anticancer therapy. Because of its availability, low cost, and lack of radiation exposure, percutaneous US has become a favorite tool to target cancer, particularly hepatic tumors. In addition, EUS-guided therapy has emerged as a promising and rapidly developing field that adds another dimension to US-guided therapy. The ability for EUS to direct therapy toward intra-abdominal cancers that can be difficult to access by percutaneous routes is a unique facet of this particular approach. In the next several years, EUS will potentially assume a significant role in cancer therapeutics, adding to its current status as an invaluable adjunct for the diagnosis and staging of malignancy. Thus both interventional radiologists and gastroenterologists have become important members of multidisciplinary teams, dedicated to improving outcomes in patients with a variety of malignancies.

REFERENCES

1. Sandhu I, Bhutani MS. Gastrointestinal endoscopic ultrasonography. Med Clin N Am 2002:86: 1289–317.
2. Ohnishi K, Ohyama N, Ito S, Fujiwara K. Small hepatocellular carcinoma: treatment with US-guided intratumoral injection of acetic acid. Radiology 1994;193:747–752.
3. Shiina S, Tagawa K, Unuma T, et al. Percutaneous ethanol injection therapy for hepatocellular carcinoma: a histopathologic study. Cancer 1991;68:1524–1530.
4. Livraghi T. Percutaneous ethanol injection of hepatocellular carcinoma: survival after 3 years in 70 patients. Ital J Gastroenterol 1992;24:72–74.
5. Livraghi T, Bolondi L, Buscarini L, et al. No treatment, resection and ethanol injection in hepatocellular carcinoma: a retrospective analysis of survival in 391 patients with cirrhosis. Italian Cooperative HCC Study Group. J Hepatol 1995;22:522–526.
6. Amin Z, Bown SG, Lees WR. Local treatment of colorectal liver metastases: a comparison of interstitial laser photocoagulation (ILP) and percutaneous alcohol injection (PAI). Clin Radiol 1993;48:166–171.
7. Livraghi T, Giorgio A, Marin G, Set al. Hepatocellular carcinoma and cirrhosis in 746 patients: long-term results of percutaneous ethanol injection. Radiology 1995;197:101–108.
8. Ebara M, Ohto M, Sugiura N, et al. Percutaneous ethanol injection for the treatment of small hepatocellular carcinoma. Study of 95 patients. J Gastroenterol Hepatol 1990;5:616–626.
9. Di Stasi M, Buscarini L, Livraghi T, et al. Percutaneous ethanol injection in the treatment of hepatocellular carcinoma. A multicenter survey of evaluation practices and complication rates. Scand J Gastroenterol 1997;32:1168–1173.
10. Koda M, Tanaka H, Murawaki Y, et al. Liver perforation: a serious complication of percutaneous acetic acid injection for hepatocellular carcinoma. Hepatogastroenterology 2000;47:1110–1112.
11. Van Hoof M, Joris JP, Horsmans Y, Geubel A. Acute renal failure requiring hemodialysis after high doses percutaneous acetic acid injection for hepatocellular carcinoma. Acta Gastroenterol Belg 1999;62:49–51.
12. Livraghi T, Goldberg SN, Lazzaroni S, et al. Small hepatocellular carcinoma: treatment with radiofrequency ablation versus ethanol injection. Radiology 1999;210:655–661.
13. Livraghi T, Goldberg SN, Lazzaroni S, et al. Hepatocellular carcinoma: radio-frequency ablation of medium and large lesions. Radiology 2000;214:761–768.
14. Rhim H, Dodd GD III. Radiofrequency thermal ablation of liver tumors. J Clin Ultrasound 1999;27:221–229.
15. Solbiati L, Ierace T, Goldberg SN, et al. Percutaneous US-guided radio-frequency tissue ablation of liver metastases: treatment and follow-up in 16 patients. Radiology 1997;202:195–203.
16. Lees WR, Gillams AR, Schumillian C, Branda H. Hypotensive anaesthesia improved the effectiveness of radiofrequency ablation in the liver (abstr). Radiology 2000;217:228.
17. de Baere T, Bessoud B, Dromain C, et al. Percutaneous radiofrequency ablation of hepatic tumors during temporary venous occlusion. AJR Am J Roentgenol 2002;178:53–59.
18. Rossi S, Garbagnati F, Lencioni R, et al. Percutaneous radio-frequency thermal ablation of nonresectable hepatocellular carcinoma after occlusion of tumor blood supply. Radiology 2000;217:119–126.
19. Lencioni R, Cioni D, Donati F, Bartolozzi C. Combination of interventional therapies in hepatocellular carcinoma. Hepatogastroenterology 2001;48:8–14.
20. Seki T, Tamai T, Nakagawa T, et al. Combination therapy with transcatheter arterial chemoembolization and percutaneous microwave coagulation therapy for hepatocellular carcinoma. Cancer 2000;89:1245–1251.
21. Curley SA, Izzo F, Ellis LM, Nicolas Vauthey J, Vallone P. Radiofrequency ablation of hepatocellular cancer in 110 patients with cirrhosis. Ann Surg 2000;232:381–391.
22. Patterson EJ, Scudamore CH, Owen DA, et al. Radiofrequency ablation of porcine liver in vivo: effects of blood flow and treatment time on lesion size. Ann Surg 1998;227:559–565.
23. Livraghi T, Solbiati L, Meloni MF, et al. Treatment of focal liver tumors with percutaneous radiofrequency ablation: complications encountered in a multicenter study. Radiology 2003;226: 441–451.
24. Goldberg SN, Gazelle GS, Compton CC, et al. Treatment of intrahepatic malignancy with radiofrequency ablation: radiologic-pathologic correlation. Cancer 2000;88:2452–2463.

25. Goldberg SN, Gazelle GS, Dawson SL, et al. Tissue ablation with radiofrequency: effect of probe size, gauge, duration, and temperature on lesion volume. Acad Radiol 1995;2:399–404.

26. Solbiati L, Goldberg SN, Ierace T, et al. Radio-frequency ablation of hepatic metastases: postprocedural assessment with a US microbubble contrast agent—early experience. Radiology 1999;211:643–649.

27. Francica G, Marone G. Ultrasound-guided percutaneous treatment of hepatocellular carcinoma by radiofrequency hyperthermia with a "cooled-tip electrode." A preliminary clinical experience. Eur J Ultrasound 1999;9:145–153.

28. Kainuma O, Asano T, Aoyama H, et al. Combined therapy with radiofrequency thermal ablation and intra-arterial infusion chemotherapy for hepatic metastases from colorectal cancer. Hepatogastroenterology 1999;46:1071–1077.

29. Goldberg SN, Gazelle GS, Mueller PR. Thermal ablation therapy for focal malignancy: a unified approach to underlying principles, techniques, and diagnostic imaging guidance. AJR Am J Roentgenol 2000;174:323–331.

30. Dodd GD 3rd, Soulen MC, Kane RA, et al. Minimally invasive treatment of malignant hepatic tumors: at the threshold of a major breakthrough. Radiographics 2000;20:9–27.

31. Gazelle GS, Goldberg SN, Solbiati L, Livraghi T. Tumor ablation with radiofrequency energy. Radiology 2000;217:633–646.

32. Dupuy DE, Goldberg SN. Image-guided radiofrequency tumor ablation: challenges and opportunities—part II. J Vasc Interv Radiol 2001;12:1135–1148.

33. Gillams AR. Thermal ablation of liver metastases. Abdom Imaging 2001;26:361–368.

34. Pavlovich CP, Walther MM, Choyke PL, et al. Percutaneous radio frequency ablation of small renal tumors: initial results. J Urol 2002;167:10–15.

35. Gervais DA, McGovern FJ, Wood BJ, Goldberg SN, McDougal WS, Mueller PR. Radio-frequency ablation of renal cell carcinoma: early clinical experience. Radiology 2000;217:665–672.

36. Dupuy DE, Zagoria RJ, Akerley W, Mayo-Smith WW, Kavanagh PV, Safran H. Percutaneous radiofrequency ablation of malignancies in the lung. AJR Am J Roentgenol 2000;174:57–59.

37. Merkle EM, Boll DT, Boaz T, et al. MRI-guided radiofrequency thermal ablation of implanted VX2 liver tumors in a rabbit model: demonstration of feasibility at 0.2 T. Magn Reson Med 1999;42:141–149.

38. Boaz TL, Lewin JS, Chung YC, et al. MR monitoring of MR-guided radiofrequency thermal ablation of normal liver in an animal model. J Magn Reson Imaging 1998;8:64–69.

39. Friedman M, Mikityopsky I, Kan A, et al. Radiofrequency ablation of cancer. Cardiovasc Intervent Radiol 2004;27:427–434.

40. Decadt B, Siriwardena AK. Radiofrequency ablation of liver tumours: systematic review. Lancet Oncol 2004;5:550–560.

41. Takamura M, Murakami T, Shibata T, et al. Microwave coagulation therapy with interruption of hepatic blood in- or outflow: an experimental study. J Vasc Interv Radiol 2001;12:619–622.

42. Ishida T, Murakami T, Shibata T, et al. Percutaneous microwave tumor coagulation for hepatocellular carcinomas with interruption of segmental hepatic blood flow. AJR J Vasc Interv Radiol 2002;13:185–191.

43. Murakami R, Yoshimatsu S, Yamashita Y, Matsukawa T, Takahashi M, Sagara K. Treatment of hepatocellular carcinoma: value of percutaneous microwave coagulation. Am J Roentgenol 1995;164:1159–1164.

44. Shimada S, Hirota M, Beppu T, et al. Complications and management of microwave coagulation therapy for primary and metastatic liver tumors. Surg Today 1998;28:1130–1137.

45. Chen Y, Chen H, Wu M, et al. [Curative effect of percutaneous microwave coagulation therapy for hepatocellular carcinoma]. Zhonghua Zhong Liu Za Zhi 2002;24:65–67.

46. Sato M, Watanabe Y, Ueda S, et al. Microwave coagulation therapy for hepatocellular carcinoma. Gastroenterology 1996;110:1507–1514.

47. Seki T, Wakabayashi M, Nakagawa T, et al. Percutaneous microwave coagulation therapy for solitary metastatic liver tumors from colorectal cancer: a pilot clinical study. Am J Gastroenterol 1999;94:322–327.

48. Gage AA. History of cryoablation. Semin Surg Oncol 1998;14:99–109.

49. Lee FT Jr, Mahvi DM, Chosy SG, et al. Hepatic cryoablation with intraoperative US guidance. Radiology 1997;202:624–632.

50. Onik G, Rubinsky B, Zemel R, et al. Ultrasound-guided hepatic cryoablation in the treatment of metastatic colon carcinoma. Preliminary results. Cancer 1991;67:901–907.

51. Silverman SG, Tuncali K, Adams DF, et al. MR imaging-guided percutaneous cryotherapy of liver tumours: initial experience. Radiology 2000;217:657–664.

52. Brewer WH, Austin RS, Capps GW, et al. Intraoperative monitoring and postoperative imaging of hepatic cryoablation. Semin Surg Oncol 1998;14:129–155.

53. Kuszyk BS, Choti MA, Urban BA, et al. Hepatic tumors treated by cryoablation: normal CT appearance. AJR Am J Roentgenol 1996;166:363–368.

54. Bilchik AJ, Wood TF, Allegra D, et al. Cryosurgical ablation and radiofrequency ablation for unresectable hepatic malignant neoplasms: a proposed algorithm. Arch Surg 2000;135:657–662; discussion 662–664.

55. Grasso A, Watkinson AF, Tibballs JM, et al. Radiofrequency ablation in the treatment of hepatocellular carcinoma—a clinical viewpoint. J Hepatol 2000;33:667–672.

56. Fong Y, Sun RL, Jarnagin W, Blumgart LH. An analysis of 412 cases of hepatocellular carcinoma at a Western center. Ann Surg 1999;229:790–800.

57. Bismuth H, Chiche L, Adam R, Castaing D, Diamond T, Dennison A. Liver resection versus transplantation for hepatocellular carcinoma in cirrhotic patients. Ann Surg 1993;218:145–151.

58. Ringe B, Pichlmayr R, Wittekind C, Tusch G. Surgical treatment of hepatocellular carcinoma: experience with liver resection and transplantation in 198 patients. World J Surg 1991;15:270–285.

59. Iwatsuki S, Starzl TE, Sheahan DG, et al. Hepatic resection versus transplantation for hepatocellular carcinoma. Ann Surg 1991;214:221–229.

60. Otto G, Heuschen U, Hofmann WJ, Krumm G, Hinz U, Herfarth C. Survival and recurrence after liver transplantation versus liver resection for hepatocellular carcinoma: a retrospective analysis. Ann Surg 1998;227:424–432.

61. Mazzaferro V, Regalia E, Doci R, et al. Liver transplantation for the treatment of small hepatocellular carcinomas in patients with cirrhosis. N Engl J Med 1996;334:693–699.

62. Greenway B. Hepatic metastases from colorectal cancer: resection or not. Br J Surg 1988;75:513–519.

63. Scheele J, Altendorf-Hofmann A, Stangle R, et al. Surgical resection of colorectal liver metastases: gold standard for solitary and radically resectable lesions [in German]. Swiss Surg 1996;Suppl 4:4–17.

64. Scheele J, Stangl R, Altendorf-Hofmann A, et al. Indicators of prognosis after hepatic resection for colorectal secondaries. Surgery 1991;110:13–29.

65. Herrera LJ, Fernando HC, Perry Y. Radiofrequency ablation of pulmonary malignant tumors in nonsurgical candidates. J Thorac Cardiovasc Surg 2003;125:929–937.

66. Lee JM, Jin GY, Goldberg SN, et al., Percutaneous radiofrequency ablation for inoperable non-small cell lung cancer and metastases preliminary report. Radiology 2004;230:125–134.

67. Kotaro Y, Susumu K, Yoshifumi S, et al., Thoracic tumors treated with CT-guided radiofrequency ablation initial experience. Radiology 2004;231:850–857.

68. Cosmo G, Vittorio M, Giuseppe C, et al., Radiofrequency ablation of 40 lung neoplasms preliminary results. AJR Am J Roentgenol 2004;183:361–368.

69. Wood BJ, Abraham J, Hvizda JL, Alexander HR, Fojo T. Radiofrequency ablation of adrenal tumors and adrenocortical carcinoma metastases. Cancer 2003;97:554–560.

70. Oto A, Bhutani M. Introduction to diagnostic ultrasonography and endosonography, in Digital Human Anatomy and Endoscopic Ultrasonography (Bhutani M, Deutsch J, eds.), London: BC Decker, 2005:13–25.

71. Eisen GM, Chutkan R, Goldstein JL, et al. Role of endoscopic ultrasonography. Gastrointest Endosc 2000;52:852–89.

72. Catalano MF, Van Dam J, Sivak MV, Jr. Malignant esophageal strictures: staging accuracy of endoscopic ultrasonography. Gastrointest Endosc 1995;41:535–539.

73. Van Dam J, Rice TW, Catalano MF, Kirby T, Sivak MV Jr. High-grade malignant stricture is predictive of esophageal tumor stage. Risks of endosonographic evaluation. Cancer 1993;71:2910–2917.

74. Wallace MB, Hawes RH, Sahai AV, Van Velse A, Hoffman BJ. Dilation of malignant esophageal stenosis to allow EUS guided fine-needle aspiration: safety and effect on patient management. Gastrointest Endosc 2000;51:309–313.

75. Eisen GM, Baron TH, Dominitz JA, et al. Guideline on the management of anticoagulation and antiplatelet therapy for endoscopic procedures. Gastrointest Endosc 2002;55:775–779.

76. Zuckerman MJ, Hirota WK, Adler DG, et al. ASGE guideline: the management of low-molecular-weight heparin and nonaspirin antiplatelet agents for endoscopic procedures. Gastrointest Endosc 2005;61:189–194.

77. Hirota WK, Petersen K, Baron TH, et al. Guidelines for antibiotic prophylaxis for GI endoscopy. Gastrointest Endosc 2003;58:475–482.
78. Erickson RA. EUS-guided FNA. Gastrointest Endosc 2004;60 *(2)*:267–729.
79. Klapman JB, Logrono R, Dye CE, Waxman I. Clinical impact of on-site cytopathology interpretation on endoscopic ultrasound-guided fine needle aspiration. Am J Gastroenterol 2003;98:1289–1294.
80. Wiersema MJ, Vilmann P, Giovannini M, Chang KJ, Wiersema LM. Endosonography-guided fine-needle aspiration biopsy: diagnostic accuracy and complication assessment. Gastroenterology 1997;112:1087–1095.
81. Chang KJ, Nguyen P, Erickson RA, Durbin TE, Katz KD. The clinical utility of endoscopic ultrasound-guided fine-needle aspiration in the diagnosis and staging of pancreatic carcinoma. Gastrointest Endosc 1997;45:387–393.
82. Erickson RA, Sayage-Rabie L, Beissner RS. Factors predicting the number of EUS-guided fine-needle passes for diagnosis of pancreatic malignancies. Gastrointest Endosc 2000;51:184–190.
83. Layfield LJ, Bentz JS, Gopez EV. Immediate on-site interpretation of fine-needle aspiration smears: a cost and compensation analysis. Cancer 2001;93:319–322.
84. Mercadante S. Celiac plexus block versus analgesics in pancreatic cancer pain. Pain 1993;52:187–192.
85. Kawamata M, Ishitani K, Ishikawa K, et al. Comparison between celiac plexus block and morphine treatment on quality of life in patients with pancreatic cancer pain. Pain 1996;64:597–602.
86. Polati E, Finco G, Gottin L, Bassi C, Pederzoli P, Ischia S. Prospective randomized double-blind trial of neurolytic coeliac plexus block in patients with pancreatic cancer. Br J Surg 1998;85:199–201.
87. Wiersema MJ, Wiersema LM. Endosonography-guided celiac plexus neurolysis. Gastrointest Endosc 1996;44:656–662.
88. Kalser MH, Barkin J, MacIntyre JM. Pancreatic cancer. Assessment of prognosis by clinical presentation. Cancer 1985;56:397–402.
89. Gress F, Schmitt C, Sherman S, Ikenberry S, Lehman G. A prospective randomized comparison of endoscopic ultrasound- and computed tomography-guided celiac plexus block for managing chronic pancreatitis pain. Am J Gastroenterol 1999;94:900–905.
90. Hoffman BJ. EUS-guided celiac plexus block/neurolysis. Gastrointest Endosc 2002;56(4 Suppl):S26–S28.
91. Levy MJ, Wiersema MJ. EUS-guided celiac plexus neurolysis and celiac plexus block. Gastrointest Endosc 2003;57:923–930.
92. Gunaratnam NT, Sarma AV, Norton ID, Wiersema MJ. A prospective study of EUS-guided celiac plexus neurolysis for pancreatic cancer pain. Gastrointest Endosc 2001;54:316–324.
93. Gress F, Schmitt C, Sherman S, Ciaccia D, Ikenberry S, Lehman G. Endoscopic ultrasound-guided celiac plexus block for managing abdominal pain associated with chronic pancreatitis: a prospective single center experience. Am J Gastroenterol 2001;96:409–416.
94. Davies DD. Incidence of major complications of neurolytic coeliac plexus block. J R Soc Med 1993;86:264–266.
95. Wong GY, Brown DL. Transient paraplegia following alcohol celiac plexus block. Reg Anesth 1995;20:352–355.
96. van Dongen RT, Crul BJ. Paraplegia following coeliac plexus block. Anaesthesia 1991;46:862–863.
97. De Conno F, Caraceni A, Aldrighetti L, et al. Paraplegia following coeliac plexus block. Pain 1993;55:383–385.
98. Eisenberg E, Carr DB, Chalmers TC. Neurolytic celiac plexus block for treatment of cancer pain: a meta-analysis. Anesth Analg 1995;80:290–295.
99. Iftikhar S, Loftus EV Jr. Gastroparesis after celiac plexus block. Am J Gastroenterol 1998;93:2223–2225.
100. Chang KJ, Nguyen PT, Thompson JA, et al. Phase I clinical trial of allogeneic mixed lymphocyte culture (cytoimplant) delivered by endoscopic ultrasound-guided fine-needle injection in patients with advanced pancreatic carcinoma. Cancer 2000;88:1325–1335.
101. Hecht JR, Bedford R, Abbruzzese JL, et al. A phase I/II trial of intratumoral endoscopic ultrasound injection of ONYX-015 with intravenous gemcitabine in unresectable pancreatic carcinoma. Clin Cancer Res 2003;9:555–561.
102. Chang K, Senzer N, Chung T, et al. A novel gene transfer therapy against pancreatic cancer (TNFerade) delivered by endoscopic ultrasound (EUS) and percutaneous guided fine needle injection (FNI). Gastrointest Endosc 2004;59:AB92.

103. Gunter E, Lingenfelser T, Eitelbach F, Muller H, Ell C. EUS-guided ethanol injection for treatment of a GI stromal tumor. Gastrointest Endosc 2003;57:113–115.
104. Barclay RL, Perez-Miranda M, Giovannini M. EUS-guided treatment of a solid hepatic metastasis. Gastrointest Endosc 2002;55:266–270.
105. Gan I, Bounds B, Brugge W. EUS-guided ethanol lavage of the pancreas is feasible and safe. Gastrointest Endosc 2004;59:AB94.
106. Lohnert M, Doniec JM, Kovacs G, Schroder J, Dohrmann P. New method of radiotherapy for anal cancer with three-dimensional tumor reconstruction based on endoanal ultrasound and ultrasound-guided afterloading therapy. Dis Colon Rectum 1998;41:169–176.
107. Doniec MJ, Loehnert MS, Kovacs G, Kremer B, Grimm HA. Rectal EUS guided HDR-brachytherapy in patients with anal and perianal malignancies. Gastrointest Endosc 2000;51:AB106.
108. Chan HH, Nishioka NS, Mino M, et al. EUS-guided photodynamic therapy of the pancreas: a pilot study. Gastrointest Endosc 2004;59:95–99.
109. Goldberg SN, Mallery S, Gazelle GS, Brugge WR. EUS-guided radiofrequency ablation in the pancreas: results in a porcine model. Gastrointest Endosc 1999;50:392–401.

11 Nanocarriers and Drug Delivery

Svetlana Gelperina, PhD

SUMMARY

Nanoparticles may serve, among other techniques, as a useful tool for achieving the main objective of regional cancer therapy: they can deliver a higher concentration of the agent to the tumor and expose the tumor to active drug for longer periods than safely possible with conventional formulations. These carriers combine many advantages, such as a potential for selective targeting and an opportunity to tailor particles with the desired characteristics offered by the versatility of polymer chemistry. This chapter describes the key issues of this research strategy relevant to the chemotherapy of cancer and provides an update on some novel targeting approaches.

Key Words: Active targeting; biodistribution; blood-brain barrier; cancer chemotherapy; drug delivery; MDR; nanoparticles; toxicity.

1. INTRODUCTION

In the past few decades, tremendous efforts have been focused on cancer chemotherapy; however, in many cases the treatment outcome for the patients remains poor. There are a number of obstacles to successful chemotherapy, such as ineffective drug access to the tumor site owing to physiological barriers (such as the blood-brain barrier) or structural abnormalities of tumor tissue, hindrance of drug penetration into the tumor cells at the cellular level (multidrug resistance), poor bioavailability (low solubility or fast degradation), or unfavorable biodistribution. As a result, high dose of the drug are needed to reach efficient concentrations in the tumor, and the antitumor effect is often

From: *Cancer Drug Discovery and Development: Regional Cancer Therapy*
Edited by: P. M. Schlag and U. S. Stein © Humana Press Inc., Totowa, NJ

achieved at the expense of deleterious side effects. This unwanted toxicity is a foresee-able consequence of an uncontrolled drug biodistribution. Indeed, cytotoxic drugs kill tumor cells but they also damage healthy cells in the body. Thus, poor specificity creates a toxicological problem and becomes a limiting factor for effective chemotherapy, with the more potent drugs tending to be more toxic.

This problem has called to life the now famous "magic-bullet concept" of drug target-ing, first formulated by Paul Ehrlich in 1908, and a number of new technologies aimed at the development of drug delivery systems. In contrast to conventional drugs subjected to an uncontrolled biodistribution, the drug delivery systems are designed with consid-eration of the specific features of the diseased organs or cells. Liposomes are the most successful and well-known example of this strategy. Another drug delivery system—nanoparticles—represents an attractive alternative. These carriers can combine many advantages of other delivery systems, such as a potential for selective targeting and an opportunity to tailor particles with the desired characteristics offered by the versatility of polymer chemistry.

The advances and pitfalls of drug targeting using nanoparticles have been covered in numerous publications over the last few years. The intention of the present chapter is to highlight some key issues of this research strategy relevant to the chemotherapy of cancer, illustrate them with selected examples and also update the reader on some novel targeting approaches. The use of nanoparticles for diagnostic purposes is beyond the scope of this review.

2. DEFINITION AND BACKGROUND

Nanoparticles for purposes of drug delivery are defined as submicron (<1 µm) colloi-dal particles. This definition includes solid nanoparticles (nanospheres) in which the active principle (drug or bioactive agent) is adsorbed, dissolved, or dispersed throughout the matrix, and nanocapsules, in which the active principle is confined to an aqueous or oily core surrounded by a polymeric wall (1). Alternatively, the drug can be covalently attached to the surface or into the matrix.

The nanoparticles are generally made from biocompatible and biodegradable materi-als, such as polymers, either natural (e.g., gelatin, albumin) or synthetic (e.g., polylactides, polyalkylcyanoacrylates) or solid lipids. In the body, the drug loaded in nanoparticles will be released from the matrix. The release mechanism is usually diffusion, assisted by matrix swelling, erosion, or degradation.

The important technological advantages of nanoparticles used as drug carriers are high stability (i.e., long shelf life), high carrier capacity (i.e., many drug molecules can be incorporated in the particle matrix), feasibility of incorporation of both hydrophilic and hydrophobic substances, and feasibility of peroral application. Owing to variable char-acteristics of the materials used for nanoparticle engineering (e.g., various rates of bio-degradation), these carriers also allow controlled (fast or sustained) drug release.

The methods for nanoparticle preparation and characterization are reviewed in refs. 2–6.

3. BIODISTRIBUTION OF NANOPARTICLES

Nanoparticles can change the fate of the drug in the body, their ultimate action being the alteration of drug biodistribution. Hence, the biodistribution study is an important milestone in the design and evaluation of the nanoparticle-based drug delivery systems.

Indeed, the biodistribution profile can predict whether nanoparticles will provide a gain in the drug therapeutic efficacy or allow decrease in toxicity. Moreover, these studies are essential for the rational design of chemotherapy experiments, particularly for planning the therapeutic schedule.

3.1. Intravenous Administration

In contrast to microspheres with a diameter of more than 1 µm, which cannot be administered systemically and have to be implanted, nanoparticles are small enough to be administered via intravascular routes and allow intracapillary passage followed by an efficient cellular uptake. In the bloodstream, conventional nanoparticles, like all colloidal carriers, are rapidly coated by plasma proteins and glycoproteins. This process, known as opsonization, is critical for the subsequent fate of the injected particles. The opsonized particles are recognized by the major defense system of the body, the mononuclear phagocyte system (MPS), as foreign particulates. They are rapidly removed from circulation by the Kupffer cells in the liver and, to a lesser extent, by macrophages of the spleen and bone marrow, as well as circulating monocytes. The uptake of nanoparticles by macrophages occurs via endocytosis, after which the particles end up in the lysosomal compartment, where they are degraded and release the drug.

Preferential uptake of nanoparticles by Kupffer cells of the liver represents a classical example of passive, although site-specific, delivery that is achieved by the physicochemical properties of the carrier and by physiological opportunity. However, in many cases, Kupffer cells are an inappropriate target; then they represent a major obstacle to the targeting of particulate carriers to the other sites and beyond the vascular compartment. Therefore, there has been growing interest in the design of colloidal carriers that upon intravenous injection avoid rapid recognition by Kupffer cells and circulate in the blood for an appropriate period.

The process of particle recognition and clearance from blood depends on their physicochemical characteristics, such as size and especially their surface properties. Hydrophobic particles are more efficiently coated with plasma components and rapidly cleared from the circulation, whereas particles with a more hydrophilic surface resist opsonization and circulate for a longer time.

The general approach for prolongation of the circulation time of colloidal particles is to reduce protein adsorption and surface opsonization by a steric surface barrier of sufficient density. Steric stabilization prevents particle recognition by macrophages, thus creating the so-called stealth effect (Stealth™ is a registered trade mark of Liposome Technology Inc.). The theory and engineering principles for the development of stealth (Kupffer cell-evading) carriers have been described in the excellent reviews of Moghimi et al. (7–9).

Generally, steric stabilization of nanocarriers in the bloodstream is achieved by physical adsorption of nonionic surfactants or amphiphilic block copolymers, such as poloxamers or poloxamines (block copolymers of poly[oxy ethylene] and poly[oxy propylene]) or by their incorporation during the production of nanoparticles. Alternatively, surface modification can be performed by covalent attachment of polyethylene glycol (PEG) chains to the surface of particles, or the particles can be formed from an amphiphilic copolymer: the hydrophobic blocks form a solid phase, whereas the hydrophilic chains extend outward and provide steric protection of the surface.

Ideally, a long-circulating carrier with adequate drug release characteristics can serve as a long-circulating drug reservoir from which the drug can be released into the vascular compartment in a continuous and controlled manner. Candidate drugs may be those with short elimination half-lives or poor bioavailability.

The prolonged circulation of the sterically stabilized particles, their ability to extend the half-life of the bound drug, and reduced liver uptake (10–20% dose vs 70–90% dose for conventional particles) have been demonstrated by many independent researchers *(10–13)*. For example, paclitaxel is an effective antitumor agent that, owing to its low solubility in water, is administered with polyethoxylated castor oil (Cremophor® EL) that causes serious side effects. The solid lipid nanoparticles (SLNs) stabilized by Pluronic® F68 or Brij® 78 allowed the slow release of paclitaxel and produced a marked increase in serum half-life compared with the free drug *(12)*. These data suggest that the use of SLNs may eliminate the need for Cremophor EL, thus improving the drug therapeutic index.

A pharmacokinetic study of doxorubicin bound to SLNs administered intravenously in rabbits demonstrated that the circulation time of the nanoparticle-bound drug was considerably increased, as were the blood and brain concentrations, whereas concentrations in other organs (liver, heart, lungs, spleen, and kidney) were decreased, compared with the drug in solution. The integral pharmacokinetic parameter, the area under curve concentration vs time (AUC), of SLN-bound doxorubicin increased with the increasing content of a stealth agent (stearic acid—PEG 2000) present in the particles *(14)*. A similar tendency was observed for other particles *(11,15)*.

It may be expected that the biological fate of the particle will depend on the structure of the steric barrier formed by a stealth agent. Indeed, it was shown that protein adsorption and phagocytic uptake of the coated nanoparticles is strongly influenced by the corona formed by PEG chains at the surface of the particles and the core composition of the particle. The extent of proteins adsorbed on the surface was governed by the conformational mobility, length, and density of PEG chains, whereas the qualitative composition of the plasma protein adsorption patterns depended more on a hydrophobicity of the core surface protected more or less by PEG chains *(16,17)*.

Covalent linking of the stealth agents to the matrix would seem a better choice than simple adsorption since in the bloodstream adsorbed agents can be easily desorbed from the surface. At the same time, it has also been shown that conventional nanoparticles injected intravenously in rats can be converted to long-circulating carriers if these rats received a bolus intravenous dose of a stealth agent (poloxamer 407 or poloxamine 908) 1 or 3 h earlier. These particles displayed resistance to phagocytosis owing to acquisition of a protective coating in the blood *(18)*.

An important observation has been made by Moghimi et al. *(19)*. It appears that a single intravenous injection of long-circulating (poloxamine 908-coated) nanoparticles dramatically affected the circulation half-life and body distribution of a second dose. This effect depends on the interval of time between the injections *(19)*. This phenomenon, also observed for liposomes, deserves further investigation, as it may have important implications for cancer therapy involving multiple dose schedules.

It should be noted that the intravenously injected particles that evade Kupffer cells in the liver are subjected to splenic filtration processes *(8,20)*. Spleen capture is especially effective for rigid particles whose size exceeds the width of the interendothelial cell slits (200–250 nm). This phenomenon offers opportunities for spleen targeting.

The above observations provide a solid basis for engineering carriers with predictable biodistribution and a pharmacologically desirable free drug profile.

3.2. Other Routes of Administration

The fate of nanoparticles after oral administration has been investigated in a number of studies (reviewed in *[21–23]*). Owing to morphological and physiological absorption barriers in the gastrointestinal tract, exploitation of this route for particulate carrier systems remains a challenging task. In general, the uptake of nanoparticles occurs: (1) by transcytosis via M cells, (2) by intracellular uptake and transport via the epithelial cells lining the intestinal mucosa, and (3) by uptake via Peyer's patches. Apart from particle size, the type and composition of the polymers used for nanoparticle preparation are crucial for successful uptake and transport across mucosal barriers. Thus, the behavior of polymeric nanoparticles in the gastrointestinal tract is influenced by their bioadhesive properties *(24)*. Mucoadhesion of nanoparticles to the gastrointestinal mucosa contributes to the absorption enhancement of the associated drug *(25)*. Bioadhesive nanoparticles with tropism for the stomach mucosa may increase the bioavailability of presystemically metabolized *(26)* or poorly soluble drugs *(27,28)*.

After interstitial or subcutaneous administration, small nanoparticles are captured by regional lymph nodes. This may be beneficial if the target is a specific lymph node or a group of them located regionally.

The drainage and lymphatic distribution of subcutaneously administered nanoparticles can be manipulated using the concept of steric stabilization. The properly engineered surface-modified nanoparticles can escape clearance by macrophages of the regional lymph nodes, reach the systemic circulation, and remain in the blood for prolonged periods *(29,30)*. When long-circulating particles, such as poloxamer-407 or poloxamine-908-coated polystyrene particles (60 nm) were injected subcutaneously into rat footpads, more than 70% of the dose drained into initial lymphatics within 2 h compared with only 20% of uncoated particles.

These observations suggest that a lymphatic delivery of the formulations based on sterically stabilized particles will be advantageous for therapeutic and diagnostic purposes (reviewed in refs. *31* and *32*).

3.3. EPR Effect: Targeting of Solid Tumors

Normally, particle escape from the vasculature is restricted to sites where the capillaries have open fenestration, as in the sinus endothelium of the liver; however, they can also extravasate into sites where the endothelium becomes permeable owing to pathological processes, as in the case of inflammation or tumor growth. The leaky vasculature at the tumor site is a critical advantage in treating cancers with nanoparticulate drugs. However, whereas hyperpermeability of tumor vessels is beneficial for transvascular transport of nanoparticles into the tumor, there are also impeding factors such as heterogeneous vascularization, unpredictable blood flow, abnormal hydrostatic pressure gradients and compression, and collapse of tumor vessels generated by tumor cell proliferation *(33,34)*.

In spite of these limitations, the intravenously injected nanoparticles and macromolecules (with a molecular weight of above 45 kDa) are able to extravasate across the leaky endothelium and accumulate in the tumor. The retention of nanoparticles (and macromolecules) in the tumor results from an impaired lymphatic drainage that is typical for neoplastic tissue. This phenomenon is called the *enhanced permeability and retention effect* (EPR effect) *(35)*. The EPR effect, initially proposed for macromolecular prodrugs, has provided a basis for the now widely accepted concept of passive drug delivery to solid tumors using both macromolecular and colloidal carriers. Therefore, in this case, site-specific (although passive) delivery is achieved owing to the physicochemical properties of a carrier and the *patho*physiological condition of a target. Accumulation of the nanoparticle-bound drugs in tumors was observed in a number of studies (e.g., refs. *36–39*).

Diffusion or convection of nanoparticles into tumor tissue vary with the tumor types and microenvironment. Hobbs et al. proposed that the transvascular transport of the particles in the tumors occurs owing to interendothelial or transendothelial open junctions rather than by endothelial phagocytosis or vesicles *(40)*. In this study, the size of the transvascular gaps in the tumors was characterized based on the size of long-circulating PEG-coated liposomes or latex particles that could extravasate from the vessels. The experimental tumors (including mammary and colorectal carcinomas, hepatomas, gliomas, and sarcomas grown subcutaneously in mice) exhibited a pore cutoff size ranging from 200 nm to 1.2 μm; most ranged between 380 and 780 nm. (For comparison, in the liver, fenestrations in the sinus endothelium are 106–175 nm in diameter.) The size was dramatically reduced when the tumor was grown intracranially.

Similar observations were reported by Lode et al. *(41)*. Uptake of the sterically stabilized poly(methyl methacrylate) nanoparticles varied in different tumor models. Immunohistological study revealed a correlation in particle uptake in the tumors with expression of vascular endothelial growth factor (VEGF), which is a marker of tumor-induced angiogenesis. The highest uptake was achieved in a subcutaneously grown B16 melanoma that was also characterized by the highest VEGF expression, whereas a negligible uptake in an intracerebral U-373 glioblastoma paralleled a lack of VEGF expression in this tumor.

Therefore, in the case of extravascular targets, such as solid tumors, the size of a carrier becomes an essential parameter: it must correlate with the pore size cutoff of a particular tumor.

4. EXPERIMENTAL CANCER CHEMOTHERAPY

Treatment of solid tumors has undoubtedly been the main research area for nanoparticles because of the advantages offered by the EPR effect (for recent reviews, *see* refs. *42–46*). Regardless of the mechanism involved, the result depends mainly on the physicochemical parameters of the delivery system. In general, long-circulating carriers have a higher probability of reaching the target if it is located outside the MPS.

4.1. Conventional and Long-Circulating Nanoparticles

Obviously, passive accumulation of conventional nanoparticles in the MPS organs may be beneficial for chemotherapy of MPS-localized tumors. Indeed, high efficacy of doxorubicin bound to biodegradable poly(alkyl cyanoacrylate) (PACA) nanoparticles was demonstrated in a murine hepatic metastases model obtained by intravenous injection of M5076 reticulosarcoma cells *(47)*. Histological examination showed that in the group treated with the nanoparticle-bound drug, both the number and the size of the tumor nodules in the liver were decreased, compared with the group treated with the drug in solution.

Interestingly, no difference in drug concentrations measured in total liver homogenates was observed between healthy and tumor-bearing animals. An in-depth biodistribution study demonstrated that although the nanoparticles did not have an affinity to the tumor tissue and were initially concentrated in Kupffer cells, hepatic tissue became an efficient reservoir of doxorubicin in the close vicinity of tumor nodules, providing prolonged release of the free drug and an effective concentration gradient favorable for its accumulation in the tumor *(48)*.

The application of stealth technology enhances the ability of nanoparticles to accumulate at the tumor site, which is a reflection of a long circulatory profile of the sterically stabilized nanoparticles. Long-circulating PEG-coated PACA nanoparticles were used for the targeting of recombinant uman tumor necrosis factor-α (rHuTNF-α) to tumor tissue. A comparative study of the pharmacokinetics and antitumor effect of rHuTNF-α in the free form and bound to conventional or PEG-coated PACA nanoparticles was conducted in mice with sarcoma-180 implanted intradermally. As expected, the highest AUC was achieved with rHuTNF-α bound to PEG-coated particles (1571 h × cpm/μL vs 571 h × cpm/μL for free rHuTNF-α), which correlated with the highest accumulation in the tumor and the most considerable tumor growth inhibition achieved by this formulation (78% inhibition vs 15% for free rHuTNF-α) *(49)*.

4.2. Resistant Cancers

A major challenge in cancer chemotherapy is multidrug resistance (MDR), which is responsible for the limited access of the drugs into the resistant cells. These cells are characterized by overexpression of specific membrane-associated proteins, known as ABC transporters, which bind undesirable molecules and pump them out of the cells. These transporters are also localized at various physiological barriers (e.g., intestine, kidney, blood-brain barrier, or blood-testis barrier) and constitute an important part of the host defense against the intracellular accumulation of toxic xenobiotics. At the same time, their presence in the membrane of cancer cells poses a formidable obstacle to effective chemotherapy. A key role of MDR in cancer has so far been attributed to P-glycoprotein (P-gp) *(50)*. A number of studies have demonstrated the therapeutic benefit of adjuvant chemotherapy using competitive P-gp inhibitors as chemosensitizers; however, this approach is often associated with high toxicity.

PACA nanoparticles display a unique ability to overcome the P-gp-related resistance of cancer cells to doxorubicin, which is a known substrate of P-gp (reviewed in ref. *51*). Thus, doxorubicin loaded in polyisobutyl cyanoacrylate nanoparticles produced considerable cytotoxic effect in the cell lines resistant to doxorubicin. It was demonstrated that contact of the particles with the cell membrane was essential for MDR reversion; however, in contrast to what was believed, internalization of the particles in the resistant cells was not required. Moreover, the intracellular accumulation and cytotoxicity of doxorubicin clearly depended on the release of the drug from the particles.

The following mechanism was proposed to explain the ability of doxorubicin loaded in PACA nanoparticles to circumvent the resistance. First, the nanoparticles adhere to cell membranes. Then adhesion is followed by the simultaneous release of the encapsulated drug and the product of polymer biodegradation (polycyanoacrylic acid), forming an ion pair that could cross the membrane without being recognized by P-gp.

The high efficacy of doxorubicin loaded in PACA nanoparticles was further demonstrated in the X/myc transgenic murine model of hepatocellular carcinoma (HCC), which was shown to overexpress the MDR-related genes *(52)*. Cytotoxicity of the nanoparticulate antibiotic evaluated by measuring the apoptosis rate of HCC cells in tumors was significantly enhanced, compared with free drug. Moreover, in this study, apoptosis induced by the nanoparticulate doxorubicin was specific and restricted to HCC tumors, since it did not enhance the apoptosis rate of noncancer hepatocytes in peritumor areas. The authors expect that higher apoptosis induced by doxorubicin loaded in PACA nanoparticles may be associated with a better outcome and overall survival of mice. However, further studies are needed to confirm this hypothesis.

A more sophisticated approach designed to improve further the efficacy of doxorubicin-loaded PACA nanoparticles in overcoming MDR involved simultaneous inhibition of P-gp using cyclosporin A. The nanoparticles were prepared so that doxorubicin was incorporated within the core of the nanoparticles, whereas cyclosporin A was located at the nanoparticle surface. In vitro experiments using a coculture of resistant cells and macrophages showed that the association of both doxorubicin and cyclosporin A within a single nanoparticle elicited the most effective growth rate inhibition of the resistant cells, whereas the doxorubicin-loaded nanoparticles by themselves can only partially overcome the MDR. The enhanced activity of the drug-loaded nanoparticles was interpreted to be a result of a synergistic effect: a high amount of cyclosporin A was released at the surface of the cell membrane, reaching the same sites as doxorubicin at the same time and thus facilitating intracellular diffusion of the drug.

So far PACA nanoparticles appear to be the only type of nanoparticle that can overcome the P-gp-related resistance to doxorubicin, owing to a the unique combination of factors, such as appropriate rates of drug release and bidegradation and the right chemistry of the counterion.

4.3. Overcoming the Blood-Brain Barrier

Systemically administered chemotherapy is often not very effective in the treatment of brain tumors. An important reason for this low efficacy is insufficient drug delivery to the tumor site owing to the presence of the blood-brain barrier (BBB), which is a complex interface that separates blood from the extracellular fluid in brain parenchyma (53,54). The structural BBB is formed by endothelial cells that line the cerebral vasculature. Compared with peripheral endothelia, these cells exhibit several fundamental differences: they are sealed together by tight junctions, they have very few fenestrations, and they display low pinocytic activity. This physical barrier restricts aqueous paracellular diffusional pathways between the blood and brain extracellular fluid. Moreover, the brain vessel endothelial cells have a high electrical resistance, which is responsible for the poor penetration of polar and ionic substances. Diffusion across the BBB is feasible for lipophilic molecules (<500 Daltons); however, accumulation of these molecules in the brain is often restricted owing to the ABC efflux transporters, such as P-gp or multidrug resistance proteins (MRPs).

The BBB function can be considerably compromised by tumor growth. As shown by tomography and magnetic resonance (MR) imaging, microvascular permeability correlates with tumor histologic grade. Whereas the vasculature of low-grade gliomas is close to normal, high-grade gliomas are characterized by both neovascularization and vascular hyperpermeability, which is similar to other solid tumors, although less pronounced (40,55–57). In contrast to normal cerebral capillaries, vessels in gliomas are tortuous and sinusoidal; they are characterized by open interendothelial and transendothelial gaps, fenestrations, and increased microvascular diameter (3–40 μm vs approx 3–5 μm for cortical capillaries) and vessel wall thickness (0.5 μm vs 0.26 μm) (58). These abnormalities contribute to an increase in nonselective transendothelial transport and microvascular permeability and, consequently, impairment of the BBB functions at the tumor site.

These features of the vascular microenvironment in gliomas have implications for the development of new drug targeting technologies. Thus, it has been hypothesized that the structural abnormalities of glioma vessels could facilitate intratumoral penetration of the stealth nanoparticles owing to the EPR effect.

This hypothesis was confirmed by the results of the comparative biodistribution study of the stealth (PEGylated) and nonstealth PACA [poly(hexadecyl cyanoacrylate)] nanoparticles in rats bearing intracranial 9L glioblastoma (59). Although both carriers were able to extravasate across the BBB at the tumor site, accumulation of the stealth particles in tumor was more than three times higher, compared with conventional particles. Moreover, a four- to eightfold higher accumulation of the PEGylated nanoparticles was also observed in parts of the brain protected by the normal BBB. This result is important since microvascular permeability in gliomas is heterogeneous and in some parts of the tumor the barrier function is retained.

In contrast, analysis of the pharmacokinetic data allowed the authors to conclude that if the mechanism of intratumoral accumulation was similar for PEGylated and non-PEGylated carriers and could be considered as a diffusion/convection process, an affinity of PEGylated particles for the normal brain was allowed by specific interaction of the PEGylated particles with the BBB endothelial cells. Therefore, the important features of the steric barrier produced by the stealth agent not only to protect the particle from opsonization thus increasing circulation time but also not to interfere with the cell membrane recognition step (10).

Interestingly, the efficacy of doxorubicin bound to these PEGylated nanoparticles in treatment of the intracranial 9L glioblastoma in rats was not improved, compared with the free drug (60). As shown by the authors, loading of the particles with doxorubicin resulted in impairment of stealth properties owing to reversion of the surface charge. Doxorubicin-loaded particles became positively charged, whereas the charge of unloaded particles was negative. The positively charged particle interacted with plasma proteins, which caused an increase in their effective size and massive accumulation in lungs and spleen, thus diverting them from brain.

As shown by extensive pharmacological studies, the nanoparticles made of polybutyl cyanoacrylate and coated with polysorbate 80 (Tween® 80) allowed brain delivery of a number of drugs normally unable to cross the BBB (e.g., loperamide, tubocurarine, dalargin, kytorphine) (61).

The effectiveness of drug delivery system based on polybutyl cyanoacrylate nanoparticles coated with polysorbate 80 was further demonstrated in rats with intracranial 101/8 glioblastomas (62). In the group treated with doxorubicin loaded in coated nanoparticles, increase in survival time reached 84%, compared with the untreated control. More than 20% animals in this group showed long-term remission; absence of tumor was confirmed by histology 6 mo post treatment. A moderate increase in survival time was also observed in the control groups treated with doxorubicin administered as a free drug in a solution of polysorbate 80 or bound to noncoated particles. Since none of these preparations was able to deliver doxorubicin to the brain of healthy animals (63), this effect is most probably explained by a higher permeability of the BBB at the tumor site that allowed entry of other formulations into the brain. It is noteworthy that clinical and histological signs of neurotoxicity were absent in this study.

The mechanism of drug transport to the brain by means of nanoparticles is not clear. The pharmacokinetic rule states that the mass of drug delivered to the brain is equally proportional to the plasma AUC and the BBB permeability coefficient (64). Indeed, enhanced brain delivery to the healthy brain by means of long-circulating nanoparticles was observed in a number of studies (10,14,65). In general and similarly to the transport of nanoparticles to other non-MPS sites, the process of brain uptake is influenced by the physicochemical parameters of the particle (e.g., size, charge, and hydrophobicty) and the chemistry and content of the surface-modifying agents. The correlation of plasma and brain concentrations suggests that the enhanced drug transport into the brain with the long-circulating nanoparticles is a result of the increased blood-brain gradient of the drug concentration.

However, prediction of brain uptake of the nanoparticle-bound drug on the basis of the circulation behavior is not always unequivocal. In contrast to the stealth nanoparticles, polybutyl cyanoacrylate particles coated with polysorbate 80 did not exhibit long-circulating behavior: the plasma AUC of doxorubicin bound to these particles was only moderately increased (by approx 70%). However, the concentration of doxorubicin in brain homogenate was very high: up to 6 µg/g. (The injected dose was 5 mg/kg; 63.)

Obviously, doxorubicin transport to the brain with polysorbate-coated nanoparticles cannot be explained by the increased blood-brain gradient. According to the pharmacokinetic rule just stated, it may be suggested that these particles increase the permeability of the BBB. However, results of the in-depth studies of Kreuter et al. provide evidence that the brain uptake of polybutyl cyanoacrylate nanoparticles coated with polysorbate 80 is not associated with an opening of the BBB caused by toxic effects (66).

Then it may be speculated that polysorbate 80-coated particles traverse the BBB via a specific mechanism. Indeed, numerous facts suggest that polybutyl cyanoacrylate nanoparticles coated with polysorbate 80 are taken up by brain capillary endothelial cells via receptor-mediated endocytosis (61,67). The following mechanism is proposed: in the bloodstream, the polysorbate coating acts as an anchor for plasma apolipoproteins E and/or B that adsorb to the surface of the particles. The nanoparticles thus mimic lipoprotein particles and interact with the lipoprotein receptors expressed in the membranes of the endothelial cells constituting the BBB; then they enter these cells via receptor-mediated endocytosis.

The results of another study suggest that the ability of polysorbate 80-coated nanoparticles to deliver drugs to the brain is not only mediated by adsorption of apolipoprotein E and/or B but probably also involves "teamwork" on the part of other apolipoproteins that prevent the hepatic uptake of the particles, thus facilitating brain delivery (68).

Other possibilities, such as transcytosis across the BBB or inhibition of the efflux mechanisms (P-gp), by the mechanism discussed above, remain to be investigated.

In fact, it is possible that different particles permit drug delivery to the brain by different pathways.

5. OPPORTUNITIES FOR ACTIVE TARGETING

Active targeting is achieved by means of a specific interaction of a homing moiety/vector with a receptor on the tumor cell surface. This is in contrast to passive targeting (discussed above) realized owing to the natural (passive) biodistribution of a carrier, which is governed by its physicochemical parameters, and the physiological (or patho-physiological) condition of a target. Various coupling methods for binding homing moieties/vectors to the nanoparticles and the related problems are summarized in ref. *69*.

Although active drug targeting using nanoparticles has not yet been extensively investigated, the proof of concept is well established. In this case also, long-circulating carriers bearing homing ligands have a higher probability of reaching the target if it is accessible from the vasculature. Several examples of successful targeting are presented below.

5.1. Targeting to the Transferrin Receptors

Membrane transferrin receptor-mediated endocytosis is an efficient cellular uptake pathway. This receptor system has been widely studied and exploited for the site-specific delivery of anticancer drugs because it is overexpressed in many tumors *(70)*. In particular, nanoparticle-based drug delivery systems with conjugated transferrin ligand or the antibodies against transferrin receptor (OX26 monoclonal antibody) have been explored in a number of studies *(71–75)*.

For example, PEG-coated biodegradable PACA nanoparticles conjugated to transferrin were used for paclitaxel delivery to S-180 solid tumors in mice *(72)*. After intravenous injection, the particles conjugated to transferrin produced a higher tumor accumulation of paclitaxel, as compared to paclitaxel in solution or bound to nonconjugated PEGylated particles. Accordingly, paclitaxel loaded in transferrin-modified particles was significantly more effective in terms of tumor growth inhibition and increase of life span.

In a murine model of prostate cancer, a single intratumoral injection of paclitaxel loaded in transferrin-conjugated nanoparticles produced a complete regression of tumor and a significantly higher survival rate, compared with nonvectorized nanoparticles or drug dissolved in Cremophor EL *(73)*. The mechanism of greater efficacy of transferrin-conjugated nanoparticles appears to be the greater cellular uptake of drug.

5.2. Targeting to the Folate Receptors

Another potential target is the folate receptor (folic acid). Folate offers many advantages as a targeting ligand: it is presumably nonimmunogenic owing to its small size, it has good stability, and it is highly specific for tumors. Elevated expression of the folate receptor has frequently been observed in various types of human cancers including ovarian, endometrial, colorectal, breast, lung, and renal cell carcinoma as well as brain metastases derived from epithelial cancers *(76)*.

A number of studies were aimed at the design of nanoparticles coupled to folic acid to target the folate-binding protein (e.g., refs. *77–80*).

Active targeting of methotrexate to KB tumor was achieved by means of acetylated dendrimer nanoparticles (<5 nm in diameter) conjugated to folic acid *(79)*. This conjugate was injected intravenously into immunodeficient mice bearing human KB tumors, which overexpress the folic acid receptor. In contrast to nontargeted carrier, folate-conjugated nanoparticles concentrated in the tumor and liver tissue over 4 d after administration. Confocal microscopy confirmed the internalization of the particles into the tumor cells. Active targeting not only increased antitumor activity of methotrexate but also markedly decreased its toxicity, thus improving the drug therapeutic index.

Efficacy of the lipophilic paclitaxel prodrug bound to SLNs that contained folate-polyethylene glycolcholesterol as a ligand was evaluated in mice bearing M109, a murine lung carcinoma that overexpresses folate receptors *(80)*. Treatment of mice with folate-targeted nanoparticles resulted in significantly higher tumor growth inhibition and animal survival compared with treatment with nontargeted SLNs or paclitaxel formulated in Cremophor EL.

5.3. Targeting the Tumor Neovasculature

Tumor growth depends on the neovasculature. Hence, mediators of angiogenesis represent potential targets for antiangiogenic therapy *(81)*. A novel approach to targeted gene therapy of tumor endothelium using nanoparticles is described by Hood et al. *(82)*. It was shown that cationic nanoparticles coupled to an integrin $\alpha_v\beta_3$-targeting ligand ($\alpha_v\beta_3$-NP) can deliver genes exclusively to the neovasculature in tumor-bearing mice with no expression in lung, liver, heart, or host vessels. Then $\alpha_v\beta_3$-NP was coupled to a mutant RAF gene, which blocks angiogenesis triggered by various growth factors but does not kill existing blood vessels. Systemic injection of these nanoparticles into tumor-bearing mice resulted in apoptosis of the tumor-associated endothelium, ultimately leading to tumor cell apoptosis. A significant regression in tumor size, with four of the six mice showing no tumor and the others with >95% reduction in tumor mass and >75% suppression in blood vessel density, was observed in this study. All the mice treated with empty targeting nanoparticles or loaded targeting nanoparticles injected with an excess of targeting ligand showed no signs of tumor growth inhibition.

6. CLINICAL TRIALS

A phase I clinical trial of doxorubicin loaded in PACA nanoparticles was conducted in 21 patients with refractory solid tumors in different localizations *(83)*. A total of 32 courses at 28-d intervals was administered at six dose levels (15–90 mg/m^2); the drug was given as an intravenous infusion. According to World Health Organization criteria, stable disease lasting 4 to 6 mo was reached only in 2/21 patients with a metastatic renal cell carcinoma and a metastatic anal squamous cell carcinoma. The low efficacy could be caused by insufficient selectivity of the formulation toward non-MPS-localized tumors.

A nanoparticulate formulation of paclitaxel based on albumin nanoparticles (ABI-007, Abraxane™) has recently been approved by the Food and Drug Administration for the treatment of metastatic breast cancer. Abraxane™ appeared to be more effective than Taxol® in terms of response rates (33 and 19%, respectively) and time to cancer progression (22 and 16 wk, respectively *(84)*. The efficacy of this formulation for the treatment of other cancers (e.g., advanced head and neck cancers and recurrent anal canal squamous cell carcinoma) has been previously demonstrated in a number of clinical studies (e.g., refs. *85–87*).

Owing to the absence of Cremophor EL as an excipient in the conventional formulation of paclitaxel (Taxol), the new formulation offers advantages in terms of safety (avoidance of hypersensitivity reactions) and morbidity (avoidance of premedication). In humans, paclitaxel plasma clearance and volume of distribution were significantly higher for the nanoparticulate drug than for Taxol, probably because of the absence of paclitaxel-sequestering Cremophor micelles *(88)*.

Preclinical studies showed a 33% greater tumor accumulation of ABI-007 compared with Taxol®. Accumulation of the nanoparticles in the tumor occurs via caveolae-mediated endocytosis in the endothelial cells of the tumor blood vessels, which is stimulated by interaction of the nanoparticle albumin with gp60 albumin receptors. Additionally, the particles find access to the tumor through the EPR effect *(84)*.

7. TOXICOLOGICAL ASPECTS

As mentioned above, the ultimate action of nanoparticles is the alteration of drug biodistribution. It is evident that the new distribution profile may influence the toxicity of the nanoparticle-bound drug. Side effects may be reduced owing to decreased access of the drug to the sites susceptible to toxicity, or, in contrast, altered distribution may generate new types of toxicity.

This assumption is illustrated by the case of doxorubicin bound to PACA nanoparticles (reviewed in ref. *3*). The quantitative parameters of acute toxicity of the nanoparticle-bound doxorubicin were similar to those of the free drug *(89)*. However, the safety profile was altered. It is known that doxorubicin displays pronounced cardiotoxicity that correlates with the peak cardiac concentration. Biodistribution studies revealed that nanoparticles produced an increase in plasma levels of doxorubicin, whereas the cardiac concentration was dramatically decreased. In accordance with the observed distribution profile, the cardiotoxicity of doxorubicin bound to nanoparticles was also reduced *(83,90)*. Inconstrast, the myelosuppressive effect of the nanoparticle-bound doxorubicin was more pronounced, which correlated with a higher concentration of the drug in the bone marrow and spleen *(91)*.

Another aspect is toxicity that could be associated with the nanocarriers themselves. This issue remains to be investigated. In this respect, the future challenge for toxicological studies is associated with understanding the ultimate fate of nanocarriers and their polymeric constituents in the body.

8. CONCLUSIONS

The data described in this chapter suggest that the nanoparticles, along with other techniques, may serve as a useful tool for achieving the main objective of regional cancer therapy: they can deliver a higher concentration of the agent to the tumor and can expose the tumor to active drug for longer periods than is safely possible with conventional formulations. This can be achieved via versatile routes. Indeed, nanoparticles can optimize drug biodistribution, reverse multidrug resistance, minimize drug side effects, or transport the drug across tight biological barriers, such as the BBB.

However, more work needs to be done to develop safe and efficient drugs to treat and perhaps prevent cancer. Obviously, an ideal drug delivery system capable of tumor targeting must be biomimetic: it must be able to travel in the body without recognition by defense systems and to use natural transport pathways to reach the target.

The rational design of long-circulating as well as target-specific nanoparticles that can avoid capture by the MPS organs relies on an understanding of the role of the different macrophage populations in the nanoparticle clearance and the nature of the scavenging properties of macrophages. More needs to be learned about the physicochemical nature of interactions between polymers and the cell surface, as well as the processes involved in trafficking the drug-loaded carriers to their cellular and intracellular targets, such as endocytic pathways, and other transport mechanisms governing the accumulation and elimination of drugs in the tumor. Adequate circulation profile and drug release characteristics must be explored along with the feasibility of specific cell/particle interactions.

Furthermore, a careful choice of adequate in vivo and in vitro models for evaluation and prediction of the therapeutic potential of the nanoparticulate drugs cannot be disregarded. Finally, the success of this technology will depend on toxicological issues that have only been marginally addressed so far.

The diversity of the targets will probably call to life a wide variety of colloidal carriers that will hopefully be developed not as competitive technologies but with the intention of producing a combinatorial delivery system for really specific tumor targeting. It can be expected that future research will concentrate on the development of vectorized delivery systems combining the advantages of the colloidal carriers, such as large payloads of a drug, with active targeting.

REFERENCES

1. Kreuter J. Nanoparticles., in Encyclopedia of Pharmaceutical Technology, vol. 10 (Swarbrick J, Boylan CJ, eds.), New York: Marcel Dekker, 1994:165.
2. Bala I, Hariharan S, Kumar MN. PLGA nanoparticles in drug delivery: the state of the art. Crit Rev Ther Drug Carrier Syst 2004;21:387–422.
3. Vauthier C, Dubernet C, Fattal E, Pinto-Alphandary H, Couvreur P. Poly(alkylcyanoacrylates) as biodegradable materials for biomedical applications. Adv Drug Deliv Rev 2003;25:519–548.
4. Couvreur P, Barratt G, Fattal E, Legrand P, Vauthier C. Nanocapsule technology: a review. Crit Rev Ther Drug Carrier Syst 2002;19:99–134.
5. Soppimath KS, Aminabhavi TM, Kulkarni AR, Rudzinski WE. Biodegradable polymeric nanoparticles as drug delivery devices. J Control Release 2001;70:1–20.
6. Wissing SA, Kayser O, Muller RH. Solid lipid nanoparticles for parenteral drug delivery. Adv Drug Deliv Rev 2004;56:1257–1272.
7. Moghimi SM, Hunter AC. Capture of stealth nanoparticles by the body's defences. Crit Rev Ther Drug Carrier Syst 2001;18:527–550.
8. Moghimi SM, Hunter AC, Murray JC. Long-circulating and target-specific nanoparticles: theory to practice. Pharmacol Rev 2001;53:283–318.
9. Moghimi SM, Szebeni J. Stealth liposomes and long circulating nanoparticles: critical issues in pharmacokinetics, opsonization and protein-binding properties. Prog Lipid Res 2003;42:463–478.
10. Calvo P, Gouritin B, Chacun H, et al. Long-circulating PEGylated polycyanoacrylate nanoparticles as new drug carrier for brain delivery. Pharm Res 2001;18:1157–1166.
11. Araujo L, Loebenberg R, Kreuter J. Influence of the surfactant concentration on the body distribution of nanoparticles. J Drug Targeting 1999;6:373–385.
12. Chen DB, Yang TZ, Lu WL, Zhang Q. In vitro and in vivo study of two types of long-circulating solid lipid nanoparticles containing paclitaxel. Chem Pharm Bull (Tokyo) 2001;49:1444–1447.
13. Redhead HM, Davis SS, Illum L. Drug delivery in poly(lactide-co-glycolide) nanoparticles surface modified with poloxamer 407 and poloxamine 908: in vitro characterisation and in vivo evaluation. J Controlled Release 2001;70:353–363.
14. Zara GP, Cavalli R, Bargoni A, Fundaro A, Vighetto D, Gasco MR. Intravenous administration to rabbits of non-stealth and stealth doxorubicin-loaded solid lipid nanoparticles at increasing concentrations of stealth agent: pharmacokinetics and distribution of doxorubicin in brain and other tissues. J Drug Target 2002;10:327–335.
15. Stolnik S, Daudali B, Arien A, et al. The effect of surface coverage and conformation of poly(ethylene oxide) (PEO) chains of poloxamer 407 on the biological fate of model colloidal drug carriers. Biochim Biophys Acta 2001;1514:261–279.
16. Gref R, Luck M, Quellec P, et al. 'Stealth' corona-core nanoparticles surface modified by polyethylene glycol (PEG): influences of the corona (PEG chain length and surface density) and of the core composition on phagocytic uptake and plasma protein adsorption. Colloids Surf B Biointerfaces 2000;18:301–313.
17. Peracchia MT, Vauthier C, Passirani C, Couvreur P, Labarre D. Complement consumption by poly(ethylene glycol) in different conformations chemically coupled to poly(isobutyl 2-cyanoacrylate) nanoparticles. Life Sci 1997;61:749–761.

18. Moghimi SM. Prolonging the circulation time and modifying the body distribution of intravenously injected polystyrene nanospheres by prior intravenous administration of poloxamine-908. A 'hepatic-blockade' event or manipulation of nanosphere surface in vivo? Biochim Biophys Acta 1997; 1336:1–6.

19. Moghimi SM, Gray T. A single dose of intravenously injected poloxamine-coated long-circulating particles triggers macrophage clearance of subsequent doses in rats. Clin Sci (Lond) 1997;93: 371–379.

20. Peracchia MT, Fattal E, Desmaele D, et al. Stealth PEGylated polycyanoacrylate nanoparticles for intravenous administration and splenic targeting. J Control Release 1999;60:121–128.

21. Jung T, Kamm W, Breitenbach A, Kaiserling E, Xiao JX, Kissel T. Biodegradable nanoparticles for oral delivery of peptides: is there a role for polymers to affect mucosal uptake? Eur J Pharm Biopharm 2000;50:147–160.

22. Florence AT, Hussain N. Transcytosis of nanoparticle and dendrimer delivery systems: evolving vistas. Adv Drug Deliv Rev 2001;50(suppl 1):S69–89.

23. Florence AT. Issues in oral nanoparticle drug carrier uptake and targeting. J Drug Target 2004;12:65–70.

24. Behrens I, Pena AI, Alonso MJ, Kissel T. Comparative uptake studies of bioadhesive and non-bioadhesive nanoparticles in human intestinal cell lines and rats: the effect of mucus on particle adsorption and transport. Pharm Res 2002;19:1185–1193.

25. Sakuma S, Sudo R, Suzuki N, et al. Behavior of mucoadhesive nanoparticles having hydrophilic polymeric chains in the intestine. J Control Release 2002;81:281–290.

26. Arbos P, Campanero MA, Arangoa MA, Irache JM. Nanoparticles with specific bioadhesive properties to circumvent the pre-systemic degradation of fluorinated pyrimidines. J Control Release 2004;16;96:55–65.

27. Yang S, Zhu J, Lu Y, Liang B, Yang C. Body distribution of camptothecin solid lipid nanoparticles after oral administration. Pharm Res 1999;16:751–757.

28. Ubrich N, Schmidt C, Bodmeier R, Hoffman M, Maincent P. Oral evaluation in rabbits of cyclosporin-loaded Eudragit RS or RL nanoparticles. Int J Pharm 2005;288:169–175.

29. Moghimi SM, Hawley AE, Christy NM, Gray T, Illum L, Davis SS. Surface engineered nanospheres with enhanced drainage into lymphatics and uptake by macrophages of the regional lymph nodes. FEBS Lett 1994;344:25–30.

30. Moghimi SM. Modulation of lymphatic distribution of subcutaneously injected poloxamer 407-coated nanospheres: the effect of the ethylene oxide chain configuration. FEBS Lett 2003;540:241–244.

31. Moghimi SM, Rajabi-Siahboomi R. Advanced colloid-based systems for efficient delivery of drugs and diagnostic agents to the lymphatic tissues. Prog Biophys Mol Biol 1996;65:221–249.

32. Nishioka Y, Yoshino H. Lymphatic targeting with nanoparticulate system. Adv Drug Deliv Rev 2001;47:55–64.

33. Jain RK. (2001) Delivery of molecular medicine to solid tumors: lessons from in vivo imaging of gene expression and function. J Control Release 2001;74:7–25.

34. Padera TP, Stoll BR, Tooredman JB, Capen D, di Tomaso E, Jain RK. Cancer cells compress intratumour vessels. Nature 2004;427:695.

35. Maeda H, Fang J, Inutsuka T, Kitamoto Y. Vascular permeability enhancement in solid tumor: various factors, mechanisms involved and its implications. Int Immunopharmacol 2003;3:319–328.

36. Yi Y, Kim JH, Kang HW, Oh HS, Kim SW, Seo MH A polymeric nanoparticle consisting of mPEG-PLA-Toco and PLMA-COONa as a drug carrier: improvements in cellular uptake and biodistribution. Pharm Res 2005; 22:200–208.

37. Miura H, Onishi H, Sasatsu M, Machida Y. Antitumor characteristics of methoxypolyethylene glycol-poly(DL-lactic acid) nanoparticles containing camptothecin. J Control Release 2004;97:101–113.

38. Lenaerts V, Labib A, Chouinard F, Rousseau J, Ali H, van Lier. Nanocapsules with a reduced liver uptake: targeting of phthalocyanines to EMT-6 mouse mammary tumor in vivo. Eur J Pharm Biopharm 1995;41:38–43.

39. Kaul G, Amiji M. Biodistribution and targeting potential of poly(ethylene glycol)-modified gelatin nanoparticles in subcutaneous murine tumor model. Drug Target 2004;12:585–591.

40. Hobbs SK, Monsky WL, Yuan F, et al. Regulation of transport pathways in tumor vessels: role of tumor type and microenvironment. Proc Natl Acad Sci USA 1998;95:4607–4612.

41. Lode J, Fichtner I, Kreuter J, Berndt A, Diederichs JE, Reszka R. Influence of surface-modifying surfactants on the pharmacokinetic behavior of ^{14}C-poly(methylmethacrylate) nanoparticles in experimental tumor models. Pharm Res 2001;18:1613–1619.

42. Moghimi SM, Hunter AC, Murray JC. Nanomedicine: current status and future prospects. FASEB J 2005;19:311–330.

43. Barratt G. Colloidal drug carriers: achievements and perspectives. Cell Mol Life Sci 2003;60:21–37.

44. Brigger I, Dubernet C, Couvreur P. Nanoparticles in cancer therapy and diagnosis. Adv Drug Deliv Rev 2002;54:631–651.

45. Brannon-Peppas L, Blanchette JO. Nanoparticle and targeted systems for cancer therapy. Adv Drug Deliv Rev 2004;56:1649–1659.

46. Feng S-S, Chien S. Chemotherapeutic engineering: application and further development of chemical engineering principles for chemotherapy of cancer and other diseases. Chem Eng Sci 2003;58: 4087–4114.

47. Chiannilkulchai N, Driouich Z, Benoit JP, Parodi AL, Couvreur P. Doxorubicin-loaded nanoparticles: increased efficiency in murine hepatic metastases. Sel Cancer Ther 1989;5:1–11.

48. Chiannilkulchai N, Ammoury N, Caillou B, Devissaguet JP, Couvreur P. Hepatic tissue distribution of doxorubicin-loaded nanoparticles after i.v. administration in reticulosarcoma M 5076 metastasis-bearing mice. Cancer Chemother Pharmacol 1990;26:122–126.

49. Li YP, Pei YY, Zhou ZH, et al. Stealth polycyanoacrylate nanoparticles as tumor necrosis factor-alpha carriers: pharmacokinetics and anti-tumor effects. Biol Pharm Bull 2001;24:662–665.

50. Lehne G. P-glycoprotein as a drug target in the treatment of multidrug resistant cancer. Curr Drug Targets 2000;1:85–99.

51. Vauthier C, Dubernet C, Chauvierre C, Brigger I, Couvreur P. Drug delivery to resistant tumors: the potential of poly(alkyl cyanoacrylate) nanoparticles. J Control Release 2003;93:151–160.

52. Barraud L, Merle P, Soma E, et al. Increase of doxorubicin sensitivity by doxorubicin-loading into nanoparticles for hepatocellular carcinoma cells in vitro and in vivo. J Hepatol 2005;42:736–743.

53. Begley DJ. Delivery of therapeutic agents to the central nervous system: the problems and the possibilities. Pharmacol Ther 2004;104:29–45.

54. Lee G, Dallas S, Hong M, Bendayan R. Drug transporters in the central nervous system: brain barriers and brain parenchyma considerations. Pharmacol Rev 2001;53:569–596.

55. Roberts HC, Roberts TP, Bollen AW, Ley S, Brasch RC, Dillon WP. Correlation of microvascular permeability derived from dynamic contrast-enhanced MR imaging with histologic grade and tumor labeling index: a study in human brain tumors. Acad Radiol 2001;8:384–391.

56. Pluen A, Boucher Y, Ramanujan S, et al. Role of tumor-host interactions in interstitial diffusion of macromolecules: cranial vs. subcutaneous tumors. Proc Natl Acad Sci U S A 2001;98:4628–4633.

57. Vajkoczy P, Menger MD. Vascular microenvironment in gliomas. Cancer Treat Res 2004; 117: 249–262.

58. Schlageter KE, Molnar P, Lapin GD, Groothuis DR. Microvessel organization and structure in experimental brain tumors: microvessel populations with distinctive structural and functional properties. Microvasc Res 1999; 58: 312–328.

59. Brigger I, Morizet J, Aubert G, et al. Poly(ethylene glycol)-coated hexadecylcyanoacrylate nanospheres display a combined effect for brain tumor targeting. J Pharmacol Exp Ther 2002;303:928–936.

60. Brigger I, Morizet J, Laudani L, et al. Negative preclinical results with stealth® nanospheres-encapsulated doxorubicin in an orthotopic murine brain tumor model. J Control Release 2004;100:29–40.

61. Kreuter J. Transport of drugs across the blood-brain barrier by nanoparticles. Curr Med Chem 2002;2:241–249.

62. Steiniger SCJ, Kreuter J, Khalansky AS, et al. Chemotherapy of glioblastoma in rats using doxorubicin-loaded nanoparticles. Int J Cancer 2004;109:159–167.

63. Gulyaev, AE, Gelperina SE, Skidan IN, et al. Significant transport of doxorubicin into the brain with Ps 80-coated nanoparticles. Pharm Res 1999; 16:1564–1569.

64. Pardridge WM. Non-invasive drug delivery to the human brain using endogeneous blood-brain barrier systems. PSTT 1999;2:49–59.

65. Yang SC, Lu LF, Cai Y, Zhu JB, Liang BW, Yang CZ. Body distribution in mice of intravenously injected camptothecin solid lipid nanoparticles and targeted effect on brain. J Control Release 1999;59:299–307.

66. Kreuter J, Ramge P, Petrov V, et al. Direct evidence that polysorbate-80-coated poly(butylcyanoacrylate) nanoparticles deliver drugs to the CNS via specific mechanisms requiring prior binding of drug to the nanoparticles. Pharm Res 2003;20:409–416.

67. Kreuter J, Shamenkov D, Petrov V, et al. Apolipoprotein-mediated transport of nanoparticle-bound drugs across the blood-brain barrier. J Drug Targeting 2002;10:317–326.

68. Gessner A, Olbrich C, Schroeder W, Kayser O, Muller RH. The role of plasma proteins in brain targeting: species dependent protein adsorption patterns on brain-specific lipid drug conjugate (LDC) nanoparticles. Int J Pharm 2001;214:87–91.

69. Nobs L, Buchegger F, Gurny R, Allemann E. Current methods for attaching targeting ligands to liposomes and nanoparticles. J Pharm Sci 2004;93:1980–1992.

70. Li H, Sun H, Qian ZM. The role of the transferrin-transferrin-receptor system in drug delivery and targeting. Trends Pharmacol Sci 2002;23:206–209.

71. Bellocq NC, Pun SH, Jensen GS, Davis ME. Transferrin-containing, cyclodextrin polymer-based particles for tumor-targeted gene delivery. Bioconjug Chem 2003;14:1122–1132.

72. Xu Z, Gu W, Huang J, et al. In vitro and in vivo evaluation of actively targetable nanoparticles for paclitaxel delivery. Int J Pharm 2005;288:361–368.

73. Sahoo SK, Ma W, Labhasetwar V. Efficacy of transferrin-conjugated paclitaxel-loaded nanoparticles in a murine model of prostate cancer. Int J Cancer 2004;112:335–340.

74. Li Y, Ogris M, Wagner E, Pelisek J, Rüffer M. Nanoparticles bearing polyethyleneglycol-coupled transferrin as gene carriers: preparation and in vitro evaluation. Int J Pharm 2003;259:93–101.

75. Olivier J-C, Huertas R, Lee HJ, Calon F, Pardridge WM. Synthesis of pegylated immunoparticles. Pharm Res 2002;19:1137–1143.

76. Sudimack J, Lee RJ. Targeted drug delivery via the folate receptor. Adv Drug Delivery Rev 2000;41:147–162.

77. Oyewumi MO, Yokel RA, Jay M, Coakley T, Mumper RJ. Comparison of cell uptake, biodistribution and tumor retention of folate-coated and PEG-coated gadolinium nanoparticles in tumor-bearing mice. J Control Release 2004;95:613–626.

78. Hattori Y, Maitani Y. Enhanced in vitro DNA transfection efficiency by novel folate-linked nanoparticles in human prostate cancer and oral cancer. J Control Release 2004;97:173–183.

79. Kukowska-Latallo JF, Candido KA, Cao Z, et al. Nanoparticle targeting of anticancer drug improves therapeutic response in animal model of human epithelial cancer. Cancer Res 2005;65:5317–5324.

80. Stevens PJ, Sekido M, Lee RJ. A folate receptor-targeted lipid nanoparticle formulation for a lipophilic paclitaxel prodrug. Pharm Res 2004;21:2153–2157.

81. Murray JC, Moghimi SM. Endothelial cells as therapeutic targets in cancer: new biology and novel delivery systems. Crit Rev Ther Drug Carrier Syst 2003;20:139–152.

82. Hood JD, Bednarski M, Frausto R, et al. Tumor regression by targeted gene delivery to the neovasculature. Science 2002; 296:2404–2407.

83. Kattan J, Droz JP, Couvreur P, et al. Phase I clinical trial and pharmacokinetic evaluation of doxorubicin carried by polyisohexylcyanoacrylate nanoparticles. Invest New Drugs 1992;10:191–199.

84. Garber K. Improved paclitaxel formulation: hints at new chemotherapy approach. J Natl Cancer Inst 2004;96:91–92

85. Ibrahim NK, Desai N, Legha S, et al. Phase I and pharmacokinetic study of ABI-007, a Cremophor-free, protein-stabilized, nanoparticle formulation of paclitaxel. Clin Cancer Res 2002;8:1038–1044.

86. Damascelli B, Cantu G, Mattavelli F, et al. Intraarterial chemotherapy with polyoxyethylated castor oil free paclitaxel, incorporated in albumin nanoparticles (ABI-007): phase II study of patients with squamous cell carcinoma of the head and neck and anal canal: preliminary evidence of clinical activity. Cancer 2001;92:2592–2602.

87. Damascelli B, Patelli GL, Lanocita R, et al. A novel intraarterial chemotherapy using paclitaxel in albumin nanoparticles to treat advanced squamous cell carcinoma of the tongue: preliminary findings. AJR Am J Roentgenol 2003;181:253–260.

88. Sparreboom A, Scripture CD, Trieu V, et al. Comparative preclinical and clinical pharmacokinetics of a cremophor-free, nanoparticle albumin-bound paclitaxel (ABI-007) and paclitaxel formulated in cremophor (Taxol). Clin Cancer Res 2005;11:4136–4143.

89. Gelperina SE, Khalansky AS, Skidan IN, et al. Toxicological studies of doxorubicin bound to polysorbate 80-coated poly(butyl cyanoacrylate) nanoparticles in healthy rats and rats with intracranial glioblastoma. Toxicol Lett 2002;126:131–141.

90. Couvreur P, Kante B, Grislain L, Roland M, Speiser P. Toxicity of polyalkylcyanoacrylate nanoparticles II: doxorubicin-loaded nanoparticles. J Pharm Sci 1982;71:790–792.

91. Gibaud S, Andreux JP, Weingarten C, Renard M, Couvreur P. Increased bone marrow toxicity of doxorubicin bound to nanoparticles. Eur J Cancer 1994;30A:820–826.

12 Local Gene Therapy for Cancer

Wolfgang Walther, PhD, Ulrike S. Stein, PhD, and Peter M. Schlag, MD, PhD

CONTENTS

INTRODUCTION
LOCAL CANCER GENE THERAPY
CONCLUSIONS
REFERENCES

SUMMARY

Cancer is an important problem in public health worldwide. Gene therapy has the potential for improved treatment of cancer patients, particularly if used in combination with other, conventional therapies. To date, many strategies of gene therapy have been explored, including correction of mutant genes, immunstimulation, prodrug activation, interference of oncogene expression, and genetically modified oncolytic viruses. Although the preclinical results of gene therapy have shown promise for some cancers, cancer gene therapy is still at an early stage of clinical development and has not yet shown a significant therapeutic benefit for patients. The main obstacles to the introduction of gene therapy for patients are poor selectivity in vector targeting, inefficient gene transfer, and great difficulties in systemic application. Owing to the complex nature of targeted vector delivery to the tumor, strategies for gene therapy have focused their efforts on the development of local gene transfer to treat tumors locally for the benefit of the patient. This is not the answer for the treatment of a metastasizing systemic disease; however, it represents an important step toward the clinical applicability of cancer gene therapy. Furthermore, local control of tumor growth and progression could contribute to better control of the disease and improved quality of life for the patient.

Key Words: Gene therapy; cancer; local treatment; vectors; therapeutic genes.

1. INTRODUCTION

1.1. Strategies for Cancer Gene Therapy

Remarkable developments and advances, particularly in the molecular biology of cancer, have provided the tools and helped to define the targets for cancer gene therapy. Such knowledge has pointed researchers' attention to the tight relationship beween a

From: *Cancer Drug Discovery and Development: Regional Cancer Therapy*
Edited by: P. M. Schlag and U. S. Stein © Humana Press Inc., Totowa, NJ

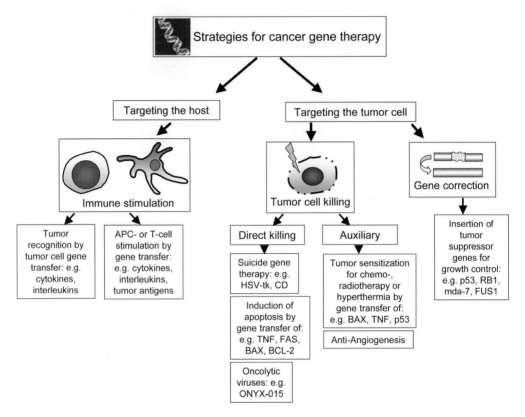

Fig. 1. Strategies used for gene therapy of cancer, which can be aimed either at the host's own immune system (to strengthen antitumor defense mechanisms), directly at the tumor for genetic correction of defined genes, or at tumor cell killing.

better understanding of tumor biology and physiology and a potential improvement in cancer gene therapy. Originally, gene therapy was defined as treatment by administration to patients of therapeutic genes or genetically modified cells. Since the first clinical gene therapy for adenosine deaminase (ADA)-deficient severe combined immunodeficiency (SCID) was initiated in 1990, 1076 gene therapy trials have been performed or are in progress worldwide (*see* www.wiley.co.uk/genmed). Access to genes of therapeutic potential and the establishment of feasible vector systems for gene transfer moved gene therapy from the lab to clinical applications, reflected by the growing number of clinical cancer gene therapy trials. Currently, more than 66% of all gene therapy trials worldwide involve cancer therapy.

Very different strategies have been developed to fight cancer; such strategies aim at either the tumor cell killing or inhibition of tumor cell growth, by directing gene therapy either to the tumor cells or to the host's own tumor defense, represented by the immune system (Fig. 1). These very different strategies imply gene repair for restoration of normal gene function of nonfunctional genes in cancer cells, the restimulation or enhancement of antitumoral activity of the patient's immune defense mechanisms against the tumor, the selective eradication of tumor cells by inducing apoptosis/ necrosis, suicide mechanisms using additive gene insertion of cell-killing genes, or the

Table 1
Strategies and Genes Used for Cancer Gene Therapy

Additive insertion of therapeutic genes
   For immunostimultion
      Cytokine genes: IFN-α, IFN-γ, IL-2, -4, -7, -10, and -12, GM-CSF, G-CSF, TNF-α
      Genes coding for costimulatory molecules or HLA determinants, e.g., B7–1, B7–2
      Genes encoding tumor antigens for tumor vaccination: CEA, PSA

   For tumor cell killing
      Suicide genes for gene-directed enzyme prodrug therapy (GDEPT): HSV-tk, CD,
         nitroreductase
      Apoptosis genes: BAX, FAS
      Multidrug resistance genes for chemoprotection in high-dose chemotherapy: MDR-1, MRP-1

   For tumor sensitization
      Genes for chemo- or radiosensitization, e.g., TNF-α, IL-2, p53, BAX

Substitution of mutated/nonfunctional genes
   Tumor suppressor genes/cell cycle regulatory genes:, e.g., RB-1, mda-7, p53, p21^{CIP1}, p16^{INK1}

Interference with gene expression
   siRNA: against growth factors and oncogenes (e.g., VEGF, c-erb2, c-fos, c-myc, K-ras)
   Ribozymes: against multidrug resistance genes (e.g., MDR-1, MRP-1)
   Antisense oligodeoxyribonucleotides (e.g., c-myc, Ha-ras, Bcl-2)

Abbreviations: CD, cytosine deaminase; CEA, carcinoembryonic antigen; G-CSF, granulocyte colony-stimulating factor; GM-CSF, granulocyte/macrophage colony stimulating factor; HLA, human lymphocyte antigen; HSV-tk, herpes simplex virus thymidine kinase; IL, interleukin; IFN, interferon; MDR1, multidrug resistance gene 1; MRP1, multidrug resistance related protein 1; PSA, prostate-specific antigen; RB-1, retinoblastoma gene 1; TNF, tumor necrosis factor; VEGF, vascular endothelial growth factor.

sensitization of tumor towards chemo- and radiotherapy or hyperthermia treatment (Fig. 1 and Table 1).

Gene correction therapy is the strategy of repairing mutated genes responsible for carcinogenesis or tumor suppression, since it is known that tumors develop as a result of an accumulation of the mutational activation of oncogenes coupled with the inactivation of tumor suppressor genes (1). Although it would appear an impossible task to repair all mutations, some of these mutations (e.g., mutated p53) are crucial for the maintenance and progression of the tumor. Therefore, correcting some of these mutations could inhibit tumor growth. Such an approach has been explored for correction of mutated p53 with wild-type (wt)-p53 to inhibit tumor growth and to induce apoptosis, which was clinically tested in a pilot study with non-small cell cancer patients (2).

In suicide gene therapy, which is also called gene-directed enzyme prodrug therapy (GDEPT), cancer cells are transduced with an enzyme-encoding gene (Table 1). This enzyme permits conversion of a nontoxic prodrug into a toxic metabolite (3). Consequently, cancer cells expressing the suicide gene are killed. In addition, surrounding cells, which do not express the suicide gene, are also killed by the *bystander effect (4,5)*. The bystander effect plays an important role in prodrug therapy. For example, significant tumor regression was observed in all mice with colorectal cancer xenografts treated with 5-fluorouracil, when only 2% of the tumor harbors cytosine deaminase (CD)-expressing cells and 98% non-CD-expressing wild-type cells (4).

Gene immune therapy is the strategy to activate an immune response against cancer cells. In the phase of cancer initiation, many transformed cells are thought to be recognized and destroyed by the host immune system. However, once cancer tissue has been established, it has escaped immune surveillance by downregulation of molecules governing the immune response, e.g., loss of class I antigen on tumor cells, lack of costimulatory signals, secretion of immunoinhibitory cytokines. To overcome these mechanisms, several strategies of gene immune therapy have been explored: (1) cytokine gene transfer to tumor cells, antigen presenting cells (APCs) or T cells; (2) co-stimulation with B7; and (3) vaccination against tumor-associated antigens (Table 1).

Despite the great variety of gene therapeutic approaches, most cancer gene therapy protocols focus on strategies to target prodrug converting enzymes as suicide genes or stimulation of antitumor immunity for tumor eradication (Table 1). In addition, during the last few years the area of tumor sensitization has received more attention. This is particularly fueled by the conviction that gene therapy can produce greater patient benefit if applied in combination with other established therapies, such as chemo- or radiotherapy, which then could lead to significant improvements in therapeutic efficacies *(6,7)* (Table 1).

1.2. Vector Systems Employed for Cancer Gene Therapy

All the different gene therapeutic strategies utilize nucleic acids as the active reagent either to express the desired proteins possessing therapeutic potential or to interfere with the expression of tumor-associated target genes at transcriptional or translational levels. The intense search for suitable vector systems to introduce genes into tumor cells led to the development of viral and nonviral vectors (Table 2). Many experimental and clinical studies have shown that selection of the right vector for a specific application is crucial to successful gene therapy. The criteria for an ideal vector include efficient and target-specific delivery of the foreign DNA into the cell nucleus, tight and regulated expression of the transgene associated with no or low toxicity and easy, inexpensive production of the vector of clinically relevant quality and at suitable quantity. During the last decade vecterology has made many advances in the improvement of transfer efficiency and selectivity of transgene expression by retargeting viral and nonviral vectors and by using tumor-specific or -inducible promoters. Particularly for virus vectors, cell-type specific promoters derived from carcinoembryonic antigen, tyrosinase, L-plastin, erbB-2, DF3/Muc1, human telomerase, caspase-8, survivin, and secretory leukoprotease inhibitor have been used to limit transgene expression to the tumor *(8–14)*. In addition, conditionally active promoters have also been used to control gene expression by physiologic conditions (hypoxia) or by chemotherapy- or radiation-induced stress *(15,16)*. Such regulable systems are of particular interest if cancer gene therapy is combined with conventional treatment modalities.

1.2.1. VIRAL VECTORS

Viral vectors are still the most efficient gene transfer vehicles; they combine an ability to infect high proportions of cells in a cell population with a great capacity for transgene insertion in their genetically modified genome *(17)*. The number of viral vector constructs possessing different features for targeted infection (high infectivity or the ability to infect resting, differentiated cell populations), safety features or cell type-specific expression is growing rapidly. Most of the current research is attempting to refine these

Table 2
Vectors and Delivery Systems for Cancer Gene Therapy

Viral vector systems[a]
  Retrovial vectors
  Adenoviral vectors
  Herpes Simplex Virus vectors
  Vaccinia Virus vectors
  Newcastle Disease Virus vector
  AAV vectors
  Measels virus
  Reovirus

Nonviral vector systems
  Liposomal systems
  Plasmid-DNA (naked DNA)
  Antisense oligonucleotides
  Ribozymes
  siRNA
  Anaerobic bacteria

[a] Includes oncolytic virus systems based on replicative viruses (e.g., ONYX-015; HSV-1).

vectors for safe and more targeted gene transfer, to express the transgenes in tumors more efficiently. This implies the reduction of potential side effects of viral vector application to humans, such as immunogenicity, toxicities, homologous recombination, or insertional mutagenesis *(18,19)*. Since cancer gene therapy is applied to a wide variety of cancers possessing very different biological characteristics, viral vectors have been adapted for specific applications. Numerous different viral vector systems have been developed for ex vivo and in vivo gene transfer, which are mainly derived from murine and human RNA and DNA viruses. The most commonly used vectors were developed from retroviruses, lentiviruses, adenovirus, herpes simplex virus, vaccinia virus, and adeno-associated virus. They possess useful characteristics for target cell infectivity, appropriate transgene capacity, and accessibility of established helper cell lines for production of recombinant virus stocks to infect target cells (Table 2). Many more different virus vector systems are under development, such as human cytomegalovirus, Epstein-Barr virus, poxviruses, and foamy virus; these have begun to enter clinical testing *(17)*.

Retroviral vectors are efficient transfer systems for introduction of foreign genes into target cells. These vectors are widely used in gene therapy (in about 25% of clinical gene therapy protocols). Retroviral vectors are derived from RNA viruses, which use reverse-transcriptase for conversion of their viral RNA genome into a double-stranded viral DNA that is then stably inserted into the host DNA. Members of this class of RNA viruses are the murine leukemia viruses (MuLVs) and the lentiviruses, which are extensively used for virus vector engineering.

Adenoviruses are most commonly used for cancer gene therapy, since these vectors achieve temporal high-level transgene expression combined with high gene transfer efficacy of the recombinant virus particles associated with broad tissue tropism in humans. Clinical protocols are being developed using adenoviral vectors for transfer of the herpes simplex virus thymidine kinase (HSV-tk) suicide gene for treatment of head and neck cancer, non-small cell lung cancer, ovarian cancer, brain tumors, and prostate cancer. Furthermore, adenoviral vectors are also employed for gene transfer of immuno-stimulatory cytokine genes such as interleukin-2 (IL-2) or granulocyte/macrophage colony-stimulating factor (GM-CSF) into tumors. Alternatively, adenovirus vectors are used for the transfer of the wild-type p53 tumor suppressor gene to induce growth arrest in tumors that are defective in normal p53 function. Apart from the use of adenovirus vectors as carriers for transgenes, the virus itself provides antitumor activity targeting tumor cells with defective p53. In this context, replication-competent vectors were generated lacking the E1B 55-kDa gene, which normally binds and inactivates wild-type p53 for efficient viral replication (20). The mutant adenovirus (ONYX-015) therefore only replicates in p53-deficient tumor cells, leading to cytopathic effects and virus spread within the tumor (21). This strategy is termed *virotherapy* and uses oncolytic viruses that are capable of virus replication, thus permitting virus spread within the tumor. Among the oncolytic viruses, HSV and reovirus vectors are also used to eradicate tumors specifically.

1.2.2. NONVIRAL VECTORS

For nonviral gene therapy, liposomal systems or naked DNA are usually used for gene delivery. The most progress has been made in the use of liposomal transfer systems, whereby DNA is complexed with cationic lipids or encapsulated in liposomal microspheres. Currently 8.6% of all gene therapy trials use liposomes for gene delivery. Many liposomal systems are in clinical testing for gene transfer, whereby lipofection is applied systemically or by local injection, or delivered as an aerosol (e.g., for gene transfer to the lungs) (24). Among these methods, the dimethylaminoethane carbamoyl-cholesterol-dioleylphosphatidyl ethanolamine (DC-cholesterol-DOPE) or dimethyl hydroxyethyl ammonium-dioleyloxy propyl trimethyl ammonium chloride (DMRIE-DOTMA) systems are widely used in clinical cancer gene therapy studies (25). They are liposomal formulations with high efficiency for cellular entry and low toxicity.

Nonviral transfer of naked DNA for gene therapy is an alternative to liposomal or viral gene transfer technologies. Currently 16% of all gene therapy trials are based on naked DNA gene transfer approaches (*see* www.wiley.co.uk/genmed). Naked DNA gene transfer is mainly used for genetic immunization, DNA vaccination, and cancer gene therapy applications. Most of this research is attempting to introduce DNA constructs, which encode proteins or peptides for induction of immune responses or result in antibody production in the host. For these intradermal, intratumoral, or intramuscular applications, naked DNA has proved to be efficient as a cancer vaccine in numerous animal models (26–31). Particularly for local delivery, different physical procedures have been employed in vitro and in vivo, such as simple needle and syringe injection, a hydrodynamics procedure, particle bombardment (by gene gun), in vivo electroporation, and jet injection (32–37).

2. LOCAL CANCER GENE THERAPY

Gene delivery is a decisive factor for successful gene therapy. Clinical cancer gene therapy trials have shown that in vivo transduction efficiency represents the major barrier for therapeutically relevant treatments and is a key factor in establishing clinically usable cancer gene therapy. A sufficiently high transduction efficiency is particularly important

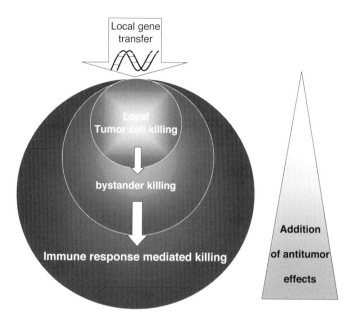

Fig. 2. Schematic representation of the concept of local cancer gene therapy. The initial local application of the viral or nonviral vector leads to local (intratumoral) expression of the therapeutic gene, which in parallel can generate an bystander effect, leading to the more efficient killing of tumor cells. Local eradication of tumor cells provokes additional responses in the host (patient), which then might augment the antitumor effects of the gene therapy.

for treatment of cancers, since unaffected surviving tumor cells can reemerge to cause recurrent disease after incomplete therapy. These serious hurdles determine the strategies for in vivo cancer gene therapy approaches. Numerous experimental and clinical efforts have clearly shown that at the current stage, systemic application of viral or nonviral gene therapy vectors is still accompanied by too many obstacles, which hinder tumor-specific vector targeting by circumventing side effects for normal tissues. Thus, local gene transfer has come into use for immunostimulatory and direct tumor cell killing strategies. Although local gene therapy cannot target a metastasizing disease (except when used for immunostimulation), such an approach is the essential first step in fulfilling the initial expectations for cancer gene therapy. This is why, in many clinical gene therapy studies, the vectors (virus particles, liposomes, naked DNA, and so on) are applied intratumorally or in close vicinity to the tumor site. The concept of an ideal local cancer gene therapy implies a local killing effect of the therapeutic gene in tight association with the bystander effect, which could then provoke additional defense mechanisms including the host's immune system (Fig. 2). Many experimental studies suggest that such a multistep concept could generate promising therapeutic effects for local disease control and the benefit of cancer patients.

2.1. Target Sites for Local Gene Therapy

The vast majority of clinical gene therapy trials are set up with the intention of stimulating an antitumor immune response. However, a second important strategy is direct tumor killing by gene therapy via suicide gene transfer, apoptosis-inducing genes, or oncolytic viruses. To achieve this, most clinical efforts employ local gene transfer by direct targeting of the tumor or tumor vicinity (Table 3). Almost 20% of all cancer gene therapy trials are using local gene transfer for viral or nonviral vectors to ensure efficient tumor-targeted transgene expression, since numerous obstacles still exist for systemically targeted gene delivery. Although retargeting of viral particles and the use of tumor-targeted liposomes show promise, the problem of unwanted gene transfer to normal tissues remains, which might generate side effects in the patient.

In this context, most clinical gene therapy treatments are given as intratumoral, peritumoral, or intraleasional applications/injections of either virus vectors, liposomal systems, or nonviral vectors. Clinical studies for breast cancer employed intratumoral/ intraleasional application of wild-type p53-expressing adenovirus or the liposomal transfer of the E1A gene to suppress tumorigenicity and to promote apoptosis in the tumor (38). Such studies have clearly shown the impact of a sufficiently high level of transgene expression for relevant antitumor effects. In a similar manner, colon cancer or liver metastases of colon cancer have been treated by local administration of the desired vector system, usually by needle injection directly into the tumor of DNA-liposome complexes, naked DNA, or adenoviruses, that express suicide (HSV-tk, CD) or tumor suppressor genes (wild-type p53).

Gene therapeutic treatment of brain tumors, in particular of malignant glioblastomas has a comparatively long history of clinical trials. Most of them stereotactically applied the vector into the tumor site or the intraleasional cavity during or shortly after surgery to eliminate remaining tumor cells (39,40). The vector applied locally for glioblastoma treatment has been retroviral, adenoviral, HSV-derived, liposomal, or genetically engineered virus producer cells, to infect the tumor cells actively in situ. Most of these approaches were used to introduce suicide (HSV-tk) expressing vectors for glioblastoma eradication. More recently, oncolytic viruses (HSV-1, ONYX-015) have been applied locally for brain tumor virotherapy (41,42). In brain tumors stereotactic application of gene therapy has generated limited but measurable success, reflected by partially extended survival and generation of stable disease (43).

Clinical gene therapy trials for non-small cell lung cancer (NSCLC) have used local instillation of DNA-liposome complexes or adenovirus, with computed tomographic guidance for flexible needle bronchoscopic injection or bronchoalveolar lavage (44,45). In a high percentage of these studies, gene transfer was used to introduce the wild-type p53 gene. Stable disease was partially achieved in NSCLC patients. More encouraging are local wild-type p53 gene transfer studies for NSCLC, in which local gene therapy is combined with radiation. Almost identical approaches are used for head and neck cancers (HNCs); these tumors are also treated locally by introducing wild-type p53-expressing nonviral vectors or adenovirus. In addition, this type of tumor has been extensively used for clinical studies of intratumoral injection of the oncolytic, replication-competent adenovirus ONYX-015 (46). Local gene therapy for HNC patients generated partial or even complete responses. The combination of local application of ONYX-015 and chemotherapy caused tumors to shrink in 25 of 30 cases treated (47). ONYX-015 has also been widely used for local treatment of ovarian and pancreatic cancers by intratumoral or intraperitoneal injections to ensure efficient infection of the tumor tissue (48,49).

Malignant melanomas are easily accessible for local gene transfer, and treatment of distant metastases is anticipated. Numerous clinical gene therapy studies have used direct intratumoral injection of nonviral DNA-liposome complexes or adenoviral vectors to express the HSV-tk suicide gene or the wild-type p53 tumor suppressor in the tumor *(50,51)*. These studies had varying success rates: low transfer efficiencies were observed. A more promising approach is the intratumoral or peritumoral injection of DNA/lipid formulations for expression of costimulatory molecules (HLA-B7, interferon-γ [IFN-γ]), which led to local tumor regression and partial or complete responses associated with increase in MAGE-A1 or tyrosinase antibodies *(52,53)*.

Among many other possible tumor entities, prostate cancer has also been preferably targeted in clinical studies by intratumoral injection gene transfer using liposomal formulations or adenovirus to express suicide (HSV-tk or fusion HSV-tk/CD) or cytokine genes. As an important parameter of this disease, reduction in serum prostate-specific antigen (PSA)-levels has been observed in several local gene therapy studies, indicating a reduction in tumor progression of treated patients *(54–56)*.

Gene therapy protocols for bladder cancer mostly use intravesical gene transfer, since this organ is easily accessible for local gene therapy. Adenovirus vectors are usually used for the expression of wild-type p53 gene or suicide genes. The major obstacle for bladder cancer gene therapy, however, is the glycosaminoglycan layer on the bladder mucosa, which can interfere with the entry of the adenovirus. Therefore, current efforts focus on modification of adenovirus fibers to improve viral infectivity *(57)*.

In contrast to the aforementioned gene transfer strategies, which use intratumoral application, ovarian cancer is mainly treated by intraperitoneal gene transfer, delivering the desired viral or nonviral (liposomal) vector system close to the tumor. Gene transfer in this tumor type has met with limited success, so recent approaches have focussed on intraperitoneal instillation of oncolytic adenovirus for improved eradication.

In the summary of clinical trials shown in Table 3, it can be seen that most studies aimed at local control of a particular tumor type by intratumoral or close-to-the-tumor gene transfer for tumor cell killing or local attraction of antitumor targeted immune responses. In this sense, local gene therapy can be defined as direct genetic intervention in the disease, primarily to achieve local control or eradication of the tumor mass.

2.2. Methods of Local Gene Delivery

Independently of the tumor entity, most clinical gene therapy studies employ local needle injection or stereotactic injection/instillation of the vector, since this methodology does not require additional technical efforts. Alternative methods of application are rarely used in clinical protocols. However, a growing arsenal of novel and efficient technologies, defined as physical delivery techniques, is being developed for local in vivo gene transfer to improve transfer efficiency and to lower the DNA load required for therapeutically relevant transgene expression *(58)* (*see* Table 4). This point is an important consideration, since for clinical application the cost and the effectiveness should be well balanced.

During the last decade, the physical gene transfer technologies came into focus as an attractive alternative for local gene delivery of nonviral but also of viral vectors. The simplest method is intratumoral needle injection of the desired vector either as naked DNA, a DNA-liposome formulation, or a viral particle. Apart from virus vectors and liposomes, it has been shown that simple needle injection is sufficient to transduce naked DNA into muscle tissue; this technique is largely inefficient for other tissues including tumors. Therefore, numerous studies have focused on the modification of this procedure for optimization of transfer efficiencies, particularly for nonviral systems *(36,59)*. This

Table 3
Clinical Use of Local Gene Transfer for Cancer Gene Therapy (as of July 2005)

Tumor entity	Site of gene transfer	Vectors used	Genes transferred
Bladder carcinoma	Intravesical transfer	Adenovirus (AdH5)	RB-1, wt-p53, HSV-tk, oncolysis[a]
		Fowl pox virus	B7.1/ICAM-1/LFA-3[b]
Brain tumors	stereotactic intratumoral	Retrovirus (RV)	HSV-tk
	Intratumoral/intracerebral	P317 RV-producer	HSV-tk
		AdH5	HSV-tk, IL-12
	Intratumoral	HSV-1, AdH5	Oncolysis
		Polio/rhinovirus	Oncolysis
Breast carcinoma	Intratumoral	DMRIE-DOPE	HLA-B7/B2 microglobulin, E1A
	Intraleasional/intratumoral	AdH5	wt-p53, B7.1, IL-12, mda-7
	Intraperitoneal/intrapleural	RV	Anti-c-myc, anti-c-fos RNA
Colon carcinoma	Intratumoral (including hepatic metastases)	Plasmid-DNA	CEA
		DMRIE-DOPE	HLA-B7/B2 microglobulin
	Intratumoral/hepatic artery	AdH5	CD, HSV-tk, wt-p53, IL-2/HSV-tk, IL-12,
	Infusion (for hepatic metastases)		TNF-α
Head/neck carcinoma	Intratumoral/intraleasional	DMRIE-DOPE	HLA-B7/B2 microglobulin
	Intratumoral	DMRIE-DOTMA	IL-12
		DC-Chol-DOPE	E1A, antisense EGF-DNA
		Plasmid-DNA	IFN-α, IL-12
		AdH5	HSV-tk, wt-p53
		Avipox virus	B7.1/ICAM-1/LF3-A
Lung carcinoma	Intratumoral	DMRIE-DOPE	wt-p53, IL-2
		AdH5	wt-p53, HSV-tk, IL-2
		RV	wt-p53, IL-2, antisense K-ras
Leptomeningeal carcinoma	Intrathecal	RV	HSV-tk

Cancer	Route	Vector	Gene/Therapy
Malignant melanoma	Intratumoral	Plasmid electroporaton	IL-12
		Plasmid-DNA	IL-12/IFN-α
		DMRI-DOPE	HLA-B7/B2 microglobulin, IL-2, IL-12
		AdH5	HSV-tk, IFN-γ, factorVII-hFc fusion gene, mda-7, wt-p53
	Intratumoral/peritumoral	RV	IFN-γ
	Intratumoral	HSV-1	Oncolysis
		Fowlpox virus	Oncolysis
Ovarian carcinoma	Intrapleural	DC-Chol-DOPE	E1A
	Intraperitoneal	PEG-PEI-cholesterol	IL-12
		RV	BRCA-1
		AdH5	HSV-tk, wt-p53, anti-erbB2 antibody cDNA, oncolysis
Pancreatic carcinoma	Intratumoral	AdH5	TNF-α, HSV-tk
Prostate cancer	Intratumoral	DMRIE-DOPE	HLA-B7/B2 microglobulin, IL-2
		RV	Antisense c-myc
		AdH5	HSV-tk, wt-p53, CD-HSV-tk fusion gene, p16, IL-12, IFN-β, TRAIL, oncolysis
		Vaccinia virus/fowlpox virus	PSA/B7.1/ICAM-1/LFA-3/GM-CSF
Renal cell carcinoma	Intratumoral	DMRIE-DOPE	HLA-B7/B2 microglobulin, IL-2
Retinoblastoma	Intraocular	AdH5	HSV-tk
Soft tissue sarcoma	Intratumoral	AdH5	TNF-α
		HSV-1	Oncolysis

Abbreviations, Ad: adenovirus; CD, cytosine deaminase; DC-chol, dimethylaminoethane carbamoyl cholesterol; DMRI, dimethyl hydroxyethyl ammonium; DOPE–dioleylphosphatidyl ethanolamine; DOTMA, dioleyloxy propyl trimethylammonium chloride; EGF, epidermal growth factor; GM-CSF, granulocyte macrophage colony stimulating factor; HLA, human lymphocyte antigen; HSV, herpes simplex virus; HSV-tk, herpes simples virus thymidine kinase; IFN, interferon; IL, interleukin; PEG, polyethylene glycol; PEI, polyethylenimine; PSA, prostate specific antigen; RV, retrovirus; TNF, tumor necrosis factor; TRAIL, TNF related apoptosis inducing ligand.

[a] Oncolysis: recombinant replication-competent viruses used for oncolytic virotherapy.

[b] Such listing represents application of gene combinations in the gene therapy trial.

Table 4
Methods for Local Gene Transfer with Potential for Use in Cancer Gene Therapy

Method of gene transfer	Vector transferred
Intratumoral needle injection	Viral vectors, DNA-liposome complexes, naked plasmid-DNA, oligonucleotides, siRNA
Hydrodynamic pressure procedure via arterial system	Naked plasmid-DNA,
Organ perfusion (intravenous vector application by venal occlusion)	Viral vectors, DNA-liposome complexes, naked DNA
In vivo electroporation	Naked plasmid-DNA
Ballistic delivery (gene-gun) for dermal, intramuscular, or intratumoral application	Naked plasmid-DNA
Jet injection for intratumoral application	Naked plasmid-DNA, DNA-liposome complexes, virus vectors, siRNA
Ultrasound-mediated delivery	Naked plasmid-DNA, DNA-liposome complexes
Laser beam transduction	Naked plasmid-DNA
Osmotic pump for continouos local application	DNA-liposome complex

resulted in the development of a the hydrodynamics-based procedure to deliver large volumes of more than 1 mL of naked DNA-containing solutions, which are either injected directly into the tissue or applied intraarterially within short periods of only a few seconds *(36,59)*. Although the efficiency of this procedure has been shown in several studies, it might be limited to the perfusion of specific organs or particular portions of the desired organ.

The use of electrical fields for gene transfer has evolved into the in vivo electroporation technology. This physical delivery technology has dramatically enhanced gene transfer efficiencies in different in vivo models and is applicable for clinical use *(58,60)*. It is mostly employed as an combination of needle injection of DNA followed by subsequent application of an electrical field to augment cellular entry of the vector. This procedure has been extensively and successfully tested for intratumoral gene transfer *(61)*.

Gene-gun, or ballistic, delivery uses DNA-coated microparticles, which are propelled into the target tissue for efficient gene transfer into different tissues. However, DNA penetration into the tissue is quite limited and therefore does not reach deeper areas. Thus most studies using ballistic delivery for nonviral gene transfer aim at immunostimulation or DNA vaccination approaches to target different areas in the skin and to affect APC populations *(62)*.

Jet injection has developed to an applicable technology. This technique allows gene transfer into different tissue types with deeper penetration of naked DNA. Jet injection is based on needleless application of fluid jets by pressurized air at high velocity into the target tissue. The energy applied to the DNA-containing fluid ensures dispersed penetration of comparatively low volumes. Because of technological improvements, this method can achieve transfer efficiencies that are comparable to in vivo electroporation or liposomal transfer systems *(37)*.

Many other new techniques for gene delivery (Table 4) might enter clinical testing soon. In addition, variations or combinations of the aforementioned physical delivery methods should help to improve transfer efficiencies.

3. CONCLUSIONS

Cancer is a complex disease and therefore cancer gene therapy is a challenging and difficult task. Despite the many obstacles in the history of cancer gene therapy, progress has been made. One major barrier is in vivo gene delivery, which was shown to have very limited transfer efficiency in clinical trials. For clinically relevant efficacy in tumor treatment, gene transfer into the tumor is decisive, for exerting tumor killing effects or generating stable disease by preventing recurrence. An analysis of current trials shows that local viral and nonviral gene transfer is presently one of the most feasible options, and therefore a high percentage of trials use this method for direct *in situ* intervention; numerous other techniques tested for systemic application lack significant tumor selectivity and transduction efficiency. Although local gene therapy will not cure a metastasizing malignancy, this approach could be beneficial for local control of tumor masses, for the rescue of vital affected organs, or to augment other, conventional therapies. In this regard, local cancer gene therapy will evolve into a valuable treatment option in a multimodality concept of cancer therapy.

REFERENCES

1. Cho KR, Vogelstein B. Genetic alterations in the adenoma-carcinoma sequence. Cancer 1992;70: 1727–1731.
2. Roth JA, Nguyen D, Lawrence DD, et al. Retrovirus-mediated wild-type p53 gene transfer to tumors of patients with lung cancer. Nature Med 1996;2:985–991.
3. Moolten FL. Drug sensitivity ("suicide") genes for selective cancer chemotherapy. Cancer Gene Ther 1994;1:279–287.
4. Huber BE, Austin EA, Richards CA, Davis ST, Good SS. Metabolism of 5-fluorocytosine to 5-fluorouracil in human colorectal tumor cells transduced with cytosine deaminase gene: significant antitumor effects when only a small percentage of tumor cells express cytosine deaminase. Proc Natl Acad Sci U S A 1994;91:8302–8306.
5. Burrows FJ, Gore M, Smiley WR, et al. Purified herpes simplex virus thymidine kinase retroviral particles: III. Characterization of bystander killing mechanisms in transfected tumor cells. Cancer Gene Ther 2002;9:87–95.
6. Rasmussen H, Rasmussen C, Lempicki M, et al. TNFerade Biologic: preclinical toxicology of a novel adenovector with a radiation-inducible promoter carrying the human tumor necrosis factor alpha gene. Cancer Gene Ther 2002;9:951–957.
7. Walther W, Stein U. Therapeutic genes for cancer gene therapy. Mol Biotechnol 1999;13:21–28.
8. Siders WM, Halloran PJ, Fenton RG. Melanoma-specific cytotoxicity induced by a tyrosinase promoter-enhancer/herpes simplex virus thymidine kinase adenovirus. Cancer Gene Ther 1998;5: 281–291.
9. Peng XY, Won JH, Rutherford T, et al. The use of the L-plastin promoter for adenoviral-mediated, tumor-specific gene expression in ovarian and bladder cancer cell lines. Cancer Res 2001;61: 4405–4413.
10. Stackhouse MA, Buchsbaum DJ, Kancharla SR, et al. Specific membrane receptor gene expression targeted with radiolabeled peptide employing the erbB-2 and DF3 promoter elements in adenoviral vectors. Cancer Gene Ther 1999;6 : 209–219.

11. Shinoura N, Saito K, Yoshida Y, et al. Adenovirus-mediated transfer of bax with caspase-8 controlled by myelin basic protein promoter exerts an enhanced cytotoxic effect in gliomas. Cancer Gene Ther 2000;7:739–748.
12. Zhu ZB, Makhija SK, Lu B, et al. Incorporating the survivin promoter in an infectivity enhanced CRAd-analysis of oncolysis and anti-tumor effects in vitro and in vivo. Int J Oncol 2005;27:237–246.
13. Song JS, Kim HP, Yoon WS, et al. Adenovirus-mediated suicide gene therapy using the human telomerase catalytic subunit (hTERT) gene promoter induced apoptosis of ovarian cancer cell line. Biosci Biotechnol Biochem 2003;67:2344–2350.
14. Maemondo M, Saijo Y, Narumi K, et al. Gene therapy with secretory leukoprotease inhibitor promoter-controlled replication-competent adenovirus for non-small cell lung cancer. Cancer Res 2004;64:4611–4620.
15. Walther W, Stein U. Cell type specific and inducible promoters for vectors in gene therapy as an approach for cell targeting. J Mol Med 1996;74:379–392.
16. Robson T, Hirst DG. Transcriptional targeting in cancer gene therapy. J Biomed Biotechnol 2003;2:110–137.
17. Walther W, Stein U. Viral vectors for gene transfer: a review of their use in the treatment of human diseases. Drugs 2000;60:249–271.
18. Lotze MT, Kost TA. Viruses as gene delivery vectors: application to gene function, target validation, and assay development. Cancer Gene Ther 2002;9:692–699.
19. El-Aneed A. An overview of current delivery systems in cancer gene therapy. J Control Release 2004;94:1–14.
20. Bischoff JR, Kirn DH, Williams A, et al. An adenovirus mutant that replicates selectively in p53-deficient human tumor cells. Science 1996;274:373–6.
21. Heise C, Sampson-Johannes A, Williams A, et al. ONYX-015, an E1B gene-attenuated adenovirus, causes tumor-specific cytolysis and antitumoral efficacy that can be augmented by standard chemotherapeutic agents. Nat Med 1997;3:639–45.
22. Varghese S, Rabkin SD. Oncolytic herpes simplex virus vectors for cancer virotherapy. Cancer Gene Ther 2002;9:967–78.
23. Norman KL, Coffey MC, Hirasawa K, et al. Reovirus oncolysis of human breast cancer. Hum Gene Ther 2002;13:641–652.
24. Orson FM, Kinsey BM, Bhogal BS, Song L, Densmore CL, Barry MA. Targeted delivery of expression plasmids to the lung via macroaggregated polyethylenimine-albumin conjugates. Methods Mol Med 2003;75:575–590.
25. Templeton NS, Lasic DD, Frederick PM, Strey HH, Roberts DD, Pavlakis GN. Improved DNA:liposome complexes for increased systemic delivery and gene expression. Nat Biotechnol 1997;15:647–652.
26. Vahlsing HL, Yankauckas M, Sawdey SH, Gromkowski M, Manthorpe M. Immunization with plasmid DNA using a pneumatic gun. J Immunol Methods 1994;175:11–22.
27. Rakhmilevich AL, Turner J, Ford MJ, et al. Gene gun-mediated skin transfection with interleukin 12 gene results in regression of established primary and metastatic murine tumors. Proc Natl Acad Sci U S A 1996;93:6291–6296.
28. Liu MA, Ulmer J B. Gene based vaccines. Mol Ther 2000;1:497–500.
29. Turner JG, Tan J, Crucian BE, et al. Broadened clinical utility of gene gun-mediated granulocyte-macrophage colony-stimulating factor cDNA-based tumor cell vaccines as demonstrated with a mouse myeloma model. Hum Gene Ther 1998;9:1121–1130.
30. Davis HL, Demeneix BA, Quantin B, Coulombe J, Whalen RG. Plasmid DNA is superior to viral vectors for direct gene transfer into adult mouse skeletal muscle. Hum Gene Ther 1993;4:733–740.
31. Heinzerling L, Feige K, Rieder S, et al. Tumor regression induced by intratumoral injection of DNA coding for human interleukin 12 into melanoma metastases in grey horses. J Mol Med 2001;78:692–702.
32. Sikes ML, O'Malley BW, Finegold MJ, Ledley FD. In vivo gene transfer into rabbit thyroid follicular cells by direct DNA injection. Hum Gene Ther 1994;6:837–844.
33. Yang N-S, Burkholder J, Roberts B, Martinell B, McCabe D. In vivo and in vitro gene transfer to mammalian cells by particle bombardment. Proc Natl Acad Sci USA 1990;87:9568–9572.
34. Aihara H, Miyazaki J-I. Gene transfer into muscle by electroporation in vivo. Nat Biotechnol 1998;16:867–870.

35. Somiari S, Glasspool-Malone J, Drabick JJ, et al. Theory and in vivo application of electroporative gene delivery. Mol Ther 2000;2:178–187.

36. Liu F, Song YK, Liu D. Hydrodynamics-based transfection in animals by systemic administration of plasmid DNA. Gene Ther 1999;6:1258–1266.

37. Walther W, Stein U, Fichtner I, Malcherek L, Lemm M, Schlag PM. Non-viral in vivo gene delivery into tumors using a novel low volume jet-injection technology. Gene Ther 2001;8:173–180.

38. Hortobagyi GN, Hung MC, Lopez-Berestein G. A Phase I multicenter study of E1A gene therapy for patients with metastatic breast cancer and epithelial ovarian cancer that overexpresses HER-2/neu or epithelial ovarian cancer. Hum Gene Ther 1998;9:1775–1798.

39. Ram Z, Culver KW, Oshiro EM, et al. Therapy of malignant brain tumors by intratumoral implantation of retroviral vector-producing cells. Nat Med 1997;3:1354–61.

40. Immonen A, Vapalahti M, Tyynela K, et al. AdvHSV-tk gene therapy with intravenous ganciclovir improves survival in human malignant glioma: a randomised, controlled study. Mol Ther 2004;10:967–972.

41. Rainov NG. A phase III clinical evaluation of herpes simplex virus type 1 thymidine kinase and ganciclovir gene therapy as an adjuvant to surgical resection and radiation in adults with previously untreated glioblastoma multiforme. Hum Gene Ther 2000;11:2389–2401

42. Chiocca EA, Abbed KM, Tatter S, et al. A phase I open-label, dose-escalation, multi-institutional trial of injection with an E1B-attenuated adenovirus, ONYX-015, into the peritumoral region of recurrent malignant gliomas, in the adjuvant setting. Mol Ther 2004;10:958–966.

43. Lawler SE, Peruzzi PP, Chiocca EA. Genetic strategies for brain tumor therapy. Cancer Gene Ther 2006;13:225–233.

44. Roth JA, Swisher SG, Merritt JA, et al. Gene therapy for non-small cell lung cancer: a preliminary report of a phase I trial of adenoviral p53 gene replacement. Semin Oncol 1998;25:33–37.

45. Swisher SG, Roth JA, Nemunaitis J, et al. Adenovirus-mediated p53 gene transfer in advanced non-small-cell lung cancer. J Natl Cancer Inst 1999;91:763–771.

46. Nemunaitis J, Khuri F, Ganly I, et al. Phase II trial of intratumoral administration of ONYX-015, a replication-selective adenovirus, in patients with refractory head and neck cancer. J Clin Oncol 2001;19:289–298.

47. Khuri FR, Nemunaitis J, Ganly I, et al. A controlled trial of intratumoral ONYX-015, a selectively-replicating adenovirus, in combination with cisplatin and 5-fluorouracil in patients with recurrent head and neck cancer. Nat Med 2000;6:879–885.

48. Heise C, Ganly I, Kim YT, Sampson-Johannes A, Brown R, Kirn D. Efficacy of a replication-selective adenovirus against ovarian carcinomatosis is dependent on tumor burden, viral replication and p53 status. Gene Ther 2000;7:1925–1929.

49. Hecht JR, Bedford R, Abbruzzese JL, et al. A phase I/II trial of intratumoral endoscopic ultrasound injection of ONYX-015 with intravenous gemcitabine in unresectable pancreatic carcinoma. Clin Cancer Res 2003;9:555–561.

50. Klatzmann D, Cherin P, Bensimon G, et al. A phase I/II dose-escalation study of herpes simplex virus type 1 thymidine kinase "suicide" gene therapy for metastatic melanoma. Study Group on Gene Therapy of Metastatic Melanoma. Hum Gene Ther 1998;9:2585–2594.

51. Dummer R, Bergh J, Karlsson Y, et al. Biological activity and safety of adenoviral vector-expressed wild-type p53 after intratumoral injection in melanoma and breast cancer patients with p53-overexpressing tumors. Cancer Gene Ther 2000;7:1069–1076.

52. Stopeck AT, Hersh EM, Akporiaye ET, et al. Phase I study of direct gene transfer of an allogeneic histocompatibility antigen, HLA-B7, in patients with metastatic melanoma. J Clin Oncol 1997;15:341–349.

53. Fujii S, Huang S, Fong TC, et al. Induction of melanoma-associated antigen systemic immunity upon intratumoral delivery of interferon-gamma retroviral vector in melanoma patients. Cancer Gene Ther 2000;7:1220–1230.

54. Herman JR, Adler HL, Aguilar-Cordova E, et al. In situ gene therapy for adenocarcinoma of the prostate: a phase I clinical trial. Hum Gene Ther 1999;10:1239–1249.

55. Freytag SO, Khil M, Stricker H, et al. Phase I study of replication-competent adenovirus-mediated double suicide gene therapy for the treatment of locally recurrent prostate cancer. Cancer Res 2002;62:4968–4976.

56. DeWeese TL, van der Poel H, Li S, et al. A phase I trial of CV706, a replication-competent, PSA selective oncolytic adenovirus, for the treatment of locally recurrent prostate cancer following radiation therapy. Cancer Res 2001;61:7464–7472.

57. Irie A. Advances in gene therapy for bladder cancer. Curr Gene Ther 2003;3:1–11.
58. Wells DJ. Gene therapy progress and prospects: electroporation and other physical methods. Gene Ther 2004;11:1363–1369.
59. Zhang G, Song YK, Liu D. Long-term expression of human alpha1-antitrypsin gene in mouse liver achieved by intravenous administration of plasmid DNA using hydrodynamics-based procedure. Gene Ther 2000;7:1344–1349.
60. Yamashita Y, Shimada M, Hasegawa H, et al. Electroporation-mediated interleukin-12 gene therapy for hepatocellular carcinoma in the mice model. Cancer Res 2001;61:1005–1012.
61. Heller LC, Coppola D. Electrically mediated delivery of vector plasmid DNA elicits an antitumor effect. Gene Ther 2002;9:1321–1325.
62. Seigne J, Turner J, Diaz J, et al. Feasibility study of gene gun mediated immunotherapy for renal cell carcinoma. J Urol 1999;162:1259–1263.

III | INDICATIONS AND RESULTS FOR DIFFERENT TUMOR ENTITIES

13 Regional Chemotherapy of Primary and Metastatic Liver Tumors

Rebecca Taylor, MD, James Tomlinson. MD, and Nancy Kemeny, MD

Contents

Summary

The rationale for hepatic arterial infusion of chemotherapy is based on the concept that most primary and metastatic liver tumors preferentially derive their blood supply from the hepatic artery, whereas normal hepatic tissue relies on the portal venous blood supply. In addition, the ability of the hepatic parenchyma to metabolize chemotherapy drugs to nontoxic metabolites offers a unique opportunity to administer highly toxic drug levels to tumor cells while minimizing systemic toxicity. Regional chemotherapy has been evaluated in both primary and metastatic hepatic malignancies with varying results. The area of most intensive research has been in the treatment of colorectal cancer because it represents the most frequent etiology of hepatic metastases. Although the response rate with newer agents used in systemic combination chemotherapy has improved, the 2-year survival is only 25 to 39%. Hepatic-arterial infusion of chemotherapy produces higher response rates, with a 2-yr survival of 50 to 60%. In patients who can undergo liver resection followed by hepatic-arterial infusion, the 2-yr survival is 85%. This chapter summarizes the pharmacological basis and technical aspects of

From: *Cancer Drug Discovery and Development: Regional Cancer Therapy*
Edited by: P. M. Schlag and U. S. Stein © Humana Press Inc., Totowa, NJ

hepatic arterial infusion, including catheter placement, infusion regimens, and the development and treatment of unique toxicities. In addition, it will review the current evidence and role of hepatic arterial infusion for all primary and secondary hepatic malignancies, with a focus on liver metastases from colorectal cancer, as this is the area of most experience and promise.

Key Words: Intraarterial infusions; liver neoplasms; colorectal neoplasms; neoplasm metastasis; hepatic artery; drug therapy; antineoplastic agents; infusion pumps, implantable.

1. INTRODUCTION

The treatment of liver metastases and primary liver cancer is an important concern in oncology. Primary hepatocellular carcinoma is diagnosed in 1 million patients per year, predominantly in eastern countries, whereas colorectal cancer is seen in 900,000 patients per year, predominantly in western countries. Surgical resection remains the optimal therapeutic option in patients with either malignancy. Hepatic arterial infusion (HAI) of chemotherapy has been employed as an alternative or combination treatment in the palliative, adjuvant, and neoadjuvant setting. The exact role of HAI in the treatment of primary and secondary hepatic neoplasms and how it will fit into current treatment strategies are still being defined.

2. RATIONALE AND ANATOMICAL BASIS OF HAI

The concept of regional chemotherapy for hepatic metastases via HAI is based on several principles. First, tumor cells from gastrointestinal malignancies, especially colorectoal cancer (CRC), spread hematogenously via the portal circulation, making the liver the first site of metastases in most patients (1). This stepwise spread of cancer from primary site to liver and from there to other organs provides an opportunity to prevent dissemination of tumor to other sites by direct treatment of hepatic metastases. Second, once hepatic metastases grow beyond 2 to 3 mm in size, they derive more than 80% of their blood supply from the hepatic artery, whereas normal hepatocytes are perfused primarily by the portal circulation (2). Infusion of chemotherapy via the hepatic artery could achieve toxic levels in tumor cells with relative sparing of normal hepatic parenchyma. Third, extraction of drug from the hepatic arterial circulation via the first-pass effect can result in high local concentrations and minimal systemic toxicity. The ideal agent should have a steep dose-response curve to maximize local antitumor activity, a high extraction rate to minimize systemic toxicity, and rapid total body clearance once infusion is discontinued. The two most commonly used agents in HAI are fluorouracil (5-FU) and fluorodeoxyuridine (FUDR). Both drugs have a steep response curve, but FUDR has a 95% hepatic extraction when given via HAI, compared with 19 to 55% for 5-FU (3). In the case of FUDR, this results in a 16-fold higher concentration in hepatic tumors, compared with venous administration. HAI of mitomycin, cisplatin, irinotecan, etoposide, and doxorubicin have all shown significantly less extraction and therefore less advantage over systemic administration (4–7). Finally, because hepatic drug uptake and metabolism are saturable processes, high drug delivery rates may exceed the hepatic capacity and diminish the regional advantage. For this reason chemotherapy is given via a slow continuous infusion to maintain a constant drug level below the hepatic capacity.

3. TECHNICAL ASPECTS OF HAI

3.1. Methods of Infusion

Several techniques are used for the delivery of HAI chemotherapy, including percu-taneously placed catheters, arterial access ports, and surgically placed implantable pumps. Early studies of HAI used a percutaneously placed hepatic artery catheter that was at-tached to an external infusion pump. These catheters were removed after each chemo-therapy session and reinserted before the next. The requirement for prolonged patient stay and bed rest during infusion, as well as the frequent complications of catheter-associated thrombosis, bleeding, infection, and migration of the catheter (5), have resulted in this technique falling out of favor. Most centers now use a totally implantable infusion pump or a subcutaneous access port with an external portable pump.

The implantable arterial port can be accessed intermittently or continuously and has a metal body with a silicone membrane that reseals after each access. Its use requires an external pump. By comparison, the implantable pump is self-contained; it is slightly larger than a pacemaker and is placed in a subcutaneous pocket at the time of surgery. Most implantable pumps have two chambers separated by titanium bellows. The inner drug chamber, containing the solution to be infused, is accessed by a central port and can hold 20 to 60 mL of fluid. The outer charging chamber contains a fluorocarbon liquid in equilibrium with its vapor phase. The vapor pressure provides the power source, exerting pressure on the bellows and forcing the fluid in the pump through a 0.22-μm bacterial filter and a flow-regulating resistance element. The flow rates of individual pumps are factory calibrated to deliver a constant set ratio, as desired. Most pumps also have a side port, which bypasses the main chamber and goes directly into the catheter.

The Medtronic Iso Med Constant-Flow pump and the Arrow-Codman model 3000 (Fig. 1) and model 3000-16 Constant Flow Infusion pump have become the most popular. The latter is available in two sizes, the original 30-mL size and the new smaller 16-mL, model 3000-16. The Codman Model 3000 pumps are available in three flow ranges. The clini-cian can select from low-, medium-, and high-flow pumps, depending on the interval desired between patient visits for pump refills and pump applications. Typically, the reservoir is filled with a 2-wk supply of chemotherapy, followed by a 2-wk infusion of heparinized saline.

The subcutaneous pump has several advantages over the port. The continuous infusion with the pump decreases the rate of hepatic artery thrombosis, and the twice monthly filling of the port allows for more convenient ambulatory treatment. In one study, the implantable pump provided 115 d of chemotherapy administration, compared with 31 and 25 d, respectively, for surgically and percutaneously placed catheters attached to an external infusion device (8). A recent single-institution retrospective comparison of pumps vs ports found a lower therapy-relevant complication rate (30% vs 47%) and a higher complication-free survival time (12.2 vs 7.3 mo) in favor of pumps (9). Doci and colleagues (10) found a much higher device failure rate in implanted ports than with implanted pumps (90% and 32%, respectively). Furthermore, the median duration of hepatic access patency was 9 mo for ports and 28 mo for implantable pumps. The latter may better maintain hepatic artery patency by means of the constant flow through the artery, thereby preventing thrombus formation at the tip of the catheter. Hepatic arterial thrombosis is reported in as many as 50% of arterial access ports, whereas in studies using implantable pumps, hepatic artery thrombosis is reported in 10 to 15% of patients (11–13).

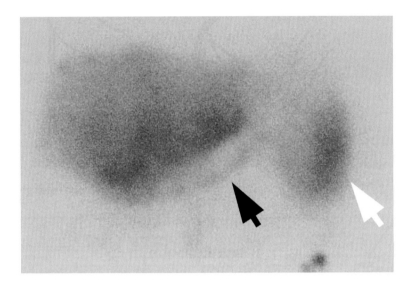

Fig. 3. [99mTc] macroaggregated albumin hepatic perfusion scans. After intravenous administration of [99mTc]-sulfur colloid to obtain baseline images, [99mTc]-macroaggregated albumin was administered via the side port of the hepatic arterial infusion pump. The dynamic image shows both liver perfusion and radiotracer uptake inferior to the liver (white arrow) and the right of the liver (black arrow), suggesting extrahepatic perfusion of the distal stomach and spleen respectively. The bright spot in the bottom right corner represents radiotracer pooling in the pump.

laparoscopy and portal node biopsy, cholecystectomy, and, increasingly, minimally invasive colon and hepatic resections. Early results suggest pump-related complications of 0 to 13%, similar to the rate reported for laparotomy (19,20). It remains to be seen whether the benefits typically ascribed to minimally invasive surgery, such as decreased pain and shorter hospitalization, will be seen following laparoscopic pump placement.

Percutaneous placement of hepatic artery catheters is advocated by some because of the reported high rate of technical success and decreased hospital stay and postoperative pain. They are, however, associated with their own complications, including peripheral artery aneurysms, tip migration, and the inability to perform a cholecystectomy. Aldrighetti et al. (21) compared percutaneous vs surgical placement of hepatic artery indwelling catheters and reported an overall incidence of device-related complications of 42.7% in the percutaneous group and 7.1% in the surgical group. This difference was attributed to a 35.7% incidence of catheter tip migration in the percutaneous group, which can be minimized by blocking the catheter in the gastroduodenal artery as opposed to leaving it free floating (22). In this study hospital stay was significantly less in the percutaneous group (1.8 vs 8.2 d), as were mean analgesic requirements.

Early pump-related complications are uncommon (5–10%) and usually technically related, including hepatic artery thrombosis, pump pocket hematomas, wound infections, underperfusion of liver, and/or extrahepatic perfusion. The 30-d mortality rate was low in two large recent series (0–0.7%) (23,24). Late complications or device malfunctions, such as catheter thrombosis or displacement, pump pocket infections, hepatic artery thrombosis, pump failure, and gastric or duodenal ulceration, have been reported in up to 30% of patients (9,23). Early pump-related complications are more likely to be salvaged than those occurring late (70% vs 30%) (25). The incidence of technical compli-

Table 1
Basic Guidelines for HAI Pump Therapy Evaluation

Preoperative evaluation
1. Rule out extrahepatic disease
   Chest X-ray
   CT chest, abdomen, and pelvis
   Colonoscopy (if metachronous)
   PET (can be considered—investigational)
2. Evaluate the hepatic vascular anatomy by celiac and superior mesenteric angiogram
   Identify gastric, duodenal, and pancreatic vessels
   Exclude patients whose liver is incompletely perfused/aberrant anatomy
   Exclude patients with portal vein thrombosis

Intraoperative evaluation by exploratory laparotomy
1. Biopsy portal and any suspicious lymph nodes
2. Place catheter in the gastroduodenal artery
3. Ligate all gastric, duodenal, and pancreatic vascular branches
4. Determine liver perfusion by fluorescein infusion into the side port

Post-operative evaluation
1. Reconfirm hepatic perfusion by macroaggregated albumin scan. Address extrahepatic
   perfusion by embolization as necessary

cations varies considerably with surgeon experience. In one study, the complication rate of pump placement was 37% for inexperienced surgeons and 6.6% for experienced surgeons (26). In a study of 544 consecutive cases of HAI pump placement, placement by a surgeon who had performed fewer than 25 earlier procedures was associated with a significantly higher rate of pump complications (31% vs 19%) (25).

4. PATIENT SELECTION AND EVALUATION

Candidates for regional therapy with HAI should have metastatic disease localized to the liver and be medically suitable for the surgical procedure. Extensive hepatic metastases (>70% replacement with tumor), moderate or severe hepatic insufficiency, and poor performance status are relative contraindications, as perioperative morbidity and mortality in those situations are high (27). Patients with portal vein thrombosis are at risk for significant hepatic ischemia and should not be considered. The preoperative evaluation should include a chest X-ray and CT scans of the chest, abdomen, and pelvis to rule out extrahepatic disease, as well as a recent colonoscopy for patients with metachronous disease (Table 1). As previously mentioned, all patients should undergo hepatic arteriography using CT angiography to define the hepatic arterial anatomy. Evidence of hepatic insufficiency and poor performance status should also be considered in the preoperative assessment.

5. ROLE OF HAI IN PRIMARY HEPATOBILIARY TUMORS

The role of regional hepatic drug delivery for primary hepatobiliary malignancies, including hepatocellular carcinoma (HCC), cholangiocarcinoma, and gallbladder cancer, has not been as extensively studied as its role in the treatment of CRC metastasis.

Table 2
Hepatic Artery Infusion (HAI) Chemotherapy Trials in HCC

Study	No. of Patients	Treatment	PR (%)	Median OS
Kinami and Miyazaki, 1978 (28)	14	HAI Mito-C	50	10 mo
Wellwood et al., 1979 (29)	28	HAI FUDR	54	NR
Olweny et al., 1980 (30)	10	HAI doxorubicin	60	NR
Cheng and Fortner, 1982 (31)	16	HAI cisplatin	19	NR
Urist, 1984 (32)	13	HAI doxorubicin	47	NR
Shildt and Stuckey, 1984 (33)	30	HAI FUDR, doxorubicin, Strepto	10	NR
Atiq et al., 1992 (34)	10	HAI FUDR, Mito-C, IFN	50	14.5 mo
Patt et al., 1994 (35)	29	HAI FUDR, LV, doxorubicin, cisplatin	41	15 mo
Carr, 1998 (36)	26	HAI Cisplatin	42	NR
Urabe et al., 1998 (37)	15	HAI MTX, 5-FU, cisplatin, IFN	47	7 mo
Okuda et al., 1999 (38)	31	HAI cisplatin, 5-FU	29	NR
Fazio and Manzoni, 2003 (39)	30	HAI Mito-C, cisplatin, 5-FU	11	8.6 mo

Abbreviations: 5-FU, 5-fluorouracil; FUDR, fluorodeoxyuridine; IFN, interferon; LV, leucovorin; Mito-C, mitomycin C; MTX, methotrepate; NR, not reported; OS, overall survival; PR, partial response.

5.1. Hepatocellular Carcinoma

Numerous small phase II trials have addressed the role of HAI chemotherapy for HCC (28–39) (Table 2). In one study, floxuridine and mitomycin were delivered via an implanted pump into the hepatic artery of patients with HCC or cholangiocarcinoma (34). Four of the eight patients with HCC achieved partial responses, and only one patient developed biliary toxicity. The median survival of all patients in the study was 14.5 mo.

Other investigators have studied the combination of the fluoropyrimidines and anthracyclines in HCC patients. In one study, patients were treated with either etoposide, Adriamycin, and Platinol (EAP) or etoposide, Platinol, and 5-FU (EDF) administered by a percutaneous catheter into the common or proper hepatic artery (40). This study reported a 50% objective partial response rate, at the expense of substantial hepatic and systemic toxicities.

HAI administration of floxuridine, leucovorin, Adriamycin, and Platinol (FLAP) (35,35), delivered through either a percutaneous catheter or an implanted pump over 4 d/cycle, produced an objective response rate of 41%, but again toxicity was substantial. Interestingly, whereas response did not appear to correlate with underlying hepatitis status, survival was significantly poorer for patients with active hepatitis B or hepatitis C, with a median survival of 7.5 mo, in contrast to 15 mo for all patients. Toxicity was also (not unexpectedly) greater in the hepatitis B- and C-positive patients.

Despite the encouraging objective response rates (as high as 60% in some of these phase I and II trials involving HAI-based therapy), these results should be interpreted with caution, since overall survival has not significantly improved relative to historic controls. It is important to keep in mind selection bias, as these patients may have represented the healthiest HCC patients. Hence, the encouraging response rates with HAI-based therapy warrant additional clinical trials to improve the poor overall survival with acceptable toxicities.

In children with unresectable hepatic malignant disease, HAI therapy with cisplatin with or without doxorubicin was a successful adjunct in altering the chances for successful liver transplantation *(41)*. In one study, 11 children received HAI therapy and achieved major reductions in α-fetoprotein, and 5 underwent successful orthotopic liver transplantation after receiving cisplatin and/or doxorubicin by HAI. Survival at 1 yr was 67% for patients with hepatoblastoma and 40% for those with hepatocellular carcinoma *(41)*.

5.2. Biliary Tract Malignancies

The role of regional therapy for biliary tract carcinomas has been addressed in small clinical trials and institutional pilot studies *(42–47)* (Table 3). The rationale for regional therapy is based on the requirement of cholangiocarcinomas for hepatic arterial blood supply. Several chemotherapeutic agents including FUDR, doxorubicin, and cisplatin have been evaluated by hepatic arterial infusion in biliary tract carcinomas. One of the earliest reported case series of biliary tract carcinomas from the Lahey Clinic describes an intriguing 60% response rate to intrahepatic chemotherapy, with 9 of 16 patients alive for longer than 1 yr and 1 patient surviving for more than 3 yr *(42)*. It is noteworthy that all these patients underwent a palliative resection with unclear tumor burden at time of initiation of therapy.

In one study of 11 patients (4 with cholangiocarcinomas and 7 with gallbladder cancers), hepatic infusion of 5-FU and mitomycin produced 7 responses but a median duration of response of only 3 mo and a median survival of 12.5 mo. Reed et al. reported seven significant regressions in nine patients with biliary carcinoma treated with intraarterial FUDR *(43)*. Melichar et al. reported a single-institution experience with HAI 5-FU-based regimens in advanced biliary tract patients, with a mean survival of 14 mo *(46)*. The heterogeneity of the patient treatments, which included subsequent therapies, complicates the interpretation of this trial. More recently, in a pilot study at Memorial Sloan-Kettering Cancer Center (MSKCC), a 43% response rate was obtained with HAI-FUDR and dexamethasone in 18 patients, 2 with HCC and 16 with cholangiocarcinoma *(48)*. Cantore et al. evaluated HAI 5-FU in nine patients with advanced biliary tract carcinomas, and reported a 55% 2-yr survival *(47)*. A recent update from this trial involving 26 patients treated with hepatic arterial epirubicin and cisplatin demonstrated a more modest response rate of 35% *(49)*. The varied experience reported with HAI-based therapy for advanced biliary tract carcinomas makes it difficult to draw uniform conclusions, but the clinical responses identified in these small trials warrant further investigation.

6. ROLE OF HAI IN METASTATIC COLORECTAL CANCER

CRC is the second leading cause of cancer-related deaths in North America and Western Europe. Because of hematogenous spread of the tumor via the portal circulation, the liver is the most common site for metastasis, with involvement in up to 60% of patients. In a third of these patients, it is the only site of metastatic disease. Prognosis is dismal for untreated patients, with median survival times of 6 to 12 mo and virtually no survivors at 5 yr *(50–52)*. For selected patients with isolated liver metastases, surgical resection is the standard of care, as this is the only modality that consistently provides long-term disease-free survival in a substantial number of patients. Reported series have

Table 3
Hepatic Artery Infusion Chemotherapy Trials in Biliary Tract Malignancies

Study	No. of Patients	Therapy	RR (%)	Median OS
Warren et al., KW 1972 *(42)*	15	HAI doxorubicin	60	NR
Smith et al., GW 1984 *(44)*	11	HAI 5-FU/Mito-C	64	12.5 mo
Makela and Kairaluoma, 1993 *(45)*	27	HAI Mito-C	48	14 mo
Melichar et al., 2002 *(46)*	32	HAI 5-FU/FA ± cisplatin	NR	14 ± 17 mo
Cantore et al., 2002 *(47)*	10	HAI epirubicin/cisplatin	70	NR
		Systemic 5-FU IVCI	55	2-yr OS
Cantore update, 2004 *(49)*	26		35	NR

Abbreviations: FA, folinic acid; 5-FU, 5-fluorouracil; IVCI, intravenous continuous infusion; Mito-C, mitomycin C, NR, not reported; OS, overall survival; RR, relative response.

described 5-yr survival rates of around 30% and 10-yr rates of around 20% *(53–56)*. Unfortunately, 65% to 80% of patients ultimately relapse, with half of the relapses occurring in the liver *(53–55,57,58)*. Moreover, only 10% of patients initially present with metastatic disease amenable to curative resection.

In the past, the principle treatment modality for patients with unresectable and/or extrahepatic disease was systemic chemotherapy with fluoropyrimidines. Treatment with 5-FU, with or without leucovorin (LV), produces a 20% response rate and 2-yr survival rate of around 20% *(59)*. More recently the addition of irinotecan and oxaliplatin to 5-FU-based regimens has resulted in superior response rates (40–50%) as well as longer median survival times (15–19.5 mo). The 2-yr survival rate, however, remains poor (25–39%), and long-term survivors are rare.

Because of the poor outcomes associated with metastatic CRC, alternative treatment strategies have been explored, including the role of regional chemotherapy to the liver. HAI has been extensively studied in patients with colorectal metastases to the liver, and this is clearly where it demonstrates the most efficacy. Its use in unresectable hepatic CRC metastases, as palliation or for neoadjuvant downstaging prior to surgery, as adjuvant therapy post R0 hepatic resection, and as prophylaxis following colonic resection to reduce the incidence of CRC hepatic metastases has been evaluated .

6.1. Palliative Hepatic Arterial Infusion for Unresectable Hepatic Metastases

There are 10 randomized trials comparing HAI with systemic therapy or best supportive care for unresectable hepatic metastases (Table 4). Eight trials compared HAI of FUDR or HAI 5-FU/LV with either i.v. FUDR, i.v. 5-FU or i.v. 5-FU/LV (Mayo or de Gramont regimen). Each trial has shown a better tumor response rate with HAI, but this has not clearly shown an improvement in overall survival.

All 10 trials showed higher response rates for HAI compared with the control arm (42–62% vs 9–25%). Although most studies demonstrated longer times to progression (TTP), overall survival (OS) times for the HAI arms were statistically significant only in the two European trials (median OS, 15 vs 11 mo *(60)* and 13.5 vs 7.5 mo *[61]*) and in the most recent Cancer and Leukemia Group B (CALGB) trial (24.4 vs 20.0 mo). In both

Table 4
Randomized Trials of Hepatic Artery Infusion (HAI) Chemotherapy for Unresectable Liver Metastases

Study	Arm	N.	No. (%) receiving assigned Rx	Crossover to HAI	Responses (CR + PR)	Median TTP (mo)	Median OS (mo)
MSKCC, 1987 (62)	HAI FUDR	48	45 (94)	Yes	50[a]	9[a]	17
	IV FUDR	51	48 (94)		20	5	12,
NCI, 1987 (63)	HAI FUDR	32	21 (66)	No	62[a]	NR	17[b]
	IV FUDR	32	29 (92)		17	NR	12[b]
NCOG, 1989 (64)	HAI FUDR	67	50 (75)	Yes	42[a]	NR	16.5
	IV FUDR	76	65 (86)		10	NR	15.8
City of Hope, 1990 (65)	HAI FUDR	31	31 (100)	Yes	55[a]	8.8	13.8
	IV 5-FU	10	10 (100)		20	7.5	11.6
NCCTG, 1990 (66)	HAI FUDR	39	33 (85)	No	48	6	12.6
	IV 5-FU/LV	35	36 (100)		12	5	10.5
French, 1992 (60)	HAI FUDR	81	70 (87)	No	44[a]	NR	15*
	IV 5-FU or BSC	82	41 (50) had 5-FU		9	NR	11
English, 1994 (61)	HAI FUDR	51	49 (96)	No	NR	NR	13.5[a]
	IV 5-FU or BSC	49	10 (20) had 5-FU		NR	NR	7.5
German, 2000 (69)	HAI FUDR	54	37 (69)	Yes	43[a]	5.9	12.7
	HAI 5-FU/LV	57	40 (70)		45	9.2	18.7
	IV 5-FU/LV	57	52 (91)		20	6.6	17.6
MRC/EORTC, 2003 (70)	HAI 5-FU/LV	145	95 (66)	No	22[c]	7.7	14.7
	IV 5-FU/LV	145	126 (87)		19	6.7	14.8
CALGB, 2003 (71)	HAI FUDR	68	59 (87)	No	48[a]	5.3	22.7[a]
	IV 5-FU/LV	67	58 (87)		25	6.8	19.8

Abbreviations: BSC, best supportive care; CR, complete response; 5-FU, 5-fluorousacil; FUDR, fluorodeoxyuridine; LV, leucovin; NR, not reported; OS, overall survival; PR, partil response; TTP, time to progression.

[a] p < 0.05
[a] Based on published Kaplan-Meier curves.
[c] Responses were calculated at a single time point (12 wk).

of the European trials the control arm included either systemic chemotherapy or best supportive care and given the currently acknowledged benefit of systemic chemotherapy over best supportive care for metastatic CRC, these two trials would not be considered to have appropriate control arms today.

Two metaanalyses of the seven original trials *(60–66)* were conducted, based on the premise that the individual trials were underpowered to detect a survival benefit. Over 600 patients were included. The Meta-Analysis Group in Cancer *(67)* confirmed the higher response rate seen with HAI (41% vs 14%). Overall, a 27% relative survival advantage was seen in the HAI arms ($p = 0.0009$) compared with the controls. When the European trials that included best supportive care were excluded, the survival advantage was 19%, but this was no longer statistically significant ($p = 0.14$). Harmantas et al. *(68)* found a 12.5% 1-yr ($p = 0.002$) and a 7.5% 2-yr ($p = 0.026$) absolute survival difference in favor of HAI over systemic chemotherapy, which persisted even when the European studies were excluded.

There are several potential reasons why the superior response rates with HAI in the individual trials did not translate into greater survival benefit. First, because patients were randomized preoperatively, technical problems with pump placement and unexpectedly high rates of extrahepatic disease discovered at laparotomy led to a substantial number of patients, assigned to HAI arms, who never received regional therapy (range 0–34%). This may have led to an underestimation of benefit using an intention-to-treat analysis was used. Second, lack of experience in certain centers and the absence of a strict, predetermined dose-reduction schema in several trials may have led to greater toxicities and fewer cycles of therapy, which may have offset any survival benefit. Finally, three trials (conducted by the MSKCC *[62]*, the Northern California Oncology Group [NCOG; *64*], and the City of Hope *[65]*) allowed crossover to HAI therapy for patients who progressed on systemic chemotherapy, further diluting any survival benefit based on intention to treat.

Since those metaanalyses, three other randomized trials of HAI have been published. The German Cooperative Group randomized 168 patients with unresectable liver metastases from CRC to HAI of FUDR, HAI of 5-FU/LV, or i.v. 5-FU/LV *(69)*. Response rates were higher in the two HAI arms, with no significant differences in time to progression (the primary end point) or overall survival among the arms. Only 70% of patients in the HAI arms actually received the assigned treatment, and 51% of patients crossed over to other arms, making interpretation of these data difficult. There was a significantly lower rate of extrahepatic progression (13% vs 41%) and a higher rate of systemic toxicity (grade 3/4 68% vs 30%) for HAI 5-FU compared with HAI FUDR, consistent with the known lower hepatic extraction of 5-FU compared with FUDR. The Medical Research Council (MRC) and the European Organization for the Research and Treatment of Cancer (EORTC) groups compared HAI 5-FU/LV with i.v. 5-FU/LV, given by the de Gramont regimen *(70)*. Crossover from the i.v. to the HAI arm was not allowed. Of 290 patients randomized, 221 (76%) received treatment as assigned, including only 66% assigned to HAI. Response rates were assessed in 183 patients at a single time point (12 wk) and were nearly identical (22% for HAI, 19% for i.v. 5-FU/LV). No differences between the arms were noted for toxicity or progression-free survival or OS. It is noteworthy that both of the above trials utilized subcutaneous ports rather than implantable pumps and had significant catheter-related problems (36% of HAI patients in the MRC/EORTC trial *[70]*) and the MRC/EORTC trial utilized 5-FU instead of FUDR.

CALGB conducted the most recently completed trial *(71)* comparing systemic 5-FU/LV via the Mayo clinic regimen (considered a standard of care at the time of the trial design) with HAI of FUDR, LV, and dexamethasone, a regimen that had produced high response rates (78%) and low toxicity (3% biliary sclerosis) in a phase II study *(72)*. No crossover was permitted. Unfortunately, only 135 patients, out of an accrual goal of 340, were randomized, in part because of delays caused by a temporary halt in production of FUDR and implantable pumps by their respective manufacturers. Most patients had >30% liver involvement (70%) and synchronous metastases (78%) and were chemotherapy naïve (97%). The response rate (48% vs 25%, $p = 0.009$) was higher in the HAI group, although TTP was not significantly different (5.3 vs 6.8 mo, $p = 0.8$), with time to hepatic progression (TTHP) better in the HAI arm (9.8 vs 7.3 mo, $p = 0.017$) and time to extrahepatic progression better in the systemic arm (7.8 vs 23.3 mo, $p = 0.0007$). The median OS time was significantly better in the HAI arm (24.4 vs 20.0 mo, $p = 0.0034$) *(71)*. The extrahepatic toxicities were also greater in the systemic group, which experienced neutropenia in 45%, stomatitis in 24%, and diarrhea in 16% compared with 2, 0, and 5% in the FUDR group, respectively. Quality of life was also improved in the HAI group, with better physical functioning (Rand-36, $p = 0.038$) and fewer symptoms (MSAS, $p = 0.017$) at 3 mo *(73)*.

Although the pharmacokinetics are not as favorable, both HAI oxaliplatin *(74–77)* and irinotecan *(78,79)* have been evaluated in phase I and II clinical trials. In a recently published French study *(74)*, 28 patients with liver-confined metastatic colonic adenocarcinoma received HAI oxaliplatin 100 mg/m^2(6-h infusion) and a systemic de Gramont schedule of 5-FU and LV. The objective response rate was 64%, with a disease-free survival of 27 mo. The most frequently reported toxicities were neutropenia and pain. A dose escalation phase I trial of HAI irinotecan in patients with unresectable liver metastases of CRC determined no dose-limiting toxicity reaching the 200 mg/m^2 maximum level *(78)*. Of the nine enrolled patients, three had partial responses (33% RR) and three had stable disease. These responses have prompted additional phase II clinical trials, to be started in the near future.

6.2. Combined HAI and Systemic Chemotherapy for Unresectable Hepatic Metastases

One observation drawn from the trials of HAI has been that, despite better control of liver metastases, the rate of (and time to) development of extrahepatic metastases has generally been similar or inferior to that seen with systemic chemotherapy. In addition, the superior rates of response and survival reported with irinotecan- and oxaliplatin-based regimens *(80–83)* have created a new standard of care for first-line treatment of metastatic CRC . It has therefore been reasoned that the combination of HAI with systemic fluoropyrimidines, oxaliplatin, or irinotecan may yield superior results than either therapy alone.

6.2.1. HAI AND SYSTEMIC 5-FU

A study of 44 patients with unresectable liver metastases compared HAI of FUDR with concurrent HAI and i.v. FUDR. A lower rate of extrahepatic spread was seen in the combination group (33% vs 61%), but response rates, toxicities, and survival were similar in the two arms *(84)*. Another single-arm study treated 40 patients with sequential HAI of FUDR and i.v. 5-FU/LV. The response rate was 62%, with a median TTP of 9 mo and a 45% incidence of extrahepatic progression *(85)*. It is noteworthy that CRC metastases to the lung, the most common site of extrahepatic spread in patients treated with HAI therapy, have been shown to express higher levels of thymidylate synthase (TS) compared with hepatic metastases *(86)*. This is clinically significant, because high TS expression has been reported to predict resistance to 5-FU therapy *(87)*, implying that combinations of HAI therapy with fluoropyrimidines may have limited efficacy in preventing extrahepatic disease.

6.2.2. HAI and Systemic Irinotecan and Oxaliplatin

Irinotecan is a topoisomerase I inhibitor with proven efficacy in first- and second-line treatment of metastatic CRC. The activity of irinotecan is not inhibited by high TS activity *(88)*; thus, combining systemic irinotecan with HAI therapy may result in better control of extrahepatic disease. In a phase I study at MSKCC, 38 patients with unresectable liver metastases received HAI of FUDR/dexamethasone and systemic irinotecan in escalating doses. All patients had been previously treated, and 16 had had prior second-line therapy with irinotecan. The regimen was well tolerated, with dose-limiting toxicities of diarrhea and myelosuppression. The response rate was 74%, median TTP was 8.1 mo, and median survival was 17.2 mo. Thirteen of 16 patients who had previously received irinotecan had partial responses *(89)*. The updated median survival is 20 mo (N. Kemeny, unpublished data).

Another nonrandomized study used HAI of FUDR with systemic irinotecan as adjuvant therapy following cytoreduction (cryotherapy, radiofrequency ablation, or partial resection) of unresectable hepatic CRC metastases. The cytoreduction was defined as cryosurgery or radiofrequency ablation and/or partial resection to treat all identifiable sites of disease. Seventy-one patients received adjuvant therapy and were compared with an historical control group receiving cytoreduction alone. TTP (19 vs 10 mo), median survival (30.6 vs 20 mo), and 2-yr survival rate (75% vs 35%) were better in the group receiving adjuvant HAI plus irinotecan *(90)*. The use of an historical control group mandates caution in interpreting these results, as surgical experience and techniques have likely improved over time. Studies of direct intra-arterial infusion of irinotecan are under way as well *(79)*, but, as significant hepatic extraction of irinotecan has not been demonstrated, it is unclear whether this approach will offer any advantage over systemic administration.

Oxaliplatin is a new cytotoxic agent with a mechanism of action similar to that of other platinum derivatives but with a different spectrum of activity and toxicity. Clinical response rates, when combined with 5-FU/LV (FOLFOX), have been greater than 50%, with a median survival of 16.2 mo in untreated patients with metastatic CRC *(82,83)*. Preliminary studies utilizing systemic oxaliplatin-based regimens combined with HAI of FUDR have demonstrated the feasibility and safety of this approach, with promising early results *(91,92)*. In the MSKCC phase I studies, 36 patients (89% previously treated) with unresectable hepatic metastases received HAI of FUDR/dexamethasone plus either systemic oxaliplatin/5-FU/LV or systemic oxaliplatin and irinotecan *(92)*. Both regimens were well tolerated, and response rates were 90 and 87%, respectively with median survival times of 36 and 22 mo. The dramatic responses seen with combination chemotherapy are demonstrated in Fig. 4. Seven patients in the systemic oxaliplatin and irinotecan group were ultimately able to undergo liver resection. Once the appropriate dosing and timing of administration have been determined, larger trials to test the efficacy and, ultimately, to compare combined HAI and systemic oxaliplatin- or irinotecan-based regimens with systemic therapy alone are warranted.

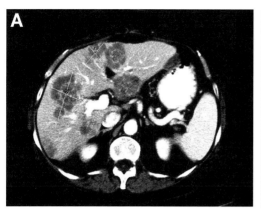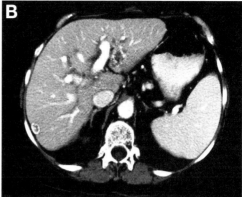

Fig. 4. Abdominal computed tomography scan of a 58-yr-old woman with metastatic olorectal cancer who progressed on systemic irinotecan, 5-FU/LV before **(A)** and after **(B)** treatment with HAI of FUDR plus systemic oxaliplatin and irinotecan.

6.3. Adjuvant Therapy After Resection of Hepatic Metastases

The best chance for cure or prolonged disease-free survival in patients with stage IV CRC with isolated liver metastases is to undergo hepatic resection. Unfortunately, even in those 20% of patients who have disease amenable to an R0 resection, hepatic recurrence develops in 30 to 60% *(93,94)*. Certainly the investigation of adjuvant therapies designed to decrease this risk of relapse is warranted.

Four reasonably sized randomized trials and two systematic reviews of adjuvant HAI have been published (Table 5). A large German Cooperative multicenter study *(95)*, randomized 226 patients to resection alone or resection plus 6 mo of HAI of 5-FU/LV given as a 5-d continuous infusion every 28 d. No systemic chemotherapy was administered in either arm, based on earlier studies demonstrating the lack of efficacy in this setting. The study was terminated early, as an interim analysis suggested a very low chance of demonstrating a survival benefit with adjuvant therapy. The impact of HAI therapy in this study is difficult to assess, as only 74% of patients assigned to HAI initiated this treatment and only 30% completed it. The low initiation rate was in large part owing to technical complications of pump placement, which in turn can be attributed to the use of subcutaneous, rather than implantable, pumps and the fact that expertise may not be as uniform in a multicenter study in which 25 centers were involved. In addition, grade 3/4 toxicities, including stomatitis and nausea/vomiting, were noted in 63% of patients receiving adjuvant therapy, most likely reflecting significant systemic absorption of 5-FU (compared with FUDR) when given via HAI. Analysis on an intention-to-treat basis demonstrated no differences in TTP, TTHP, or median OS, whereas when patients were analyzed "as treated," TTHP (45 vs 23 mo) and TTP or death (20 vs 12.6 mo) were better in the HAI arm.

In an American Intergroup study (ECOG/SWOG) *(96)* 109 patients were randomized to resection alone or resection followed by four cycles of HAI of FUDR and infusional systemic 5-FU, followed by eight more cycles of systemic 5-FU. Patients with more than three liver metastases or extrahepatic disease at laparotomy were taken off the study, and pumps were not placed. Therefore, only 80 of 109 patients were actually included in the

Table 5
Randomized Trials of Adjuvant Hepatic Artery Infusion (HAI) Chemotherapy After Complete Resection of Liver Metastases

	Study and arms					
	German, 1998 (95)		MSKCC, 1999 (97)		Intergroup, 2002 (96)	
Parameter	HAI FUDR + IV 5-FU/LV	No Rx	HAI FUDR IV 5-FU	IV 5-FU/LV	HAI 5-FU/LV	No Rx
No.	113	113	74	82	53	56
No. (%) receiving assigned tx	84 (74)	100 (88)	68 (92)	76 (93)	30 (57)	45 (80)
Median TTP (mo)	20	12.6	37.4[a]	17.2	37[b]	18[b]
Median OS (mo)	44.8	39.7	72.2	59.3	63.7	49.7
2-yr PFS (%)	NR	NR	57	42	46	25
2-yr HPFS (%)	67	63	90[a]	60	67[a]	43
2-year OS (%)	(1.5-yr HPFS) 62[b]	(4-yr HPFS) 65[b]	86[a]	72	62	53

Abbreviations: 5-FU, 5-fluorousacil; FUDR, fluorodeoxyuridine; HPFS, hepatic progression-free survival; LV, leucovorin; MSKCC, Memorial Sloan-Kettring Cancer Center; NR, not reported; OS, overal survival; PFS, progression-free survival; TTP, time to progression.

[a] $p < 0.05$.
[b] Based on published Kaplan-Meier curves.

study. When patients were analyzed as treated ($n = 75$), 4-yr disease-free survival (46% vs 25%, $p = 0.04$) and 4-yr hepatic disease-free survival (67% vs 43%, $p = 0.03$) were better in the adjuvant therapy arm. Currently, 5-yr survival is 60% vs 45% favoring adjuvant therapy (M.M. Kemeny, personal communication).

In a study done at the MSKCC *(97)*, 156 patients with resected hepatic metastases were randomized to 6 mo of systemic 5-FU/LV or systemic 5-FU/LV plus HAI of FUDR/ dexamethasone. The primary end points were 2-yr overall survival and progression-free survival. Forty percent of patients had received prior adjuvant chemotherapy following resection of their primary CRC, and 15% had received prior chemotherapy as treatment for metastatic disease. Randomization was performed intraoperatively after complete resection of metastases, and patients were stratified based on the number of metastases and prior treatment history. Ninety-two percent of patients received treatment as assigned. The 2-yr survival rate was 86% in the combined-therapy group vs 72% for systemic therapy alone ($p = 0.03$), with median survivals of 72.2 and 59.3 mo, respectively. The 2-yr hepatic progression-free survival (HPFS) rate was 90% for combined therapy and 60% for monotherapy ($p < 0.001$), with a trend toward a superior 2-year overall progression-free survival rate (57% vs 42%, $p = 0.07$) and median TTP of 37.4 and 17.2 mo, respectively. Toxicities were moderate, with 39% of patients in the combined therapy group requiring hospitalization for diarrhea, neutropenia, mucositis, or small bowel obstruction, compared with 22% of the monotherapy group ($p = 0.02$). There were no significant differences between the groups in therapy-related deaths (one combined, two monotherapy) and in biliary sclerosis requiring stents (four combined, two monotherapy). Recently an update of this study was published with a median follow-up of 10.3 yr *(98)*. The overall progression-free survival is now significantly greater in the combined group compared with the monotherapy group (31.3 vs 17.2 mo, $p = 0.02$) with 10-yr overall survival rates of 41.1% and 27.2%, respectively (Fig. 5). Using the clinical risk score for predicting recurrence after hepatic resection defined by Fong et al. *(55),** outcomes were significantly better with combined therapy as compared with monotherapy in patients with a clinical risk score of 3 to 5 (Fig. 6).

A Greek study by Lygidakis et al. *(99)* randomized 122 patients following an R0 resection for colorectal metastases in the liver to either the combination of HAI and systemic chemoimmunotherapy (mitomycin C and 5-FU/LV both i.v. and by HAI plus interleukin-2 [IL-2] by HAI alone) or the same regimen given only systemically. At 2 yr, significantly fewer patients in the HAI group had developed recurrent disease (34% vs 52%, $p = 0.002$), and significantly more patients were alive (92% vs 75%, $p < 0.05$). These same authors have previously published a smaller study *(100)* (40 patients) with a similar treatment protocol (including splenic artery infusion of interferon-γ), which also demonstrated a significant improvement in median survival (11 vs 30 mo, $p < 0.001$). Although these studies use different and more varied agents for HAI, they are based on the same principle of regional therapy to maximize therapeutic dose and minimize systemic side effects.

---

* Clinical risk score for predicting recurrence after hepatic resection for metastatic colorectal cancer (assigning one point for each of the following: node-positive primary, disease-free interval from primary to metastasis >12 mo, more than one hepatic metastasis, largest hepatic tumor >5 cm, and carcinoembryonic antigen (CEA) level >200 ng/mL).

Overall Survival

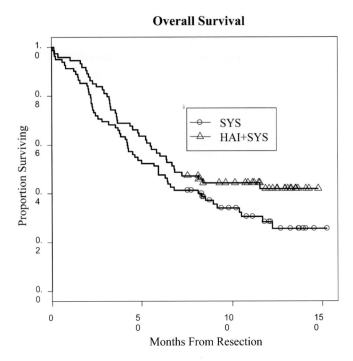

Fig. 5. Kaplan-Meier estimates of overall survival in the groups assigned to either hepatic artery infusion (HAI) plus systemic chemotherapy (SYS) or systemic chemotherapy alone. The estimated median survival was 72.2 mo in the combined-therapy group (29 of 74 patients died) and 59.3 mo in the monotherapy group (38 of 82 patients died).

Current and future studies will explore regimens that combine HAI chemotherapy with FUDR and systemic chemotherapy with newer agents such as irinotecan or oxaliplatin. A recent phase I/II study of adjuvant HAI with floxuridine and dexamethasone with intravenous irinotecan following resection of hepatic metastases from colon cancer demonstrated the safety and feasibility of this regimen *(101)*. The maximum tolerated dose of irinotecan was 200 mg/m^2 every other week with FUDR and dexamethasone for 14 d a month. With a median follow-up of 40 mo, the 2-yr survival rate was 89%. The National Surgical Adjuvant Breast and Bowel Project (NSABP) group will start a trial of HAI plus systemic oxaliplatin and capecitabine vs systemic alone.

At the present time the survival rates with HAI combined with systemic chemotherapy after hepatic resection approach 86% at 2-yr. This compares favorably with the survival with adjuvant systemic therapy alone (72%) and with historical 2-yr survival for patients treated with resection alone (55–70%). It is anticipated that combination therapies that include the newer and more efficacious chemotherapeutics will even further improve the survival rates after hepatic resection for stage IV colon cancer *(53–55,57,58,102)*.

6.4. Neoadjuvant Treatment Prior to Resection for Patients with Unresectable Hepatic Metastases

Neoadjuvant chemotherapy has many justifications in patients with hepatic metastases from CRC. It has the potential to render previously unresectable patients resectable, treats

Overall Survival

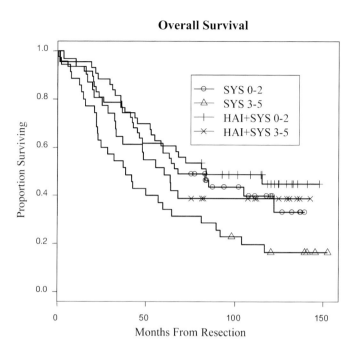

Fig. 6. Kaplan-Meier estimates of overall survival in the groups assigned to either hepatic artery infusion (HAI) plus systemic chemotherapy (SYS) or systemic chemotherapy alone with stratification based on the preoperative clinical risk score. Using the clinical risk score for predicting recurrence after hepatic resection defined by Fong et al. *(55)* outcomes were significantly better with combined therapy compared with monotherapy in patients with a higher clinical risk scores (3 to 5).

micrometastatic disease early, and is an in vivo test of chemoresponsiveness to a particular agent. A number of trials have demonstrated the ability of neoadjuvant systemic chemotherapy to render 3 to 41% of patients resectable *(103–113)*. Those patients who undergo complete resection have a median survival between 30 and 60 mo *(105,107)*.

Neoadjuvant regional therapy with HAI has also demonstrated favorable results (Table 5). Most of the regional chemotherapy trials have used either FUDR or FU. Clavien et al. *(114)*, using HAI FUDR with or without LV, induced resectability in six (26%) of 23 previously treated patients (including 20 previously treated with irinotecan). The actuarial survival rates at 3 yr were 84% for responders to neoadjuvant therapy compared with 40% for nonresponders. At MSKCC, 36 pretreated patients with extensive liver metastases received HAI FUDR and dexamethasone plus oxaliplatin and irinotecan or oxaliplatin and 5-FU/LV systemic chemotherapy in a phase I trials *(92)*. The study population in this trial had a high preoperative clinical risk score *(55)* with a number of patients who had more than four metastases, metastases greater than 5 cm in size, more than 25% liver involvement with tumor, a CEA level greater than 10 ng/dL, and previous chemotherapy exposure. Even so, the overall objective response rate was 88%, resulting in complete gross resection of tumor in 7 (33%) of the 21 patients in the oxaliplatin and irinotecan group and a median survival of 36 mo for patients in this group *(92)*.

A number of trials have also evaluated HAI FU. Elias et al. *(115)* identified 14 (5.8%) of 239 patients (unspecified number of CRC and non-CRC patients) who were rendered resectable when treated with FU-based HAI. After a mean follow-up of 36 mo after HAI, five of the nine patients were free of disease. Milandri et al. *(116)* treated 36 patients with FU-based HAI (including 13 chemotherapy-naive patients who also received systemic therapy), and 4 patients (11%) became resectable. The survival of the three patients who underwent resection ranged from 24 to more than 39 mo and was superior to the survival of 13 mo seen for all 36 patients. Noda et al. *(117)* treated 51 patients with HAI FU and oral uracil and tegafur and achieved a response rate of 78%, rendering 31 patients resectable. Eight patients chose to continue HAI therapy without surgery and had a 5-yr survival rate of 0%, whereas the 24 resected patients had a 5-yr survival rate of 42%.

Link et al. *(118)* evaluated 168 patients treated using four HAI regimens, with two arms containing FUDR only and the other two arms containing FU-based chemotherapy. The overall resection rate was 5% ($n = 9$), but despite similar response rates in all arms, the resected patients were all from the FU-containing arms. The median survival for all patients in the two FUDR groups was 20.8 mo, compared with 19.8 mo for FU/LV alone and 27.4 mo for the combination of FU/LV, mitoxantrone, and mitomycin. In the nine patients who underwent resection, seven patients were alive at 2 to 58 mo after resection. No specific details were provided on the baseline extent of disease in patients or on their performance status. A possible explanation for the poor results seen with HAI FUDR in this trial may be related to discrepancies in the baseline characteristics of the patients. Sclerosing cholangitis or liver cirrhosis was seen in 0% to 25% of the FUDR treated patients compared with 0% in the FU-treated patients and may also have prevented liver resection in the FUDR group. Meric et al. *(147)* also used HAI FUDR- or FU-based therapy to render 22 (4.4%) of 383 patients resectable. There are no details on the response rates or baseline characteristics of the 383 patients, and so an explanation for the low resection rate is difficult, although the authors suggest that it may be because many of their patients had already experienced disease progression on prior chemotherapy. As a result of alternating treatments and crossover, no analysis was made on the relative merits of HAI FUDR vs HAI FU.

Neoadjuvant HAI maximizes drug exposure to the liver and so seems to be an ideal choice for neoadjuvant therapy. It has demonstrated high response rates in both the first- and second-line settings. Although the results from neoadjuvant HAI trials are provocative, it is impossible to compare these trials with neoadjuvant systemic chemotherapy trials because of the heterogeneity in the study populations. Current data support the use of either neoadjuvant HAI or systemic chemotherapy, and randomized trials will be required to determine the optimal approach.

The encouraging results for HAI in the treatment of colorectal metastases to the liver have led investigators to evaluate the benefit of prophylactic HAI to the liver following resection of a colorectal primary. Sadahiro et al. randomized 316 stage II and III patients to surgery plus continuous 5-FU by HAI for 3 wk or surgery alone *(119)*. In addition, systemic adjuvant chemotherapy was administered at the treating physician's discretion. At 59 mo there was a significant decrease in the frequency of hepatic metastases (4% vs 15%) but not extrahepatic metastases. The decrease in hepatic metastases resulted in a significant improvement in OS (89% vs 76% at 5 yr). This result is provocative but warrants further evaluation, particularly in light of new regimens for adjuvant systemic therapy for primary CRC.

Table 6
MSKCC Guidelines for Fluorodeoxyuridine (FUDR) Fose Modification

Aspartate aminotransferase

Reference value (ref)[a]	≤50 U/L	>50U/L	
Current value[b]	0 to <3 × ref	0 to <2 × ref	100%
	3 to <4 × ref	2 to <3 × ref	80%
	4 to <5 × ref	3 to <4 × ref	50%
	≥5 × ref	≥4 × ref	*Hold*
If held, restart when:	<4 × ref	<3 × ref	50% of last dose given

Alkaline phosphatase

Reference value (ref)	≤90 U/L	>90 U/L	
Current value	0 to <1.5 × ref	0 to <1.2 × ref	100%
	1.5 to >2 × ref	1.2 to 1.5 × ref	50%
	≥2 × ref	≥1.5 × ref	*Hold*
If held, restart when:	<1.5 × ref	<1.2 × ref	25% of last dose given

Total bilirubin

Reference value (ref)	≤1.2 mg/dL	>1.2 mg/dL	
Current value	0 to <1.5 × ref	0 to <1.2 × ref	100%
	1.5 to <2 × ref	1.2 to <1.5 × ref	50%
	≥2 × ref	≥1.5 × ref	*Hold*
If held, restart when:	<1.5 × ref	<1.2 × ref	25% of last dose given

[a] Reference value is the value obtained on the day patient received the last FUDR dose.

[b] Current value is the value obtained at pump emptying or on the day of planned treatment (whichever is higher).

7. TOXIC EFFECTS OF HAI AND THEIR MANAGEMENT

Because of its high extraction rate by the liver, HAI of FUDR alone is rarely associated with systemic side effects such as myelosuppression, stomatitis, nausea, vomiting, or diarrhea. If diarrhea does occur, perfusion of the bowel should be suspected *(120)*. The most common toxicities are peptic ulceration, chemical hepatitis, and biliary sclerosis. Ulceration or inflammation of the stomach or duodenum usually results from inadvertent perfusion and drug delivery to these organs. Persistent abdominal pain, melena, or diarrhea in patients on HAI therapy mandates prompt holding of therapy and endoscopic evaluation. Upper GI ulceration is diagnosed by endoscopy of the stomach and duodenum, with concomitant injection of methylene blue by the pump side port. Immediate deep staining of the ulcerated site warrants an angiographic search for the vessel causing the misperfusion *(18)*.

Chemical hepatitis refers to an elevation in liver enzymes or bilirubin and is the most common dose-limiting toxicity associated with HAI therapy with FUDR, occurring in 42% of patients in the randomized trials *(17)*. Liver enzymes and bilirubin should be monitored every 2 wk while the patient is on therapy, and strict guidelines regarding dose reductions and/or cessation should be followed (Table 6). The hepatic toxicity may be a direct effect of the chemotherapy, which, at this concentration, caused pericholoangitis and fibrosis of the biliary tree. In the early stages of toxicity, liver function abnormalities resolve when the drug is withdrawn. These patients may develop biliary strictures, most commonly at the site of hepatic bile duct bifurcation, but strictures may also appear in the common bile duct or intrahepatic radicals *(121)*. Radiographically, the strictures resemble idiopathic sclerosing cholangitis, and the diagnosis is made by endoscopic retrograde cholangiopancreatography, which helps to exclude metastatic lesions as a cause of strictures. This complication is usually associated with FUDR, not 5-FU, with an incidence of 3 to 26% in randomized trials *(17)*. Patients with progressive jaundice require endoscopic retrograde cholangiopancreatography to distinguish this finding from malignant strictures and to provide palliative stenting if possible. Cholecystitis can develop in 33% of patients *(121)*; however, this is no longer a problem now that cholecystectomy is routinely performed at the time of pump placement.

Attempts have been made to reduce the hepatic toxic effects of floxuridine by adding dexamethasone to the infusion mixture. In a randomized study of floxuridine with dexamethasone vs floxuridine alone, the former group showed a smaller rise in bilirubin (9%) than those receiving floxuridine alone (30%) ($p = 0.07$) *(122)*. Although the addition of dexamethasone was not associated with a significant increase in the amount of floxuridine that could be administered, response rate and survival were better in the patients treated with floxuridine plus dexamethasone than in those given floxuridine alone (71% and 23 mo vs 45% and 16 mo, respectively).

8. ROLE OF HAI IN HEPATIC METASTASES FROM NONCOLONIC PRIMARY TUMOR TYPES

There is limited HAI experience in the treatment of hepatic metastases from a number of tumor types including melanoma, sarcoma, and gastric, pancreatic, and breast cancers, with variable results. Regional HAI treatment of patients with liver metastases from breast cancer has induced significant antitumor activity in a number of case reports *(123–126)*, but unfortunately any treatment effect is overshadowed by the systemic nature of this disease *(127)*. A similar conclusion can be drawn for patients with isolated hepatic metastases form pancreatic cancer *(128)*. HAI in patients with isolated hepatic metastases from gastric cancer, however, may improve prognosis in those patients who attain an objective response to the therapy *(129)*. In a single case report of hepatic metastases from sarcoma, none of the six patients responded to therapy, and disease progressed in all cases *(130)*.

There is relatively more experience with metastatic cutaneous or uveal melanoma, localized to the liver, in which HAI treatment with agents such as doxorubicin *(131)*, carboplatin *(132)*, fotemustine alone *(133)* or in combination with carboplatin, fotemustine, and/or dacarbazine plus cisplatin *(134)* has achieved response rates as high as 40 to 50%. In these series of reports, the only significant toxicity was myelosuppression, and HAI preserved the patients' quality of life.

9. NOVEL STRATEGIES USING HAI CHEMOTHERAPY

A new approach combines HAI with hemofiltration; this allows the administration of high doses of drugs to the tumor while filtering the venous effluent blood coming from the tumor to limit systemic exposure *(135)*. During the procedure, the cytotoxic drugs are injected into the arterial supply of the tumor and the venous blood coming from the tumor bed undergoes hemofiltration to extract the cytotoxic drug from the systemic blood *(136)*.

This procedure is currently considered in patients with unresectable liver metastases from CRC in whom first-line chemotherapy has been unsuccessful and in patients with unresectable hepatic malignancies *(137)*.

Another interesting treatment strategy exploits the fact that the *p53* gene is commonly defective or deleted in colorectal cancer. A selectively replicating adenovirus, Onyx-015, displays tumor selectivity for *p53* mutant cells. In a phase I study, this virus was given by HAI to 11 patients with metastatic CRC to the liver, in combination with infusional 5-FU/LV. Fevers with rigors were observed in all patients, but none experienced dose-limiting toxicity. Antitumor activity was demonstrated in combination with fluorouracil and leucovorin in all three patients treated at viral doses of $>6 \times 10^{11}$ plaque-forming units *(138)*. Other studies have also evaluated Onyx-015 with modest but promising results *(139,140)*. The regional delivery via HAI of newer oncolytic viruses, including herpes virus NV1020 *(141)* and vesicular stomatitis virus *(142)*, is currently being evaluated in humans and animal models.

Alternatively, a strategy to reintroduce the defective p53 gene into cancer cells has been explored. Gene therapy of colorectal liver metastases with a replication-defective recombinant adenovirus (SCH58500) encoding wild-type *p53* via HAI has been investigated in phase I and II studies *(143,144)*. Single-dose *p53* administration into the hepatic artery was safe, and the regional delivery results in significant transgene expression. Although these studies were designed to determine safety and dosing, results regarding tumor response and survival have been disappointing.

The value of molecular markers to predict response to fluorouracil-based intraarterial therapy has also been studied. TS was shown to predict response and resistance to HAI chemotherapy in patients with colorectal liver metastases *(145,146)*. Patients with low activity of TS were 4.1 times more likely to respond to fluorouracil-based chemotherapy than patients with high activities of this enzyme. In the CALGB study, low TS and *p53* expression predicted better outcome in a subset of 45 patients in whom these were measured *(73)*.

Finally, the advent of new biological therapy with recombinant humanized monoclonal antibodies to the epidermal growth factor receptor and the vascular endothelial cell growth factor have changed the treatment algorithm for therapy of stage IV colon cancer. These therapies, combined with HAI, will certainly be studied in the near future.

10. CONCLUSIONS

The benefit of using HAI over systemic chemotherapy in primary hepatic tumors and hepatic metastases other than colon cancer is unclear, with evidence from small, nonrandomized studies. Conversely, HAI chemotherapy appears to be beneficial in the multimodal therapy of stage IV colon cancer with isolated hepatic metastases in a number of randomized clinical trials. The results of combination chemotherapy trials with newer agents may see HAI emerge as a pivotal component in the evolving treatment of colorectal hepatic metastases.

REFERENCES

1. Weiss L, Grundmann E, Torhorst J, et al. Haematogenous metastatic patterns in colonic carcinoma: an analysis of 1541 necropsies. J Pathol 1986;150:195–203.
2. Breedis C, Young G. The blood supply of neoplasms in the liver. Am J Pathol 1954;30:969–977.

3. Ensminger WD, Rosowsky A, Raso V, et al. A clinical-pharmacological evaluation of hepatic arterial infusions of 5-fluoro-2'-deoxyuridine and 5-fluorouracil. Cancer Res 1978;38:3784–3792.

4. Ensminger WD, Gyves JW. Clinical pharmacology of hepatic arterial chemotherapy. Semin Oncol 1983;10:176–182.

5. Ensminger WD. Intrahepatic arterial infusion of chemotherapy: pharmacologic principles. Semin Oncol 2002;29:119–125.

6. Van Groeningen CJ, Van der Vijgh WJ, et al. Phase I clinical and pharmacokinetic study of 5 day CPT-11 hepatic arterial infusion (HAI) chemotherapy. Proc Am Soc Clin Oncol 1997; 1997. p. 768.

7. van Tellingen O, Kuck MT, Vlasveld LT, Rodenhuis S, Nooijen WJ, Beijnen JH. Unchanged pharmacokinetics of etoposide given by intra-arterial hepatic infusion as compared with i.v. infusion. Cancer Chemother Pharmacol 1996;38:387–390.

8. Yasuda S, Noto T, Ikeda M, et al. [Hepatic arterial infusion chemotherapy using implantable reservoir in colorectal liver metastasis]. Gan To Kagaku Ryoho 1990;17:1815–1819.

9. Heinrich S, Petrowsky H, Schwinnen I, et al. Technical complications of continuous intra-arterial chemotherapy with 5-fluorodeoxyuridine and 5-fluorouracil for colorectal liver metastases. Surgery 2003;133:40–48.

10. Doci R, Bignami P, Quagliuolo V, et al. Continuous hepatic arterial infusion with 5-fluorodeoxyuridine for the treatment of colorectal metastases. Reg Cancer Treat 1990;3:13–18.

11. Hohn DC, Rayner AA, Economou JS, Ignoffo RJ, Lewis BJ, Stagg RJ. Toxicities and complications of implanted pump hepatic arterial and intravenous floxuridine infusion. Cancer 1986;57:465–4670.

12. Rougier P, Ducreux M, Pignon JP, et al. Prognostic factors in patients with liver metastases from colorectal carcinoma treated with discontinuous intra-arterial hepatic chemotherapy. Eur J Cancer 1991;27:1226–1230.

13. Schneebaum S, Walker MJ, Young D, Farrar WB, Minton JP. The regional treatment of liver metastases from breast cancer. J Surg Oncol 1994;55:26–31; discussion 2.

14. Allen PJ, Stojadinovic A, Ben-Porat L, et al. The management of variant arterial anatomy during hepatic arterial infusion pump placement. Ann Surg Oncol 2002;9:875–880.

15. Daly JM, Kemeny N, Oderman P, Botet J. Long-term hepatic arterial infusion chemotherapy. Anatomic considerations, operative technique, and treatment morbidity. Arch Surg 1984;119:936–941.

16. Elias D, Lasser P, Rougier P. A simplified surgical technical procedure for intra-arterial chemotherapy in secondary liver cancer. Experience in 50 patients. Eur J Surg Oncol 1987;13:441–448.

17. Skitzki JJ, Chang AE. Hepatic artery chemotherapy for colorectal liver metastases: technical considerations and review of clinical trials. Surg Oncol 2002;11:123–135.

18. Bloom AI, Gordon RL, Ahl KH, et al. Transcatheter embolization for the treatment of misperfusion after hepatic artery chemoinfusion pump implantation. Ann Surg Oncol 1999;6:350–358.

19. Cheng J, Hong D, Zhu G, Swanstrom LL, Hansen PD. Laparoscopic placement of hepatic artery infusion pumps: technical considerations and early results. Ann Surg Oncol 2004;11:589–597.

20. Urbach DR, Hansen PD. Laparoscopic placement of a continuous hepatic artery infusion pump. Semin Laparosc Surg 2000;7:140–147.

21. Aldrighetti L, Arru M, Angeli E, et al. Percutaneous vs surgical placement of hepatic artery indwelling catheters for regional chemotherapy. Hepatogastroenterology 2002;49:513–517.

22. Elias D, de Baere T, Sideris L, Ducreux M. Regional chemotherapeutic techniques for liver tumors: current knowledge and future directions. Surg Clin North Am 2004;84:607–625.

23. Curley SA, Chase JL, Roh MS, Hohn DC. Technical considerations and complications associated with the placement of 180 implantable hepatic arterial infusion devices. Surgery 1993;114:928–935.

24. Kemeny N, Sigurdon E. Intra-arterial Chemotherapy for Liver Tumors, 2nd ed. New York: Churchill Livingstone; 1994.

25. Allen PJ, Nissan A, Picon AI, et al. Technical complications and durability of hepatic artery infusion pumps for unresectable colorectal liver metastases: an institutional experience of 544 consecutive cases. J Am Coll Surg 2005;201:57–65.

26. Campbell KA, Burns RC, Sitzmann JV, Lipsett PA, Grochow LB, Niederhuber JE. Regional chemotherapy devices: effect of experience and anatomy on complications. J Clin Oncol 1993;11:822–826.

27. Koea JB, Kemeny N. Hepatic artery infusion chemotherapy for metastatic colorectal carcinoma. Semin Surg Oncol 2000;19:125-134.

28. Kinami Y, Miyazaki I. The superselective and the selective one shot methods for treating inoperable cancer of the liver. Cancer 1978;41:1720–1727.

29. Wellwood JM, Cady B, Oberfield RA. Treatment of primary liver cancer: response to regional chemotherapy. Clin Oncol 1979;5:25–31.
30. Olweny CL, Katongole-Mbidde E, Bahendeka S, Otim D, Mugerwa J, Kyalwazi SK. Further experience in treating patients with hepatocellular carcinoma in Uganda. Cancer 1980;46:2717–2722.
31. Cheng EW, Fortner J. Regional intra-arterial infusion of cisplatin in primary liver cancer: a phase II trial. ASCO 1982.
32. Urist MB. Intra-arterial chemotherapy for hepatoma using Adriamycin administered by an implantable infusion pump. ASCO 1984.
33. Shildt RB, Stuckey W. Hepatic artery infusion (HAI) with 5-FUDR, Adriamycin and Streptozocin in unresectable hepatoma. ASCO 1984.
34. Atiq OT, Kemeny N, Niedzwiecki D, Botet J. Treatment of unresectable primary liver cancer with intrahepatic fluorodeoxyuridine and mitomycin C through an implantable pump. Cancer 1992;69: 920–924.
35. Patt YZ, Charnsangavej C, Yoffe B, et al. Hepatic arterial infusion of floxuridine, leucovorin, doxorubicin, and cisplatin for hepatocellular carcinoma: effects of hepatitis B and C viral infection on drug toxicity and patient survival. J Clin Oncol 1994;12:1204–1211.
36. Carr B. Effects of ciapltin (DDP) intensity on hepatocellular carcinoma responses and survival in 57 patients. ASCO 1998.
37. Urabe T, Kaneko S, Matsushita E, Unoura M, Kobayashi K. Clinical pilot study of intrahepatic arterial chemotherapy with methotrexate, 5-fluorouracil, cisplatin and subcutaneous interferon-alpha-2b for patients with locally advanced hepatocellular carcinoma. Oncology 1998;55:39–47.
38. Okuda K, Tanaka M, Shibata J, et al. Hepatic arterial infusion chemotherapy with continuous low dose administration of cisplatin and 5-fluorouracil for multiple recurrence of hepatocellular carcinoma after surgical treatment. Oncol Rep 1999;6:587–591.
39. Fazio N, Manzoni S. Hepatic arterial infusion using a percutaneous temporary catheter in patients with advanced primary liver carcinoma. ASCO 2003.
40. Yodono H, Sasaki T, Tarusawa K, Midorikawa H, Saito Y, Takekawa SD. Arterial infusion chemotherapy for advanced hepatocellular carcinoma using EPF and EAP therapies. Cancer Chemother Pharmacol 1992;31(Suppl):S89-S92.
41. Gerber DA, Arcement C, Carr B, Towbin R, Mazariegos G, Reyes J. Use of intrahepatic chemotherapy to treat advanced pediatric hepatic malignancies. J Pediatr Gastroenterol Nutr 2000;30:137–144.
42. Warren KW, Mountain JC, Lloyd-Jones W. Malignant tumors of the bile-ducts. Br J Surg 1972;59: 501–505.
43. Reed ML, Vaitkevicius VK, Al-Sarraf M, et al. The practicality of chronic hepatic artery infusion therapy of primary and metastatic hepatic malignancies: ten-year results of 124 patients in a prospective protocol. Cancer 1981;47:402–409.
44. Smith GW, Bukowski RM, Hewlett JS, Groppe CW. Hepatic artery infusion of 5-fluorouracil and mitomycin C in cholangiocarcinoma and gallbladder carcinoma. Cancer 1984;54:1513–1516.
45. Makela JT, Kairaluoma MI. Superselective intra-arterial chemotherapy with mitomycin for gallbladder cancer. Br J Surg 1993;80:912–915.
46. Melichar B, Cerman J Jr, Dvorak J, et al. Regional chemotherapy in biliary tract cancers—a single institution experience. Hepatogastroenterology 2002;49:900–906.
47. Cantore M, Rabbi C, Guadagni S, Zamagni D, Aitini E. Intra-arterial hepatic chemotherapy combined with continuous infusion of 5-fluorouracil in patients with metastatic cholangiocarcinoma. Ann Oncol 2002;13:1687–1688.
48. Danso M, Jarnagin WR, Muruganandham M, et al. Hepatic arterial infusion (HAI) therapy in patients with unresectable primary liver cancer: use of dynamic contrast enhanced MRI to evaluate response. ASCO 2005; (abstract 4129).
49. Mambrini AFG, Pennucci C. Intra-arterial hepatic chemotherapy combined with systemic infusion of 5-FU in patients with advanced biliary tract cancers. ASCO 2004; 14S (abstract 4197).
50. Bengtsson G, Carlsson G, Hafstrom L, Jonsson PE. Natural history of patients with untreated liver metastases from colorectal cancer. Am J Surg 1981;141:586–589.
51. Finan PJ, Marshall RJ, Cooper EH, Giles GR. Factors affecting survival in patients presenting with synchronous hepatic metastases from colorectal cancer: a clinical and computer analysis. Br J Surg 1985;72:373–377.
52. de Brauw LM, van de Velde CJ, Bouwhuis-Hoogerwerf ML, Zwaveling A. Diagnostic evaluation and survival analysis of colorectal cancer patients with liver metastases. J Surg Oncol 1987;34:81–86.

53. Nordlinger B, Guiguet M, Vaillant JC, et al. Surgical resection of colorectal carcinoma metastases to the liver. A prognostic scoring system to improve case selection, based on 1568 patients. Association Française de Chirurgie. Cancer 1996;77:1254–12562.

54. Jamison RL, Donohue JH, Nagorney DM, Rosen CB, Harmsen WS, Ilstrup DM. Hepatic resection for metastatic colorectal cancer results in cure for some patients. Arch Surg 1997;132:505–510; discussion 11.

55. Fong Y, Fortner J, Sun RL, Brennan MF, Blumgart LH. Clinical score for predicting recurrence after hepatic resection for metastatic colorectal cancer: analysis of 1001 consecutive cases. Ann Surg 1999;230:309–318; discussion 18–21.

56. Abdalla EK, Vauthey JN, Ellis LM, et al. Recurrence and outcomes following hepatic resection, radiofrequency ablation, and combined resection/ablation for colorectal liver metastases. Ann Surg 2004;239:818–825; discussion 25–27.

57. Scheele J, Stangl R, Altendorf-Hofmann A. Hepatic metastases from colorectal carcinoma: impact of surgical resection on the natural history. Br J Surg 1990;77:1241–1246.

58. Fegiz G, Ramacciato G, Gennari L, et al. Hepatic resections for colorectal metastases: the Italian multicenter experience. J Surg Oncol Suppl 1991;2:144–154.

59. Modulation of fluorouracil by leucovorin in patients with advanced colorectal cancer: evidence in terms of response rate. Advanced Colorectal Cancer Meta-Analysis Project. J Clin Oncol 1992;10:896–903.

60. Rougier P, Laplanche A, Huguier M, et al. Hepatic arterial infusion of floxuridine in patients with liver metastases from colorectal carcinoma: long-term results of a prospective randomized trial. J Clin Oncol 1992;10:1112–1118.

61. Allen-Mersh TG, Earlam S, Fordy C, Abrams K, Houghton J. Quality of life and survival with continuous hepatic-artery floxuridine infusion for colorectal liver metastases. Lancet 1994;344:1255–1260.

62. Kemeny N, Daly J, Reichman B, Geller N, Botet J, Oderman P. Intrahepatic or systemic infusion of fluorodeoxyuridine in patients with liver metastases from colorectal carcinoma. A randomized trial. Ann Intern Med 1987;107:459–465.

63. Chang AE, Schneider PD, Sugarbaker PH, Simpson C, Culnane M, Steinberg SM. A prospective randomized trial of regional vs systemic continuous 5-fluorodeoxyuridine chemotherapy in the treatment of colorectal liver metastases. Ann Surg 1987;206:685–693.

64. Hohn DC, Stagg RJ, Friedman MA, et al. A randomized trial of continuous intravenous vs hepatic intraarterial floxuridine in patients with colorectal cancer metastatic to the liver: the Northern California Oncology Group trial. J Clin Oncol 1989;7:1646–1654.

65. Wagman LD, Kemeny MM, Leong L, et al. A prospective, randomized evaluation of the treatment of colorectal cancer metastatic to the liver. J Clin Oncol 1990;8:1885–1893.

66. Martin JK Jr, O'Connell MJ, Wieand HS, et al. Intra-arterial floxuridine vs systemic fluorouracil for hepatic metastases from colorectal cancer. A randomized trial. Arch Surg 1990;125:1022–1027.

67. Reappraisal of hepatic arterial infusion in the treatment of nonresectable liver metastases from colorectal cancer. Meta-Analysis Group in Cancer. J Natl Cancer Inst 1996;88:252–258.

68. Harmantas A, Rotstein LE, Langer B. Regional vs systemic chemotherapy in the treatment of colorectal carcinoma metastatic to the liver. Is there a survival difference? Meta-analysis of the published literature. Cancer 1996;78:1639–1645.

69. Lorenz M, Muller HH. Randomized, multicenter trial of fluorouracil plus leucovorin administered either via hepatic arterial or intravenous infusion vs fluorodeoxyuridine administered via hepatic arterial infusion in patients with nonresectable liver metastases from colorectal carcinoma. J Clin Oncol 2000;18:243–254.

70. Kerr DJ, McArdle CS, Ledermann J, et al. Intrahepatic arterial vs intravenous fluorouracil and folinic acid for colorectal cancer liver metastases: a multicentre randomised trial. Lancet 2003;361:368–373.

71. Kemeny N, Hollis R. Hepatic arterial infusion (HAI) vs systemic therapy for hepatic metastases from colorectal cancer; a CALGB randomized trial of efficacy, quality of life (QOL), cost effectiveness, and molecular markers. Proc Am Soc Clin Oncol 2003; 252a (abstract).

72. Kemeny N, Conti JA, Cohen A, et al. Phase II study of hepatic arterial floxuridine, leucovorin, and dexamethasone for unresectable liver metastases from colorectal carcinoma. J Clin Oncol 1994;12:2288–2295.

73. Kemeny N, Niedzwiecki D, Hollis DR, et al. Final analysis of hepatic arterial infusion (HAI) versus systemic therapy for hepatic metastases from colorectal cancer; a CALGB randomized trial of efficacy, quality of life (QOL), cost effectiveness, and molecular markers. ASCO; 2005; abstract 183.

74. Ducreux M, Ychou M, Laplanche A, et al. Hepatic arterial oxaliplatin infusion plus intravenous chemotherapy in colorectal cancer with inoperable hepatic metastases: a trial of the gastrointestinal group of the Federation Nationale des Centres de Lutte Contre le Cancer. J Clin Oncol 2005;23: 4881–4887.

75. Boige V, Lacombe S, De Baere T. Hepatic arterial infusion oxaliplatin with intravenous 5-FU and folinic acid in non-resectable liver metastasis colorectal cancer (abstract). Proc Am Soc Clin Oncol 2003; 291a.

76. Kern W, Beckert B, Lang N, et al. Phase I and pharmacokinetic study of hepatic arterial infusion with oxaliplatin in combination with folinic acid and 5-fluorouracil in patients with hepatic metastases from colorectal cancer. Ann Oncol 2001;12:599–603.

77. Tomirotti M, Pallavicine E, Tacconi F. First-line activity of hepatic arterial infusion of oxaliplatin and systemic chemotherapy with leucovorin plus 5-fluorouracil in metastatic colorectal cancer: preliminary data of a multicenter study. Proc Am Soc Clin Oncol 2002; 135b.

78. Vogl T. A phase I study of hepatic arterial infusion of irinotecan in patients with inoperable liver metastases of colorectal cancer. ASCO 2004.

79. van Riel JM, van Groeningen CJ, Kedde MA, et al. Continuous administration of irinotecan by hepatic arterial infusion: a phase I and pharmacokinetic study. Clin Cancer Res 2002;8:405–412.

80. Douillard JY, Cunningham D, Roth AD, et al. Irinotecan combined with fluorouracil compared with fluorouracil alone as first-line treatment for metastatic colorectal cancer: a multicentre randomised trial. Lancet 2000;355:1041–1047.

81. Saltz LB, Cox JV, Blanke C, et al. Irinotecan plus fluorouracil and leucovorin for metastatic colorectal cancer. Irinotecan Study Group. N Engl J Med 2000;343:905–914.

82. de Gramont A, Figer A, Seymour M, et al. Leucovorin and fluorouracil with or without oxaliplatin as first-line treatment in advanced colorectal cancer. J Clin Oncol 2000;18:2938–2947.

83. Tournigand C, Louvet C, Quinaux E. FOLFIRI followed by FOLFOX vs FOLFOX followed in metastatic colorectal cancer (MCRC): final results of a phase II study. Proc Am Soc Clin Oncol 2001; 124a.

84. Safi F, Bittner R, Roscher R, Schuhmacher K, Gaus W, Beger GH. Regional chemotherapy for hepatic metastases of colorectal carcinoma (continuous intraarterial vs continuous intraarterial/intravenous therapy). Results of a controlled clinical trial. Cancer 1989;64:379–387.

85. O'Connell MJ, Nagorney DM, Bernath AM, et al. Sequential intrahepatic fluorodeoxyuridine and systemic fluorouracil plus leucovorin for the treatment of metastatic colorectal cancer confined to the liver. J Clin Oncol 1998;16:2528–2533.

86. Gorlick R, Metzger R, Danenberg KD, et al. Higher levels of thymidylate synthase gene expression are observed in pulmonary as compared with hepatic metastases of colorectal adenocarcinoma. J Clin Oncol 1998;16:1465–1469.

87. Leichman CG, Lenz HJ, Leichman L, et al. Quantitation of intratumoral thymidylate synthase expression predicts for disseminated colorectal cancer response and resistance to protracted-infusion fluorouracil and weekly leucovorin. J Clin Oncol 1997;15:3223–3229.

88. Saltz LB, Danenberg K, Paty P. High thymidylate synthase (TS) expression does not preclude activity of CPT-11 in colorectal cancer (CRC). Proc Am Soc Clin Oncol 1998; 281a.

89. Kemeny N, Gonen M, Sullivan D, et al. Phase I study of hepatic arterial infusion of floxuridine and dexamethasone with systemic irinotecan for unresectable hepatic metastases from colorectal cancer. J Clin Oncol 2001;19:2687–2695.

90. Litvak DA, Wood TF, Tsioulias GJ, et al. Systemic irinotecan and regional floxuridine after hepatic cytoreduction in 185 patients with unresectable colorectal cancer metastases. Ann Surg Oncol 2002;9:148–155.

91. Pancera G, Garassino MC, Beretta GD, et al. A feasibility study of combined hepatic arterial infusion (HAI) with FUDR and systemic chemotherapy (SYS) with FOLFOX-4 in advanced colorectal cancer (CRC). Proc Am Soc Clin Oncol 2002; 105b (abstract).

92. Kemeny N, Jarnagin W, Paty P, et al. Phase I trial of systemic oxaliplatin combination chemotherapy with hepatic arterial infusion in patients with unresectable liver metastases from colorectal cancer. J Clin Oncol 2005;23:4888–4896.

93. Ballantyne GH, Quin J. Surgical treatment of liver metastases in patients with colorectal cancer. Cancer 1993;71(12 suppl):4252–4266.

94. Lehnert T, Otto G, Herfarth C. Therapeutic modalities and prognostic factors for primary and secondary liver tumors. World J Surg 1995;19:252–263.

95. Lorenz M, Muller HH, Schramm H, et al. Randomized trial of surgery vs surgery followed by adjuvant hepatic arterial infusion with 5-fluorouracil and folinic acid for liver metastases of colorectal cancer. German Cooperative on Liver Metastases (Arbeitsgruppe Lebermetastasen). Ann Surg 1998;228: 756–762.

96. Kemeny MM, Adak S, Gray B, et al. Combined-modality treatment for resectable metastatic colorectal carcinoma to the liver: surgical resection of hepatic metastases in combination with continuous infusion of chemotherapy—an intergroup study. J Clin Oncol 2002;20:1499–1505.

97. Kemeny N, Huang Y, Cohen AM, et al. Hepatic arterial infusion of chemotherapy after resection of hepatic metastases from colorectal cancer. N Engl J Med 1999;341:2039–2048.

98. Kemeny NE, Gonen M. Hepatic arterial infusion after liver resection. N Engl J Med 2005;352: 734–735.

99. Lygidakis NJ, Sgourakis G, Vlachos L, et al. Metastatic liver disease of colorectal origin: the value of locoregional immunochemotherapy combined with systemic chemotherapy following liver resection. Results of a prospective randomized study. Hepatogastroenterology 2001;48:1685–1691.

100. Lygidakis NJ, Ziras N, Parissis J. Resection vs resection combined with adjuvant pre- and postoperative chemotherapy—immunotherapy for metastatic colorectal liver cancer. A new look at an old problem. Hepatogastroenterology 1995;42:155–161.

101. Kemeny N, Jarnagin W, Gonen M, et al. Phase I/II study of hepatic arterial therapy with floxuridine and dexamethasone in combination with intravenous irinotecan as adjuvant treatment after resection of hepatic metastases from colorectal cancer. J Clin Oncol 2003;21:3303–3309.

102. van Ooijen B, Wiggers T, Meijer S, et al. Hepatic resections for colorectal metastases in The Netherlands. A multiinstitutional 10-year study. Cancer 1992;70:28–34.

103. Bismuth H, Adam R, Levi F, et al. Resection of nonresectable liver metastases from colorectal cancer after neoadjuvant chemotherapy. Ann Surg 1996;224:509–520; discussion 520–522.

104. Adam R, Avisar E, Ariche A, et al. Five-year survival following hepatic resection after neoadjuvant therapy for nonresectable colorectal. Ann Surg Oncol 2001;8:347–53.

105. Giacchetti S, Itzhaki M, Gruia G, et al. Long-term survival of patients with unresectable colorectal cancer liver metastases following infusional chemotherapy with 5-fluorouracil, leucovorin, oxaliplatin and surgery. Ann Oncol 1999;10:663–669.

106. Wein A, Riedel C, Kockerling F, et al. Impact of surgery on survival in palliative patients with metastatic colorectal cancer after first line treatment with weekly 24-hour infusion of high-dose 5-fluorouracil and folinic acid. Ann Oncol 2001;12:1721–1727.

107. Alberts S, Donhoe J, Mahoney M. Liver resection after 5-fluorouracil, leucovorin and oxaliplatin for patients with metastatic colorectal cancer (MCRC) limited to the liver: A North Central Cancer Treatment Group (NCCTG) phase II study. Proc Am Soc Clin Oncol 2003; 263 (abstr 1053).

108. Gaspar E, Artigas V, Montserrat E. Single centre study of L-OHP/5-FU/LV before liver surgery in patients with NOT optimally resectable colorectal cancer isolated liver metastases. Proc Am Soc Clin Oncol 2003; 353 (abstr 1416).

109. Delaunoit T, Krook J, Sargent D. Chemotherapy-allowed resection of metastatic colorectal cancer: a cooperative group experience. ASCO Gastrointest Cancers Symp 2004:138 (abstr 96).

110. Falcone A, Masi G, Cupini S. Surgical resection of metastases (mts) after biweekly chemotherapy with irinotecan, oxaliplatin and 5-fluororacil/leucovorin (FOLFOXIRI) in initially unresectable metastatic colorectal cancer (MCRC). Proc Am Soc Clin Oncol 2004; 258 (abstr 3553).

111. De La Camara J, Rodriguez J, Rotellar F. Triplet therapy with oxaliplatin, irinotecan, 5-fluorouracil and folinic acid within a combined modality approach in patients with liver metastases from colorectal cancer. Proc Am Soc Clin Oncol 2004; 268 (abstr 3591).

112. Quenet F, Nordlinger B, Rivoire M. Resection of previously unresectable liver metastases from colorectal cancer (LMCRC) after chemotherapy (CT) with CPT-11/L-OHP/LV5FU (Folfirinox): a prospective phase II trial. Proc Am Soc Clin Oncol 2004; 273 (abstr 3613).

113. Pozzo C, Basso M, Cassano A, et al. Neoadjuvant treatment of unresectable liver disease with irinotecan and 5-fluorouracil plus folinic acid in colorectal cancer patients. Ann Oncol 2004;15:933–939.

114. Clavien PA, Selzner N, Morse M, Selzner M, Paulson E. Downstaging of hepatocellular carcinoma and liver metastases from colorectal cancer by selective intra-arterial chemotherapy. Surgery 2002;131:433–442.

115. Elias D, Lasser P, Rougier P, Ducreux M, Bognel C, Roche A. Frequency, technical aspects, results, and indications of major hepatectomy after prolonged intra-arterial hepatic chemotherapy for initially unresectable hepatic tumors. J Am Coll Surg 1995;180:213–219.

116. Milandri C, Calzolari F, Giampalma E, et al. [Combined treatment of inoperable liver metastases from colorectal cancer]. Tumori 2003;89(4 suppl):112–114.
117. Noda M, Yanagi H, Yoshikawa R. Second-look hepatectomy after pharmacokinetic modulating chemotherapy (PMC) combination with hepatic arterial 5FU infusion and oral UFT in patients with unresectable hepatic colorectal metastases. Proc Am Soc Clin Oncol 2004; 304 (abstr 3739).
118. Link KH, Pillasch J, Formentini A, et al. Downstaging by regional chemotherapy of non-resectable isolated colorectal liver metastases. Eur J Surg Oncol 1999;25:381–388.
119. Sadahiro S, Suzuki T, Ishikawa K, et al. Prophylactic hepatic arterial infusion chemotherapy for the prevention of liver metastasis in patients with colon carcinoma: a randomized control trial. Cancer 2004;100:590–597.
120. Kemeny N, Fata F. Hepatic-arterial chemotherapy. Lancet Oncol 2001;2:418–428.
121. Kemeny MM, Battifora H, Blayney DW, et al. Sclerosing cholangitis after continuous hepatic artery infusion of FUDR. Ann Surg 1985;202:176–181.
122. Kemeny N, Seiter K, Niedzwiecki D, et al. A randomized trial of intrahepatic infusion of fluorodeoxyuridine with dexamethasone vs fluorodeoxyuridine alone in the treatment of metastatic colorectal cancer. Cancer 1992;69:327–334.
123. Fujito T, Maeura Y, Matsuyama J, et al. [A case of multiple liver metastases from breast cancer in which we confirmed disappearance of cancer cells after hepatic resection following hepatic arterial infusion chemotherapy]. Gan To Kagaku Ryoho 2002;29:2354–2357.
124. Iwamoto S, Gon G, Nohara T, Iwamoto M, Kobayashi T, Tanigawa N. [A case of liver metastasis of breast cancer successfully treated with paclitaxel infusion into the hepatic artery: an attempt of once weekly regimen]. Gan To Kagaku Ryoho 2002;29:917–920.
125. Chino Y, Suzuki Y, Ubukata N, Yoshihara K, Tani T, Ogata M. [Hepatic infusion of docetaxel using PEIT for a patient with stage IV breast cancer]. Gan To Kagaku Ryoho 2001;28:1897–1899.
126. Hara S, Hashizume S, Itoyanagi N, et al. [A case of hepatic arterial infusion chemotherapy for multiple liver metastasis from breast cancer]. Gan To Kagaku Ryoho 1997;24:1809–1812.
127. Elias D, Maisonnette F, Druet-Cabanac M, et al. An attempt to clarify indications for hepatectomy for liver metastases from breast cancer. Am J Surg 2003;185:158–164.
128. Ishii H, Furuse J, Nagase M, et al. Hepatic arterial infusion of 5-fluorouracil and extrabeam radiotherapy for liver metastases from pancreatic carcinoma. Hepatogastroenterology 2004;51:1175–1178.
129. Melichar B, Voboril Z, Cerman J Jr, et al. Hepatic arterial infusion chemotherapy in gastric cancer: a report of four cases and analysis of the literature. Tumori 2004;90:428–434.
130. Melichar B, Voboril Z, Nozicka J, et al. Hepatic arterial infusion chemotherapy in sarcoma liver metastases: a report of 6 cases. Tumori 2005;91:19–23.
131. Hwu WJ, Salem RR, Pollak J, et al. A clinical-pharmacological evaluation of percutaneous isolated hepatic infusion of doxorubicin in patients with unresectable liver tumors. Oncol Res 1999;11:529–537.
132. Cantore M, Fiorentini G, Aitini E, et al. Intra-arterial hepatic carboplatin-based chemotherapy for ocular melanoma metastatic to the liver. Report of a phase II study. Tumori 1994;80:37–39.
133. Leyvraz S, Spataro V, Bauer J, et al. Treatment of ocular melanoma metastatic to the liver by hepatic arterial chemotherapy. J Clin Oncol 1997;15:2589–2595.
134. Salmon RJ, Levy C, Plancher C, et al. Treatment of liver metastases from uveal melanoma by combined surgery-chemotherapy. Eur J Surg Oncol 1998;24:127–130.
135. Taton G, Ghanem G, Pandin P, et al. First results of a clinical pilot study on intraarterial chemotherapy with hemofiltration of locally advanced gastrointestinal cancers. Acta Chir Belg 1996;96:206–210.
136. Palumbo G, Pantaleoni GC, Guadagni S. Pharmacokinetic of intraarterial mitomycin C with extra corporeal detoxification in humans. Clin Ter 1999;150:209–214.
137. Pingpank JF, Libutti SK, Chang R, et al. Phase I study of hepatic arterial melphalan infusion and hepatic venous hemofiltration using percutaneously placed catheters in patients with unresectable hepatic malignancies. J Clin Oncol 2005;23:3465–3474.
138. Reid T, Galanis E, Abbruzzese J, et al. Intra-arterial administration of a replication-selective adenovirus (dl1520) in patients with colorectal carcinoma metastatic to the liver: a phase I trial. Gene Ther 2001;8:1618–1626.
139. Habib NA, Sarraf CE, Mitry RR, et al. E1B-deleted adenovirus (dl1520) gene therapy for patients with primary and secondary liver tumors. Hum Gene Ther 2001;12:219–226.
140. Heise C, Sampson-Johannes A, Williams A, McCormick F, Von Hoff DD, Kirn DH. ONYX-015, an E1B gene-attenuated adenovirus, causes tumor-specific cytolysis and antitumoral efficacy that can be augmented by standard chemotherapeutic agents. Nat Med 1997;3:639–645.

141. Ruan DT, Warren RS. Liver-directed therapies in colorectal cancer. Semin Oncol 2005;32:85–94.
142. Shinozaki K, Ebert O, Woo SL. Eradication of advanced hepatocellular carcinoma in rats via repeated hepatic arterial infusions of recombinant VSV. Hepatology 2005;41:196–203.
143. Habib NA, Hodgson HJ, Lemoine N, Pignatelli M. A phase I/II study of hepatic artery infusion with wtp53-CMV-Ad in metastatic malignant liver tumors. Hum Gene Ther 1999;10:2019–3204.
144. Venook AP, Bergsland EK, Ring E. Gene therapy of colorectal liver metastases using recombinant adenovirus encoding wildtype p53 (SCH58500) via hepatic arterial infusion: a phase I study. Proc Am Soc Clin Oncol 1998; 431c.
145. Kornmann M, Link KH, Lenz HJ, et al. Thymidylate synthase is a predictor for response and resistance in hepatic artery infusion chemotherapy. Cancer Lett 1997;118:29–35.
146. Davies MM, Johnston PG, Kaur S, Allen-Mersh TG. Colorectal liver metastasis thymidylate synthase staining correlates with response to hepatic arterial floxuridine. Clin Cancer Res 1999;5:325–328.
147. Meric F, Pratt YZ, Curley SA, et al. Surgery after downstaging of unresectable hepatic tumors with intra-arterial chemotherapy. Ann Surg Oncol 2000;7(7):490–495.

14 Focal Liver Ablation Techniques in Primary and Secondary Liver Tumors

Giuseppe Garcea, MD, and David P. Berry, MD

CONTENTS

SUMMARY

Focal ablative techniques are promising tools in the treatment of unresectable primary and secondary liver tumors. Despite a lack of randomized controlled trials, early data suggest that these methods are effective and well-tolerated, with an acceptable complication rate. This chapter, an overview of established and experimental ablative methods, as well as clinical results reported thus far.

Key Words: Liver ablation; PEI; PAAI; radiofrequency ablation; high-intensity focused ultrasound; interstitial laser photocoagulation; microwave ablation; electrolysis; cryoablation.

1. INTRODUCTION

Primary hepatocellular carcinoma (HCC) is the fifth most common malignancy, with an increasing incidence in the Western world, secondary to the increasing prevalence of hepatitis C *(1–3)*. The liver is also the most common site for blood-borne metastases, particularly for malignancies arising in organs drained by the portal circulation. Colorectal carcinoma is the second most common cause of death in developed countries *(4)*, and up

From: *Cancer Drug Discovery and Development: Regional Cancer Therapy*
Edited by: P. M. Schlag and U. S. Stein © Humana Press Inc., Totowa, NJ

to 25% of patients will have metastatic spread to the liver at the time of diagnosis. A further 25% will develop metastases at a later date, and this progressive involvement of the liver may be the major or sole factor determining survival *(4a)*.

Liver resection is the accepted gold standard of treatment for liver tumors. Unfortunately, only 10 to 20% of patients with colorectal liver metastases are candidates for hepatic resection *(5)*. The resectability rate for HCC is about 20 to 30% in noncirrhotic liver but is reduced in patients with cirrhotic liver *(6,7)*. Hence, in any cohort of patients with primary or secondary tumors, most will be unsuitable for curative resection, owing to the presence of extrahepatic disease, the anatomical distribution of their lesions, or their tumor burden—at least 20% of normal functioning liver must remain following resection to avoid fulminant postoperative liver failure *(8)*. These considerations have led to considerable interest in nonresectional modalities of treatment for primary and secondary liver tumors, of which focal ablation techniques form a significant part.

2. OVERVIEW

The attraction of focal ablative techniques in patients unsuitable for resectional surgery is that they allow the destruction of the tumor deposits while preserving as much functional liver tissue as possible. Tumor destruction is achieved by injection of a cytotoxic or corrosive agent such as in percutaneous ethanol or acetic acid injection (PEI, PAAI); indirect generation of cytotoxic intermediaries such as electrolysis; heating such as radiofrequency ablation (RFA), interstitial laser photocoagulation (ILP), hot saline injection, or microwave coagulation therapy (MCT); mechanical shock or cavitation high-intensity focused ultrasound (HIFU) or freezing such as cryoablation (Fig. 1).

The success and applicability of any ablative techniques can be assessed by several desirable properties (Fig. 2). A predictable cell-killing action is required, to ensure that reproducible tumor ablation is produced in consecutive patients. A dose response is also needed, to allow the ablation of varying sized tumors. This killing zone produced by varying doses must also be predicable in its size and shape. To avoid damage to adjacent structures, the killing zone must not spread beyond the target area. The ability to monitor, in real time, the spread of the killing zone from the applicator is also necessary, as the cell destruction caused by some ablative techniques may not be immediately apparent. Other desirable, but perhaps not essential, qualities include ease of application (ideally percutaneously or laparoscopically), a manageable delivery time of the cell-killing modality, the ability to ablate multiple tumors simultaneously, and the lack of a systemic response following ablation. The degree to which both established and experimental ablation methods comply with these properties will probably be the major determinant in their long-term clinical application.

3. PERCUTANEOUS ETHANOL INJECTION

PEI is a well-established technique for tumor ablation and was first described for the treatment of HCC by Suguira et al. in 1983 *(9)*. The technique involves passing a 22-gage Chiba needle into the tumor mass under local anesthetic, using ultrasound (US) or computed tomography (CT) guidance. Ethanol (99.5 or 95%) is injected into the deepest aspect of the tumor, and injection is continued while the needle is slowly withdrawn. This ensures uniform and adequate dispersion of ethanol into the tumor mass. The needle is left in position for several minutes after injection, to prevent leakage of ethanol along the

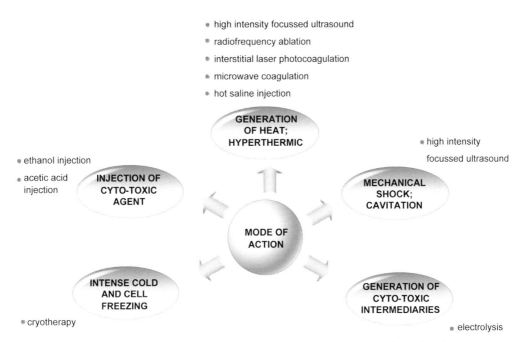

Fig. 1. Main focal liver ablative techniques and main mechanism of action

needle track. Following injection of ethanol, 1 to 2 mL of local anesthetic is also injected to minimize any pain post procedure. PEI is usually performed in several sessions on an outpatient basis or as single session under general anesthesia *(10)*. The number of injections needed for complete ablation of a tumor is approximately twice the lesion diameter in centimeters *(11)*.

The injected alcohol usually spreads in a 1- to 3-cm radius around the tip of needle, and injection is stopped when significant leakage outside the lesion is detected. The amount of alcohol needed to ablate a lesion is dependent on tumor consistency, vascularity, internal septae, areas of tumor necrosis (which provide a path of preferential alcohol diffusion), and the presence of tumor capsule (which contains the alcohol but also prevents it from reaching areas of extracapsular tumor *(12)*). The formula $V = (4/3)\pi(r+0.5)^3$ (where V in mL is the volume of ethanol and r (cm) is the radius of the lesion) is used by some centers to calculate the total volume of ethanol to be administered. An extra 0.5 mL is added to provide a margin of normal tissue ablation and ensure complete tumor destruction *(13)*. The microbubbles within the ethanol form an echogenic blush on US, allowing real-time monitoring during injection to ensure adequate perfusion of ethanol into the tumor *(14)*. CT scanning post procedure demonstrates a low-density uniform lesion that marks the area of liver necrosis *(15)*. Gelfoam powder or steel coils can be used to mark the part of the lesion that has been injected; alternatively, videotape can be used to record the injection for future reference *(13,16,17)*.

Ethanol acts through two mechanisms. The injected alcohol diffuses into neoplastic cells and causes dehydration and coagulative necrosis, followed by fibrosis. Second, the injected ethanol enters the microcirculation around the tumor and induces necrosis of endothelial cells, platelet aggregation and thrombosis of capillaries. The resulting tissue ischemia causes further tumor cell death *(18)*. Contrast-enhanced Doppler US can be

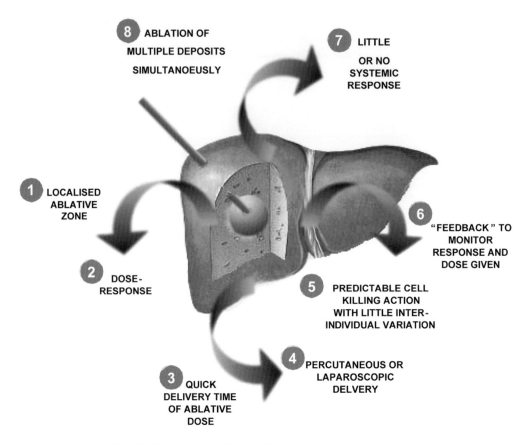

Fig. 2. Desirable qualities of focal liver ablation methods.

used to assess changes in tumor vascularity following PEI, with a reported 92% sensitivity and 100% specificity in identifying residual tumor *(19)*.

3.1. Results of PEI in the Treatment of Hepatocellular Cancer

PEI appears most efficacious in the treatment of HCC. HCC nodules have a soft consistency and are usually surrounded by firm cirrhotic liver. As a result, ethanol diffuses easily and selectively into the lesion, and further spread of ethanol is limited by the change in consistency of the surrounding liver tissue. PEI has been described as achieving complete necrosis in HCC nodules less than 3 cm in diameter *(20,21)*.

The efficiency of tumor killing by PEI appears to be, at least partly, size dependent. This and the difficulties of injecting large volumes of ethanol under local anesthetic have, until recently, limited PEI to small tumors. However, reports suggest that larger tumors, over 8 cm, can be treated safely using a single injection under general anesthesia. Volumes of up to 40 mL can be used on an outpatient basis *(22,23)* and up to 210 mL under general anesthesia *(17)*. Fructose 1,6-diphosphate and glutathione can be employed to neutralize the systemic effects of injected alcohol. If residual tumor is present, it is usually found in nests around the main lesion, along the edge of the lesion, or within the main tumor mass, where it is protected from the PEI by the presence of septae *(24)*. An alternative application of PEI, recently described, is its use to obliterate tumor-feeding vessels for very large HCC tumors *(25)*.

The results of PEI in HCC are summarized in Table 1 *(10,15,24,26–35)*. Early survival rates for PEI in tumors less than 5 cm range from 80 to 100%. For tumors larger than 5 cm, short-term survival following the first year have a poorer outcome of 72%, although 2- to 3-yr survival rates are similar in both groups. Prognostic factors that have been identified following PEI include tumor diameter less than 3 cm *(36)*, pretreatment α-fetoprotein levels, multiple tumors, and the presence of a tumor capsule *(24,31,33,36)*.

In addition to tumor burden, baseline liver function plays an important part in determining prognosis. Reports show a clear difference in survival between patients with Child's A, Child's B, and Child's C cirrhosis; with Child's C cirrhosis and the presence of portal vein thrombosis having the poorest outcome *(29)*. Other scoring systems used to predict survival are the Cancer of the Liver Italian Program score (CLIP), the Barcelona Clinic Liver Cancer score (BCLC), and Okuda scoring systems. The BCLC scoring system has been shown to give the best prediction of prognosis in patients with early disease undergoing PEI *(37)*. Recurrence rates following PEI are variable ranging from 40 to 81% after 5 yr (Table 1). These recurrences frequently occur in sites other than the tumor site following PEI, probably reflecting the multifocal pathology of HCC in cirrhotic livers.

Long-term survival following PEI is uniformLy poor, with most studies reporting a 30% survival at 5 yr (Table 1). Retrospective studies of PEI vs palliative treatment show a clear survival advantage *(38)* of up to 33% vs 14% in the untreated group *(30)*.

Although PEI is preferable to palliative treatment in the management of HCC, it may not be a superior treatment to resectional surgery or liver transplantation. Some data suggest that for larger HCC tumors, above 2 to 3 cm in diameter, resection surgery may offer better long-term outcomes and lower recurrence rates that for PEI alone *(34,39)*. The survival benefit of surgery over PEI has been found to be consistent despite the severity of the patients' cirrhosis. This notion is further supported by recent retrospective evidence from an Italian study, which has shown that 5- and 10-yr survival rates are better in patients who have undergone liver transplantation for early HCC than in patients who have undergone PEI *(40)*. Survival rates were 25.3 and 18.0% at 5 and 10 yr, respectively, in the PEI group, compared with 84.6 and 82.2%, respectively, in the transplant group. This survival benefit persisted in spite of the degree of liver impairment. The role of PEI among other available treatments for HCC is suggested in Fig. 3 *(41)*.

3.1.1. PEI in Combination with Other Regional Techniques

PEI has been combined with other regional techniques in an attempt to improve efficacy. Transarterial catheter embolization (TACE) has been used in conjunction with PEI and has been found to result in improved survival compared with PEI alone *(42)*. Intraarterial injection of ethanol in to the feeding artery of HCC tumors should, in theory, allow a more complete and selective spread of the ablative agent. The use of percutaneous intraarterial ethanol injection (PIAEI), has been advocated in the ablation of large HCC lesions. PIAEI, either alone, or in combination with PEI, has proved efficacious in the ablation of large HCCs (9 cm in diameter) *(43)*; however, it is associated with an increased risk of serious complications.

The ablative effect of RFA following PEI appears to be increased by the injection of alcohol, resulting in consistently larger lesions in fewer sessions, although long-term

Table 1
Results of Percutaneous Etanol Injection (PEI) in Hepatocellular Carcinoma (HCC)

Study and year	No. of patients	Tumor Size (cm)	Survival Rate (%)							3–5-Yr Recurrence (%)
			1 Yr	2 Yr	3 Yr	4 Yr	5 Yr	6 Yr	7 Yr	
Omata et al., 2004 (35)	524	3	—	—	79.4	—	64.7	—	45.1	—
		3	—	—	55.2	—	33.8	—	23.8	—
Lencioni et al., 2003 (26)	102	3–5	100	98	—	—	—	—	—	—
Yammamoto et al., 2001 (27)	39	3–5	100	—	82	—	—	—	—	59
Lin et al., 1999 (28)	47	≤3	85	75	61	39	—	—	—	79
Livraghi et al., 1998 (29)	108	5–8.5	72	65	57	44	—	—	—	—
Orlando et al., 1997 (30)	35	≤4	100	87	71	71	—	—	—	—
Castellono et al., 1997 (33)	71	≤5	89	54	24	—	—	—	—	81
Lencioni et al., 1995 (31)	82	≤5	96	87	68	51	32	24	—	40
Isobe et al., 1994 (32)	37	≤5	95	81	70	—	—	—	—	40
Ebara et al., 1993 (15)	162	≤3	95.9	—	60.5	—	36.9	—	21.7	63
Castellano et al., 1993 (34)	30	≤4	83	66	55	34	—	—	—	65
Shiina et al., 1993 (24)	146	≤2	79	64	46	38	38	—	—	60
Livraghi et al., 1992 (10)	162	≤5	90	80	63	—	—	—	—	—

[a] Randomized controlled trial of PEI vs radiofrequency ablation (RFA).

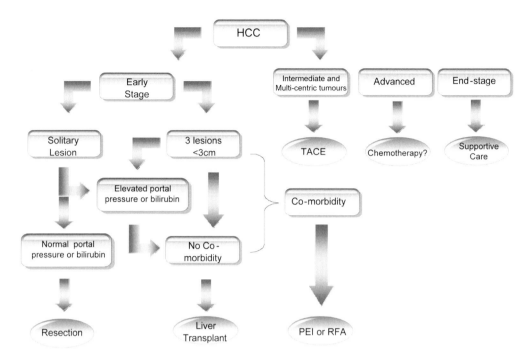

Fig. 3. Role of percutaneous techniques, such as percutaneous ethanol injection (PEI) in the management of hepatocellular carcinoma (HCC). RFA, radiofrequency ablation; TACE, transarterial catheter embolization. (Adapted from ref. *41*.)

survival data are lacking *(44,45)*. RFA may supersede PEI in the ablation of HCC. Two studies have demonstrated that RFA results in a 10% increase in complete ablation rate compared with PEI *(26)* alone and a reduction in local recurrence *(46)*. One of the largest comparisons between PEI and RFA examined 524 patients undergoing 1230 PEI treatments and 629 patients undergoing 1372 RFA treatments; in the RFA group demonstrated a 5 to 8% better survival *(35)*.

3.2. Results of PEI in Metastatic Liver Deposits

Unlike HCC, colorectal metastatic lesions are far more difficult to destroy by PEI. The injected alcohol tends to spread into the softer adjacent normal liver parenchyma, rather than staying within the hard tumor tissue, through which it diffuses in an inhomogeneous and irregular fashion *(47)*. There are few data relating the results of PEI for metastatic tumors. Complete necrosis of tumors has only been observed in 52 to 56% of lesions *(48,49)*, and progression of disease has occurred in a series of eight patients undergoing PEI *(50)*. Lesions that have the greatest response are small (2-cm) endocrine metastases, and the 3-yr survival for these patients has been reported as 39% *(49)*. PEI of metastatic liver deposits remains experimental and should not be the treatment of choice over resection or alternative ablative techniques.

3.3. Complications and Contraindications for PEI

Most patients experience some degree of pain or discomfort following PEI, either right upper quadrant or shoulder tip in location *(51)*. Pyrexia following PEI is also common.

Major complications are uncommon, occurring in 0.7 to 3% of patients *(38,49)*, and include hepatic infarction, intraperitoneal bleeding, pneumothorax, ascites, hemobilia, portal vein thrombosis, and cholangitis *(31,38,51,52)*. Deaths related to PEI have occurred secondary to massive hepatic necrosis and portal vein thrombosis *(53,54)*. Perhaps unsurprisingly, the complication rate following the more aggressive single session treatment is higher, with a recent report suggesting a 4.6% procedure-related mortality *(17)*. Long-term complications of PEI include a reported case of bile duct stricture *(55)* and needle tract implantation of HCC, which has been noted in less than 1% of cases *(56)*. Common to all percutaneous liver puncture techniques, PEI is contraindicated in severe thrombocytopenia and clotting dyscrasias. Very large tumors (> 8.5 cm in diameter) are also considered a relative contraindication to PEI, as is a preexisting thrombosis in the portal vein and ascites.

4. PERCUTANEOUS ACETIC ACID INJECTION

The principles of using acetic acid in tumor ablation are the same as in PEI. However, owing to its greater necrotizing power, smaller volumes of acetic acid are required in fewer injections to achieve the same therapeutic effect. Acetic acid will, therefore, not only destroy tumors more efficiently but will also break down internal septae, thereby enhancing its effects *(57)*. In PAAI, 50% acetic acid is substituted for ethanol, but the technique is otherwise unchanged. The main risk of acetic acid injection is leak of acetic acid outside the tumor into bile ducts, portal veins, and hepatic veins *(58)*. Presumably, the ability of acetic acid to breakdown internal septae also renders it more able to breach the tumor capsule frequently found in HCCs. CT fluoroscopy can be employed to monitor the distribution of acetic acid and hence minimize these sequelae. Persistent retention of acetic acid, as monitored by US, following injection is associated with complete tumor ablation and correlates with favorable tumor response *(59)*.

4.1. Results of PAAI in HCC

Ohnishi et al. *(60)* reported a randomized controlled trial that compared PAAI with PEI and found a lower recurrence rate (8% for PAAI vs 37% for PEI) and superior 2-yr survival rate (92% for PAAI vs 63% for PEI) in favor of PAII. A smaller study looking at 18 patients *(61)* showed no recurrence in 17 patients after 29-mo follow-up. More recently, a prospective study comparing PAAI and PEI in 63 patients found that both techniques were equally effective with a 1- and 3-yr survival of 81 and 46% in the PEI group and 84 and 51% in the PAAI groups *(62)*. Recurrence rates at 1 and 3 yr were also similar. PAAI did display the advantage that fewer injection sessions were needed to achieve the same results.

Another study comparing TACE and PAAI found that for small tumors (<3 cm) there was no difference in survival between the two techniques *(63)*. However, for patients with HCCs over 3 cm in diameter, TACE resulted in significantly better survival than PAAI *(63)*. Combining TACE with PAAI has been associated with an increased therapeutic effect over and above using PAAI alone. In a prospective study of 33 patients, a TACE/PAAI combination resulted in 96.7, 86.6, 51.3, and 33.3%, 1-, 2-, 3-, and 4-yr survival compared with 66.7, 44.4, 16.7, and 0% in patients receiving TACE alone *(64)*. These observations have been further supported by other reports demonstrating a survival advantage with TACE/PAAI therapy over PAAI alone in patients with HCC over 3 cm in diameter *(65)*.

4.2. Complications of PAAI

The widespread reluctance to adopt PAAI stems from several severe complications recorded, despite the limited data on PAAI. These include hepatic wedge infarction, fatal hepatic failure (61), liver perforation (66), and severe renal failure (67). These complications are secondary to systemic absorption of acetic acid and its necrotizing power following injection. More data are needed on the use of PAAI before valid conclusions regarding its safety and efficacy can be drawn.

5. OTHER PERCUTANEOUS INJECTION TECHNIQUES

Two other injection techniques are briefly mentioned here. Percutaneous injection of alkaline solutions has been assessed in animal models against PEI and PAAI. An alkaline solution of dilute sodium hydroxide has been shown to be more effective than ethanol in cell killing but less effective than acetic acid (68). Its primary advantage over PAAI is a much better survival rate (100% vs 50%) with no damage to other organs because the toxic effect of acetic acid on other organs has been avoided. However, no clinical data exist as yet validating its use in human subjects.

Hot saline injection (HSI) therapy has been proposed as a way of overcoming distal and local toxic effects following injection of cytodestructive agents. The method of tumor killing is heat destruction, causing coagulative necrosis. The method of fluid instillation is identical to those already described; however, because hot saline is used to destroy the tumor, as it cools, it becomes physiological saline, so that the complications associated with ethanol and acetic acid toxicity should not occur.

The first human trial of HSI was reported by Honda et al. in 1994 (61). Twenty patients with HCCs smaller than 3 cm were injected with hot saline. During a 2- to 36-mo follow-up period, no local recurrence was seen. Yoon et al. reported on a series of 29 patients with large HCCs (mean diameter 7 cm) (62). Initial regression rate at 3 mo was 42%, with a median survival of 10 mo and no complications. More recently, Araki et al. reported on a series of 17 patients in whom complete tumor ablation was achieved using HSI, as demonstrated by CT scanning (69). Magnetic resonance imaging (MRI) scanning can be used to assess the temperature gradient during HSI and hence can be employed to monitor the spread of saline, to ensure adequate distribution throughout the lesion (70). Although HSI appears to be safe and very well tolerated, the short follow-ups and small numbers of studies published so far do not allow for accurate survival conclusions to be made. However, HSI may be a feasible alternative for large HCCs.

6. RADIOFREQENCY ABLATION

RFA is an electrosurgical technique utilizing high-frequency alternating current to heat tissues, leading to thermal coagulation. When cells are heated above 45°C, cellular proteins denature and cell membranes lose their integrity as their lipid component melts (71). RFA is well-established for many symptomatic cardiac arrhythmias because of its ability to create localized necrotic lesions in the cardiac conducting system. During RFA, a high frequency alternating current (350–500 kHz) flows from the uninsulated tip of an electrode into the tissue. Ionic agitation is produced in the tissue around the electrode tip as the ions attempt to follow the direction of the alternating current, and it is this agitation which results in frictional heating in the tissue around the electrode (72,73). The size and shape of the necrotic RFA lesion has been shown to be dependent on the probe gage, length of the exposed tip, probe temperature and duration of treatment *(72–75)*. A recent report studying RFA in vivo in a pig model also suggests that local blood flow is a strong predictor of lesion dimensions by reducing lesion size *(76)*.

Theoretically, it should be possible to create lesions of 1.6 × 8 cm with a single probe *(72,74)*; however, this has not been the case in vivo because lesion uniformity breaks down when the length of the probe tip exceeds 3 cm, thereby limiting the actual lesion size to a maximum diameter of 3.6 cm. Modifications such as multiple probes *(77)* and saline enhancement *(78)* have been described to achieve lesions of approximately 4 cm in diameter. This has led to the advancement of the *expandable wet electrode*, whereby hypertonic saline solution is infused at the same time as RFA to obtain larger ablated volumes of liver *(79,80)*. Abolishing the vascular inflow, via the Pringle maneuver, during RFA can also produce larger lesions (mean diameter 3.4 cm) with a faster warm-up time and also a more spherical lesion in place of the characteristic elliptical shape *(81)*. Balloon occlusion of the hepatic artery has also been shown to have a similar effect in increasing the size of the lesion produced with RFA *(82)*. Cooling the tip of the RFA needle prevents charring of liver tissue around the needle and thereby allows a higher power to be used, which results in a larger hyperthermic lesion.

Percutaneous RFA has been described under general or local anesthesia *(75,78)*, along with a laparoscopic approach *(83)*. Usually, a 15- to 21-gage RF probe with a 2- to 3-cm tip exposure is positioned into the lesion. A monopolar RF generator serves as the energy source, and a grounding pad is placed on the patient's thigh *(75,78)*. RF treatment is often based on intraprocedural temperature monitoring to determine the thermal lesion produced. The probes may be repositioned during treatment to achieve complete tumor ablation in one treatment session. During treatment under US control, a gradually enlarging elliptical lesion can be seen with ill-defined margins *(74)*. These appearances persist up to several months after treatment, and this heterogeneity precludes the distinction between ablated tumor and residual disease.

Even with CT or MR follow-up, the appearances of the residual disease or ablated tumor may be indistinguishable from one another, and this represents perhaps the biggest disadvantage with RFA. In clinical practice, the CT Hounsfield unit of density can be used to gage the extent of tissue necrosis following ablation. Absence of increased Hounsfield unit density, following contrast injection, indicates necrotic tissue; viable tissue shows an increase in Hounsfield unit density *(84)*. More recently, fluorescence spectroscopy has been trialled in porcine models, which could be used to detect hepatocellular thermal damage in real time and hence ensure adequate tumor ablation *(85)*. Other techniques currently under development include ultrasonagraphic assessment of microbubble contrast agents through the liver, known as hepatic transit time (HTT). Since the HTT is markedly reduced in patients with liver metastases, normalization of HTT could be used as a means of monitoring successful RFA *(86)*. Positron emission tomography (PET) scanning can also be employed in surveillance post RFA with a higher sensitivity than CT alone *(87)*. However, a significant drawback is the limited access many centers have, at present, to these technologies.

6.1. Results of RFA in Liver Tumors

Radiofrequency is rapidly increasing in popularity as the technique of choice in ablating liver tumors. Since 1995, more than 50 publications have described the results of RFA in primary liver tumors and colorectal hepatic metastases. Table 2 summarizes these data *(88–129)*. Local recurrence rates following RFA vary from 0 to 34% and the best results appear to be observed in tumors of 3.0 cm or less. Survival data following ablation suffer from short follow-up periods, with no study, to date, giving follow-up data beyond 3 yr for RFA in colorectal hepatic metastases. As previously discussed, RFA appears to achieve more complete tumor eradication than PEI for HCC, despite a higher complication rate (12.7% vs no complications for the PEI cohort) *(46)*. Tateishi et al. recently reported on a large series of 664 patients with HCC undergoing 1000 RFA treatments *(129)*. This large study would appear to confirm both the safety of RFA (4.0% major complication rate) and the efficacy of RFA (54.3% 5-yr survival for first-time patients), over PEI.

In comparison with cryotherapy, RFA appears to be safer and more effective at eradicating tumors, with a complication rate of 3.3% vs 40.7% and a recurrence rate of 2.2% vs 13.6% *(100)*. When RFA is compared with microwave coagulation therapy, there is an equivalent complication and therapeutic effect; however, RFA was found to be superior because tumor ablation could be achieved in fewer sessions *(130)*.

RFA has also been shown to be cost effective when compared with palliative treatments for both HCC and liver metastases *(131)*. The European Organization for Research and Treatment of Cancer (EORTC) and national Cancer Research Network (NCRN) endorsed randomized-controlled CLOCC trial is currently recruiting patients and comparing chemotherapy with chemotherapy and RFA, in patients with unresectable hepatic disease in the absence of extrahepatic disease. The study will end in 2006 and should answer the question as to whether ablation confers any survival advantage to patients over chemotherapy alone. To date, when compared with liver resection for the treatment of metastatic hepatic tumors, resection has been more effective in terms of Quality of Life and cost effectiveness *(132)*, and so resection will remain the mainstay of disease control for the foreseeable future.

Significant confounding factors in the evaluation of RFA are the short follow-up times and the difficulty in assessing the presence of viable tumor in the surrounding tissue following ablation. Factors that determine survival following RFA include the location of tumors (centrally placed tumors have a higher recurrence), tumor number, and tumor size (>4–5 cm). These factors probably relate to the efficacy of achieving complete tumor eradication, if the tumor burden is very high or if the access is technically difficult *(125,133–135)*. Young age and poor differentiation of tumor cells have also been implicated in poor prognosis *(133)*. The approach used in RFA may also affect outcome. Although percutaneous ablation has been shown to be advantageous over other ablation approaches in terms of reduced postoperative pain, shorter hospitalization, and reduced costs *(136)*, some reports suggest that the percutaneous approach may result in a higher recurrence than the laparoscopic or open approach *(135)*, at 53% vs 23.0% and 6.0%, respectively *(125)*.

New techniques for increasing the size of the ablated lesion may improve the ability to eradicate larger liver tumors. These include expandable tips, venous occlusion, and increasing the perfusion rate of cooled-tip catheters. Using these methods, tumors above 4 cm can be treated with an 80 to 95% eradication rate *(97,123,137–140)*. With the use of an umbrella-shaped probe and a 200-W generator, 100% destruction of very large colorectal metastases (up to 10 cm) was achieved in a series of 30 patients *(141)*.

Table 2
Results of Radiofrequency Ablation (RFA) in Primary and Secondary Hepatic Tumors

Study	Tumor size (cm)	Type of tumor — HCC or other	Type of tumor — Colorectal metastases	Needle type	Approach	Mean follow-up (mo)	Local recurrence rate (%)
Tateishi et al., 2005 (129)	3.4	664	—	Cooled-tip	Perc	5 yr	Survival of 53 mo
Gillams et al., 2005 (128)	—	Other 25	—	—	Perc	21	
Miyamoto et al., 2004 (127)	5.2	—	4	—	Open	12.7	n = 1
Kurshinoff et al., 2002 (125)	4.0	11	34	Cooled-tip expandable	Open 17 Lap 13 Perc 15	12 12	Open = 6% Lap = 23% Perc = 53%
Kosari et al., 2002 (124)	3.2	27	18	Cooled-tip expandable	Open 20 Lap 21 Perc 11	19.5	7.7
Ianitti et al., 2002 (123)	5.2	HCC 30 Other 41	52	Cooled-tip expandable	Open 33 Lap 3 Perc 87	20.0	—
Elias et al., 2002 (121)	2.1	HCC 5 Other 13	29	Cooled-tip expandable	Perc	14.0	9.0
Chan et al., 2002 (120)	2.1	—	—	Expandable needle	—	5.0	5.0
Berber et al., 2002 (119)	2.3	Other 34	—	Expandable needle	Lap	19.0	13.0
Morimoto et al., 2002 (126)	3.0	26	—	Expandable needle	Perc	6.0	8.0
Hosida et al., 2002 (122)	2.2	45	—	—	Perc	—	—
Machi et al., 2001 (117)	3.6	HCC 18 Other 3	25	Expandable needle	—	20.0	8.8

Chung et al., 2001 (112)	2.6	HCC 4 Othr 17	6	Expandable needle	Lap	14.0	15.0
Bewles et al., 2001 (111)	3.0	HCC 25 Other 12	39	Expandable needle	—	15.0	9.0
Podnos et al., 2001 (118)	3.1	12	—	Expandable needle	Lap	7.4	8.3
Llovett et al., 2001 (116)	2.8	32	—	Cooled tip	Perc	10.0	12.5
Lin et al., 2001 (115)	2.6	40	—	Expandable needle	Perc	16.6	21.0
Ideda et al., 2001 (114)	3.0	23	—	Cooled-tip	Perc	12.0	15.0
De Sio et al., 2001 (113)	3.8	35	—	Cooled-tip	Perc	—	—
Wood et al., 2000 (110)	2.0	—	—	—	—	9.0	18.0
Siperstein et al., 2000 (109)	0.5–1.0	—	—	Expandable needle	Lap	—	28
Huppert et al., 2000 (107)	1.3–3.0	—	—	Cooled-tip	Perc	11.0	7.0
Holtkamp et al., 2000 (106)	1.2–4.7	—	—	Cooled-tip	Perc	7.0	—
De Baere et al., 2000 (104)	0.5–4.2	—	68	Cooled-tip	Open 21 Perc 47	13.0	9.0
Bilchik et al., 2000 (102)	2/0	—	—	Expandable needle	Open 26 Lap 26 Perc 16	16.0	2.8
Livraghi et al., 2000 (108)	5.4	114	—	Cooled-tip	Perc	10.0	—
Goletti et al., 2000 (105)	4.0	7	—	Cooled-tip	Lap	6.0	10.0
Burley et al., 2000 (103)	2.8–4.6	110	—	Cooled-tip	Open 31 Lap 31 Perc 76	19.0	3.6

(continued)

241

Table 2 (Continued)

Study	Tumor size (cm)	HCC or other	Colorectal metastases	Type of tumor — Needle type	Type of tumor — Approach	Mean follow-up (mo)	Local recurrence rate (%)
Scudamore et al., 1999 (101)	2.9	—	10	Expandable needle	Perc	10.0	—
Pearson et al., 1999 (100)	3.6	Hcc 34 Othr 12	46	Expandable needle	Open	15.0	2.2
Jiao et al., 1999 (98)	—	HCC 8 Other 10	17	Cooled-tip	—	10.0	14.0
Cushieri et al., 1999 (96)	15.0	2	8	Expandable needle	Lap	13.0	0.0
Curley et al., 1999 (95)	3.4	HCC 48 Other 14	61	Expandable needle	Open 92 Perc 13	15.0	1.8
Livraghi et al., 1999 (99)	2.3	42	—	Cooled-tip	Perc	10.0	—
Francica et al., 1999 (97)	2.8	15	—	Cooled-tip	Perc	15.0	0.0
Buscarini et al., 1999 (94)	5.2	14	—	Expandable needle	Perc	13.0	0.0
Allgaier et al., 1999 (93)	3.2	12	—	Expandable needle	Perc	5.0	0.0
Rossi et al., 1998 (92)	2.9	23	14	Expandable needle	Perc	10.0	5.0
Lencioni et al., 1998 (91)	1.3–5.1	Other 5	24	Cooled-tip	Perc	6.5	12.0
Rossi et al., 1995 (88)	3.0	24	—	Straight needle	Perc	24.0	8.5
Solbiati et al., 1997 (90)	1.3–5.1	Other 7	22	Cooled-tip	Perc	12.0	34.0
Rossi et al., 1996 (89)	2.2	Other 39	11	Cooled-tip	Perc	22.0	5.0

Abbreviations: Lap, laparoscopic; Perc, percutaneous.

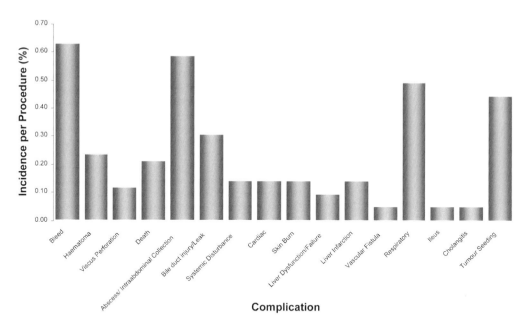

Fig. 4. Complications following radiofrequency ablation (RFA) from 4302 procedures between 1996 and 2005. Isolated case reports are not included in data series.

6.2. Complications of RFA

Figure 4 summarizes the overall complications from over 4000 RFA procedures between 1996 and 2005 *(88–129)*. Bleeding and hepatic/intraabdominal abscesses are the main complications following RFA. Needle tract seeding by tumor cells has been exclusively reported following RFA for HCCs and would appear to be a significant problem in this group of patients. A wide range of respiratory problems have also been reported including effusions, hemothoraces, pneumothoraces, and diaphragmatic paralysis. Complications such as vascular fistulae, bile duct strictures/leaks, and viscus perforation would appear to be a consequence of failing to control the ablative lesions, hence leading to damage to adjacent structures. Overall, RFA is safe and well tolerated, with a per procedure mortality of only 0.21%.

7. HIGH-INTENSITY FOCUSED ULTRASOUND

HIFU is unique in that it is an extracorporeal, transcutaneous method of tissue ablation. The use of sound waves of much higher amplitude than those used in a diagnostic setting, along with a concave US transducer, results in selective, targeted delivery of higher energy, without the possibility of damage to intervening tissues *(142)* (Fig. 5). In HIFU, the sound waves are focused in the same way that a magnifying glass is used to focus sunlight. HIFU exerts its effects primarily by heating; the sound waves are absorbed by the target organ, and the heat generated leads to coagulative necrosis in the tissues *(142)*.

Another mechanism by which HIFU can exert its effect is by cavitation of the target organ. Cavitation describes the mechanism whereby tissue destruction occurs by mechanical shock and free radical formation. The threshold at which cavitation occurs is determined by the probe frequency, the sound wave intensity, and the impedance

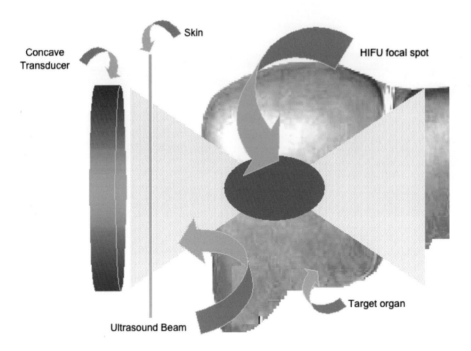

Fig. 5. Schematic diagram of high-intensity focused ultrasound (HIFU).

characteristics of the tissue. Although cavitation causes more rapid tissue destruction, it is less controllable than heating; hence the latter effect of HIFU has been mostly used for tumor ablation *(142)*. There is also evidence that HIFU results in coagulative necrosis in tumor vessels *(143)* and activates aggregation and adhesion of platelets *(144)*. These changes in the tumor microvasculature could be critical as a secondary cause of tumor death *(145)*. The hemostatic effect of HIFU could also be useful in obtaining hemostasis in the liver following tumor destruction and so reduce bleeding complications *(146)*.

HIFU has been performed in animal models using a concave transducer to focus the beam with a frequency range of 1 to 4 MHz and peak intensity of 100 to 1500 W/cm^2 for 1 to 10 s *(147,148)*. Encouraging early results were obtained in animal studies with improved survival rates following HIFU *(142,149)*. Total treatment times for HIFU vary from 1 h to up to 5 h for a 10-cm tumor. A potential problem in the application of HIFU is patient movement during the procedure. The natural ultrasonic "scatters" in biological tissue can be used as markers to track the motion of the target area. A real-time feedback of the HIFU beam can then be achieved, so its ablative effect can be concentrated only on the tumor *(150)*. In vivo studies have used iodized oil to increase the temperature, and hence the size of the lesion created by HIFU, resulting in better survival *(151)*. A split-focus transducer has also been trialled in pig models to give a lesion three to four times larger than a single-spot focus for the same acoustic power *(152)*.

7.1. Results of HIFU in Humans

Trials of HIFU in humans are limited at present. The earliest application of HIFU in humans resulted in no visible effect in one patient and extensive tissue laceration and only patchy necrosis in the other *(153)*. Wu et al. reported in 2004 on results from HIFU in

55 patients with HCCs ranging from 4 to 14 cm in diameter *(154)*. Follow-up imaging showed a reduction in tumor size in all patients, with normalization of α-fetoprotein levels in 34% of patients. Another Chinese study in 100 patients with liver tumors found that HIFU alleviated symptoms in 86.6% of patients and lowered α-fetoprotein levels by 50% in 65% of patients *(155)*. CT and MRI scanning post ablation revealed reduction in tumor size in all patients. One study employing HIFU for tumors followed by liver resection found that the tumor was completely eradicated in all 30 cases *(145)*. Another study has, however, reported recurrence rates following HIFU as high as 10% *(156)*.

There are no comparative trials of HIFU over liver resection or other better established ablation modalities. A randomized trial of TACE plus HIFU over TACE alone found that combination therapy resulted in better 1-yr survival (42.9% vs 0%, respectively) for 26 patients with advanced HCC *(157)*. Complications recorded included skin burns, liver laceration, and peripheral nerve injuries *(153,156)*. HIFU lesions are very sharply demarcated, with a border of only several cell layers between normal and destroyed tissue *(145)*. This sharp demarcation, coupled with accurate targeting techniques, could allow treatment of deep-seated tumors close to structures that have rendered them in-operable. However, more trials of HIFU are needed before any conclusions regarding its clinical validity can be drawn.

8. INTERSTITIAL LASER PHOTOCOAGULATION

ILP is another method of causing tissue destruction by heating, thereby inducing coagulative necrosis. ILP was introduced by Bown in 1983 and involves local delivery of laser light via flexible fibers. The biological response of tissue following the absorption of laser light results in several different thermal effects. At 40 to 45°C, heating and enzyme denaturation occurs. At temperatures of 60 to 140°C, cell shrinkage, hyperchromasia, membrane rupture, and protein denaturation results. At higher temperatures, from 300 to 1000°C, vaporization and carbonization occurs *(158–160)*. Coagulation is defined as the irreversible thermal damage of tissue proteins at temperatures between 55 and 95°C. ILP uses laser light at low power (typically 3–15 W) with exposure times of 3 to 20 min. It is the conversion of the absorbed light energy into heat that is responsible for tissue necrosis. The absorption of light may occur directly, or after scattering of the light in the treated tissue. The latter results in greater tissue penetration and more uniform energy distribution *(161,162)*.

The low absorption and high scatter characteristics of the Neodymium: yttrium-aluminum-garnet laser (Nd:YAG), which has a wavelength of 1064 nm, maximize tissue penetration and the uniformity of energy distribution *(162)*. Heat conduction and convection extend the area of necrosis beyond the area of light penetration *(163)*. The size of the resultant lesions is dependent on the fiber position within the tumor and the temperature gradient created by the amount of power, as well as duration of exposure. Increasing the power (the most important variable) and exposure time during ILP increases the area of necrosis *(164)*. In addition, the use of multiple synchronous fibers can also increase the lesion size to as large as 5 cm *(165,166)*. Blood flow along portal vessels acts as a "heat sink," and it has been found that occluding portal vessels results in larger lesions *(167–170)*. A similar effect can be achieved with hepatic arterial embolization using degradable starch microspheres *(171)*. Carbonization at the tip of the lesion is best avoided, as this tissue limits the penetration of light into the surrounding tissue, resulting in local temperature accumulation *(160)*. With cylindrical, diffusing tips, homogenous light emission can be distributed throughout the surrounding tissue, which results in larger lesions with less interlesion variation *(169,172)*.

The first clinical report of ILP treatment was in 1985 by Hashimoto et al. *(173)*, who treated patients with both liver metastases and HCC at laparotomy. This study used a YAG laser with a bare tip, at low power (5 W) and long exposure times. The study proved the feasibility of the technique without major complications. In 1991, Huang et al. *(174)* modified the technique to avoid carbonization at the tip. In 1989, Steger et al. *(175)* introduced the percutaneous technique, and several groups have since modified this. ILP is now usually performed percutaneously under US control, although a recent report of MRI-guided ILP appears very encouraging *(176)*.

Although variations in technique exist, the most widely employed method of tumor ablation is to place one or more 19-gage needles into the deepest aspect of the tumor under US control. The number of needles required relates to the tumor size. Each needle is then exchanged for an optical fiber tip, which is coupled to a laser source, resulting in heating of the tumor. The tips can be repositioned during treatment to allow complete tumor ablation, but multiple sessions are often required for lesions over 3 cm. Energy per metastasis can vary from 1000 to 34,000 J, depending on the size of the lesion *(47)*. When a diffusing fiber is used, it can be connected to microthermocouples to monitor the temperature. The fiber is introduced into the center of the tumor, which is heated until the temperature at the lesion edge reaches either 60°C or 45°C for 15 min *(162)*. Real-time noninvasive imaging is poor, although on-line monitoring with T1-weighted turbo fast low-angle shot (FLASH) MRI demonstrates a "dark rim" around the edge of the tumor, which is accurate in predicting necrosis in 85% of cases *(177)*.

8.1. Results of ILP in Liver Tumors

Table 3 summarizes the results of ILP in liver tumors *(47,162,174,178–185)*. The percentage of tumors in which ILP achieves complete destruction varies from as low as 60% but up to 98%. In keeping with other ablative treatments that rely on heating, it would appear that ILP is best suited to lesions below 3 cm *(180,183,186)*. Monitoring in real time of the lesions produced by ILP has also been reported as problematic *(185)*, and this could be a factor in the wide variation of complete necrosis rates observed with ILP. There is evidence from animal studies that biliary structures may interfere with the therapeutic effect of ILP by acting as a heat sink and are the focus of local recurrence *(187)*.

Vogl et al. are responsible for the largest reported series of ILP. Their results suggest that there is clinical potential in ILP, with results that approach those following liver resection *(178,179,188)*. Vogl et al. have achieved local control of tumors of 97% after 6 mo of follow-up, with a cumulative survival rate of 45% *(179)*. In their later report, the same group described 2 and 5-yr survival rates of 74 and 30%, respectively, in patients with hepatic metastases *(178)*. The patients included in this study all had fewer than five tumors, each smaller than 5 cm, with no extrahepatic spread. Comparisons of ILP with other focal ablative treatments are limited. One study by Amin et al. *(47)* compared ILP with PAI and found ILP to be superior in the treatment of colorectal liver metastases. Comparisons between ILP and RFA are problematic, because of the differing methodology and study protocols employed by different groups. At present, the emerging data suggest that ILP may offer equivalent treatment potential to RFA, despite its less wide-

Table 3

Results from Interstitial Laser Photocoagulation (ILP) of Liver Tumor

Group and year	No. of Patients	Type of lesion treated		% of Tumors in which full necrosis achieved	Extent of partial tumor necrosis achieved in remaining tumors	Survival rate	Local recurrence rate (%)
		HCC	Colorectal metastases				
Vogl et al., 2002 (178)	899	—	—	—	—	74 and 35% at 3 and 5 yr, respectively	—
Vogl et al., 2001 (179)	676	16	376 CRC 122 Breast mets 162 Other mets	—	—	63% at 28 mo	5.0
Pacella et al., 2001 (180)	74	74	—	97	—	15% 5-yr survival	8.7
Gillams and Lees, 2000 (181)	69	—	69	—	63	22% 5-yr survival	—
Giorgio et al., 2000 (182)	104	77	27	82 of HCC 77 of mets	—	—	—
Caspani et al., 1997 (183)	35	15	20	77.5	—	—	—
Gillams et al., 1997 (184)	55	—	55	16	38% partial response	—	—
Tranberg et al., 1996 (185)	10	5	7	42	50% necrosis in remaining tumors	—	50
Amin et al., 1993 (47)	22	—	22	52	87% of remaining tumors achieved over 50% necrosis	—	—
Nolsoe et al., 1993 (162)	11	—	11	75	—	—	36
Huang et al., 1991 (174)	5	5	—	20	—	—	33

Abbreviations: CRC, colorectal cancer; HCC, hepatocellular carcinoma; mets, metastases.

spread clinical use. One cause of concern regarding ILP is the large variation in recurrence rates, ranging from 8 to 50% (Table 3). This could be partly owing to problems in monitoring ILP lesions in real time, as discussed in the previous paragraph. It may be that with increasing experience in ILP that these figures will fall to the recurrence rates of between 5 and 8%, as reported by other groups *(178,180)*.

8.2. Complications of ILP

Complications are infrequently reported following ILP. Pain and fever are common. Other minor complications are pleural effusion, subcapsular hematoma, paralytic ileus, and one case of gastric hemorrhage *(47,182)*. Pretreatment liver function is important, as ILP can cause severe deterioration in liver function assays, and one death has been reported in a patient with Childs C cirrhosis *(182)*. ILP in larger tumors could be associated with a higher complication rate. Tranberg et al. *(185)* reported a death from multiple organ failure following ILP of an 8-cm tumor Animal models have also demonstrated the presence of gas formation in vascular structures during ILP *(189)*. In a clinical setting, it is theoretically possible that the presence of intracardiac gas in a patient with a patent foramen ovale could lead to a paradoxical embolus. No biliary complications have been reported following ILP, the most common complication appearing to be intrahepatic abscess formation and subcapsular hematoma (reported in some series as up to 2%). In spite of the above complications, ILP appears to be a well-tolerated procedure, with a complication rate of approximately 4.7% and mortality rate of 0.3% in over 2500 ILP procedures *(178)*.

9. MICROWAVE COAGULATION THERAPY

Since its introduction in 1979 by Tabuse *(190)*, MCT has been used at laparotomy *(191)*, laparoscopically *(192)*, percutaneously *(193)*, and thorascopically *(194)*. MCT is another hyperthermic technique relying on the conversion of energy to heat, to destroy tumors. During treatment, 2450-MHz microwaves polarize water molecules secondary to the rapidly alternating electromagnetic radiation. As the water molecules follow the changing polarity of the field, heat is generated from within the tissue, resulting in coagulative necrosis and hemostasis. Tissue coagulation occurs in a spindle-shaped configuration around the monopolar field *(195)*. MCT creates a predictable and reproducible area of tissue necrosis, and it can ablate the tumor capsule and so destroy any surrounding extracapsular invasion. Similar to HIFU, MCT appears to produce a hemostatic effect on surrounding tissues, at least theoretically, reducing the risk of hemorrhage post procedure *(191)*.

Percutaneous MCT is performed under US control and local anesthetic. The microwave electrode is positioned in the lesion under US guidance, and microwaves are administered at 60 W for 60 to 120 s *(195)*. For large lesions, a sequential technique with multiple needles has been developed *(196)*. This technique uses 80 W of power for 60 s to create a lesion of 2 cm in diameter; by overlapping these lesions, large ablation areas can be achieved. Real-time US monitoring demonstrates that the lesion becomes hypoechoic immediately following treatment *(195)*, giving quick and accurate feedback regarding the size of the lesion. New microwave tips are currently under development, which can produce much larger lesions (3–6 cm) in diameter without the need for overlapping *(197)*. These lesions can be produced very rapidly, within 3 min, with a high degree of consistency in interlesion formation.

Larger ablated lesions can also be achieved by selectively blocking the blood flow to the liver *(198,199)*. Both hepatic artery and venous occlusion result in larger lesions, but venous occlusion appears to have a greater effect on lesion size than arterial occlusion alone *(200)*. Multiple microwave probes have been used successfully to result in synergistically larger zones of coagulation necrosis *(201)*. Distal effects of MCT beyond the anatomical ablation zone have also been observed. Local changes in immune cell function may also contribute to tumor killing *(202)*, and activation of caspase-3 has been noted beyond the ablated zone with induction of cell apoptosis, resulting in an expansion of the tumor-killing field *(203)*. Percutaneous lesions appear teardrop-shaped on CT scan, whereas intraoperative lesions are round *(204)*. The ease of monitoring lesion size coupled with the rapidity of ablation are two major advantages over other types of therapy currently being developed.

9.1. Results of MCT in Liver Tumors

Table 4 summarizes data following MCT for liver tumors in humans *(205–215)*. Survival after 3 yr appears encouraging, at 43 to 98%, with a 5-yr survival of around 20%. Local recurrence varies, from 0 to 33%, with most studies reporting a local recurrence rate of approximately 10% *(216)*. There is some evidence that the efficiency of tumor ablation varies according to tumor size. Ohmoto et al. *(217)* reported on the results of percutaneous MCT in 17 tumor nodules and found complete remission in 80% of tumors below 2 cm, with only 71% of tumors above 2 cm showing complete destruction *(217)*. The largest series of percutaneous MCT treatment is currently by Dong et al., whose group reports 5-yr survival rates approaching 60%, which compare favorably against 5-yr survival following PEI and RFA for HCC *(207)*. Tumor grade, number of metastases, and tumor size have all been isolated as prognostic factors following MCT for colorectal hepatic metastases *(216)*.

Shibata et al. *(218)* randomLy assigned 30 patients with colorectal liver metastases to resection or treatment with MCT. All patients included in the study had multiple liver metastases. The group found the 3-yr survival following MCT or resection to be comparable, 14 and 23%, respectively, and the mean survival times from treatment to be 27 mo in the resection group and 24 mo in MCT group. This suggests that, at least for multiple liver metastases, MCT is comparable to liver resection. Seki et al. *(212)*, compared MCT with PEI in the treatment of HCC. The overall 5-yr survival rates for well-differentiated HCCs were no different between the groups, 70% for MCT and 78% for PEI. However, MCT was significantly better in the moderately and poorly differentiated HCCs, with 5-yr survival rate of 78% compared with 38% with PEI.

9.2. Complications of MCT

Complication rates of 14% for HCCs and 20% for metastases have been reported following MCT *(194)*. Pneumothorax following the procedure is a relatively common finding, having been reported in three independent series looking at a total of 120 patients *(193,194,219)*; other complications include liver and lung abscess, biliary fistula, portal vein thrombosis, hepatic failure, biloma, hemorrhage, and tumor cell dissemination into the peritoneal cavity and along the needle track *(193,194,214,219–224)*. The complication rate is related to the size of the tumor treated, rising significantly in tumors over 4 cm *(194)*. The induction of artificial ascites or hydrothorax has been attempted to reduce the risk of distal heating effects, but this practice has not been adopted widely *(225)*.

Table 4

Results Following Microwave Coagulation Therapy (MCT) for Liver Tumors

Group and year	Type of lesion HCC	Type of lesion CRC mets	Method of MCT delivery	Period of follow-up	Local recurrence rate (%)	Survival rate (if applicable) (%) 1 Yr	2 Yr	3 Yr	4 Yr	5 Yr
Xu et al., 2004 (205)	54	—	Percutaneous	1–3 yr	7.1	—	—	—	—	—
Morita et al., 2004 (206)	—	52	23 Laparotomy 4 Percutaneous 25 Combined with resection	5 yr	—	—	—	—	—	20 Laparotomy 24 Percutaneous 24 Combined with resection
Dong et al., 2003 (207)	234	—	Percutaneous	5 yr	—	92.7	81.6	72.9	66.4	56.7
Liang et al., 2003 (207)	—	74	Percutaneous	5 yr	—	91.4	59.5	46.4	29	29
Chen et al., 2002 (208)	—	52	Percutaneous	12 mo	6	—	—	—	—	—
Itamoto et al., 2001 (209)	33	—	Percutaneous	4 yr	—	94	78	78	62	—
Lu et al., 2001 (210)	50	—	Percutaneous	3 yr	8	96	83	73	—	—
Seki et al., 2000 (211)	24	—	Percutaneous	3 yr	14.3	—	—	92	—	—
Seki et al., 1999 (212)	15	—	Percutaneous	38 mo	0	—	—	—	—	—
Beppu et al., 1998 (213)	54	40	Percutaneous	5 yr	33 HCC 14 CRC mets	—	—	63 HCC 43 mets	—	38 HCC 33 mets
Matsukawa et al., 1997 (214)	20	7	Percutaneous	Mean of 18 mo	—	83.1	68.7	—	—	—
Sato et al., 19966 (215)	19	—	12 Laparotomy 5 Laparoscopic 2 Thorascopic	37 mo	10	—	—	—	—	—

Abbreviations: CRC, colorectal cancer; HCC, hepatocellular carcinoma; mets, metastases.

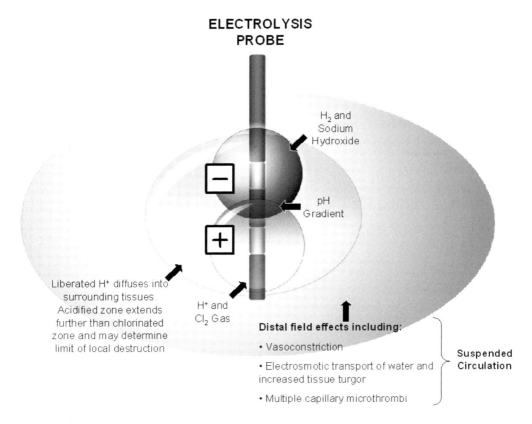

**ELECTROLYSIS
PROBE**

H$_2$ and
Sodium
Hydroxide

pH
Gradient

Liberated H⁺ diffuses into
surrounding tissues.
Acidified zone extends
further than chlorinated
zone and may determine
limit of local destruction

H⁺ and
Cl$_2$ Gas

Distal field effects including:

• Vasoconstriction

• Electrosmotic transport of water and
increased tissue turgor

• Multiple capillary microthrombi

**Suspended
Circulation**

Fig. 6. Local and distant field effects of electrolysis.

Although MCT is usually well tolerated even in cirrhotic patients, it may have a negative impact on survival in patients with very poor hepatic reserve *(226)*.

10. ELECTROLYSIS

Electrolysis is a novel treatment that uses direct current (DC) to produce tissue destruction *(227)*, with the volume of tissue necrosis produced being proportional to the electrolytic dose *(227,228)*. Direct currents (80–100 mA) are passed between two electrodes inserted into liver tissue. Electrolysis induces tissue necrosis by producing chlorine and hydrogen ions (H+) ions at the anode and hydrogen gas and sodium hydroxide at the cathode *(227,229)*, thereby creating a pH gradient (Fig. 6). The electrode products, hydrogen chloride (HCl) and chlorine gas (Cl$_2$), have been noted to be toxic to tissue *(229)*. Thermal necrosis plays no role in electrolytic ablation *(227,230,231)*. There are also many distal field effects, which include an electrophoretically induced cascade reaction causing intracellular disintegration of neoplastic tissue, the formation of eddy currents, and activation of the immune system *(231,232)*. Immune system activation involves the activation of macrophages, with the ability to destroy neoplastic cells selectively, and the accumulation of leukocytes in the cathode field by extravazation through spaces between endothelial cells *(231,232)*.

Electrolysis also results in local ischemia in the region of liver undergoing ablation by one of several mechanisms *(231,232)*. Activation of endothelial redox proteins leads to the destruction of blood cells and formation of multiple capillary microthromboses. The superimposed electric field over the liver capillaries also causes strong segmental contraction of the arterial ends by stimulating podocytes. This vasospasm is so intense that erythrocytes are unable to pass. In addition, the electroosmotic transport of water toward the cathodic field increases the local tissue turgor and further impedes blood flow. The combination of these distal field effects results in vascular obstruction and a suspended circulation. This secondary ischemia is a significant contributor to tumor killing.

Much of the preliminary data evaluating electrolysis has been obtained from small rodent models *(233)*; however, because of the small size of these models, the translation of the results into human livers was problematic. Porcine models have been used more recently because pig liver is similar in size and physiology to human liver. Electrolysis produces a dose-dependent and predictable response *(234)* in the porcine model. In rabbits, liver necrosis was produced at a rate of 2.4 cm^3 per 100 C *(235)*; in rats, liver necrosis was produced at a rate of 2.8 cm^3 per 100 C *(233)*. Its safety when used adjacent to vascular structures appears promising. Electrolysis next to the hepatic vein resulted in some intravascular gas but no damage to the vessel itself *(236)*. Unlike other ablative techniques, electrolysis is not accompanied by any evidence of a systemic response, as measured by tumor necrosis factor-α ad interleukin-8 serum levels in porcine models *(237)*.

The size of the lesion produced by electrolysis can be varied by increasing the "dose" of current administered and also by placing the electrodes a greater distance apart *(233)*. Data from porcine models have shown that lesions of up 8 cm in diameter can be produced by a combination of multiple electrodes and hepatic inflow occlusion, via the Pringle maneuver *(238,239)*. Electrolysis creates a pH gradient in liver tissue, and real-time monitoring of the pH changes have been shown to predict accurately the degree of liver damage produced during electrolysis *(240)*. Currently, the biggest disadvantage to electrolysis is the length of time required to obtain liver destruction, with 3 h of ablation time required to produce an 8-cm lesion.

10.1. Results of Electrolysis in Patients

There are few data regarding electrolysis in humans. An isolated case of one patient, who had no histological evidence of recurrence 12 mo following electrolytic ablation of a liver metastases, was reported by Berry et al. in 2000 *(241)*. A further series of five patients exists from 2002 *(236)*, which demonstrated that electrolysis was well-tolerated and that following treatment the lesion had been completely ablated. A series of nine patients, with a mean follow-up of 9 mo, showed that seven patients had no evidence of local recurrence on CT follow-up; median survival post electrolysis was 17 (range, 9–24) mo *(242)*. A multicenter prospective randomized controlled trial of liver resection vs liver resection with electrolytic ablation is currently in progress in Australia and the United Kingdom; until the results of this trial are known, the value of electrolysis in a clinical setting remains to be seen. No complications have been recorded with electrolysis thus far, but more clinical data are needed.

11. CRYOTHERAPY

Cryotherapy involves rapid freezing of tissue to subzero temperatures, which results in ice formation in the extracellular space and cellular damage by dehydration and destruction of normal cellular structures *(243)*. A probe, cooled with liquid nitrogen or argon is inserted into the tumor mass under US control. The ice ball produced is monitored using US, where it can be seen as a growing hyperechoic lesion *(244)*. Acoustic shadowing and loss of signal may compromise visualization of the cryolesion circumference. MRI provides a clear delineation of the cryolesion circumference and is being increasingly used to monitor cryoablation *(245)*. A further refinement of this technique incorporates three-dimensional MRI scanning to provide a quantitative assessment of the technical success of cryotherapy *(246)*. Cryotherapy is normally undertaken at laparotomy, although percutaneous and laparoscopic methods have also been described *(247,248)*. Postprocedure follow-up normally incorporates contrast-enhanced CT. The normal postcryotherapy appearance within the liver appears similar to a hepatic infarct or abscess, which makes detection of postprocedure complications problematic. In addition to a direct cell destruction effect, cryotherapy also stimulates an immune system-mediated antitumor response, thereby enhancing its tumor-killing action *(249)*.

Large ice balls are required for ablation of even small hepatic tumors, as only parts of the ice ball harbor temperatures adequate for tumor ablation. Ice balls of $4.9 \times 2.2 \times 2.2$ cm can normally be produced with one cryoprobe *(250)*; however, with the use of multiple probes, these ablated lesions can be increased to $6.0 \times 4.9 \times 5.6$ cm *(250)*. Huang et al. *(251)*, increased their ablated lesion volume by four times with the use of multiple probes. Cell necrosis can also be enhanced by using multiple freeze-thaw cycles *(249,252)*. Hepatic vascular inflow occlusion has been attempted in porcine models *(252)* and has been found to result in cryolesions nearly 200% larger than those induced without inflow occlusion *(253)*. In addition, the lesions produced by cryoablation in this manner were more geometrical and predictable. Vascular occlusion can also be employed in treating lesions lying near the vena cava. Ordinarily, the heat sink effect produced by blood flow within hepatic veins makes ablation of tumors in this vicinity problematic. With total vascular exclusion, however, these lesions can be treated with no significant vascular complications in animal models *(254)*.

11.1. Cryotherapy and Liver Tumors

Table 5 summarises results following cryoablation for primary and secondary liver tumors *(102,255–267)*. Most published cryoablation series have relatively short follow-up periods. Median survival following cryoablation ranges from 8 to 30 mo, with most studies reporting median survival of over 24 mo. Five-year survival appears to be around 30% regardless of the type of tumor treated. Local recurrence rates vary widely between groups; some studies report local recurrence rates of around 50%. This may reflect the growing concern that intraprocedural monitoring of the cryolesion is vital in achieving consistent and complete ablation of liver tumors.

Cryotherapy has been used in conjunction with liver resection, to ensure adequate resection margins and to reduce the tumor load, rendering liver resection possible. This combination of treatments has been found to achieve similar 5-yr survival rates, compared with tumors that were suitable for resection without cryotherapy (37% vs 36%, respectively) *(268)*. This finding is supported by other studies that have found equivalent survival rates between patients undergoing primary liver resection and those with tumors rendered operable by the combination of cryotherapy and resection *(269–271)*.

Cryotherapy has also been successfully combined with hepatic artery chemotherapy for colorectal hepatic metastases with improved survival of up to twofold in some reports

Table 5
Results Following Cryotherapy for Liver Tumors

Group and year	Type of lesion		Method of delivery	Median survival (mo)	Local recurrence (%)	Long-term survival (%)			
	HCC	Colorectol mets				1 Yr	2 Yr	3 Yr	5 Yr
Mala et al., 2004 (256)	—	19	19 Percutaneously 5 Laparotomy 3 Laparoscopically	—	44	—	48	—	—
Seifert et al., 2002 (257)	6	65	Laparotomy	28	20	—	—	38	30
Sheen et al., 2002 (258)	—	57	Laparotomy	22	—	—	—	—	—
Shimonov et al., 2002 (259)	8	10	Laparoscopy	32	—	—	—	—	—
Ruers et al., 2001 (255)	—	30	—	32	—	—	61	—	—
Bilchik et al., 2000 (102)	—	180 Colorectal 60 Other	—	28	22.8				
Chung et al., 2001 (260)	—	14	Laparotomy	42	—	—	—	—	—
Seifert et al., 2000 (261)	—	49	Laparotomy	29	16	—	—	—	—
Shaprio et al., 1998 (262)	—	5 Carcinoid mets	Laparotomy	—	—	60	40	20	—
Zhou et al., 1998 (263)	245	—	Laparotomy	—	—	78.4	—	54.1	39.8
Weaver et al., 1998 (264)	138	—	Laparotomy	30	35	85[a]	60[a]	40[a]	20[a]
Hewitt et al., 1998 (265)	—	20	Laparotomy	32	35	88	60	—	—
Junginer et al., 1998 (266)	—	29	Laparotomy	—	24	—	—	—	—
Weaver et al., 1995 (267)	—	43	Laparotomy	26	—	62	—	—	—

Abbreviations: CRC, colorectal cancer; HCC, hepatocellular carcinoma; mets, metastases.
[a]Figures taken from survival graph.

(272–275). Other combination treatments reported include cryotherapy with PEI for HCC (with a 1-yr survival of 78%) *(276)*, and cryotherapy following TACE (with a reported 41% complete eradication of tumor and normalization of tumor markers) *(277)*.

Tumor size appears to influence the efficacy of cryotherapy. For colorectal hepatic metastases, tumor diameter over 3 cm is associated with a shorter disease-free interval at the cryosite *(256,278–280)*. For primary HCC, Zhou et al. *(263)* found that HCCs under 5 cm had a better 5-yr survival (55.4% vs 39.8%). Other favorable prognostic factors include a low carcinoembryonic antigen level before the procedure, no intraoperative blood transfusion, and tumor grade *(281)*. The percentage fall in CEA following cryoablation is also related to survival *(282,283)*.

11.2. Complications of Cryotherapy

The overall complication rate following cryotherapy has been reported at 27% *(260)* with a postprocedure mortality of 0 to 1.4% *(102,255–267)*. Hemorrhage may occur following cryotherapy, usually because of cracking of the liver parenchyma during freeze-thaw cycles. This bleeding is exacerbated by the transient thrombocytopenia and coagulopathy following cryotherapy *(284)*. Other complications reported are small bowel obstruction, pleural effusions, liver abscess, bile leaks, biliary fistulas, and bilomas *(284–286)*. Hypothermia has been reported intraoperatively, which can be avoided by warming body compartments. Right-sided pleural effusions and pyrexia are commonly observed in almost all patients; these usually require only supportive management, although drainage of large effusions is occasionally required.

Perhaps the most feared complication following cryoablation is the phenomenon of cryoshock. This appears to be a systemic inflammatory response that complicates 1% of all cryotherapy procedures, with a mortality rate of 18.2% *(287)*. Cryoshock appears to be mediated via the release of the proinflammatory cytokines interleukin-6 and tumor necrosis factor *(288)*, and there is evidence from animal models that its severity may be related to the size of the tumor lesion treated *(251)*. These systemic responses have also been observed following RFA; in porcine models, however, the release of serum inflammatory markers and pneumonitis is much more substantial following cryoablation *(289)*.

12. CONCLUSIONS

The field of focal ablative treatments has seen a rapid expansion over the last three decades. Even so, there is tangible lack of randomized controlled trials comparing focal ablation over regional/systemic chemotherapy or against other ablative methods. The CLOCC trial described in Subheading 6.1. is the first large prospective randomized trial of an ablative technique; it should at least answer the question as to whether these techniques confer any survival benefit to patients. Many reported studies also suffer from short follow-up periods and small numbers. This confusion is heightened by the combination treatments currently being employed, whereby one ablation method is combined with another, or with liver resection. A further confounding factor is that with increased anesthetic and surgical experience, the definition of what constitutes an inoperable tumor burden in the liver is also changing. Staged liver resections are currently being described for traditionally inoperable liver metastases, with 100% 1-yr survival *(290)*, comparing favorably with the ablative methods described above. There is no doubt that increasing surgical confidence combined with focal ablative methods will offer huge benefits for patients with traditionally poor prognosis secondary to their tumor burden. However, the exact role that each treatment modality will play in the future has yet to be determined.

REFERENCES

1. El-Serag HB, Mason AC. Rising incidence of hepatocellular carcinoma in the United States. N Engl J Med 1999;340:745–750.
2. El-Serag HB, Mason AC. Risk factors for the rising rates of primary liver cancer in the United States. Arch Intern Med 2000;160:3227–3230.
3. Taylor-Robinson SD, Foster GR, Arora S, Hargreaves S, Thomas HC. Increase in primary liver cancer in the UK, 1979–94. Lancet 1997;350:1142–1143.
4. Boring CC, Squires TS, Tong MS. Cancer statistics. CA Cancer J Clin 1994;44:7–26.
4a. National Cancer Institute. Cancer statistics review 1973–1987. NIH publication no. 90-279. Bethesda, MD: National Cancer Institute, 1990.
5. Scheele J, Stang R, Altendorf-Hofmann A, Paul M. Resection of colorectal liver metastases. World J Surg 1995;19:59–71.
6. Tranberg KG. Percutaneous ablation of liver tumors. Best Pract Res Clin Gastroenterol 2004;18:125–145.
7. Farmer DG, Rosove MH, Shaked A, Busuutil RW. Current treatment modalities for hepatocellular carcinoma. Ann of Surg 1994;219:236–247.
8. Stone HH, Long WD, Smith RB 3rd, Haynes CD. Physiologic considerations in major hepatic resections. Am J Surg 1969;117:78–84.
9. Sugiura NT, K. Ohto, M. Treatment of small hepatocellular carcinoma by percutaneous injection of ethanol into tumor with real-time ultrasound scanning. Acta Hepatol Jpn 1983;24:920.
10. Livraghi T, Bolondi L, Lazzaroni S, et al. Percutaneous ethanol injection in the treatment of hepatocellular carcinoma in cirrhosis. A study on 207 patients. Cancer 1992;69:925–929.
11. Giorgio A, Tarantino L, de Stefano G, et al. Ultrasound-guided percutaneous ethanol injection under general anesthesia for the treatment of hepatocellular carcinoma on cirrhosis: long-term results in 268 patients. Eur J Ultrasound 2000;12:145–154.
12. Bartolozzi C, Lencioni R. Ethanol injection for the treatment of hepatic tumors. Eur Radiol 1996;6:682–696.
13. Shiina S, Tagawa K, Unuma T, et al. Percutaneous ethanol injection therapy of hepatocellular carcinoma: analysis of 77 patients. AJR Am J Roentgenol 1990;155:1221–1226.
14. De Sanctis JT, Goldberg SN, Mueller PR. Percutaneous treatment of hepatic neoplasms: a review of current techniques. Cardiovasc Intervent Radiol 1998;21:273–296.
15. Ebara M, Kita K, Nagato Y, Yoshikawa M, Sugiura N, Ohto M. [Percutaneous ethanol injection (PEI) for small hepatocellular carcinoma]. Gan To Kagaku Ryoho 1993;20:884–888.
16. Sheu JC, Huang A, Chen DS, Sung JL, Yang PM. Small hepatocellular carcinoma: intratumor ethanol treatment using new needle and guidance systems. Radiology 1987;163:43–48.
17. Livraghi T, Giorgio A, Marin G, et al. Hepatocellular carcinoma and cirrhosis in 746 patients: long-term results of percutaneous ethanol injection. Radiology 1995;197:101–108.
18. Erce C, Parks RW. Interstitial ablative techniques for hepatic tumors. Br J Surg 2003;90:272–289.
19. Bartolozzi C, Lencioni R, Ricci P, Paolicchi A, Rossi P, Passariello R. Hepatocellular carcinoma treatment with percutaneous ethanol injection: evaluation with contrast-enhanced color Doppler US. Radiology 1998;209:387–393.
20. Shiina S, Tagawa K, Unuma T, et al. Percutaneous ethanol injection therapy for hepatocellular carcinoma. A histopathologic study. Cancer 1991;68:1524–1530.
21. Vilana R, Bruix J, Bru C, Ayuso C, Sole M, Rodes J. Tumor size determines the efficacy of percutaneous ethanol injection for the treatment of small hepatocellular carcinoma. Hepatology 1992;16:353–357.
22. Lee MJ, Mueller PR, Dawson SL, et al. Percutaneous ethanol injection for the treatment of hepatic tumors: indications, mechanism of action, technique, and efficacy. AJR Am J Roentgenol 1995;164:215–220.
23. Elgindy N, Lindholm H, Gunven P. High-dose percutaneous ethanol injection therapy of liver tumors. Patient acceptance and complications. Acta Radiol 2000;41:458–463.

24. Shiina S, Tagawa K, Niwa Y, et al. Percutaneous ethanol injection therapy for hepatocellular carcinoma: results in 146 patients. AJR Am J Roentgenol 1993;160:1023–1028.
25. Rustemovic N, Vucelic B, Opacic M, et al. Palliative treatment of hepatocellular carcinoma with percutaneous ethanol injection using tumor's feeding artery occlusion under the ultrasonic Doppler guidance. Coll Antropol 2004;28:781–791.
26. Lencioni R, Algaier HP, Cioni D, Olschewksi M, Dreibert P, Crocetti L. Small hepatocellular carcinoma in cirrhosis: randomized controlled comparison of radiofrequency thermal ablation vs percutaneous ethanol injection. Radiology 2003;228:235–420.
27. Yammamoto J, Oka M, Shimada K, et al. Treatment strategy for hepatocellular carcinoma: comparison of long-term results after percutaneous ethanol injection therapy and surgical resection. Hepatology 2001;34:707–713.
28. Lin SM, Lin DY, Lin CJ. Percutaneous ethanol injection therapy in 47 cirrhotic patients with hepatocellular carcinoma 5 cm or less: a long-term result. Int J Clin Pract 1999;53:257–262.
29. Livraghi T, Benedini V, Lazzaroni S, Meloni F, Torzilli G, Vettori C. Long term results of single session percutaneous ethanol injection in patients with large hepatocellular carcinoma. Cancer 1998;83:48–57.
30. Orlando A, Cottone M, Virdone R, et al. Treatment of small hepatocellular carcinoma associated with cirrhosis by percutaneous ethanol injection. A trial with a comparison group. Scand J Gastroenterol 1997;32:598–603.
31. Lencioni R, Bartolozzi C, Caramella D, et al. Treatment of small hepatocellular carcinoma with percutaneous ethanol injection. Analysis of prognostic factors in 105 Western patients. Cancer 1995;76:1737–1746.
32. Isobe H, Sakai H, Imari Y, Ikeda M, Shiomichi S, Nawata H. Intratumor ethanol injection therapy for solitary minute hepatocellular carcinoma. A study of 37 patients. J Clin Gastroenterol 1994;18:122–126.
33. Castellano L, Calandra M, Del Vecchio Blanco C, de Sio I. Predictive factors of survival and intrahepatic recurrence of hepatocellular carcinoma in cirrhosis after percutaneous ethanol injection: analysis of 71 patients. J Hepatol 1997;27:862–870.
34. Castells A, Bruix J, Bru C, et al. Treatment of small hepatocellular carcinoma in cirrhotic patients: a cohort study comparing surgical resection and percutaneous ethanol injection. Hepatology 1993;18:1121–116.
35. Omata M, Tateishi R, Yoshida H, Shiina S. Treatment of hepatocellular carcinoma by percutaneous tumor ablation methods; ethanol injection therapy and radiofrequency ablation. Gastrenterology 2004;127:S159–S66.
36. Mazzanti R, Arena U, Pantaleo P, et al. Survival and prognostic factors in patients with hepatocellular carcinoma treated by percutaneous ethanol injection: a 10-year experience. Can J Gastroenterol 2004;18:611–618.
37. Grieco A, Pompili M, Caminiti G, et al. Prognostic factors for survival in patient with early intermediate hepatocellular carcinoma undergoing non-surgical therapy: comparison of Okuda, CLIP and BCLC staging systems in a single Italian center. Gut 2005;54:328–329.
38. Livraghi T, Bolondi L, Buscarini L. No treatment, resection and ethanol injection in hepatocellular carcinoma; a retrospective analysis of survival in 391 patients with cirrhosis. Italian Coperative Study Group. J Hepatol 1995;22:522–526.
39. Arii S, Yamaoka Y, Futagawa S. Results of surgical and nonsurgical treatment for small-sized hepatocellular carcinomas: a retrospective and nationwide survey in Japan. The Liver Study Group of Japan. Hepatology 2000;32:1224–1229.
40. Andriulli A, de Sio L, Solmi L, et al. Survival of cirrhotic patients with early hepatocellular carcinoma treated by percutaneous ethanol injection or liver transplantation. Liver Transplant 2004;10:1355–1363.
41. Blum HE. Treatment of hepatocellular carcinoma. Best Pract Res Clin Gastroenterol 2005;19:129–145.
42. Koda M, Muruwaki Y, Mitsuda A. Combination therapy with transarterial catheter embolisation and percutaneous ethanol injection alone for patients with small hepatocellular carcinoma: a randomized controlled study. Cancer 2001;92:1516–1524.
43. Seror O, N'Kontchou G, Haddar D, et al. Large infiltrative hepatocellular carcinomas: treatment with percutaneous intraarterial ethanol injection alone or in combination with percutaneous ethanol injection. Radiology 2004;234:299–309.

44. Poggi G, Gatti C, Teragni C, Delmonte A, Bernardo C. Radiofrequency ablation combined with percutaneous ethanol injection in the treatment of hepatocellular carcinoma and portal vein neoplastic thrombosis. Anticancer Res 2004;24:2419–2421.

45. Shankar S, van Sonnenberg E, Morrison PR, Tuncali K, Silverman SG. Combined radiofrequency ablation and alcohol injection for percutaneous hepatic tumor ablation. AJR Am J Roentol 2004;183:1425–1429.

46. Livraghi T, Goldberg SN, Lazzaroni S, Meloni F, Sublimate L, Gazelle GS. Small hepatocellular carcinoma: treatment with radio-frequency ablation vs ethanol injection. Radiology 1999;210: 655–661.

47. Amin Z, Bown SG, Lees WR. Local treatment of colorectal liver metastases: a comparison of interstitial laser photocoagulation (ILP) and percutaneous alcohol injection (PAI). Clin Radiol 1993;48:166–171.

48. Livraghi T, Vettori C, Lazzaroni S. Liver metastases: results of percutaneous ethanol injection in 14 patients. Radiology 1991;179:709–712.

49. Giovannini M, Seitz JF. Ultrasound-guided percutaneous alcohol injection of small liver metastases. Results in 40 patients. Cancer 1994;73:294–297.

50. Mazziotti A, Grazi GL, Gardini A, et al. An appraisal of percutaneous treatment of liver metastases. Liver Transplant Surg 1998;4:271–275.

51. Redvanly RD, Chezmar JL, Strauss RM, Galloway JR, Boyer TD, Bernardino ME. Malignant hepatic tumors: safety of high-dose percutaneous ethanol ablation therapy. Radiology 1993;188:283–285.

52. Lencioni R, Caramella D, Bartolozzi C. Hepatocellular carcinoma: use of color Doppler US to evaluate response to treatment with percutaneous ethanol injection. Radiology 1995;194:113–118.

53. Lencioni R, Cioni D, Uliana M, Bartolozzi C. Fatal thrombosis of the portal vein following single-session percutaneous ethanol injection therapy of hepatocellular carcinoma. Abdom Imaging 1998;23:608–610.

54. Taavitsainen M, Vehmas T, Kauppila R. Fatal liver necrosis following percutaneous ethanol injection for hepatocellular carcinoma. Abdom Imaging 1993;18:357–359.

55. Koda M, Okamoto K, Miyoshi Y, Kawasaki H. Hepatic vascular and bile duct injury after ethanol injection therapy for hepatocellular carcinoma. Gastrointest Radiol 1992;17:167–9.

56. Ishii H, Okada S, Okusaka T, et al. Needle tract implantation of hepatocellular carcinoma after percutaneous ethanol injection. Cancer 1998;82:1638–1642.

57. Huo C, Chen SC, Chang WY, Chen CH. Comparison of necrotic characteristics and benefits between 50% acetic acid and pure ethanol in local hepatic injection: a study in rats. Kaohsiung J Med Sci 1999;15:414–418.

58. Arrive L, Rosmorduc O, Dahan H, et al. Percutaneous acetic acid injection for hepatocellular carcinoma: using CT fluoroscopy to evaluate distribution of acetic acid mixed with an iodinated contrast agent. AJR Am J Roentgenol 2003;180:159–162.

59. Huo TI, Huang YH, Wu JC, Lee PC, Chang FY, Lee SD. Persistent retention of acetic acid is associated with complete tumor necrosis in patients with hepatocellular carcinoma undergoing percutaneous acetic acid injection. Scand J Gastroenterol 2004;39:168–173.

60. Ohnishi K. Comparison of percutaneous acetic acid injection and percutaneous ethanol injection for small hepatocellular carcinoma. Hepatogastroenterology 1998;45(suppl 3):1254–1258.

61. Liang HL, Yang CF, Pan HB, et al. Small hepatocellular carcinoma: safety and efficacy of single high-dose percutaneous acetic acid injection for treatment. Radiology 2000;214:769–74.

62. Huo TI, Huang YH, Wu JC, Lee PC, Chang FY, Lee SD. Comparison of percutaneous acetic acid injection and percutaneous ethanol injection for hepatocellular carcinoma in cirrhotic patients; a prospective study. Scand J Gastroenterol 2003;38:770–778.

63. Huo T, Huang YH, Wu JC, et al. Comparison of transarterial catheter embolisation and percutaneous acetic acid injection as the primary loco-regional therapy for unresectable hepatocellular carcinoma. a prospective survey. Aliment Pharmacol Ther 2004;19:1301–1308.

64. Chen HB, Huang YH, Dai DL, et al. Therapeutic effect of transcatheter arterial chemoembolisation and percutaneous injection of acetic acids on primary liver cancer. Hepatobiliary Pancreatic Dis Int 2004;3:55–57.

65. Huo TI, Huang YH, Wu JC, et al. Sequential transarterial chemoembolisation and percutaneous acetic acid injection therapy vs repeated percutaneous acetic acid injection for unresectable hepatocellular carcinoma; a prospective study. Ann Oncol 2003;14:1648–1653.

66. Koda M, Tanaka H, Murawaki Y, et al. Liver perforation: a serious complication of percutaneous acetic acid injection for hepatocellular carcinoma. Hepatogastroenterology 2000;47:1110–1112.

67. Van Hoof M, Joris JP, Horsmans Y, Geubel A. Acute renal failure requiring hemodialysis after high dose percutaneous acetic acid injection for hepatocellular carcinoma. Acta Gastroenterol Belg 1999;62:49–51.

68. Tamai T, Seki T, Imamura M, et al. Percutaneous injection of a low-concentration alkaline solution targeting hepatocellular carcinoma. Oncol Rep 2000;7:719–723.

69. Arakii Y, Hukano M, Urabe M, et al. Hepatocellular carcinoma treated by percutaneous hot saline injection. Oncol Rep 2004;12:569–571.

70. Okuda S, Kuroda K, Oshio K, et al. MR-based temperature monitoring for hot saline injection therapy. J Magn Reson Imaging 2000;12:330–338.

71. Lounsberry WG, V. Linke, C. The early histological changes following electrocoagulation. Gastrointest Endosc 1995;41:68–60.

72. Goldberg SN, Gazelle GS, Dawson SL, Rittman WJ, Mueller PR, Rosenthal DI. Tissue ablation with radiofrequency: effect of probe size, gage, duration, and temperature on lesion volume. Acad Radiol 1995;2:399–404.

73. McGahan JP, Browning PD, Brock JM, Tesluk H. Hepatic ablation using radiofrequency electrocautery. Invest Radiol 1990;25:267–270.

74. Goldberg SN, Gazelle GS, Halpern EF, Rittman WJ, Mueller PR, Rosenthal DI. Radiofrequency tissue ablation: importance of local temperature along the electrode tip exposure in determining lesion shape and size. Acad Radiol 1996;3:212–218.

75. Solbiati L, Ierace T, Goldberg SN, et al. Percutaneous US-guided radio-frequency tissue ablation of liver metastases: treatment and follow-up in 16 patients. Radiology 1997;202:195–203.

76. Patterson EJ, Scudamore CH, Owen DA, Nagy AG, Buczkowski AK. Radiofrequency ablation of porcine liver in vivo: effects of blood flow and treatment time on lesion size. Ann Surg 1998;227: 559–565.

77. Goldberg SN, Gazelle GS, Dawson SL, Rittman WJ, Mueller PR, Rosenthal DI. Tissue ablation with radiofrequency using multiprobe arrays. Acad Radiol 1995;2:670–674.

78. Livraghi T, Goldberg SN, Monti F, et al. Saline-enhanced radio-frequency tissue ablation in the treatment of liver metastases. Radiology 1997;202:205–210.

79. Curley SA, Izzo F, Ellis LM, Nicolas Vauthey J, Vallone P. Radiofrequency ablation of hepatocellular cancer in 110 patients with cirrhosis. Ann Surg 2000;232:381–391.

80. Miao Y, Ni Y, Yu J, Zhang H, Baert A, Marchal G. An ex vivo study on radiofrequency tissue ablation: increased lesion size by using an "expandable-wet" electrode. Eur Radiol 2001;11:1841–1847.

81. Scott DJ, Fleming JB, Watumull LM, Lindberg G, Tesfay ST, Jones DB. The effect of hepatic inflow occlusion on laparoscopic radiofrequency ablation using simulated tumors. Surg Endosc 2002;23:23.

82. Yamasaki T, Kurokawa F, Shirahashi H, Kusano N, Hironaka K, Okita K. Percutaneous radiofrequency ablation therapy for patients with hepatocellular carcinoma during occlusion of hepatic blood flow. Comparison with standard percutaneous radiofrequency ablation therapy. Cancer 2002;95: 2353–2360.

83. Buscarini L, Rossi S, Fornari F, Di Stasi M, Buscarini E. Laparoscopic ablation of liver adenoma by radiofrequency electrocautery. Gastrointest Endosc 1995;41:68–70.

84. Beber E, Foroutani A, Garland A. Use of CT Hounsfield unit density to identify ablated tumor after laparoscopic radiofrequency ablation of liver tumors. Br J Surg 2000;14:799–804.

85. Anderson CD, Li WC, Beckham J, et al. Fluorescence spectroscopy accurately detects irreversible cell damage during radiofrequency ablation. Surgery 2004;136:524–531.

86. Zhou W, Strobel D, Haensler J, Bernatik T. Hepatic transit time: indicator of the therapeutic response to radiofrequency ablation of liver tumors. Br J Radiol 2005;78:433–436.

87. Blokhuis TJ, van der Schaaf MC, van den Tol MP, Comans EF, Manoliu RA, van der Sijp JR. Results of radiofrequency ablation of primary and secondary liver tumors: long term follow-up with computed tomography and positron emission tomography-18F-deoxofluoroglucose scanning. Scand J Gastroenterol 2004;241:93–97.

88. Rossi S, Stasi M, Buscarini E. Percutaneous radiofrequency interstitial thermal ablation in the treatment of small hepatocellular carcinoma. Cancer J Sci Am 1995;1:73–77.

89. Rossi S, Di Stasi M, Buscarini E. Interstitial thermal ablation in the treatment of hepatic cancer. AJR Am J Roentgenol 1996;167:759–768.

90. Solbiati L, Goldberg SN, Ierace T. Hepatic metastases: percutaneous radiofrequency ablation with cooled-tip electrodes. Radiology 1997;205:367–373.

91. Lencioni R, Goletti O, Armillota N. Radiofrequency thermal ablation of liver metastases with a cooled-tip electrode needle: results of a pilot clinical trial. Eur Radiol 1998;8:1205–1211.

92. Rossi S, Buscarini E, Garbagnati F. Percutaneous treatment of small heaptic tumors by an expandable RF electrode needle. AJR Am J Roentgenol 1998;170:1015–1022.

93. Allgaier HP, Deibert P, Zuber I. Percutaneous radiofrequency interstitial thermal ablation of small hepatocellular carcinoma. Lancet 1999;353:1676–1677.

94. Buscarini L, Buscarini E, Di Stasi M. Percutaneous radiofrequency ablation combined with transcatheter arterial embolisation in the treatment of large hepatocellular carcinoma. Ultraschall Med 1999;20:47–53.

95. Curley SA, Izzo F, Delrio P. Radiofrequency ablation of unresectable primary and metastatic hepatic malignancies: results in 123 patients. Am Surg 1999;230:1–8.

96. Cushieri A, Bracken J, Bony L. Initial experience with laparoscopic ultrasound-guided radiofrequency thermal ablation of hepatic tumors. Endoscopy 1999;31:318–321.

97. Francica G, Marone G. Ultrasound-guided percutaneous treatment of hepatocellular carcinoma by radiofrequency hyperthermia with a "cooled-tip needle." A preliminary clinical experience. Eur J Ultrasound 1999;210:145–153.

98. Jiao LR, Hansen PD, Havlik R. Clinical short-term results of radiofrequency ablation in primary and secondary liver tumors. Am J Surg 1999;177:303–306.

99. Livraghi T, Goldberg SN, Lazzaroni S. Small hepatocellular carcinoma: treatment with radiofrequency ablation vs ethanol injection. Radiology 1999;210:655–661.

100. Pearson AS, Izzo F, Fleming RY. Intraoperative radiofrequency ablation or cryoablation for hepatic malignancies. Am J Surg 1999;178:592–599.

101. Scudamore CH, Lee SI, Patterson EJ. Radiofrequency ablation followed by resection of malignant liver tumors. Am J Surg 1999;177:411–417.

102. Bilchik AJ, Wood TF, Allegra D. Cryosurgical ablation and radiofrequency ablation for unresectable hepatic malignant neoplasms. A proposed algorithm. Arch Surg 2000;135:657–664.

103. Burley SA, Izzo F, Ellis LM. Radiofrequency ablation of hepatocellular cancer in 110 patients with cirrhosis. Ann of Surg 2000;232:381–391.

104. De Baere T, Elias D, Dromain C. Radiofrequency ablation of 100 hepatic metastases with a mean follow-up of more than 1 year. AJR Am J Roentgenol 2000;175:1619–1625.

105. Goletti O, Lencioni R, Armillota N. Laparoscopic radiofrequency thermal ablation of hepato-carcinoma: preliminary experience. Surg Laparosc Endosc Percutan Tech 2000;10:284–290.

106. Holtkamp W, Muller W. Ultrasonically controlled percutaneous high frequency thermotherapy of liver tumors with perfused needle electrodes. Z Gastroenterol 2000;38:221–227.

107. Huppert PE, Trubenbach J, Schick F. MRI-guided percutaneous radiofrequency ablation of hepatic neoplasms—first technical and clinical experience. Rofo Fortschr Geb Rontgenstr Neuen Bildgbeb Verfahr 2000;172:692–700.

108. Livraghi T, Goldberg SN, Lazzaroni S. Hepatocellular carcinoma: radiofrequency ablation of medium and large lesions. Radiology 2000;214:761–768.

109. Siperstein A, Garland A, Engle K. Laparoscopic radiofrequency ablation of primary and metastatic liver tumors. Technical considerations. Surg Endosc 2000;14:400–405.

110. Wood TF, Rose DM, Chung M. Radiofrequency ablation of 231 unresectable hepatic tumors: indications, limitations and complications. Ann Surg Oncol 2000;7:593–600.

111. Bewles BJ, Machi J, Limm WLM. Safety and efficacy of radiofrequency thermal ablation in advanced liver tumors. Arch Surg 2001;136:864–869.

112. Chung M, Wood TF, Tsioulias GJ. Laparoscopic radiofrequency ablation of unresectable hepatic malignancies: a phase II trial. Surg Endosc 2001;15:1020–1026.

113. De Sio I, Castellano L, Girolamo V, al. Tumor dissemination after radiofrequency ablation of hepatocellular carcinoma. Hepatology 2001;34:609–610.

114. Ikeda M, Okada S, Ueno H. Radiofrequency ablation and percutaneous ethanol injection in patients with small hepatocellular carcinoma; a comparative study. Jpn J Clin Oncol 2001;31:322–326.

115. Lin HK, Choi D, Lee WJ. Hepatocellular carcinoma treated with percutaneous radiofrequency ablation: evaluation with follow-up multiphase helical CT. Radiology 2001;221:447–454.

116. Llovet JM, Vilana R, Bru C. Increased risk of tumor seeding after percutaneous radiofrequency ablation for single hepatocellular carcinoma. Hepatology 2001;33:1124–1129.

117. Machi J, Uchida S, Sumida K. Ultrasound-guided radiofrequency thermal ablation of liver tumors: percutaneous, laparoscopic and open surgical approaches. J Gastrointest Surg 2001;5:477–489.

118. Podnos YD, Henry G, Ortiz JA. Laparoscopic ultrasound with radiofrequency ablation in cirrhotic patients with hepatocellular carcinoma; technique and technical considerations. Am Surg 2001;67: 1181–1184.

119. Berber E, Flesher N, Siperstein AE. Laparoscopic radiofrequency ablation of neuroendocrine liver metastases. World J Surg 2002;26:985–990.

120. Chan RP, Asch M, Kachura J. Radiofrequency ablation of malignant hepatic neoplasms. Can Assoc Radiol 2002;53:272–278.

121. Elias D, De Baere T, Smayra T. Percutaneous radiofrequency thermoablation as an alternative to surgery for the treatment of liver tumor recurrence after hepatectomy. Br J Surg 2002;89:752–756.

122. Hosida Y, Shiratori Y, Koike T. Hepatic volumetry to predict adverse events in percutaneous ablation of hepatocellular carcinoma. Hepatogastroenterology 2002;49:451–455.

123. Iannitti DA, Dupuy DE, Mayo-Smith WW, Murphy B. Hepatic radiofrequency ablation. Arch Surg 2002;137:422–427.

124. Kosari K, Gomes M, Hunter D, al. e. Local intrahepatic and systemic recurrence patterns after radiofrequency ablation of hepatic malignancies. J Gastrointest Surg 2002;6:255–263.

125. Kurshinoff BW, Ota DM. Radiofrequency ablation of liver tumors; influence of technique and tumors size. Surgery 2002;132:605–612.

126. Morimoto M, Sufimori K, Shirato K. Treatment of hepatocellular carcinoma with radiofrequency ablation: radiologic-histologic correlation during follow-up periods. Hepatology 2002;35:1467–1475.

127. Miyamoto N, Tsuji K, Sakurai Y, et al. Percutaneous radiofrequency ablation for unresectable large hepatic tumors during hepatic blood flow occlusion in four patients. Clin Radiol 2004;59:812–818.

128. Gillams AR, Cassoni A, Conway G, Lees W. Radiofrequency ablation of neuroendocrine liver metastases: the Middlesex experience. Abdom Imaging 2005;30:435–441.

129. Tateishi R, Shiina S, Teratani T, et al. Percutaneous radiofrequency ablation for hepatocellular carcinoma. An analysis of 1000 cases. Cancer 2005;103:1201–1209.

130. Shibata T, Limuro Y, Yamamoto Y. Small hepatocellular carcinoma: comparison of radio-frequency ablation and percutaneous microwave coagulation therapy. Vasc Intervent Radiol 2001;2001:331–337.

131. Shetty SK, Rosen MP, Raptopoulos V, Goldberg SN. Cost-effectiveness of percutaneous radiofrequency ablation for malignant hepatic neoplasms. J Vasc Interv Radiol 2001;12:823–833.

132. Gazelle GS, McMahon PM, Beinfeld MT, Halpern EF, Weinstein MC. Metastatic colorectal carcinoma: cost-effectiveness of percutaneous radiofrequency ablation vs that of hepatic resection. Radiology 2004;233:729–739.

133. Yu HC, Cheng JS, Lai KH, et al. Factors for early tumor recurrence of single small hepatocellular carcinoma after percutaneous radiofrequency ablation therapy. 2005;14:1439–1444.

134. Berber E, Pelly R, Siperstein A. Predictors of survival after radiofrequency thermal ablation of colorectal cancer metastases to the liver; a prospective study. J Clin Oncol 2005;23:1358–1364.

135. Choy PY, Koea J, McCall J, Holden A, Osbourne M. The role of radiofrequency ablation in the treatment of primary and metastatic tumors of the liver: initial lessons learned. N Z Med J 2002;115:U128.

136. Crucitti A, Danza FM, Pirulli PG, et al. Radiofrequency thermal ablation (RFA) of liver tumors: open surgical or percutaneous approaches. J Chemother 2004;16:82–85.

137. de Baere T, Bessoud B, Dromain C, et al. Percutaneous radiofrequency ablation of hepatic tumors during temporary venous occlusion. AJR Am J Roentgenol 2002;178:53–59.

138. Poggi G, Gatti C, Cupella F, Fiori M, Avanza F, Baldi M. Percutaneous US-guided radiofrequency ablation of hepatocellular carcinomas: results in 15 patients. Anticancer Res 2001;21:739–742.

139. Nicoli N, Casaril A, Marchiori L, et al. Intraoperative and percutaneous radiofrequency thermal ablation in the treatment of hepatocellular carcinoma. Chir Ital 2000;52:29–40.

140. Frieser M, Haensler J, Schaber S, et al. Radiofrequency ablation of liver tumors: how to enlarge the necrotic zones. Eur J Surg Res 2004;36:357–361.

141. Mahnken AH, Tacke J, Bucker A, Gunther RW. [Percutaneous radiofrequency ablation of liver malignancies: first experience with a 200-W radiofrequency generator]. Rofo Fortschr Geb Rontgenstr Neuen Bildgeb Verfahr 2002;174:216–223.

142. Yang R, Reilly CR, Rescorla FJ, et al. High-intensity focused ultrasound in the treatment of experimental liver cancer. Arch Surg 1991;126:1002–1009; discussion 9–10.

143. Wu F, Chen WZ, Bai J, et al. Tumor vessel destruction resulting from high-intensity focused ultrasound in patients with solid malignancies. Ultrasound Med Biol 2002;28:535–542.

144. Poliachik SL, Chandler WL, Mourad PD, Ollos RJ, Crum LA. Activation, aggregation and adhesion of platelets exposed to high-intensity focused ultrasound. Ultrasound Med Biol 2001;27:1567–1576.

145. Wu F, Chen WZ, Bai J, et al. Pathological changes in human malignant carcinoma treated with high-intensity focused ultrasound. Ultrasound Med Biol 2001;27:1099–1106.

146. Vaezy S, Martin R, Crum L. High intensity focused ultrasound: a method of hemostasis. Echocardiography 2001;18:309–315.

147. Yang R, Sanghvi NT, Rescorla FJ, et al. Extracorporeal liver ablation using sonography-guided high-intensity focused ultrasound. Invest Radiol 1992;27:796–803.

148. Chapleton JP, Sibille A., Abou-el-Fadil F., Theillere Y., Cthignol D. Extracorporeal selective focused destruction of hepatic tumors by high intensity ultrasound in rabbits bearing VX-2-carcinoma. Min Invas Ther 1992;10:125–131.

149. Linke CA, Carstensen EL, Frizzell LA, Elbadawi A, Fridd CW. Localized tissue destruction by high-intensity focused ultrasound. Arch Surg 1973;107:887–891.

150. Pernot M, Tanter M, Fink M. 3-D real-time motion correction in high-intensity focused ultrasound therapy. Ultrasound Med Biol 2004;9:1239–1249.

151. Cheng SQ, Zhou XD, Tang ZY, Yu Y, Bao SS, Qian DC. Iodized oil enhances the thermal effect of high-intensity focussed ultrasound. J Res Clin Oncol 1997;123:639–644.

152. Satsaki K, Azuma T, Kawabata K, Shimoda S, Koku E, Umemura S. Effect of split-focus approach on producing larger coagulation in swine liver. Ultrasound Med Biol 2003;29:591–599.

153. Vallancien G, Harouni M, Veillon B, Mombet A, Brisset J, Bougaran J. Focused extracorperal pyotherapy. J Endourol 1992;6:173–181.

154. Wu F, Wang ZB, Chen WZ, et al. Extracorporeal high intensity focused ultrasound ablation in the treatment of patients with large hepatocellular carcinoma. Ann Surg Oncol 2004;11:1061–1069.

155. Li CX, Xu JL, Jiang ZY, et al. Analysis of clinical effect of high-intenstiy focused ultrasound in liver cancer. World J Gastroenterol 2004;10:2201–2204.

156. Chen W, Wang Z, Wu F, et al. [High intensity focused ultrasound alone for malignant solid tumors]. Zhonghua Zhong Liu Za Zhi 2002;24:278–281.

157. Jin CB, Wu F, Wang ZB, Chen WZ, Zhu H. High intensity focused ultrasound therapy combined with transcatheter arterial chemoembolisation for advanced hepatocellualar carcinoma. Zhonghua Zhong Liu Za Zhi 2003;25:401–403.

158. Thomsen S. Pathologic analysis of photothermal and photomechanical effects of laser-tissue interactions. Photochem Photobiol 1991;53:825–835.

159. Hunter JG, Dixon JA. Lasers in cardiovascular surgery—current status. West J Med 1985;142:506–510.

160. Welch AJ, Motamedi M, Rastegar S, LeCarpentier GL, Jansen D. Laser thermal ablation. Photochem Photobiol 1991;53:815–823.

161. Murer L, Marijnessen J, Star W. Improvements in the design of linear photodynamic therapy. Phys Med Biol 1997;42:1461–1464.

162. Nølsoe CP, Torp-Pedersen S, Burcharth F, et al. Interstitial hyperthermia of colorectal liver metastases with a US-guided Nd-YAG laser with a diffuser tip: a pilot clinical study. Radiology 1993;187:333–337.

163. Svaasand LO, Boerslid T, Oeveraasen M. Thermal and optical properties of living tissue: application to laser-induced hyperthermia. Lasers Surg Med 1985;5:589–602.

164. Sturesson C. Interstitial laser-induced thermotherapy: influence of carbonization on lesion size. Lasers Surg Med 1998;22:51–57.

165. Wyman DR. Selecting source locations in multifiber interstitial laser photocoagulation. Lasers Surg Med 1993;13:656–663.

166. Heiterkamp J, van Hillegersberg R, Sinofsky E, Ijzermans J. Interstitial Nd:YAG laser coagulation using simultaneous multiple fiber application with an optical beam splitter: importance of mutual fiber distance.

167. Heisterkamp J, van Hillegersberg R, de Man RA, et al. [Treatment of non-resectable liver tumors with percutaneous interstitial laser coagulation while interrupting blood circulation to the liver]. Ned Tijdschr Geneeskd 2000;144:1542–1548.

168. Heisterkamp J, van Hillegersberg R, Mulder PG, Sinofsky EL, JN IJ. Importance of eliminating portal flow to produce large intrahepatic lesions with interstitial laser coagulation. Br J Surg 1997;84: 1245–1248.
169. Heisterkamp J, van Hillegersberg R, Sinofsky E, JN IJ. Heat-resistant cylindrical diffuser for interstitial laser coagulation: comparison with the bare-tip fiber in a porcine liver model. Lasers Surg Med 1997;20:304–309.
170. Heisterkamp J, van Hillegersberg R, Zondervan PE, JN IJ. Metabolic activity and DNA integrity in human hepatic metastases after interstitial laser coagulation (ILC). Lasers Surg Med 2001;28:80–86.
171. Germer CT, Isbert C, Albrecht D. Laser-induced thermotherapy combined with heaptic arterial embolisation in the treatment of liver tumors in a rat tumor model. Ann of Surg 1999;230:55–62.
172. Moller PH, Lindberg L, Henriksson PH, Persson BR, Tranberg KG. Temperature control and light penetration in a feedback interstitial laser thermotherapy system. Int J Hypertherm 1996;12:49–63.
173. Hashimoto D, Takami M, Idezuki Y. In depth radiation therapy by YAG laser for malignant tumors of the liver under ultrasound imaging. Gastrenterology 1985;88:1633.
174. Huang G, Wang T, Sheu J. Low power laser thermia for the treatment of small hepatocellular carcinoma. Eur J Cancer 1991;27:1622–1627.
175. Steger AC, Lees WR, Walmsley K, Bown SG. Interstitial laser hyperthermia: a new approach to local destruction of tumors. BMJ 1989;299:362–365.
176. Vogl TJ, Mack MG, Straub R, Roggan A, Felix R. Magnetic resonance imaging-guided abdominal interventional radiology: laser-induced thermotherapy of liver metastases. Endoscopy 1997;29: 577–583.
177. Vogl TJ, Muller PK, Hammerstingl R, et al. Malignant liver tumors treated with MR imaging-guided laser-induced thermotherapy: technique and prospective results. Radiology 1995;196:257–65.
178. Vogl TJ, Straub R, Eichler KC. Malignant liver tumors treated with MR imaging-guided laser-induced thermotherapy: experience with complications in 899 patients. Radiology 2002;225:367–377.
179. Vogl TJ, Eichler KC, Straub R. Laser-induced thermotherapy of malignant liver tumors: general principles, equipment, procedures, side effects, complications and results. Eur J Ultrasound 2001;13:117–127.
180. Pacella CM, Bizzarri G, Magnolfi F, et al. Laser thermal ablation in the treatment of small hepatocellular carcinoma: results in 74 patients. Radiology 2001;221:712–720.
181. Gillams AR, Lees WR. Survival after percutaneous, image-guided, thermal ablation of hepatic metastases from colorectal cancer. Dis Colon Rectum 2000;43:656–661.
182. Giorgio A, Tarantino L, de Stefano G, et al. Interstitial laser photocoagulation under ultrasound guidance of liver tumors: results in 104 treated patients. Eur J Ultrasound 2000;11:181–188.
183. Caspani B, Cecconi P, Bottelli R, Della Vigna P, Ideo G, Gozzi G. [The interstitial photocoagulation with laser light of liver tumors]. Radiol Med (Torino) 1997;94:346–354.
184. Gillams AR, Brookes J, Hare C. Follow up of patients with metastatic liver lesions treated with interstitial laser therapy. Br J Cancer 1997;196:31.
185. Tranberg KG, Moller PH, Hannesson P, Stenram U. Interstitial laser treatment of malignant tumors: initial experience. Eur J Surg Oncol 1996;22:47–54.
186. Pacella CM, Bizzarri G, Ferrari FS, et al. [Interstitial photocoagulation with laser in the treatment of liver metastasis]. Radiol Med (Torino) 1996;92:438–447.
187. Prudhomme M, Rouy S, Tang J, Landgrebe J, Delacretaz G, Godlewski G. Biliary structures lead to tumor recurrences after laser-induced interstitial thermotherapy. Lasers Surg Med 1999;24:269–275.
188. Vogl TJ, Muller PK, Straub R, Roggan A, Felix R. Percutaneous MRI-guided laser-induced thermotherapy for hepatic metastases for colorectal cancer. Lancet 1997;350:29.
189. Malone DE, Lesiuk L, Brady AP, Wyman DR, Wilson BC. Hepatic interstitial laser photocoagulation: demonstration and possible clinical importance of intravascular gas. Radiology 1994;193:233–237.
190. Tabuse K. A new operative procedure of hepatic surgery using a microwave tissue coagulator. Nippon Geka Hokan 1979;48:160–172.
191. Tabuse K, Katsumi M. Application of a microwave tissue coagulator to hepatic surgery the hemostatic effects on spontaneous rupture of hepatoma and tumor necrosis. Nippon Geka Hokan 1981;50: 571–579.
192. Watanabe Y, Sato M, Abe Y, et al. Laparoscopic microwave coagulo-necrotic therapy for hepatocellular carcinoma: a feasible study of an alternative option for poor-risk patients. J Laparoendosc Surg 1995;5:169–175.

193. Seki T, Wakabayashi M, Nakagawa T, et al. Ultrasonically guided percutaneous microwave coagulation therapy for small hepatocellular carcinoma. Cancer 1994;74:817–825.
194. Shimada S, Hirota M, Beppu T, et al. Complications and management of microwave coagulation therapy for primary and metastatic liver tumors. Surg Today 1998;28:1130–1137.
195. Murakami R, Yoshimatsu S, Yamashita Y, Matsukawa T, Takahashi M, Sagara K. Treatment of hepatocellular carcinoma: value of percutaneous microwave coagulation. AJR Am J Roentgenol 1995;164:1159–1164.
196. Sato M, Watanabe Y, Kashu Y, Nakata T, Hamada Y, Kawachi K. Sequential percutaneous microwave coagulation therapy for liver tumor. Am J Surg 1998;175:322–324.
197. Strickland AD, Clegg PJ, Cronin NJ, et al. Experimental study of large-volume microwave ablation in the liver. Br J Surg 2002;89:1003–1007.
198. Takamura M, Murakami T, Shibata T, et al. Microwave coagulation therapy with interruption of hepatic blood in- or outflow: an experimental study. J Vasc Interv Radiol 2001;12:619–622.
199. Ishida T, Murakami T, Shibata T, et al. Percutaneous microwave tumor coagulation for hepatocellular carcinomas with interruption of segmental hepatic blood flow. J Vasc Interv Radiol 2002;13:185–191.
200. Shibata T, Morita T, Okuyama M, Kitada M, Shimano T, Ishida T. [Comparison of percutaneous microwave coagulation area under interruption of hepatic arterial blood flow with that under hepatic arterial and venous blood flow for hepatocellular carcinoma]. Gan To Kagaku Ryoho 2002;29: 2146–2148.
201. Wright AS, Lee FT, Jr., Mahvi DM. Hepatic microwave ablation with multiple antennae results in synergistically larger zones of coagulation necrosis. Ann Surg Oncol 2003;10:275–283.
202. Zhang J, Dong B, Liang P, et al. Significance of changes in local immunity in patients with hepatocellular carcinoma after percutaneous microwave coagulation therapy. Chin Med J (Engl) 2002;115:1367–1371.
203. Ohno T, Kawano K, Sasaki A, Aramaki M, Yoshida T, Kitano S. Expansion of an ablated site and induction of apoptosis after microwave coagulation therapy in rat liver. J Hepatobiliary Pancreat Surg 2001;8:360–366.
204. Mitsuzaki K, Yamashita Y, Nishiharu T, et al. CT appearance of hepatic tumors after microwave coagulation therapy. AJR Am J Roentgenol 1998;171:1397–1403.
205. Xu H, Yie X, Lu MD. Ultrasound-guided percutaneous thermal ablation of hepatocellular carcinoma using microwave and radiofrequency ablation. Clin Radiol 2004;59:53–61.
206. Morita T, Shibata T, Okuyama M, et al. [Clinicopathological analysis of two patients with local recurrence after microwave coagulation therapy for liver metastases from colorectal cancer]. Gan To Kagaku Ryoho 2002;29:2234–2237.
207. Dong B, Liang P, Yu X, et al. Percutaneous sonographically guided microwave coagulation therapy for hepatocellular carcinoma: results in 234 patients. AJR Am J Roentgenol 2003;180:1547–1555.
208. Chen Y, Chen H, Wu M, et al. [Curative effect of percutaneous microwave coagulation therapy for hepatocellular carcinoma]. Zhonghua Zhong Liu Za Zhi 2002;24:65–67.
209. Itamoto T, Asahara T, Kohashi T, et al. [Percutaneous microwave coagulation therapy for hepatocellular carcinoma]. Gan To Kagaku Ryoho 1999;26:1841–1844.
210. Lu MD, Chen JW, Xie XY, et al. Hepatocellular carcinoma: US-guided percutaneous microwave coagulation therapy. Radiology 2001;221:167–172.
211. Seki T, Wakabayashi M, Nakagawa T, et al. Percutaneous microwave coagulation therapy for solitary metastatic liver tumors from colorectal cancer: a pilot clinical study. Am J Gastroenterol 1999;94: 322–327.
212. Seki T, Wakabayashi M, Nakagawa T, et al. Percutaneous microwave coagulation therapy for patients with small hepatocellular carcinoma: comparison with percutaneous ethanol injection therapy. Cancer 1999;85:1694–1702.
213. Beppu T, Ogawa M, Matsuda T, et al. [Efficacy of microwave coagulation therapy (MCT) in patients with liver tumors]. Gan To Kagaku Ryoho 1998;25:1358–1361.
214. Matsukawa T, Yamashita Y, Arakawa A, et al. Percutaneous microwave coagulation therapy in liver tumors. A 3-year experience. Acta Radiol 1997;38:410–415.
215. Sato M, Watanabe Y, Ueda S, et al. Microwave coagulation therapy for hepatocellular carcinoma. Gastroenterology 1996;110:1507–1514.
216. Liang P, Dong B, Yu D, et al. Prognostic factor for percutaneous microwave coagulation therapy of hepatic metastases. AJR Am J Roentgenol 2003;181:1319–1325.

217. Ohmoto K, Miyake I, Tsuduki M, et al. Percutaneous microwave coagulation therapy for unresectable hepatocellular carcinoma. Hepatogastroenterology 1999;46:2894–2900.

218. Shibata T, Niinobu T, Ogata N, Takami M. Microwave coagulation therapy for multiple hepatic metastases from colorectal carcinoma. Cancer 2000;89:276–284.

219. Abe T, Shinzawa H, Wakabayashi H, et al. Value of laparoscopic microwave coagulation therapy for hepatocellular carcinoma in relation to tumor size and location. Endoscopy 2000;32:598–603.

220. Takahashi Y, Shibata T, Shimano T, et al. [A case report of intra-thoracic biliary fistula after percutaneous microwave coagulation therapy]. Gan To Kagaku Ryoho 2000;27:1850–1853.

221. Morimoto O, Nagano H, Sakon M, et al. Liver abscess formation after microwave coagulation therapy applied for hepatic metastases from surgically excised bile duct cancer: report of a case. Surg Today 2002;32:454–457.

222. Kojima Y, Suzuki S, Sakaguchi T, et al. Portal vein thrombosis caused by microwave coagulation therapy for hepatocellular carcinoma: report of a case. Surg Today 2000;30:844–848.

223. Sato M, Tokui K, Watanabe Y, et al. Generalized intraperitoneal seeding of hepatocellular carcinoma after microwave coagulation therapy: a case report. Hepatogastroenterology 1999;46:2561–2564.

224. Matsumoto K, Beppu T, Ishiko T, Doi K, Ogawa M. [Liver and lung abscess after thoracoscopic microwave coagulation therapy for hepatocellular carcinoma]. Gan To Kagaku Ryoho 2002;29: 2225–2228.

225. Shimada S, Hirota M, Beppu T, et al. A new procedure of percutaneous microwave coagulation therapy under artificial hydrothorax for patients with liver tumors in the hepatic dome. Surg Today 2001;31:40–44.

226. Okano H, Shiraki K, Inoue H, et al. Laparoscopic microwave coagulation therapy for small hepatocellular carcinoma on the liver surface. Oncol Rep 2002;9:1001–1004.

227. David SL, Absolom DR, Smith CR, Gams J, Herbert MA. Effect of low level direct current on in vivo tumor growth in hamsters. Cancer Res 1985;45:5625–5631.

228. Samuelsson L. Electrolysis and surgery in experimental tumors in the rat. Acta Radiol Diagn 1981;22:129–131.

229. Berendson J, Simonsson D. Electrochemical aspects of treatment of tissue with direct current. Eur J Surg Suppl 1994;574:111–115.

230. Heiberg E, Nalesnik WJ, Janney C. Effects of varying potential and electrolytic dosage in direct current treatment of tumors. Acta Radiol 1991;32:174–177.

231. Nordenstrom BE. The paradigm of biologically closed electric circuits (BCEC) and the formation of an International Association (IABC) for BCEC systems. Eur J Surg Suppl 1994;574:7–23.

232. Nordenstrom BE. Survey of mechanisms in electrochemical treatment (ECT) of cancer. Eur J Surg Suppl 1994;574:93–109.

233. Robertson GS, Wemyss-Holden SA, Dennison AR, Hall PM, Baxter P, Maddern GJ. Experimental study of electrolysis-induced hepatic necrosis. Br J Surg 1998;85:1212–1216.

234. Wemyss-Holden SA, Robertson GS, Dennison AR, Vanderzon PS, Hall PM, Maddern GJ. A new treatment for unresectable liver tumors: long-term studies of electrolytic lesions in the pig liver. Clin Sci (Lond) 2000;98:561–567.

235. Samuelsson L, Olin T, Berg NO. Electrolytic destruction of lung tissue in the rabbit. Acta Radiol Diagn 1980;21:447–454.

236. Wemyss-Holden SA, Berry DP, Robertson GS, Dennison AR, De La MHP, Maddern GJ. Electrolytic ablation as an adjunct to liver resection: safety and efficacy in patients. Aust N Z J Surg 2002;72: 589–593.

237. Berry DP, Garcea G, Chung C, et al. Systemic reaction following electrolytic treatment of pig livers in vivo. Aust N Z J Surg 2004;74:586–590.

238. Berry DP, Garcea G, Vanderzon P, et al. Augmenting the ablative effect of liver electrolysis: using multiple electrodes and the Pringle maneuver. J Invest Surg 2004;17:105–112.

239. Teague BD, Court FG, Morrison CP, Kho M, Wemyss-Holden S, Maddern GJ. Electrolytic liver ablation is not associated with evidence of a systemic inflammatory response syndrome. Br J Surg 2003;91:178–183.

240. Finch JG, Fosh B, Anthony A, et al. Liver electrolysis: pH can reliably monitor the extent of hepatic ablation in pigs. Clin Sci (Lond) 2002;102:389–395.

241. Berry DP, Dennison AR, Ward R, Maddern GJ. Electrolytic ablation of colorectal liver metastases: 1-year histological patient follow-up. Dig Surg 2000;17:518–519.

242. Fosh BG, Finch JG, Lea M, et al. Use of electrolysis as an adjunct to liver resection. Br J Surg 2002;89:999–1002.
243. Ravikumar TS, Steele GD Jr. Hepatic cryosurgery. Surg Clin North Am 1989;69:433–440.
244. Cuschieri A, Crosthwaite G, Shimi S, et al. Hepatic cryotherapy for liver tumors. Development and clinical evaluation of a high-efficiency insulated multineedle probe system for open and laparoscopic use. Surg Endosc 1995;9:483–489.
245. Mala T, Aurdal L, Frich L, et al. Liver tumor ablation: a commentary on the need of improved procedural monitoring. Technol Cancer Res Treat 2004;3:85–91.
246. Silverman SG, Sun MR, Tuncali K, et al. Three-dimensional assessment of MRI-guided percutaneous cryotherapy of liver metastases. AJR Am J Roentgenol 2004;183:707–712.
247. Schuder G, Pistorius G, Schneider G, Feifel G. Preliminary experience with percutaneous cryotherapy of liver tumors. Br J Surg 1998;85:1210–1211.
248. Heniford BT, Arca MJ, Iannitti DA, Walsh RM, Gagner M. Laparoscopic cryoablation of hepatic metastases. Semin Surg Oncol 1998;15:194–201.
249. Hamad GG, Neifeld JP. Biochemical, hematologic, and immunologic alterations following hepatic cryotherapy. Semin Surg Oncol 1998;14:122–128.
250. Silverman SG, Tuncali K, Adams DF, et al. MR imaging-guided percutaneous cryotherapy of liver tumors: initial experience. Radiology 2000;217:657–664.
251. Huang A, McCall JM, Weston MD, et al. Phase I study of percutaneous cryotherapy for colorectal liver metastasis. Br J Surg 2002;89:303–310.
252. Kollmar O, Richter S, Schilling MK, Menger MD, Pistorius G. Advanced hepatic tissue destruction in ablative cryosurgery: potentials of intermittent freezing and selective vascular inflow occlusion. Cryobiology 2004;48:263–272.
253. Mala T, Firch L, Aurdal L, et al. Hepatic vascular inflow occlusion enhances tissue destruction during cryoablation of porcine liver. J Surg Res 2003;115:265–271.
254. Jungraithmayr W, Szarynski M, Neeff H, et al. Significance of total vascular exclusion for hepatic cryotherapy: an experimental study. J Surg Res 2004;116:32–41.
255. Ruers TJM, Joosten J, Jager GJ, Wobbes T. Long-term results in treating colorectal metastases with cryosurgery. Br J Surg 2001;88:844–849.
256. Mala T, Edwin B, Mathisen O, et al. Cryoablation of colorectal liver metastases: minimally invasive tumor control. Scand J Gastroenterol 2004;39:571–578.
257. Seifert JK, Heintz A, Junginger T. [Cryotherapy for primary and secondary liver tumors]. Zentralbl Chir 2002;127:275–281.
258. Sheen AJ, Poston GJ, Sherlock DJ. Cryotherapeutic ablation of liver tumors. Br J Surg 2002;89:1396–1401.
259. Shimonov M, Shechter P, Victoria F, Ada R, Henri H, Czerniak A. [Laparoscopic cryoablation of liver tumors]. Harefuah 2002;141:414–417, 500.
260. Chung MH, Ye W, Ramming KP, Bilchik AJ. Repeat hepatic cryotherapy for metastatic colorectal cancer. J Gastrointest Surg 2001;5:287–293.
261. Seifert JK, Achenbach T, Heintz A, Bottger TC, Junginger T. Cryotherapy for liver metastases. Int J Colorectal Dis 2000;15:161–166.
262. Shapiro RS, Shafir M, Sung M, Warner R, Glajchen N. Cryotherapy of metastatic carcinoid tumors. Abdom Imaging 1998;23:314–317.
263. Zhou XD, Tang ZY. Cryotherapy for primary liver cancer. Semin Surg Oncol 1998;14:171–174.
264. Weaver ML, Ashton JG, Zemel R. Treatment of colorectal liver metastases by cryotherapy. Semin Surg Oncol 1998;14:163–170.
265. Hewitt PM, Dwerryhouse SJ, Zhao J, Morris DL. Multiple bilobar liver metastases: cryotherapy for residual lesions after liver resection. J Surg Oncol 1998;67:112–116.
266. Junginger T, Seifert JK, Weigel TF, Heintz A, Kreitner KF, Gerharz CD. [Cryotherapy of liver metastases. Initial results]. Med Klin 1998;93:517–523.
267. Weaver ML, Atkinson D, Zemel R. Hepatic cryosurgery in treating colorectal metastases. Cancer 1995;76:210–214.
268. Rivoire M, De Cian F, Meeus P, Negrier S, Sebban H, Kaemmerlen P. Combination of neoadjuvant chemotherapy with cryotherapy and surgical resection for the treatment of unresectable liver metastases from colorectal carcinoma. Cancer 2002;95:2283–2292.
269. Finlay IG, Seifert JK, Stewart GJ, Morris DL. Resection with cryotherapy of colorectal hepatic metastases has the same survival as hepatic resection alone. Eur J Surg Oncol 2000;26:199–202.

270. Seifert JK, Morris DL. Cryotherapy of the resection edge after liver resection for colorectal cancer metastases. Aust N Z J Surg 1998;68:725–728.

271. Gruenberger T, Jourdan JL, Zhao J, King J, Morris DL. Reduction in recurrence risk for involved or inadequate margins with edge cryotherapy after liver resection for colorectal metastases. Arch Surg 2001;136:1154–1157.

272. Preketes A, Caplehorn JR, King J, Clingan PR, Ross WB, Morris DL. Effect of hepatic artery chemotherapy on survival of patients with hepatic metastases from colorectal carcinoma treated with cryotherapy. World J Surg 1995;19:768–771.

273. Morris DL, Horton MD, Dilley AV, Walters A, Clingan PR. Treatment of hepatic metastases by cryotherapy and regional cytotoxic perfusion. Gut 1993;34:1156–1157.

274. Allen-Mersh TG, Earlam S, Fordy C, Abrams K, Houghton J. Quality of life and survival with continuous hepatic-artery floxurinde infusion for colorectal liver metastases. Lancet 1994;344:1255–1260.

275. Rougier P, Laplanche A, Hughuier M, May JM, Ollivier JM, Escat J. Hepatic arterial infusion of floxuridine in patients with liver mestases from colorectal carcinoma; long-term results of a prospective randomized trial. J Clin Oncol 1992;10:1112–1118.

276. Xu KC, Nil LZ, He WB, Guo ZQ, Hu YZ, Juo JS. Percutaneous cryoablation in combination with ethanol injection for unresectable hepatocellular carcinoma. World J Gastroenterol 2003;9:2686–2689.

277. Qian GJ, Chen H, Wu MC. Percutaneous cryoablation after chemoembolisation of liver carcinoma: a report of 34 cases. Hepatobiliary Pancreatic Dis Int 2003;2:520–524.

278. Seifert JK, Junginger T, Morris DL. [Diameter of metastases is decisive for local treatment outcome of cryotherapy of colorectal liver metastases]. Langenbecks Arch Chir Suppl Kongressbd 1998;115:1455–1457.

279. Seifert JK, Morris DL. Indicators of recurrence following cryotherapy for hepatic metastases from colorectal cancer. Br J Surg 1999;86:234–240.

280. Adam R, Akpinar E, Johann M, Kunstlinger F, Majno P, Bismuth H. Place of cryosurgery in the treatment of malignant liver tumors. Ann Surg 1997;225:39–38; discussion 48–50.

281. Seifert JK, Junginger T. Prognostic factors for cryotherapy of colorectal liver metastases. Eur J Surg Oncol 2004;30:34–40.

282. Preketes AP, King J, Caplehorn JR, Clingan PR, Ross WB, Morris DL. CEA reduction after cryotherapy for liver metastases from colon cancer predicts survival. Aust N Z J Surg 1994;64:612–614.

283. Morris DL, Ross WB, Iqbal J, McCall J, King J, Clingan PR. Cryoablation of hepatic malignancy. An evaluation of tumor marker data and survival in 110 patients. GI Cancer 1996;1:247–251.

284. Wallis CB, Coventry DM. Anaesthetic experience with laparoscopic cryotherapy. A new technique for treating liver metastases. Surg Endosc 1997;11:979–981.

285. Iannitti DA, Heniford T, Hale J, Grundfest-Broniatowski S, Gagner M. Laparoscopic cryoablation of hepatic metastases. Arch Surg 1998;133:1011–1015.

286. Soon PS, Glenn D, Jorgensen J, Morris DL. Fluorodeoxyuridine causes bilomas after hepatic cryotherapy. J Surg Oncol 1998;69:45–50.

287. Seifert JK, Morris DL. World survey on the complications of hepatic and prostate cryotherapy. World J Surg 1999;23:109–113; discussion 13–14.

288. Seifert JK, Stewart GJ, Hewitt PM, Bolton EJ, Junginger T, Morris DL. Interleukin-6 and tumor necrosis factor-alpha levels following hepatic cryotherapy: association with volume and duration of freezing. World J Surg 1999;23:1019–1026.

289. Ng KK, Lam CM, Poon RT, et al. Comparison of systemic responses of radiofrequency ablation, cryotherapy and surgical resection in a porcine liver model. Ann Surg Oncol 2004;11:650–657.

290. Garcea G, Polomenovi N, O'Leary E, Lloyd TD, Dennison A, Berry DP. Two-stage liver resection and chemotherapy for bilobar liver metastases. Eur J Surg Oncology 2004;30:759–764.

15

Regional Therapy for Peritoneal Surface Malignancy

Yehuda Skornick, MD
and Paul H. Sugarbaker, MD

CONTENTS

SUMMARY

Carcinomatosis has been in the past a universally fatal manifestation of gastrointestinal cancer. It has also carried a nearly lethal prognosis in ovarian cancer. It remains the major site of treatment failure with these diseases. A review of the natural history of carcinomatosis from the world literature was undertaken. The rationale, technology, and results of treatment using peritonectomy and perioperative intraperitoneal chemotherapy represents an essential part of the treatment. Small-volume residual disease must be treated by chemotherapy and hyperthermia. To apply these treatments properly, selection of patients using prognostic indicators is necessary. The results of treating patients who have peritoneal mesothelioma, pseudomyxoma peritonei, and carcinomatosis from colorectal cancer indicate that progress in the curative management of carcinomatosis has been made. Peritoneal surface dissemination of cancer can no longer be equated with a terminal condition. A multidisciplinary approach to treatment

From: *Cancer Drug Discovery and Development: Regional Cancer Therapy*
Edited by: P. M. Schlag and U. S. Stein © Humana Press Inc., Totowa, NJ

employing surgery and regional chemotherapy has created a new standard of care for this pattern of cancer dissemination.

Key Words: Carcinomatosis; cytoreductive surgery; peritonectomy; intraperitoneal chemotherapy; colorectal cancer; appendiceal cancer; peritoneal mesothelioma.

1. INTRODUCTION

Samson first described peritoneal carcinomatosis in 1931 *(1)*. Since then, it has remained a therapeutic dilemma. This process represents an advanced form of intraabdominal and pelvic malignancies, which is commonly associated with a grim prognosis *(2)*. The prognosis mainly relates to the histopathology of the primary tumor. However, infiltration of the visceral and parietal peritoneum with tumor is a major source of severe morbidity and mortality and is therefore regarded as a preterminal condition.

Traditionally, carcinomatous patients have undergone palliative procedures aimed at preventing or overcoming complications, which almost inevitably arise, particularly future formation of bowel obstruction and debilitating abdominal ascites.

The oncologist's approach to this condition has begun to change in recent years. Instead of palliation, cytoreductive surgery is performed, combined with perioperative intraperitoneal hyperthermic chemotherapy. The modern goal is curative management of carcinomatosis. This multimodality therapy has been described and has shown promise in several large studies *(3–6)*. The treatment paradigm is now an attempt to bring about long-term survival of patients with peritoneal carcinomatosis with an acceptable rate of morbidity and mortality.

2. ORIGIN OF PERITONEAL CARCINOMATOSIS

In a few unusual malignancies, peritoneal surface malignancy has the peritoneum as the primary site. Papillary ovarian adenocarcinoma is associated with peritoneal tumor deposits *(7)*. Peritoneal mesothelioma is also a primary peritoneal malignancy *(8)*. More commonly, diffuse peritoneal surface malignancy is the result of intraperitoneal dissemination from abdominal or pelvic primary tumors like stomach, pancreas, small bowel, colon, appendix, and ovary. Peritoneal spread is the natural history of ovarian cancer, with 65% of patients showing carcinomatosis at the time of diagnosis. To a lesser extent in colorectal cancer, carcinomatosis is observed with diagnosis of the primary in 10 to 15% of patients. In colorectal cancers, similarities between peritoneal carcinomatosis and liver secondaries allow oncologists to regard the peritoneum as an intraabdominal structure that can, like the liver, be resected with curative intent when disseminated disease has occurred. Peritoneal spread may also occur as a result of locoregional recurrence after resection of primary tumors like cancers of the stomach, pancreas, and colon.

Large-volume peritoneal involvement presenting with the primary tumor is commonly seen in pseudomyxoma peritonei. The extensive intraabdominal gelatinous tumor is associated with benign adenoma or mucous adenocarcinoma of the appendix *(9)*. In this condition peritoneal spread represents only a regional, rather than systemic, dissemination of the primary tumor.

The mechanism by which primary tumors spread to the peritoneum has been well characterized. The intraperitoneal tumor cells can arise from intraabdominal tumors that have involved the bowel wall and penetrated the serosal membrane. The free intraperitoneal tumor cells may adhere to the peritoneal surfaces *(10)*. Basement membrane invasion, angiogenesis, tumor establishment, and progression are enhanced by the presence of growth factors, cytokines, and metalloproteases. Inflammatory response at the site of a tumor implant recruits macrophages and platelets that promote angiogenesis *(11–13)*.

Based on this model of peritoneal cancer dissemination, surgery alone for the treatment of peritoneal carcinomatosis may paradoxically provide an environment that is favorable for continued peritoneal cancer progression. We have previously described the *tumor cell entrapment hypothesis (14)*, which postulates the pathways that lead to peritoneal surface dissemination during surgery: (1) tumor cell shedding owing to tumor penetration of visceral serosal membranes, (2) leakage of tumor cells from transected lymphatics and blood vessels, (3) release of malignant cells from the primary tumor owing to intraoperative manipulations, (4) fibrin entrapment of tumor cells on traumatized peritoneal surfaces, and (5) progression of tumor growth through the release of growth factors.

Prevention of tumor cell entrapment is the rationale supporting the use of perioperative intraperitoneal chemotherapy as an adjunctive treatment modality.

3. RATIONALE FOR PERITONECTOMY PROCEDURES

Peritonectomy procedures are necessary if one is to treat peritoneal surface tumors successfully with curative intent. The procedure is used in the areas of sizable cancer progression in an attempt to leave the patient with only microscopic residual disease. In addition to stripping of the peritoneal surfaces, small tumor nodules are removed using electroevaporation. Involvement of the visceral peritoneum frequently requires resection of a portion of the stomach, small intestine, or colorectum.

3.1. Location of Peritoneal Surface Malignancies

Peritoneal surface malignancies tend to involve the visceral peritoneum at three definite sites *(15)*. These are sites where the bowel is anchored to the retroperitoneum and peristalsis results in less motion of the visceral peritoneal surface. The sigmoid colon has a non-mobile portion as it comes up out of the pelvis; therefore it frequently requires resection. A complete pelvic peritonectomy involves stripping of the abdominal side walls, the peritoneum overlying the bladder, the cul-de-sac, and the rectosigmoid colon.

The ileocecal region is another area where there is a limited mobility. Resection of the terminal ileum and a small portion of the right colon are often necessary in cytoreductive surgery. The third site often requiring special attention is the antrum of the stomach. The antrum is fixed to the retroperitoneum at the pylorus. Tumor coming into the foramen of Winslow accumulates in the subpyloric space and may cause intestinal obstruction as a result of gastric outlet obstruction. Occasionally tumor in the lesser omentum will cause a confluence of disease on the lesser curvature of the stomach and encasement of the left gastric artery. Complete resection in these cases requires total gastrectomy including the left gastric artery *(16)*.

4. ELECTROEVAPORATIVE SURGERY

Peritonectomy and visceral organ resections using scissors or knife dissection results in a large volume of small vessel bleeding. Electrosurgical dissection minimizes small vessel bleeding and leaves a margin of heat necrosis that is devoid of viable malignant cells *(17)*. Electroevaporation of tumor and normal tissue at the margins of resection not only reduces the likelihood of persistent disease but also minimizes blood loss. Electroevaporation is achieved by using a 3-mm ball-tipped electrosurgical hand piece (Valleylab, Boulder, CO). The instrument is placed at the interface of tumor and normal tissues while the focal point for further dissection is placed on strong traction. The electrosurgical generator is used on pure cut at high voltage. The ball-tipped electrode is used cautiously for tumor removal on tubular structures like ureters, small bowel, and colon, to avoid heat necrosis and fistula formation.

5. PERITONECTOMY PROCEDURES FOR COMPLETE CYTOREDUCTION

The abdomen is opened by a long midline incision extending from the xiphoid to the symphysis pubis. A careful assessment of the abdominal cavity is performed. The small bowel and the stomach are inspected for tumor nodules. A massive involvement of the stomach may require gastrectomy and small bowel segmental resection. A decision has to be made as to whether complete cytoreduction is likely to be achievable prior to embarking on irreversible, high-risk procedures.

Complete cytoreduction involves six peritonectomy procedures *(6)*, in the following order:

1. Greater omentectomy with splenectomy.
2. Stripping of the left hemidiaphragm.
3. Stripping of the right hemidiaphragm.
4. Cholecystectomy and lesser omentectomy.
5. Distal gastrectomy (antrectomy).
6. Pelvic peritonectomy with resection of the rectosigmoid by anterior resection.

Involvement of the parietal peritoneum on the anterior and lateral abdominal wall may require additional excision. A right hemicolectomy is usually performed in pseudo-myxoma peritonei owing to the concentration of disease around the ileocecal region. However, not all patients require all six peritonectomies described. All depends on whether complete cytoreduction has been achieved.

6. PERIOPERATIVE INTRAPERITONEAL CHEMOTHERAPY

In patients with carcinomatosis, extensive removal of the peritoneum without intraperitoneal chemotherapy will allow tumor cells to become implanted beneath the peritoneal surface of the abdomen and pelvis. As these deeply implanted cancer cells progress, they may contribute to obstruction of vital structures such as the ureter, common bile duct, or even gastric outlet. Therefore aggressive perioperative intraperitoneal chemotherapy should be planned as part of an operative intervention for carcinomatosis.

The fundamental objective of delivering chemotherapeutic agents directly into the peritoneum is to maximize the dose intensity of the drug to tumor cells while minimizing their systemic toxicity. This is accomplished by using large doses of high-molecular-weight chemotherapy agents that can take advantage of the unique physiology of the peritoneum *(18)*. The peritoneal-plasma barrier consists of the peritoneal fluid and the peritoneum itself. The peritoneum is composed of an outer layer of mesothelial cells, a basement membrane, and an interstitium, which contains bundles of collagen fibrils and abundant capillaries. Lymphatic vessels are found primarily in the peritoneum of the diaphragm and the omentum.

Experimental models revealed the ability of the peritoneal-plasma barrier to maintain a high drug concentration gradient between the intraabdominal cavity and plasma *(19,20)*. It was also demonstrated that the peritoneal clearance of an agent is inversely proportional to the square root of its molecular weight *(21)*. The retention of high concentrations of chemotherapy administered by the intraperitoneal route results in reduced systemic toxicity compared with intravenous administration at equivalent doses. The therapeutic dose of many cytotoxic agents may be escalated when they are given by intraperitoneal administration.

6.1. Hyperthermia

Hyperthermia has been shown to possess antitumor effects. The direct cytotoxic effect of hyperthermia has been attributed to its ability to destabilize cell membranes and induce changes in the cellular cytoskeleton *(22)*. Elevation of intraperitoneal temperature has also been shown to enhance the cytotoxicity of various therapeutic agents *(23)*. Increased blood flow associated with moderate hyperthermia has been suggested as one reason for this synergy *(24)*. It has also been shown that heat increases the diffusion of chemotherapy agents into the tumor nodules *(25)*. Currently, the use of temperatures between 41.0° and 42.50°C has become an integral part of intraoperative intraperitoneal chemotherapy. Since awake patients tolerate elevated intraabdominal temperatures poorly, the application of hyperthermia can only be performed intraoperatively, when the patients are under general anesthesia. The intraperitoneal chemotherapy starts with heated mitomycin C (15 mg/m^2) or cisplatin (50 mg/m^2) and doxorubicin (15 mg/m^2) at approximately 42°C in 3 L of peritoneal dialysis solution. During the open methodology of heated intraperitoneal chemotherapy, manual distribution of the heat and the cytotoxic drugs are made possible through the surgeon's double-gloved hand. In the postoperative period intraperitoneal 5-fluorouracil (5-FU) at 600 mg/m^2 or paclitaxel at 20 mg/m^2/d for 5 d is administered.

7. INTRAOPERATIVE ASSESSMENT OF CARCINOMATOSIS

For most tumor types, the likelihood of complete cytoreduction is dependent on the extent of carcinomatosis. In carcinomatous patients this is a determinant of resectability and survival.

The peritoneal cancer index (PCI) is a quantitative prognostic indicator of carcinomatosis *(26)*. It is a quantitative assessment of both cancer distribution and cancer implant size throughout the abdomen and pelvis (Fig. 1). To determine the PCI, two transverse planes and two sagittal planes divide the abdomen into nine abdominopelvic regions numbered in a clockwise direction with 0 at the umbilicus and 1 defining the space beneath the right hemidiaphragm. Regions 9 and 10 define the upper and lower portions of the jejunum, and regions 11 and 12 define the upper and lower portions of the ileum.

Lesion size refers to the greatest diameter of the implants on the peritoneal surface. In the presence of many implants within the abdominopelvic region, the greatest diameter of the largest implants is measured and recorded. Implants are scored as lesion size 0 through 3 (LS-0 to LS-3). LS-0 means that no implants are seen, after complete lysis of all adhesions and complete inspection of all peritoneal surfaces. LS-1 refers to implants

Peritoneal Cancer Index

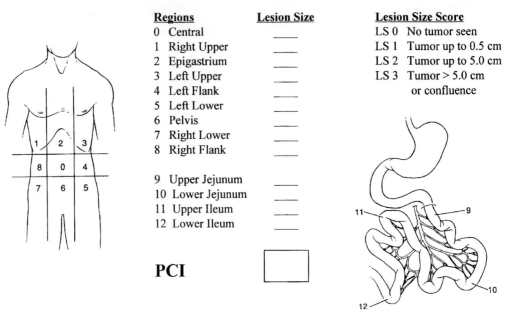

Regions	Lesion Size	Lesion Size Score
0 Central	____	LS 0 No tumor seen
1 Right Upper	____	LS 1 Tumor up to 0.5 cm
2 Epigastrium	____	LS 2 Tumor up to 5.0 cm
3 Left Upper	____	LS 3 Tumor > 5.0 cm
4 Left Flank	____	or confluence
5 Left Lower	____	
6 Pelvis	____	
7 Right Lower	____	
8 Right Flank	____	
9 Upper Jejunum	____	
10 Lower Jejunum	____	
11 Upper Ileum	____	
12 Lower Ileum	____	

PCI

Fig. 1. Peritoneal cancer index (PCI).

up to 0.5 cm in diameter. LS-2 indicates that nodules are 0.5 cm up to 5 cm. LS-3 refers to implants 5 cm or greater in diameter. A confluence of cancerous implants is scored as LS-3. The lesion size assessment is then combined with the distribution assessment for each region, which can be summated as a numerical score, ranging from 0 to 39. PCI is a useful tool for quantitating the extent of peritoneal surface malignancy and thereby estimating survival in most diseases with carcinomatosis. An exception to the usefulness of this index is the adenomucinosis type of pseudomyxoma and cystic mesothelioma. In these noninvasive diseases, a PCI of 39 can be converted to a PCI of 0 by cytoreductive surgery. With invasive cancers, PCI has no prognostic implications in the presence of nonresectable tumor mass, even with a low PCI. In this situation there will not be a complete cytoreduction. However, in most patients, a low PCI is associated with a lower tumor load and may identify a case with a greater likelihood of complete surgical cytoreduction.

Assessment of the completeness of cancer resection (CCR) is assessed by the surgeon at the end of the procedure: CCR-0 indicates that no macroscopic residual tumor remained, CC-1 that no residual nodule greater than 2.5 mm in diameter remained, and CC-2 that the diameter of residual nodules is 2.5 mm to 2.5 cm. CC-3 indicates tumor nodules greater than 2.5 cm and a layering of unresected cancer at any site *(27)*.

8. RESULTS OF COMBINED TREATMENT
FOR PERITONEAL MESOTHELIOMA

The incidence of pleural and peritoneal mesothelioma has been rising worldwide since 1970. Peritoneal mesothelioma represents about one-fifth to one-third of all forms of mesothelioma *(28–30)*. There seems little doubt that asbestos exposure is linked to the

Table 1
Treatment Data on 68 Patients with Peritoneal Mesothelioma

Variable		No. of patients	Median survival (mo)[a]	p value[b]
Peritoneal cancer index	0–28	42	67.4	0.046
	29–39	25	26.1	
Completeness of cytoreduction score	0–2	41	67	0.003
	3	27	26	
Perioperative chemotherapy	Yes	58	35	NS
	No	10	NR	
Metastasis	Yes	7	15	0.005
	No	61	55	
Second-look surgery	Yes	17	89	NS
	No	51	55	
Status				
No evidence of disease		22	NR	
Alive with disease		18	NR	
Dead of disease		22	13	

Abbreviations: NR, median survival not yet reached; NS, no statistically significant.
[a] Survival was measured from time of diagnosis.
[b] Log-rank test.

development of malignant pleural mesothelioma (31). Some would consider it a significant etiologic factor in peritoneal mesothelioma. The Washington Cancer Institute study
has shown that although there was a strong relationship between asbestos exposure and
peritoneal mesothelioma in men, there was no such relationship among women (32).
Other differences in peritoneal mesothelioma between men and women will be discussed
later in this section when the response to therapy is described.

Sixty-eight patients with peritoneal mesothelioma were treated at the Washington
Cancer Institute (33). Increased abdominal girth was the most common symptom reported
by those patients. The second most common initial symptom or sign was abdominal pain.
Loss of weight and a new onset of hernia were common among men and were much less
in women. Definitive diagnosis of peritoneal mesothelioma is traditionally a significant
problem. Long delays in definitive diagnosis delay the definitive treatment.

Obtaining fluid from these patients rarely provides the proper cytologic diagnosis. An
additional problem concerns the distinction of peritoneal mesothelioma from carcinomatosis of another origin (34). Laparoscopy and/or laparotomy with biopsy were required
of almost all the patients. The interventional radiologists or laparoscopic surgeons should,
however, be very careful in searching for a diagnosis by an invasive test (35). This tumor
is extremely efficient in its ability to implant within a needle tract, laparoscopy port site,
or abdominal incisions.

The results of treatment at the Washington Cancer Institute (33) are shown in Table 1.
For men, the mean interval between diagnosis and treatment was 6.9 mo compared with
22.1 mo for women.

The PCI and the completeness of cytoreduction score were quantitative prognostic
indicators that were statistically significant predictors of survival (33). The completeness

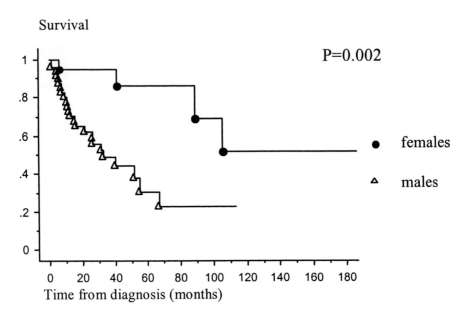

Fig. 2. Kaplan-Meier survival curve of the 21 female (circles) and 47 male (triangles) patients with peritoneal mesothelioma treated at the Washington Cancer Institute between 1989 and 2003. $p = 0.002$.

of cytoreduction score was 0–2 in 41 patients and 3 in 27 patients, with median survivals of 67 and 26 mo, respectively.

The Kaplan-Meier distribution of 21 female patients treated in this group is shown in Fig. 2. These results are statistically significantly different, with a p-value of 0.002, from the survival distribution in men. The reason is not readily apparent. However, the longer interval between diagnosis and definitive treatment in women, the lack of relationship with asbestos, the diagnosis as an incidental finding, and less weight loss suggests less disruption of function and a less aggressive disease process in women.

Of 68 patients, there were 16 patients with grade III to IV complications, giving an overall morbidity rate of 23.5%. Persistent bile leak from the liver surface, small bowel fistula, and intraabdominal bleeding required reoperations. There were five perioperative deaths (7%), three from sepsis and two from pulmonary embolism.

9. RESULTS OF COMBINED TREATMENT FOR PSEUDOMYXOMA PERITONEI

Pseudomyxoma peritonei (PMP) is a rare condition that presents at laparotomy with "jelly belly" (36). It is characterized by copious production of mucinous ascites that fills the peritoneal cavity. Although mostly diagnosed at laparotomy, increasingly the diagnosis is made, prior to laparotomy, by awareness of the condition and advances in cross-sectional imaging. Most authorities acknowledge that PMP predominantly originates in the appendix in men, which is also the commonest site of origin in women, although synchronous disease is also found in the ovary in most women with PMP (37,38).

The appendix as a primary cancer site for seeding of the peritoneal surface is somewhat unique *(39–42)*. Appendix cancer is usually of low biological aggressiveness. Rarely does it involve lymph nodes and almost never metastasizes to the liver. The pathologist sees these mucinous adenocarcinomas as minimally invasive in that they do not penetrate tissues. Appendiceal malignancy causes peritoneal dissemination early in the natural history of the disease. The tumor, usually characterized as an appendiceal adenoma, enlarges so that the walls of the appendix are stretched to a bursting point. As the malignancy progresses, the walls of the appendix leak tumor cells into the peritoneal cavity. The mucus provides the fluid for widespread dissemination of the tumor cells to specific anatomical sites within the abdomen. Peritoneal fluid is absorbed on the undersurface of the right hemidiaphragm through the lymphatic lacunae and on the greater and lesser omental surfaces through lymphoid aggregates. Other sites are within the pelvis, beneath the right lobe of the liver, in the right retrohepatic space, at the ligament of Treitz, and in the abdominal gutters. The small bowel, which is active in peristalsis nearly all the time, prevents noninvasive tumor deposits from implanting on its surface. The stomach and large bowel are variably involved. This distribution phenomenon makes cytoreductive surgery possible, with a nearly complete removal of all cancer from the abdominal cavity. TRegional chemotherapy will prevent the large number of residual tumor cells remaining after cytoreductive surgery from implanting in the traumatized peritoneal surfaces and causing progressing disease at a later time.

PMP is usually an unexpected finding at laparotomy for suspected appendicitis, or peritonitis, or ovarian mass. However in an increasing number of patients the diagnosis is suspected at imaging alone, particularly based on the classical features on computed tomography (CT) *(43,44)*. Tumor markers are measured; based on the CA-125 in women, and the carcinoembryonic antigen (CEA) levels in either sex, many patients are erroneously diagnosed as having advanced ovarian cancer or metastatic intestinal adenocarcinoma. A delay in diagnosis is common, and many patients are diagnosed with irritable bowel syndrome for a number of years prior to definitive diagnosis.

As described treatment consists of maximal surgery combined with maximal regional chemotherapy, two therapies that are blended together into a single treatment plan *(6,17,45)*. Traditionally, in PMP, mitomycin C has been given at operation, followed by 4 to 5 d of postoperative intraperitoneal 5-FU. Newer agents, particularly platinum-based therapies, are currently being evaluated.

Figure 3 shows survival rates by completeness of cytoreduction. Survival differences were significant, with a p value of <0.0001. Patients who left the operating room after cytoreductive surgery with tumor nodules <2.5 mm in diameter remaining were much more likely to survive long term than were those with an incomplete cytoreduction *(42)*. There was also a significant difference in survival between patients with adenomucinosis and those with mucinous adenocarcinoma. A noninvasive histopathology is extremely important in selecting patients who are most likely to benefit from this treatment strategy. The mortality rate in this group was 2%. The overall grade III/IV morbidity was 27%. Pancreatitis (7.1%) and fistula formation (4.7%) were the major complications. No mortality was associated with the adjuvant chemotherapy administration.

Table 2 reviews the experience of various centers with cytoreductive surgery and perioperative intraperitoneal chemotherapy in patients with mucinous appendiceal tumors with peritoneal dissemination *(42,46–47)*.

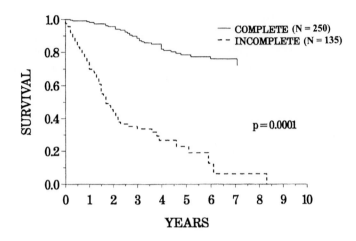

Fig. 3. Peritoneal surface malignancy of the appendix: survival by cytoreduction.

10. RESULTS OF COMBINED THERAPY FOR PERITONEAL CARCINOMATOSIS FROM COLORECTAL CANCER

At initial diagnosis of colon cancer, the peritoneal surface is involved by tumor in 10 to 15% of patients *(52,53)* and is the second most common site for recurrence after so-called curative colorectal cancer resection. Phase II studies from a series of experienced cancer treatment centers showed that with combined therapy, approximately 30% of patients with peritoneal carcinomatosis can be cured of this otherwise deadly manifestation *(54)*. Also, a prospective phase III study showed that the standard of care offered a 12-mo median survival in this group of patients. With cytoreductive surgery and intraperitoneal mitomycin C chemotherapy, this survival was increased to 22 mo *(55)*. Finally, Glehen and colleagues, in a multiinstitutional study, collected 503 patients who had colorectal cancer and who were treated with this new combined management plan *(50)*. In patients who had a complete cytoreduction, 32% were alive and well at 5 yr (Fig. 4). All these results are in marked contrast to the natural history studies that record an approximate 6 mo of survival in this group of patients *(2,53,57)*. Even with modern chemotherapy, a recent report shows that the survival of colorectal cancer patients with carcinomatosis is limited to about 6 months *(57)*. The conclusion from all these clinical data is that combined treatment is an option to be considered in carcinomatosis from gastrointestinal cancer and that a wider application of this new management strategy needs to be explored.

11. CONCLUSIONS

The current state-of-the-art treatment of peritoneal carcinomatosis and primary peritoneal surface malignancy is described in this chapter. The applications concern a wide variety of abdominal and pelvic malignancies. PMP syndrome should no longer be managed by serial debulking but by cytoreductive surgery with peritonectomy procedures to achieve a disease-free status, followed by perioperative intraperitoneal chemotherapy. A major proportion of these patients should be cured. Peritoneal mesothelioma represents a similar condition for which combined therapy should be considered the

Table 2
Literature Review of Cytoreductive Surgery and Perioperative Intraperitoneal Chemotherapy as a Treatment for Mucinous Appendiceal Tumors With Peritoneal Dissemination

Author and year	Institution	References	No. of Patients	Method	Survival (%) 3-yr	Survival (%) 5-yr	Morbidity (%)	Mortality (%)
Sugarbaker and Chang, 1999	Washington, DC	42	385	MMC	74	63	27	2.70
Deraco, 2004	Milan	46	33	Cisplatin/MMC	NA	96	33	3
Guner, 2004	Hanover	47	28	Cisplatin/MMC/5-FU	NA	75	36	7
Loungnarath, 2005	Lyon	48	27	Cisplatin/MMC	80	50	44	0
Murphy, 2006	Basingstake	49	123	MMC/5-Fu	NA	75	21	5
Smeek, 2006	Amsterdam	50	103	MMC	71	60	NA	NA
Stewart, 2006	Winston Salem	51	110	MMC	59	53	38	4

Abbreviations: 5-FU, 5-fluorouracil; MMC, mitomycin C; NA, not available.

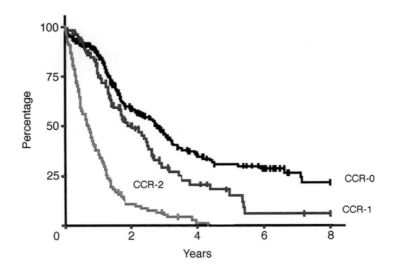

Fig. 4. Actuarial survival of 506 patients who had cytoreductive surgery combined with perioperative intraperitoneal chemotherapy, according to the completeness of cancer resection (CCR). CCR-0 = no residual disease; CCR-1 = nodule < 5.0 mm; CCR-2 = nodule 5.0 mm.

standard of practice. With this treatment, previous survival rates of 10% at 1 yr have been extended to 90% survival at 1 yr with approximately 50% 5-yr survival. Patients with colon cancer at high risk for peritoneal seeding or patients with small to moderate volumes of peritoneal surface dissemination should be treated. Multiple investigators have demonstrated survival rates of approximately 30% at 5 yr in these patients.

The use of perioperative intraperitoneal chemotherapy and its modalities needs to be validated by randomized studies. A comparison of the intraperitoneal route with the most modern systemic polychemotherapy after maximal cytoreductive surgery is warranted.

REFERENCES

1. Sampson J. Implantation peritoneal carcinomatosis of ovarian origin. Am J Pathol 1931;7:423–443.
2. Sadeghi B, Arvieux C, Glehen O, et al. Peritoneal carcinomatosis from non-gynecologic malignancies: results of the EVOCAPE 1 multi-centric prospective study. Cancer 2000;88:358–363.
3. Rossi CR, Foletto M, Mocellin S, et al. Hyperthermic intraoperative intraperitoneal chemotherapy with cisplatin and doxorubicin in patients who undergo cytoreductive surgery for peritoneal carcinomatosis and sarcomatosis: phase I study. Cancer 2002;94:492–499.
4. Witkamp AJ, de Bree E, Kaag MM, et al. Extensive cytoreductive surgery followed by intra-operative hyperthermic intraperitoneal chemotherapy with mitomycin-C in patients with peritoneal carcinomatosis of colorectal origin. Eur J Cancer 2001;37:979–984.
5. Eilber FC, Rosen G, Forscher C, Nelson SD, Dorey FJ, Eilber FR. Surgical resection and intraperitoneal chemotherapy for recurrent abdominal sarcomas. Ann Surg Oncol 1999;6:645–650.
6. Sugarbaker PH. Peritonectomy procedures. Surg Oncol Clin North Am 2003;12:703–727.
7. Eltabbakh GH, Werness BA, Piver S, Blumenson LE. Prognostic factors in extraovarian primary peritoneal carcinoma. Gynecol Oncol 1998;71:230–239.
8. Mohamed F, Sugarbaker PH. Peritoneal mesothelioma. Curr Treat Options Oncol 2002;3:375–386.
9. Wirtzfed DA, Rodriguez-Bigas M, Weber T, Petrelli NJ. Disseminated peritoneal adenomucinosis: a critical review. Ann Surg Oncol 1999;:797–801.

10. Weiss L. Metastatic inefficiency: intravascular and intraperitoneal implantation of cancer cells, in Peritoneal Carcinomatosis: Principles of Management (Sugarbaker PH, ed.), Boston: Kluwer Academic; 1996:1–12.

11. Weiss L. Metastatic inefficiency: intravasculat and intraperitoneal implantation of cancer cells. Cancer Treat Res 1996;82:1–12.

12. Chang C, Werb Z. The many faces of metalloproteases: cell growth, invasion, angiogenesis and metastasis. Trend Cell Biol 2001;11:537–543.

13. Crowther M, Brown NJ, Bishop ET, Lewis CE. Microenvironmental influence on macrophage regulation of angiogenesis in wounds and malignant tumors. J Leukoc Biol 2001;70:478–490.

14. Sugarbaker PH. Management of peritoneal-surface malignancy: the surgeon's role. Langenbecks Arch Surg 1999;384:576–587.

15. Carmignani CP, Sugarbaker TA, Bromley CM, Sugarbaker PH. Intraperitoneal cancer dissemination: mechanism of the patterns of spread. Metastases Rev 2003;22:465–472.

16. Sugarbaker PH. Total gastrectomy with diverting jejunoseomy for complete cytoreduction of 36 patients with pseudomyxoma peritonei syndrome. Br J Surg 2002;89:208–212.

17. Sugarbaker PH. Laser-mode electrosurgery, in Peritoneal Xarcinomatosis: Principles of Management (Sugarbaker PH, ed.), Boston: Kluwer, 1996:375–385.

18. Jacquet P, Sugarbaker PH. Peritoneal-plasma barrier, in Peritoneal Carcinomatosis: Principles of Management (Sugarbaker PH, ed.), Boston: Kluwer, 1996:53–63.

19. Dedrick RL. Theoretical and experimental bases of intraperitoneal chemotherapy. Semin Oncol 1985;12(3 suppl 4):1–6.

20. Flessner MF, Fenstermacher JD, Dedrick RL, Blasberg RG. A distributed model of peritoneal-plasma transport: tissue concentration gradients. Am J Physiol 1985;248(3 pt 2):F425–435.

21. Dedrick RL, Myers CE, Bungay PM, DeVita VT Jr. Pharmacokinetic rationale for peritoneal drug administration in the treatment of ovarian cancer. Cancer Treat Rep 1978;62:1–11.

22. Armour EP, McEachern D, Wang Z, Corry PM, Martinez A. Sensitivity of human cells to mild hyperthermia. Cancer Res 1993;53:2740–2744.

23. Los G, Sminia P, Wondergem J, et al. Optimisation of intraperitoneal cisplatin therapy with regional hyperthermia in rats. Eur J Cancer 1991;27:472–477.

24. Hildebrandt B, Wust P, Ahlers O, et al. The cellular and molecular basis of hyperthermia. Crit Rev Oncol Hematol 2002;43:33–56.

25. van de Vaart PJ, van der Vange N, Zoetmulder FA, et al. Intraperitoneal cisplatin with regional hyperthermia in advanced ovarian cancer: pharmacokinetics and cisplatin-DNA adduct formation in patients and ovarian cancer cell lines. Eur J Cancer 1998;34:33–56.

26. Jacquet P, Sugarbaker PH. Clinical research methodologies in diagnosis and staging of patients with peritoneal carcinomatosis, inPeritoneal Carcinomatosis: Principles of Management (Sugarbaker PH, ed.), Boston: Kluwer Acadenic, 1996:359–374.

27. Jacquet P, Sugarbaker PH. Current methodologies for clinical assessment of patients with peritoneal carcinomatosis. J Exp Clin Cancer Res 1996;15:49–58.

28. Shridhar KS, Doria R, Raub WA Jr, Thurer RJ, Saldana M. New strategies are needed in diffuse malignant mesothelioma. Cancer 1992;70:2969–2979.

29. Antman K, Shemin R, Ryan L, et al. Malignant mesothelioma: prognostic variables in a registry of 180 patients, the Dana-Farber Cancer Institute and Brigham and Women's Hospital experience over two decades, 1965–1985. J Clin Oncol 1988;6:147–153.

30. Ascensio JA, Goldblatt P, Thomford NR. Primary malignant peritoneal mesotheliomas. A report of seven cases and a review of the litrature. Arch Surg 1990;125:477–481.

31. Wagner JC, Sleegs CA, Marchand P. Diffuse pleural mesothelioma and asbestos exposure in the North Western Cape Province. Br J Ind Med 1960;17:260–271.

32. Acherman YIZ, Welch LS, Bromley CM Sugarbaker PH. Clinical presentation of mesothelioma. Tumori 2003;89:269–273.

33. Sugarbaker PH, Welch LS, Mohamed F, Glehen O. A review of peritoneal mesothelioma at the Washington Cancer Institute. Surg Oncol Clin North Am 2003;12:605–621.

34. Alcorn KW, Yan H, Shmookler BM, et al. Differential diagnosis of the simultaneous occurrence of colon carcinoma and peritoneal mesothelioma by immunohistichemistry. Surg Rounds 2000;23: 411–417.

35. Jacquet P, Sugarbaker PH. Influence of wound healing on gastrointestinal cancer recurrence. Wounds 1995;7:40–47.
36. Fann JI, Vierra M, Fisher D, et al. Pseudomyxoma peritonei. Surg Gynecol Obstet 1993;177:441–447.
37. Hinson FL, Ambrose NS. Pseudomyxoma peritonei. Br J Surg 1998;85:1332–1339.
38. Sherer DM, Abulafia O, Eliakim R. Pseudomyxoma peritonei: a review of current literature. Gynecol Obstet Invest 2001;51:73–80.
39. Sugarbaker PH, Ronnett BM, Archer A, et al. Pseudomyxoma peritonii syndrome. Adv Surg 1997;30:233–280.
40. Ronnett BM, Zahn CM, Kurman RJ, et al. Disseminated peritoneal adenomucunosis and peritoneal mucinous carcinomatosis. Am J Surg Path 1995;19:1390–1408.
41. Sugarbaker PH. Pseudomyxoma peritonei: a cancer whose biology is characterized by a redistribution phenomenon. Ann Surg 1994;219:109–111.
42. Sugarbaker PH, Chang D. Result of treatment of 385 patients with peritoneal surface spread of appendiceal malignancy. Ann Surg Oncol 1999;6:727–731.
43. Archer AG, Sugarbaker PH, Jelinek JS. Radiology of peritoneal carcinomatosis, in Peritoneal Carcinomatosis: Principles of Management (Sugarbaker PH, ed.), Boston: Kluwer, 1996:263–288.
44. Jacquet P, Jelinek J, Sugarbaker PH. Abdominal computed tomographic scan in the selection of patients with nucinous peritoneal carcinomatosis for cytoreductive surgery. J Am Coll Surg 1995; 181:530–538.
45. Sugarbaker PH. Intraperitoneal Chemotherapy and Cytoreductive Surgery: Manual for Physicians and Nurses, 3rd ed. Grand Rapids, MI: Ludann, 1998.
46. Deraco M, Baratti D, Inglese MG, et al. Peritonectomy and intraperitoneal hyperthrmic perfusion (IPHP): a strategy that has confirmed its efficacy in patients with pseudomyxoma peritonei. Ann Surg Oncol 2004;11:393–398.
47. Guner Z, Schmidt U, Dahlke MH, et al. Cytoreductive surgery and intraperitoneal chemotherapy for pseudomyxoma peritonei. Int J Coloretal Dis 2005;20:155–160.
48. Loungnarath R, Causeret S, Bossard N, et al. Cytoreductive surgery with intraperitoneal chemo-hyperthermia for the treatment of pseudomyxoma peritonei: a prospective study.Dis Colon Rectum 2005;48:1372–1379.
49. Murphy EM, Sexton R, Moran BJ. Early results of surgery in 123 patients with pseudomyxoma peritonei from a perforated appendiceal neoplasm. Dis Colon Rectum 2006;50:37–42.
50. Smeenk RM, Verwaal VJ, Antonini N, Zoetmulder FAN. Survival analysis of pseudomyxoma peritonei patients treated by cytoreductive surgery and hyperthrmic intraperitoneal chemotherapy. Ann Surg 2007;245:104–109.
51. Stewart JH 4th, Shen P, Russell GB, et al. Appendiceal neoplasms with peritoneal dissemination: outcomes after cytoreductive surgry and intraperitoneal hyperthermic chemotherapy. Ann Surg Oncol 2006;13:624–634.
52. Dawson LE, Russell AH, Tong D, et al. Adenocarcinoma of the sigmoid colon: sites of initial dissemination and clinical pattern of recurrence following surgery alone. J Surg Oncol 1983;22:95–99.
53. Chu DZ, Lang NP, Thompson C, et al. Peritoneal carcinomatosis in nongynecologic malignancy: a prospective study of prognostic factors. Cancer 1989;63:364–367.
54. Glehen O, Gilly FN, Sugarbaker PH. New perspectives in the management of colorectal cancer: what about peritoneal carcinomatosis? Scand J Surg 2003;92:178–179.
55. Verwaal VJ, van Ruth S, de Bree E, van Slooten GW, et al. Randomized trial of cytoreduction and hyperthermic intraperitoneal chemotherapy versus systemic chemotherapy and palliative surgery in patients with peritoneal carcinomatosis of colorectal cancer. J Clin Oncol 2003;21:3737–3743.
56. Glehen O, Kwiatkowsky F, Sugarbaker PH, et al. Cytoreductive surgery combined with perioperative intraperitoneal chemotherapy for the management of peritoneal carcinomatosis from colorectal cancer: a multi-institutional study. J Clin Oncol 2004;22:3284–3292.
57. Jayne DG, Fook S, Loi C, et al. Peritoneal carcinomatosis from colorectal cancer. Br J Surg 2002;89:1545–1550.

16 Malignant Peritoneal Mesothelioma

David P. Mangiameli, MD, Steven K. Libutti, MD, James F. Pingpank, MD, and H. Richard Alexander, MD

Summary

Malignant peritoneal mesothelioma (MPM) is an incurable disease. It represents approximately 15% of all mesotheliomas and has a male predominance. It has a known relationship to asbestos, but most patients present with no known history of exposure. Simian virus 40 (SV40) exposure is potentially another risk factor, although the relationship is not entirely supported. Patients usually present with vague symptoms. Diagnosis is usually made on the basis of a CT scan and percutaneous or open biopsy. The disease remains confined to the abdominal cavity until very late in the disease course. Ascites is a frequent sign; morbidity and mortality are usually a consequence of disease progression within the abdominal cavity. Systemic chemotherapy and radiation have not yet been shown to have much influence over the natural history of the disease. In selected patients, surgical cytoreduction with intraoperative hyperthermic peritoneal chemotherapy is associated with long-term survival. A summary of clinical experience with surgical cytoreduction and intraoperative intraperitoneal chemotherapy for MPM is presented.

Key Words: Peritoneal mesothelioma; mesothelioma; surface malignancy; cytoreduction; tumor debulking; peritoneal perfusion; intraperitoneal chemotherapy; regional therapy; asbestos.

From: *Cancer Drug Discovery and Development: Regional Cancer Therapy*
Edited by: P. M. Schlag and U. S. Stein © Humana Press Inc., Totowa, NJ

1. INTRODUCTION

Malignant peritoneal mesothelioma (MPM) is a rare primary neoplasm of the abdominal serosa. It has a morbid course that, if untreated, invariably leads to death. Patients usually become symptomatic by virtue of their abdominal tumor burden and ascites. Diagnosis typically involves a laparoscopy or laparotomy, and untreated patients can anticipate a life expectancy of 6–12 mo. Owing to the rarity of the disease, the pathogenesis, diagnosis, and management have been surrounded by debate. Historically, the interpretation of various treatment approaches has suffered from small patient numbers, and poor outcomes have been reported; however, over the last decade, a more efficacious therapy has been validated in selected patients. This treatment includes surgical debulking followed by intraperitoneally delivered hyperthermic chemotherapy. It has led to a median survival of 4 to 8 yr and for those who are candidates, remains the treatment of choice *(1,2)*. Investigational efforts continue to define screening strata further, optimize technical application, and determine the utility of other adjuvant treatments. Unfortunately, most patients still die as a consequence of regional tumor progression.

2. EPIDEMIOLOGY

Mesothelioma may arise from the pleura, peritoneum, pericardium, or tunica vaginalis testes. Despite management disparities between differing sites of primary mesothelioma, few epidemiologic studies stratify by the site of origin. The Public Health Agency of Canada showed primary pleural mesothelioma to be ninefold more common than peritoneal mesothelioma in men and threefold more common in women *(3)*. Primary peritoneal mesothelioma accounts for 10 to 15% of all mesotheliomas *(4)*, a diagnosis that, regardless of primary location, carries an incidence of 1/100,000 and a male predominance four- to fivefold over that of women *(5)*. The U.S. National Cancer Institute organizes data from a group of large tumor registries in the country. This database, collectively termed the Surveillance Epidemiology and End Results (SEER), presently represents approximately 26% of the American population. Based on the SEER data, it is likely that the United States is experiencing a waning of overall incidence *(6)*. The decline is presumably owing to a national ban on asbestos. If the decline continues, as is expected, this will be one of the few examples in cancer epidemiology in which environmental rehabilitation and awareness have translated into a change in a disease incidence. In developed countries, asbestos has lost most of its utility. Unfortunately, marketing and sales remain strong from large mining countries to targeted developing areas, such as from Canada to Asian and African countries *(7)*.

3. RISK FACTORS

3.1. Asbestos

There is a confirmed relationship between asbestos exposure and the development of mesothelioma, although most patients present with no history of exposure. This link, in the setting of a low incidence, makes the diagnosis a sensitive marker for the overall health effects of asbestos. The relationship underscores an environmental and occupational risk that has led the disease to be the focus of medical research and tort reform.

Asbestos is a generic name for a group of fibrous minerals, all of which convey exposure risk for mesothelioma, lung cancer, and pulmonary asbestosis. Russia, China, and Canada are presently its major producers. The two most clinically relevant forms of asbestos are chrysotile and crocidolite. Chrysotile, the most ubiquitously encountered form, makes up nearly 95% of the world's production. Crocidolite, although not as common, carries a two- to fourfold increase in its ability to cause mesothelioma, relative to alternate forms of asbestos. All fibers carry equal abilities to cause lung cancer *(8)*.

The translation of asbestos exposure into disease is associated with the extent of exposure and the time interval since first exposure. The latency period of asbestos-induced mesothelioma is approximately 30 yr. An analysis of major published cohorts estimates that peritoneal mesothelioma risk is proportional to the square of cumulative exposure. This contrasts pleural mesothelioma risk, which rises less than linearly, with the cumulative asbestos dose *(9)*. Camus et al. investigated nonoccupational exposure and showed the development of pleural cancer to have a relative risk (RR) of 7.63 in mining areas relative to nonmining areas in people with no occupational risk *(10)*. As one would expect, occupational risk has an even more profound relationship with disease formation. McDonald and McDonald *(11)* defined the RR of developing pleural or peritoneal mesothelioma based on the type of occupation. RR ranged from 2.6 in construction workers to 46.1 in those who worked with insulation. Importantly, insulation workers and those employed in asbestos manufacturing and production (occupations with the highest overall RR) had an increased percent of peritoneal mesothelioma. In fact, 44.2% of mesotheliomas that arose in this group originated as a primary peritoneal malignancy *(11)*. This led to the debated concept that peritoneal mesothelioma induced by asbestos is generally related to a higher cumulative dose than its pleural counterpart. There is no physical evidence to explain a mechanism for the relationship.

3.2. Simian Virus 40

Even though the link between asbestos and mesothelioma is evident, the fact remains most people with mesothelioma have no history of exposure and even among those heavily exposed, less than 5% will go on to develop the disease. This has led investigators to pursue other possible etiologies. Simian virus 40 (SV40) is a DNA virus naturally found in some species of monkeys. A third of almost 100 million polio vaccines manufactured between 1955 and 1961 were contaminated with the virus. Rhesus monkey kidney cells were used to prepare the vaccine until SV40 was identified as a tumorigenic virus in rodents in 1961. Vaccines already made were disseminated through 1963 *(12)*. SV40 is presently being implicated as a carcinogen in the development of several cancers. One of the best supported examples is that of mesothelioma *(13)*.

Human mesothelial malignant transformation via SV40 has been shown to occur in vitro. In fact, rates of transformation are frequently at $1/10^3$ cells. This occurs with low rates of apoptosis, which accelerates the transformation rate *(14)*. Mesothelial immortality is brisk and is facilitated by direct activation of telomerase *(15)*. Altogether, SV40 has been shown in vitro to inactivate tumor suppressors (p53 and Rb) and to activate telomerase and growth factor receptors. Despite molecular investigation, the cause and effect in vivo has not been shown. This shifts more of the burden onto epidemiologic data, which thus far have been problematic, partly because of the inherently low incidence of mesothelioma. The epidemiologic data also suffer the inability to show which subjects were and were not exposed to vaccine-delivered virus, as opposed to those subject to ambient viral contact, which is known to occur. SV40 is likely to have carcinogenic activity in vivo, although this has not been supported epidemiologically. The public health risk remains to be defined.

3.3. Miscellaneous

There is a report of genetic susceptibility increasing the incidence of mesothelioma in a family cluster from two villages in central Turkey (16). The pedigree consisted of 526 people with 22 nuclear families. Fifty percent of offspring were affected, and all affected offspring had affected parents. The male-to-female ratio in this cluster was 1 to 26, clearly an atypical pathogenicity.

There are also case reports of radiation predisposing to mesothelioma. Although instances of mesothelioma arising in irradiated fields are reported, no causal relationship has been established or supported by any epidemiologic evidence (17,18).

4. PATHOLOGY

4.1. Gross and Surgical Pathology

MPM is a rare primary malignancy of the mesothelial lining of the abdominal cavity. It is typically a disease of adults, but childhood cases have been reported (19–21). MPM is histologically identical to pleural mesothelioma and has similar proliferative tendencies. Grossly, the tumors are disseminated throughout the peritoneal cavity. Depending on the extent of progression, the lesions may range from diffuse subcentimeter grayish hard nodules to large nodular masses that can replace the omentum, circumferentially encase bowel, invade solid organs, and defunctionalize the mesentery and diaphragm. Tumors may have a gelatinous consistency, depending on the hyaluronic acid content, and as they progress they interrupt peritoneal lymphatics and weep exudative fluid from their surface. This results in the notorious ascites, which is often the dominant source of morbidity. MPM may infrequently extend into the chest; when it does, it is a late finding. Although MPM may metastasize to abdominal and pelvic lymph nodes, distant metastasis is uncommon. There is no uniformly accepted staging system for MPM, and untreated patients usually succumb in less than 12 mo.

Although core needle biopsy may occasionally result in a diagnosis, it should be avoided if possible, owing to the routine inadequacy of the specimen and the propensity for this tumor to seed needle tracts or trocar sites (1). Most cases require open biopsy. It is imperative that an ample amount of nonfrozen tissue be sent for permanent sectioning, because freezing of a specimen may alter its immunophenotype and subsequently preclude diagnosis (22). It is also important to include a rim of normal tissue so the absence, presence, and extent of invasion can be defined. True stromal invasion is the single most important parameter that allows the distinction between benign mesothelial proliferations and MPM (Fig. 1) (23). A finding of diffuse involvement or omental caking would leave most oncologists uncomfortable with a benign diagnosis, and further diagnostic tests may be performed.

4.2. Histology

MPM is most commonly divided into three histologic subtypes: epithelial, biphasic, and sarcomatoid. Biphasic mesothelioma is defined as a specimen that has both epithelial and sarcomatous components, each contributing more than 10% to the overall histology. Studies have looked at large series of specimens and determined that 62 to 76% were

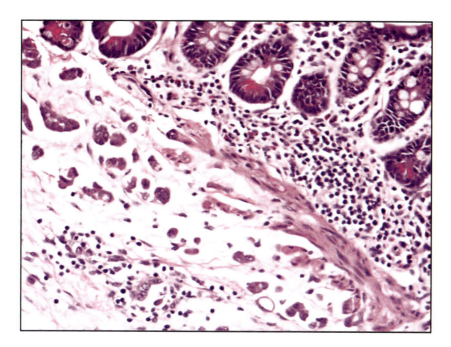

Fig. 1. Stromal invasion by a malignant peritoneal mesothelioma (H&E, original magnification ×400).

epithelial, 22 to 27% biphasic, and 2 to 11% sarcomatoid *(24,25)*. These three subtypes encompass further delineated subgroups, which include tubulopapillary/papillary, adenomatoid, and desmoplastic mesothelioma. Figure 2 shows examples of common histologies. Multicystic and well-differentiated papillary mesotheliomas are not considered to be malignant.

Papillary serous carcinoma is a primary neoplasm of the peritoneum but is not likely of mesothelial origin. It is not entirely understood but can most rationally be described as a tumor that arises from ovarian epithelial rests that are remnants of the ovary's descent into the pelvis. Any of the pelvic adnexa may, in fact, be a source of these cells; however, the mesothelial lining as a source remains an unlikely candidate. These tumors are histologically, immunophenotypically, and clinically distinct from mesothelioma, but they are similar to epithelial carcinomas of the ovary (Table 1).

The sarcomatoid subtype of MPM conveys a survival disadvantage. Sugarbaker et al. *(1)* showed that a combined papillary and epithelial subgroup had a median survival of 55 mo compared with a combined sarcomatoid and biphasic subgroup, which had a median survival of 13 mo ($p = 0.002$). The study involved a regional treatment of all patients ($n = 68$) on a clinical protocol *(1)*. Additionally, Feldman et al. *(2)* published findings on 49 patients receiving similar therapy. This cohort was divided into four histologic types subsequently separated into two grades, adenomatoid/tubulopapillary (low grade) and epithelioid/sarcomatoid (high grade). This analysis showed that low-grade lesions had a progression-free ($p = 0.039$) and overall survival benefit ($p = 0.041$) *(2)*. These two studies show that not only does a sarcomatous component affect survival untowardly but that the papillary and adenomatoid subgroup is independently favorable.

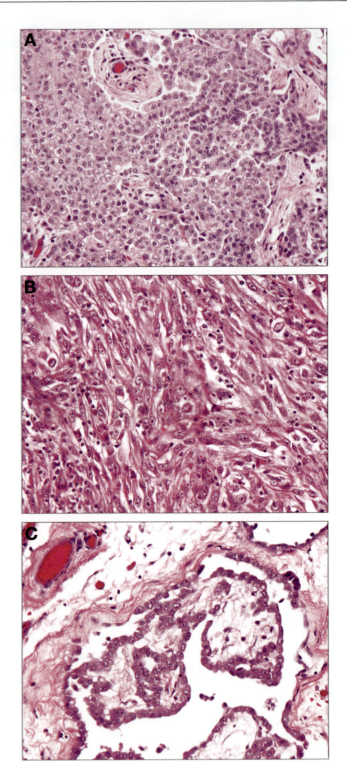

Fig. 2. (**A**) Epithelioid, (**B**) sarcomatoid, and (**C**) tubulopapillary subtypes of peritoneal mesothelioma (H&E, original magnification ×400).

Table 1
Immunohistochemistry[a]

	Mesothelioma (%)	Nonovarian/ nonrenal adenocarcinoma (%)	Serous carcinoma of the peritoneum (%)
Positive markers			
Thrombomodulin	49–100	6–77	2–35
Cytokeratin 5/6	53–100	0–7	5–33
Calretinin	42–100	0–10	0–10
WT-1	72–100	0–25	83–86
EMA	73–100	25–83	100
Negative markers			
MOC-31	0–50	58–100	62–96
B72.3	2–48	81	72–100
Ber-EP4	0–26	85–100	87–100
CA19–9	0–33	100	66
S-100	2–11	31	31–100
BG8	0–23	93–100	87
E-Cadherin	0–50	83–100	90
CEA	0–10	90–100	13–26
Leu-M1 (CD15)	0–6	58–100	30–80
Vimentin	26–40	16–40	33
c-KIT	0	NA	52

[a] Percentages represent percentage of reactive specimens in referenced literature. NA, not available. Data from refs. *1, 30, 31*, and *46–52*.

4.3. Pathologic Diagnosis

The first challenge of tissue analysis lies in the distinction between benign and malignant specimens. Cytologic fluid analysis has virtually no utility in the diagnosis of this disease. It has a low yield and does not allow for visualization of invasion. Histologic evidence of true invasion is the defining parameter in the diagnosis of malignant or benign lesions. Several issues complicate this distinction. First, mesothelial cells are frequently subject to entrapment in adhesions, fat lobules, and inflammatory tissue. This phenomenon may falsely lead one to a conclusion of invasion. Pelvic adnexae are notorious for granulomatous and adhesive mesothelial entrapment, owing to the intense inflammatory conditions frequently found. Also, cells in ascites or local effusions can sediment onto a mesothelial surface that biopsied, resembles a mesothelial proliferation that has subserosal invasion *(23)*. Atypia and necrosis are more common in malignant tumors but are not sensitive or specific in making the distinction between benign and malignant mesothelium *(22)*. The difficulty in this determination was shown after the U.S.-Canadian Mesothelioma Reference Panel reviewed 217 cases. There was virtually total agreement on mesothelial origin but disagreement regarding malignancy in 22% of the cases *(23)*. Recently, immunohistochemical labeling of telomerase has been shown to differentiate benign from malignant mesothelium. This pattern of expression is promising and is still under evaluation *(26–28)*.

Histochemistry is useful in differentiating MPM from other surface malignancies. MPM produces large amounts of hyaluronic acid, in contrast to adenocarcinomas. This distinction is easily made with the use of colloidal iron or alcian blue and hyaluronidase. Another differentiating feature is the presence or absence of neutral mucins. The determination is performed with periodic acid Schiff (PAS) stain and diastase. MPM is invariably devoid of neutral mucin *(22,24,29)*.

Most pathologists regard immunohistochemistry (IHC) as the most important ancillary technique in differentiating MPM from other cancers. Unfortunately, there is no one marker that confirms the diagnosis. Panels of antibodies must be used to achieve a confident diagnosis. Recommendations are limited by the fact that antibodies from different proprietors have different sensitivities to a given marker *(30)*. Additionally, a narrow- or broad-spectrum antibody against the same marker may create different immunophenotypes for similar tissues. Regardless of the hurdles, most MPM is identifiable. Each lab must evaluate its own panel of markers to determine relative sensitivities. Table 1 shows the published percent of cases that are reactive for markers, given various tumor types. It is important to consider that some of these studies are not specific for the site of primary mesothelioma.

Markers are divided into positive and negative categories depending on the predominant reactivity for mesothelioma. Generally speaking, cytokeratin 5/6, calretinin, and WT-1 are the most useful positive markers, whereas CEA, Ber-EP4, LeuM1, and BG8 tend to be the most useful negative markers. When mesothelioma is extremely dedifferentiated or if it is a desmoplastic variant, ultrastructural analysis via electron microscopy may be beneficial, although rarely indicated.

It has been traditionally accepted that there is no significant difference in the immunophenotype of pleural and peritoneal mesothelioma. However, after analysis of 24 peritoneal and 9 pleural cases, immunohistochemical reactivity for epidermal growth factor receptor (EGFR) was found in 92% of peritoneal and 33% of pleural mesotheliomas ($P = 0.0004$) *(31)*. This is a lower expression of EGFR by pleural mesothelioma than previously described *(32)*. Confirmatory studies still need to be completed.

5. CLINICAL PRESENTATION

MPM has no sign or symptom that is specific for its diagnosis. Instead, its manifestations are related to ascites or large tumor burden. Some patients are diagnosed incidentally, after inquiry into an unrelated process such as infertility. Studies have estimated the median age of presentation to be between 40 and 65 *(33)*. Unfortunately, owing to the indolent progression of nonspecific symptoms, many patients present with advanced disease.

Abdominal distension is the most frequent initial symptom. It commonly begets early satiety, dysphagia, and shortness of breath, which contribute to weight loss and overall inanition. Abdominal distension may also manifest as a new or worsening abdominal wall hernia, whose repair may lead to the coincidental diagnosis of mesothelioma. Increased abdominal girth is the presenting symptom in 56 to 82% of patients *(1,34)*. Increased girth does not portend a poor prognosis; however, weight loss independently may be a poor prognostic sign *(1)*. Pain is the second most common initial symptom, found in 27 to 58% of patients *(1,34–36)*. Most patients who present describe a diffuse nonspecific pain, although a small minority may present with an acute abdomen. In patients who present acutely, mesothelioma is usually a secondary finding in the setting of an alternate source of pain, such as appendicitis, cholecystitis, peptic ulcer disease, and so on. Mesothelioma can also cause intermittent intestinal obstruction, which can present as intestinal colic. Additionally, up to a third of patients present after palpable discovery of an abdominal mass (35,37).

The initial physical exam is not specific for the diagnosis, although there is a tendency for common findings among patients. Abdominal distension with weight loss is relatively common at presentation and although not specific to mesothelioma should raise suspicion of malignancy. Although not specific to mesothelioma, the combination of these signs is relatively common at presentation. Shifting dullness is a known finding of ascites and may also be present. Inguinal adenopathy and the presence of an abdominal mass may present on initial exam, but not in most cases.

Serum chemistries and markers have no value in establishing a diagnosis. The literature has also failed to show their benefit in following disease status. Hyaluronan, CA-125, α-fetoprotein (AFP), carcinoembiyonic antigen (CEA), and tissue polypeptide antigen (TPA) have been evaluated, and although some patients have elevated levels concordant with disease progression, sensitivities and specificities remain low (34,38–40). Unfortunately, these conclusions likely are a result of underpowered evaluations rather than lack of utility. A significant group of our patients have increasing or decreasing levels of CA-125 associated with progression or regression of clinical tumor burden. This association can only be validated if the patients have levels drawn at multiple evaluation time points. In the subgroup that shows correlation, the CA-125 level is an important tool for patient surveillance.

Patients typically undergo a range of radiologic studies during the workup of their signs and symptoms. Unfortunately, there are no radiographic studies that yield pathognomic information. Instead, there is usually vague evidence of a surface malignancy from an unknown primary site. Evidence of a surface malignancy in the absence of hepatic metastasis may suggest mesothelioma. The most common radiographic finding is ascites. It is found with imaging in 60 to 100% of presenting patients (34,41). Both abdominal CT and ultrasound demonstrate sensitivity in detecting ascites. Other frequent findings are omental caking/thickening, peritoneal changes, liver scalloping, diaphragm involvement, foreshortening of the mesentery, and/or bowel wall thickening (Fig. 3). Table 2 shows published frequencies of positive CT findings.

6. MANAGEMENT

6.1. Basis for Treatment Approach

Until recently, there has been no uniform consensus on the treatment of MPM. Various treatment modalities have been applied, but owing to the rarity of the disease, most accounts are anecdotal. To dilute the experience even further, some of the reports are not specific for peritoneal primary disease. Although this is not as much a consideration with regard to the data that inform pathologic diagnosis, pleural and peritoneal mesotheliomas are entirely different management entities. The disparity in management is largely a result of the different anatomic considerations that may or may not permit various regional therapies. Additionally, survival data used to evaluate the treatment modalities may partially reflect manifestation differences between peritoneal and pleural disease sites.

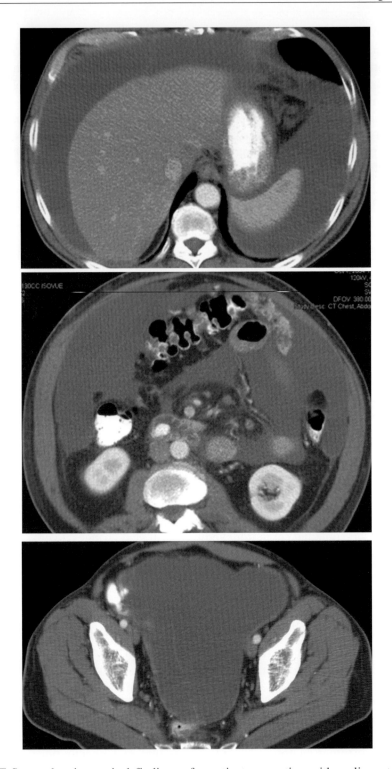

Fig. 3. CT Scans showing typical findings of a patient presenting with malignant peritoneal mesothelioma. (**A**) Medial displacement of the liver. (**C**) Compression of the rectosigmoid in the pelvis. (**B**) Diffuse ascites and shortened mesentery owing to malignant infiltration of tissues.

Table 2
Abdominal CT

Initial CT findings	Frequency (%)
Ascites	60–100
Omental involvement	66–91
Peritoneal changes	73–88
Diaphragm or liver surface involvement	77–82
Small bowel or mesentery involvement	60–82
Pleural changes[a]	23–80
Pleural effusion[a]	17–20
Abdominal adenopathy	12–27
Discrete masses	12–20

[a] Some studies additionally used plain radiographs for interpretation.
Data from refs. *34*, *41–43*, and *45*.

Systemic chemotherapy has not had great efficacy in patients with MPM. Antman et al. *(42)* reported results in 23 patients. Unfortunately, this was a small series whose subjects received a heterogeneous group of treatments that included multiple types and regimens of systemic chemotherapy, surgical cytoreduction, and/or external beam radiation *(42)*. Three of the eight patients who survived longer than 12 mo from diagnosis received chemotherapy alone. The series was the only real tabulated experience as of 1983 and remained the basis for treatment by oncologists for over a decade. Other small series evaluating systemic chemotherapy followed, and all failed to show a plausible utility *(43)*.

The overwhelming majority of patients with MPM ultimately succumb to complications related to tumor progression in the peritoneal cavity. It is, therefore, intuitive sense that an effective regional therapy would translate into a survival advantage. The most favorable and sound survival data to date have arisen from aggressive surgical cytoreduction (tumor debulking) followed by immediate continuous hyperthermic intraperitoneal chemotherapy (CHPP). Median overall survival with this treatment is reported to be 56 to 92 mo from the time of therapy. The data have proved reproducible and form the basis of present-day management.

6.2. Operative Screening

Owing to the low incidence of MPM, this unique population should be managed at an institution that has experience with CHPP and that is actively collecting data. A careful patient selection process and a consistent treatment regimen are important considerations in gauging outcome. To optimize outcomes, preoperative and intraoperative patient stratification remains crucial. Feldman et al. *(2)* did an analysis of factors associated with outcomes in 49 patients with MPM undergoing CHPP. They showed survival data that significantly identified several prognostically important parameters. Cox model analysis additionally showed that deep invasion and age greater than 60 yr were independent factors associated with shortened survival. Patients who had a history of a prior debulking procedure also had a progression-free and overall survival advantage. This finding may be a result of selection bias but more likely reflects the indolent biology of tumor represented in that cohort. Overall, patients with MPM treated with cytoreduction followed by immediate hyperthermic intraperitoneal chemotherapy (cisplatin) had a median progression-free and overall survival of 17 and 92 mo, respectively. Acherman and coworkers reviewed prognostic parameters in 51 patients receiving similar therapy *(44)*. Their experience yielded an overall median survival of 56 mo. They identified initial weight loss and male gender to be negative prognostic variables.

Histology, invasion depth, age, weight loss, and, potentially, gender may be important for stratifying patients into groups that are more or less likely to benefit from surgical therapy. Because completeness of cytoreduction is associated with better outcome, patient selection is an important consideration. Yan et al. evaluated the preoperative CT scan of 30 patients with MPM *(45)*. They reviewed 39 radiographic parameters and their association to completeness of resection. Presence of a lesion >5 cm in the epigastric region and loss of intestinal or mesenteric architecture were both independent predictors of inadequate surgical cytoreduction. No patients in the study were adequately resected if both parameters were present. Additionally, the absence of both parameters was associated with a 94% chance of adequate cytoreduction. In addition to radiographic criteria, surgical experience with cytoreduction and peritonectomy procedures is also an important factor.

Procedures left to the surgeon's discretion are numerous and include splenectomy, small and large bowel resections, enterostomy creation, diaphragm resection with primary or prosthetic repair, hysterectomy, salpingectomy, oopherectomy, and gastrectomy. The procedure is associated with an operative mortality of 3 to 5% and a reported morbidity of 23 to 25%. Published findings in 48 patients defined the most frequent perioperative complications to be wound infection (6%), fascial dehiscence (4%), pleural effusion (4%), prolonged ileus (4%), and catheter sepsis (4%) *(2)*. Additional complications with lower incidence include the development of enterocutaneous fistula, small bowel obstruction, pneumothorax, prolonged mechanical ventilation, acute renal failure, hematologic toxicity, pancreatitis, and abdominal wall herniation.

There has been investigation into delayed intraperitoneal chemotherapy. This treatment is administered through an indwelling intraperitoneal Tenckhoff catheter that is placed at the time of surgical cytoreduction. A chemotherapeutic agent is typically infused within the first 2 postoperative weeks and has been associated with hematologic toxicity in the form of cytopenia. This maneuver has not been shown to be of any definitive benefit and is still considered investigational.

6.3. Operative Management

Preoperatively, the patient undergoes standard bowel preparation and is kept on deep venous thrombosis prophylaxis. At operation, the abdomen is systematically inspected for extent and distribution of tumor burden. This includes appreciation of all four quadrants and the pelvis. It is important to note that each patient and tumor distribution will differ markedly, and this description of techniques is a general guideline, meant to convey the diversity of procedures that this population requires. The sequence and content of procedures may be different depending on the individual needs of the patient.

The greater omentum is usually a site of bulky disease. An omentectomy should be done to facilitate access to other areas of the abdomen. The supra- and subpyloric regions may then be debulked with electrocautery and blunt dissection, and distal gastrectomy

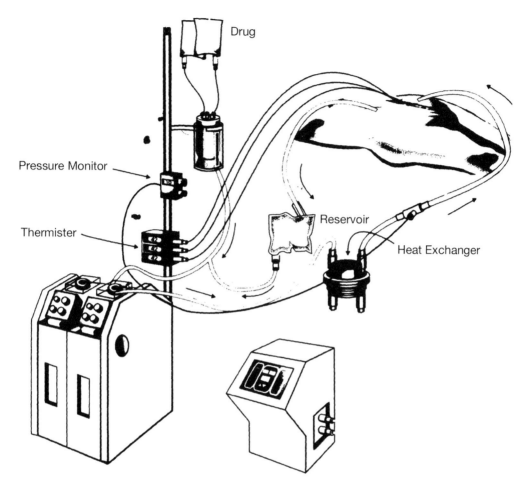

Fig. 4. Schema of perfusion circuit showing the catheters positioned in the abdomen, the reservoir, the roller pump, and the heat exchanger.

may be performed in some cases. Systematic peritoneal stripping is used to extirpate parietal peritoneal disease. The small bowel and mesenteric implants are treated with ball cautery of surface lesions. Circumferential or deeply invasive disease should be resected if possible, as they remain high-risk sites of mechanical obstruction. It is imperative that the anatomy be defined as the surgeon proceeds into the pelvis. The ureters can be obscured by tumor-laden peritoneum and are prone to iatrogenic injury. The dependency of the cul de sac of Douglas makes it an inevitable site for tumor implantation. Depending on the tumor burden of the female genital system, a total abdominal hysterectomy with bilateral salpingo-oophorectomy should be considered. If the rectosigmoid colon is circumferentially involved, a low anterior resection may be performed and protected by a loop ileostomy.

After the debulking is complete, the perfusion catheters are placed. Large-bore inflow and outflow catheters are placed; the inflow catheter is positioned over the dome of the liver and the outflow catheter is placed in the pelvis (Fig. 4). Subperitoneal temperature probes are placed on both sides of the abdomen and in the pelvis. The abdominal fascia

Table 3
Clinical and Pathology Characteristics
in Patients with Malignant and Peritoneal Mesothelioma

Characteristic	No. of patients	%
Total number	49	
Sex		
Women	21	
Men	28	
Age (yr)		
Range	16–76	
Mean	49	
Median	47	
Prior chemotherapy		
None	41	84
Paclitaxel and cisplatin	8	16
Prior surgery		
Exp lap and LOA	18	37
Tumor debulking and/or organ resection	7	14
None	24	49
Histologic type[a]		
High grade	30	64
Epithelioid	26	
Sarcomatoid	4	
Low grade	17	36
Tubulopapillary	16	
Adenomatoid	1	

Abbreviations: Exp lap, exploratory laparotomy; LOA, lysis of adhesions.
[a] Sufficient tissue for detailed histologic analysis was available in 47 patients.

is closed with a running, water-tight, full-thickness suture. The inflow and outflow catheters are connected to and complete a circuit that has a roller pump, reservoir, and heat exchanger in-line. The circuit is turned on and a perfusate of 0.9% sodium chloride at a flow rate of 1.5 L/min is used to warm the abdomen to 41 to 43°C. The high flow rate is necessary to generate hyperthermic temperatures within the peritoneal tissues. The total volume of perfusate may range from 4 to 6 L. The chemotherapeutic agent being used is then added to the circuit. To optimize the distribution of perfusate and disrupt the tendencies of laminar flow, the abdomen is manually agitated for the entire 90 min of perfusion. The abdomen is then drained of all perfusate, and the midline incision is reopened, followed by removal of the perfusion catheters. Inspection of the abdomen and pelvis is again performed, and the laparotomy is closed in the usual fashion.

7. OUTCOMES OF THE NCI EXPERIENCE

At the National Institutes of Health, National Cancer Institute, Surgery Branch, we have a phase II treatment protocol available for patients with MPM. The treatment includes a best effort surgical debulking (cytoreduction), followed by a hyperthermic peritoneal perfusion with cisplatin. After surgical recovery, the patient receives an adjunct dose of paclitaxel and 5-FU through an indwelling intraperitoneal catheter, usually placed

Table 4
Operative and Perfusion Data

	No. of patients	%
Operative procedure		
Exp lap and LOA	10	17
Cytoreduction and omentectomy	25	51
Cytoreduction and organ resection	14	29
Cisplatin dose (mg)		
Mean	450	
Range	330–816	
Operative time (h)		
Mean	6.5	
Range	4–11.3	
Peritoneal temperature (°C)		
Mean	41	
Range	38.3–43	
Perfusion flow rate (mL/min)		
Mean	1500	
Range	1000–2000	
Residual disease status		
RD 0: complete debulking	7	14
RD 1: <100 lesions, all <5 mm	16	33
RD 2: >100 lesions or any >5 mm	20	41
RD 3: any lesion size >1 cm	6	12
Postoperative intraperitoneal dwell	35	72
No dwell	14	28
Dwell regimen (mg)		
5-Fluorouracil		
Mean dose	1,425	
Range	1038–2100	
Paclitaxel		
Mean dose	208	
Range	98–300	
Follow-up time (mo)		
Mean	36	
Range	2–93+	
Potential follow-up time (mo)		
Mean	28.3	
Range	1–106	

Abbreviations: Exp lap, exploratory laparotomy; LOA, lysis of adhesions.

at the time of perfusion. We have published our experience based on the first 49 patients and describe here a summary of our findings (2).

Patient characteristics are shown in Table 3. It is worth noting that 16% of the study subjects had had prior chemotherapy and 51% had had prior laparotomy; this includes 14% who underwent some form of previous surgical debulking. Almost two-thirds of those on the protocol had high-grade histology. A subsequent analysis of the operative data (Table 4) showed the rate of complete resection to be around

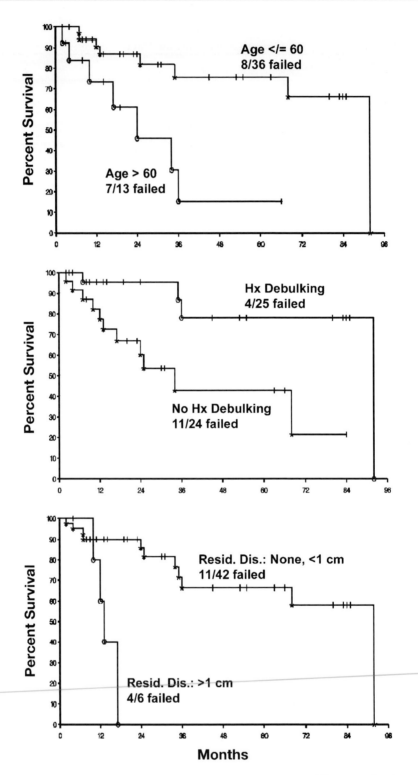

Fig. 5. Effects of (**A**) age, (**B**) history (Hx) of previous debulking, and (**C**) status of residual disease (resid. dis.) after surgical cytoreduction on overall survival after treatment.

Pre-CHPP

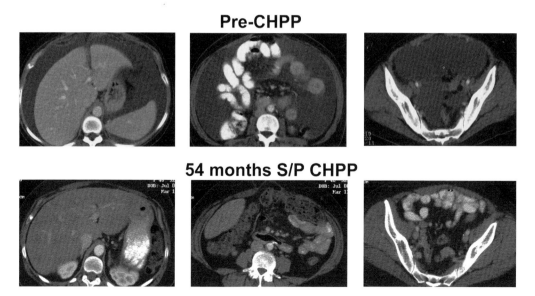

54 months S/P CHPP

Fig. 6. Pretreatment and 54-mo post-treatment (surgical cytoreduction and hyperthermic intraperitoneal chemotherapy [CHPP]) CT scans of a patient who presented with symptomatic malignant ascites secondary to mesothelioma.

14%. Additionally, postoperative intraperitoneal dwell chemotherapy was given to 72% of the cohort.

Overall, there were 18 complications in 12 patients, a surgical complications rate of about 25%. Operative morbidity was dominated by wound complications. Significant chemotherapy-related abnormalities were not typical. There were perturbations in serologic liver, renal, and hematologic tests, but none translated into clinical consequence.

At a median potential follow-up of 28.3 mo, the progression-free survival (PFS) and overall survival (OS) were 17 and 92 mo, respectively (Figs. 5 and 6). Of the 26 patients who suffered from symptomatic ascites preoperatively, 15 had complete resolution, for an actuarially determined median interval of 25.3 mo. It is also worth noting that 11 of the 15 were not completely resected. This implies that the perfusion component of therapy may independently have palliative benefit.

A search for adverse prognostic variables was performed with univariate analysis and Cox regression (Table 5). The results showed that a lack of prior debulking and the presence of deep invasion indicate poorer PFS and OS. The analysis also showed that age greater than 60 yr and inability to undergo complete resection convey adverse prognostic value to OS.

8. CONCLUSIONS

MPM is a rare condition with morbidity and mortality that result from disease progression within the abdominal cavity. Certain clinical and pathological parameters appear to be associated with aggressive or indolent tumor biology. There is currently considerable interest in regional therapeutic approaches, the most common being a combined modality

Table 5
Adverse Prognostic Significance of
Clinicopathologic Variables Based on Cox Proportional Hazards Model Alanysis

End point	Variable (in terms of poor prognosis)	Parameter estimate	SE	p	Hazard ratio	95% Cl
PFS	No previous debulking vs debulking	1.55	0.43	0.0003	4.7	2.02–10.9
	Deep invasion vs no deep invasion	1.28	0.44	0.003	3.6	1.53–8.48
OS	Age >60 vs ≤60 years	1.29	0.61	0.034	3.65	1.10–12.1
	No previous debulking vs debuling	1.67	0.8	0.036	5.33	1.12–25.4
	Deep invasion vs no deep invasion	1.44	0.71	0.041	4.24	1.06–16.9
	Residual disease >1 cm vs none <1 cm	1.75	0.82	0.032	5.76	1.16–28.5

Abbreviations: PFS, progression-free survival; OS, overall survival.

approach using operative tumor cytoreduction and intraoperative hyperthermic chemotherapy. Several centers have reported durable progression-free and overall survival in selected patients undergoing this treatment. Nevertheless, recurrence and eventual disease progression are the rule, and ongoing efforts to understand the molecular biology of the disease and identify new targets for intervention will be necessary to move toward a cure for this condition.

ACKNOWLEDGEMENTS

This research was supported in part by the Intramural Research Program of the NIH, National Cancer Institute, Center for Cancer Research.

REFERENCES

1. Sugarbaker PH, Welch LS, Mohamed F, Glehen O. A review of peritoneal mesothelioma at the Washington Cancer Institute. Surg Oncol Clin North Am 2003;12:605–621, xi.
2. Feldman AL, Libutti SK, Pingpank JF, et al. Analysis of factors associated with outcome in patients with malignant peritoneal mesothelioma undergoing surgical debulking and intraperitoneal chemotherapy. J Clin Oncol 2003;21:4560–4567.
3. Cancer Surveillance. 2005. Ref Type: Internet Communication
4. Antman K, Shemin R, Ryan L, et al. Malignant mesothelioma: prognostic variables in a registry of 180 patients, the Dana Farber Cancer Institute and Brigham and Women's Hospital experience over two decades, 1965–1985. J Clin Oncol 1988;6:147–153.
5. SEER. Cancer Statistics Review—Mesothelioma fast stats. 2005.
6. Weill H, Hughes JM, Churg AM. Changing trends in US mesothelioma incidence. Occup Environ Med 2004;61:438–441.
7. Zellos L, Christiani DC. Epidemiology, biologic behavior, and natural history of mesothelioma. Thorac Surg Clin 2004;14:469–77, viii.
8. Landrigan PJ. Asbestos—still a carcinogen. N Engl J Med 1998;338:1618–1619.
9. Hodgson JT, Darnton A. The quantitative risks of mesothelioma and lung cancer in relation to asbestos exposure. Ann Occup Hyg 2000;44:565–601.
10. Camus M, Siemiatycki J, Meek B. Nonoccupational exposure to chrysotile asbestos and the risk of lung cancer. N Engl J Med 1998;338:1565–1571.
11. McDonald AD, McDonald JC. Malignant mesothelioma in North America. Cancer 1980;46:1650–1656.
12. Simian Virus 40 (SV 40), Polio Vaccine, and Cancer. 5 A.D.

13. Carbone M, Kratzke RA, Testa JR. The pathogenesis of mesothelioma. Semin Oncol 2002;29:2–17.
14. Carbone M, Pass HI, Miele L, Bocchetta M. New developments about the association of SV40 with human mesothelioma. Oncogene 2003;22:5173–5180.
15. Foddis R, De Rienzo A, Broccoli D, et al. SV40 infection induces telomerase activity in human mesothelial cells. Oncogene 2002;21:1434–1442.
16. Roushdy-Hammady I, Siegel J, Emri S, Testa JR, Carbone M. Genetic-susceptibility factor and malignant mesothelioma in the Cappadocian region of Turkey. Lancet 2001;357:444–445.
17. Austin MB, Fechner RE, Roggli VL. Pleural malignant mesothelioma following Wilms' tumor. Am J Clin Pathol 1986;86:227–230.
18. Sanders CL, Jackson TA. Induction of mesotheliomas and sarcomas from "hot spots" of 239 PuO 2 activity. Health Phys 1972;22:755–759.
19. Powell JE, Stevens MC, Stiller CA. Clustering of childhood peritoneal mesothelioma in the Midlands, UK. Lancet 1995;345:66–67.
20. Kelsey A. Mesothelioma in childhood. Pediatr Hematol Oncol 1994;11:461–462.
21. Niggli FK, Gray TJ, Raafat F, Stevens MC. Spectrum of peritoneal mesothelioma in childhood: clinical and histopathologic features, including DNA cytometry. Pediatr Hematol Oncol 1994;11:399–408.
22. Corson JM. Pathology of mesothelioma. Thorac Surg Clin 2004;14:447–460.
23. Churg A, Colby TV, Cagle P, et al. The separation of benign and malignant mesothelial proliferations. Am J Surg Pathol 2000;24:1183–1200.
24. Suzuki Y. Diagnostic criteria for human diffuse malignant mesothelioma. Acta Pathol Jpn 1992;42:767–786.
25. Kannerstein M, Churg J. Peritoneal mesothelioma. Hum Pathol 1977;8:83–94.
26. Dhaene K, Hubner R, Kumar-Singh S, Weyn B, Van Marck E. Telomerase activity in human pleural mesothelioma. Thorax 1998;53:915–918.
27. Dhaene K, Wauters J, Weyn B, Timmermans JP, Van Marck E. Expression profile of telomerase subunits in human pleural mesothelioma. J Pathol 2000;190:80–85.
28. Kumaki F, Kawai T, Churg A, et al. Expression of telomerase reverse transcriptase (TERT) in malignant mesotheliomas. Am J Surg Pathol 2002;26:365–370.
29. Rosai J. Rosai and Ackerman'sSurgical Pathology. 9th ed. Edinburgh-London-New York: Mosby-Elsevier; 2004.
30. Ordonez NG. Value of calretinin immunostaining in differentiating epithelial mesothelioma from lung adenocarcinoma. Mod Pathol 1998;11:929–933.
31. Trupiano JK, Geisinger KR, Willingham MC, et al. Diffuse malignant mesothelioma of the peritoneum and pleura, analysis of markers. Mod Pathol 2004;17:476–481.
32. Dazzi H, Hasleton PS, Thatcher N, Wilkes S, Swindell R, Chatterjee AK. Malignant pleural mesothelioma and epidermal growth factor receptor (EGF-R). Relationship of EGF-R with histology and survival using fixed paraffin embedded tissue and the F4, monoclonal antibody. Br J Cancer 1990;61:924–926.
33. Averbach AM, Sugarbaker PH. Peritoneal mesothelioma: treatment approach based on natural history. Cancer Treat Res 1996;81:193–211.
34. Kebapci M, Vardareli E, Adapinar B, Acikalin M. CT findings and serum CA 125 levels in malignant peritoneal mesothelioma: report of 11 new cases and review of the literature. Eur Radiol 2003;13:2620–2626.
35. Antman KH. Clinical presentation and natural history of benign and malignant mesothelioma. Semin Oncol 1981;8:313–320.
36. van Gelder T, Hoogsteden HC, Versnel MA, de Beer P, Vandenbroucke JP, Planteydt HT. Malignant peritoneal mesothelioma: a series of 19 cases. Digestion 1989;43:222–227.
37. Antman KH, Blum RH, Greenberger JS, Flowerdew G, Skarin AT, Canellos GP. Multimodality therapy for malignant mesothelioma based on a study of natural history. Am J Med 1980;68:356–362.
38. Hedman M, Arnberg H, Wernlund J, Riska H, Brodin O. Tissue polypeptide antigen (TPA), hyaluronan and CA 125 as serum markers in malignant mesothelioma. Anticancer Res 2003;23:531–536.
39. Dahl IM, Solheim OP, Erikstein B, Muller E. A longitudinal study of the hyaluronan level in the serum of patients with malignant mesothelioma under treatment. Hyaluronan as an indicator of progressive disease. Cancer 1989;64:68–73.
40. Frebourg T, Lerebours G, Delpech B, et al. Serum hyaluronate in malignant pleural mesothelioma. Cancer 1987;59:2104–2107.

41. Ros PR, Yuschok TJ, Buck JL, Shekitka KM, Kaude JV. Peritoneal mesothelioma. Radiologic appearances correlated with histology. Acta Radiol 1991;32:355–358.
42. Antman K, Pomfret F, Aisner J, et al. Peritoneal mesothelioma: natural history and response to chemotherapy. J Clin Oncol 1983;1:386.
43. Plaus WJ. Peritoneal mesothelioma. Arch Surg 1988;123:763–766.
44. Acherman YI, Welch LS, Bromley CM, Sugarbaker PH. Clinical presentation of peritoneal mesothelioma. Tumori 2003;89:269–273.
45. Yan TD, Haveric N, Carmignani CP, Chang D, Sugarbaker PH. Abdominal computed tomography scans in the selection of patients with malignant peritoneal mesothelioma for comprehensive treatment with cytoreductive surgery and perioperative intraperitoneal chemotherapy. Cancer 2005;103: 839–849.
46. Ordonez NG. Role of immunohistochemistry in distinguishing epithelial peritoneal mesotheliomas from peritoneal and ovarian serous cacinomas. Am J Surg Pathol 1998;22:1203–1214.
47. Ordonez NG. The immunohistochemical diagnosis of epithelial mesothelioma. Hum Pathol 1999;30:313–323.
48. Roberts F, Harper CM, Downie I, Burnett RA. Immunohistochemical analysis still has a limited role in the diagnosis of malignant mesothelioma. A study of thirteen antibodies. Am J Clin Pathol 2001;116:253–262.
49. Attanoos RL, Webb R, Dojcinov SD, Gibbs AR. Value of mesothelial and epithelial antibodies in distinguishing diffuse peritoneal mesothelioma in females from serous papillary carcinoma of the ovary and peritoneum. Histopathology 2002;40:237–244.
50. Ordonez NG. Value of thyroid transcription factor-1, E-cadherin, BG8, WT1, and CD44S immunostaining in distinguishing epithelial pleural mesothelioma from pulmonary and nonpulmonary adenocarcinoma. Am J Surg Pathol 2000;24:598–606.
51. Politi E, Kandaraki C, Apostolopoulou C, Kyritsi T, Koutselini H. Immunocytochemical panel for distinguishing between carcinoma and reactive mesothelial cells in body cavity fluids. Diagn Cytopathol 2005;32:151–155.
52. Ruan Q, Hu Y. Immunophenotypings of malignant epithelial mesothelioma and their roles in the differential diagnosis. J Huazhong Univ Sci Techn Med Sci 2004;24:112–115.

17 Regional Therapy of Pancreatic Cancer

Hiroshi Yoshida, MD, Yasuhiro Mamada, MD, Nobuhiko Taniai, MD, Yoshiaki Mizuguchi, MD, Tetsuya Shimizu, MD, Yoshiharu Nakamura, MD, Takayuki Aimoto, MD, Eiji Uchida, MD, and Takashi Tajiri, MD

CONTENTS

SUMMARY

Pancreatic cancer is a major cause of cancer death. Despite impressive advances in early hospital mortality and morbidity rates, overall, the chance of long-term survival is extremely low. Surgical treatment is currently the only potentially curative strategy for pancreatic cancer, but surgery alone cannot guarantee a cure. Regional therapy, such as regional chemotherapy or radiation, has been widely used in patients with advanced pancreatic cancer, with some success in controlling the cancer locally. The rationale for regional chemotherapy of pancreatic cancer is to enhance cellular drug uptake. There are various techniques of regional therapy, such as chemoembolization, arterial or portal venous infusion, hyperthermia, radiation, and gene therapy. This article reviews English reports of regional therapy for pancreatic cancer cited in the Medline database of Pubmed up to July 2005.

Key Words: Regional therapy; pancreatic cancer; celiac trunk infusion; hypoxic abdominal perfusion; radiation; hyperthermia.

From: *Cancer Drug Discovery and Development: Regional Cancer Therapy*
Edited by: P. M. Schlag and U. S. Stein © Humana Press Inc., Totowa, NJ

1. INTRODUCTION

Pancreatic cancer is a major cause of cancer death. Despite impressive advances in early hospital mortality and morbidity rates, overall, the chance of long-term survival is extremely low. Surgical treatment is currently the only potentially curative strategy for pancreatic cancer, but surgery alone cannot guarantee a cure. Regional therapy, such as regional chemotherapy or radiation, has been widely used in patients with advanced pancreatic cancer, with some success in controlling the cancer locally. The rationale for regional chemotherapy of pancreatic cancer is to enhance cellular drug uptake. It is of key importance in chemotherapy to apply a high enough concentration of the drug to the tumor locally to overcome drug resistance, without increasing systemic toxicity at the same time. Studies suggest that intraarterial infusion (regional chemotherapy) will avoid the first-pass effect of chemotherapy and direct a higher concentration of the drug locally to the tumor cell membrane.

This article reviews English reports of regional therapy for pancreatic cancer cited in the Medline database of Pubmed up to July 2005.

2. TECHNIQUES OF REGIONAL CHEMOTHERAPY

2.1. Antitumor Agents

Chemotherapy is a therapeutic modality for the neoadjuvant or adjuvant treatment of operable pancreatic cancer or the treatment of inoperable pancreatic cancer. Various antitumor agents have been used in chemotherapy for the treatment of pancreatic cancer—examples are 5-fluorouracil (5-FU), mitomycin C (MMC), cisplatin, Adriamycin, epirubicin, mitoxantrone, folinic acid, methotrexate, paclitaxel, cytarabin, bromodeoxyuridine, melphalan, streptozotocin, and gemcitabine. Gemcitabine is the most active single agent for pancreatic cancer and is also a potent radiation sensitizer (1).

Lygidakis et al. (2) performed adjuvant regional immunotherapy, with interleukin-2, in patients with pancreatic cancer who had undergone pancreatic resection.

2.1.1. Chemoembolization

Reducing or completely blocking blood flow can increase drug exposure at the tumor site, and thus drug uptake. The regional concentration of the cytostatic drug is inversely related to the regional arterial blood flow, i.e., the lower the blood flow, the higher the regional drug concentration and vice versa (3). In addition, the systemic drug concentration is decreased because of a reduced drug washout from the tumor.

Numerous trials have been performed in an attempt to achieve this, by injecting embolizing agents such as gelatin sponge particles (Gelfoam, Upjohn, Kalamazoo, MI), Lipiodol (Lipiodol Ultrafluide, Laboratoire Guerbet, Aulnay-sous-Bois, France), or degradable starch microspheres (Spherex, Pharmacia, Sweden).

Embolization with Gelfoam results in tumor necrosis and possible increased cytotoxicity of the infused antitumor agent. However, long-lasting or permanent vascular occlusion leads to unacceptable morbidity, jeopardizing repeated applications, especially when this procedure is used for the treatment of pancreatic cancer.

Therefore, a requirement of chemoembolization is that the particles of the embolizing agent should be small enough to lodge in precapillary vessels. This will allow a more homogenous distribution throughout the entire organ. It will also permit repeated application, thanks to blocking of blood flow that is short term and predictable, ensuring that regional adverse effects are minimal. Both Spherex and Lipiodol meet these criteria.

Other trials have been carried out using a transarterial infusion of styrene maleic acid neocarzinostatin ([SMANCS] Yamanouchi Pharmaceutical, Tokyo, Japan) and Lipiodol, which has a characteristic anti–tumor effect on hepatocellular carcinoma *(4–6)*. Neocarzinostatin (NCS) is a proteinaceous antitumor antibiotic (M_r 11,700) obtained from the culture filtrate of *Streptomyces carzinostaticus*. A lipophilic high-molecular-weight derivative of NCS designated as SMANCS was prepared by chemical conjugation of a copolymer of styrene and maleic acid (SMA) and NCS *(7)*. Lipiodol is a lympho-graphic contrast medium and acts as a carrier for SMANCS. When a homogeneous suspension of SMANCS and Lipiodol is administered intraarterially, the Lipiodol blocks blood flow and prolongs drug release.

2.2. Arterial or Portal Venous Infusion

Drugs with a high hepatic first-pass or total body clearance are preferable for use in regional chemotherapy. [0] These drugs have less adverse effects because hepatic metabolism decreases the systemic drug concentration of the infused drugs. If these types of drugs are used during the selective application of antitumor agents to the tumor, high regional drug concentrations can be obtained without the ensuing side effects of a comparable systemic treatment.

Branches of the celiac trunk and the superior mesenteric artery provide the arterial blood supply to the pancreas. In an investigation of the distribution of the pancreatic blood supply, a strictly separated blood supply to the head and the rest of the pancreas was found in 33% of the cases examined. In most cases, anastomosis between the pancreatic head and the rest of the pancreas was discovered *(8,9)*. Celiac trunk infusion allows perfusion of the pancreas and the liver (the most common site of metastasis from pancreatic cancer) with high-dose chemotherapy.

The usual process followed in studies was to insert a catheter into the selected artery either under angiographic guidance or during laparotomy.

For the process that was carried out under angiographic guidance, a catheter was inserted into the femoral artery using the Seldinger technique and advanced into the abdominal aorta. The catheter was placed in the celiac trunk *(10–18)* and connected to the infusion device. It was usually left in this position for the entire cycle of chemotherapy.

Certain studies involved a transcatheter splenic artery embolization followed by placement of the catheter into the splenic artery. In these studies, ^{99m}Tc-MAA-DTPA was then injected into the catheter. In the angiographic image, the body and tail of the pancreas were clearly visible and the spleen was partially visible. Highly concentrated antitumor agents could then be delivered to the unresectable cancer in the body and tail of the pancreas *(19,20)*.

For the process that was carried out during laparotomy, authors reported several different locations for insertion of the chemotherapy catheter: the splenic artery *(21–24)*; both the hepatic artery and the portal vein *(25–27)*; the portal vein *(28)* alone; the superior mesenteric artery through the jejunal arterial branch *(2,23)*; or the gastroduodenal artery *(24)*.

2.2.1. HEMOFILTRATION

In one study, a filtration catheter was inserted into the vena cava to reduce systemic drug exposure during regional intraarterial chemotherapy. The tip of the catheter was

cancer, who had undergone an extended pancreatectomy. The cumulative survival rates after 5 yr were 41% for patients who had undergone adjuvant liver perfusion chemotherapy and 25% for patients who had not.

Nakayama et al. *(28)* performed adjuvant liver perfusion chemotherapy via the portal vein using 5-FU directly after pancreatectomy for advanced pancreatic cancer. The study found that for patients who did not demonstrate intratumoral dihydropyrimidine dehydrogenase (DPD), liver perfusion chemotherapy with 5-FU was an effective adjuvant therapy for pancreatic cancer.

6.3. Other Arterial Infusions

Bayar et al. *(21)* performed regional chemotherapy from the splenic artery in patients with unresectable pancreatic cancer. The median survival was 8 mo.

Ohigashi et al. *(24)* selectively placed catheters into the splenic artery and/or into the gastroduodenal artery during laparotomy. Then 50 to 100 mg of methotrexate mixed with 10 μg of angiotensin-II was infused via the catheters, with the aim of increasing blood flow in the tumor tissue and decreasing blood flow to the nontumor tissues. Simultaneously, a bolus i.v. infusion of 5-FU (500 mg) was given. At 1 d after each chemotherapy, leucovorin (30 mg) was given orally. The median survival period was 14 mo in the patients with unresectable pancreatic cancer.

Lygidakis et al. *(23)* implanted two arterial catheters at the end of the operative procedure, the first into the splenic artery (positioned after ligation, near the origin of the splenic artery at the celiac trunk and pointing toward the spleen) and the second through a side arterial branch of the middle colic artery into the superior mesenteric artery. Adjuvant chemotherapy was performed by infusing antitumor agents from the catheters in the splenic artery and the branch of the superior mesenteric artery. Median survival was significantly greater (30 mo) in the regional chemotherapy group than in the control group (16.8 mo).

The same team *(2)* also carried out a prospective randomized study to evaluate the long-term results of adjuvant locoregional chemoimmunotherapy in patients with advanced pancreatic cancer who had undergone pancreatic resection. They divided 128 patients into three groups. Group A ($n = 40$) patients underwent surgical resection alone. For Group B ($n = 45$) patients, an arterial catheter was advanced, under fluoroscopic control, into the superior mesenteric artery, via a side arterial branch of the jejunal artery. Group B patients then received adjuvant chemotherapy consisting of gemcitabine, carboplatin, mitoxantrone, MMC, 5-FU, and folinic acid. Group C ($n = 43$) patients were implanted with the same kind of arterial catheter but were administered interleukin-2 in Lipiodol as an adjuvant locoregional chemoimmunotherapy . During the initial surgical exploration, all patients underwent pancreatic resection. The 2- and 5-yr survival figures were 29 and 0% for group A, 52 and 10% for group B, and 65 and 18% for group C. The respective percentages for disease-free survival were 20 and 0% for group A, 35 and 7% for group B, and 58 and 11% for group C. They concluded that, when applied regionally, combined chemoimmunotherapy is simple, safe, and effective. This type of therapy substantially prolongs overall survival and improves disease-free survival compared with either surgical resection alone or with combined surgical resection and adjuvant regional chemotherapy.

Kouloulias et al. *(22)* performed neoadjuvant chemotherapy plus radiation in patients with unresectable pancreatic cancer. During laporotomy, they carried out intraoperative regional chemotherapy with 5-FU from the splenic artery. They also performed hyperthermia. The median survival for patients in this study was 18.5 mo.

Separate study teams performed transcatheter splenic artery embolization *(33)* prior to placing a catheter into the splenic artery, in patients with unresectable pancreatic cancer *(19,20)*. SMANCS-Lipiodol (an antitumor agent plus carrier and embolizing agent) was then injected into the splenic artery. Computed tomography taken immediately after injection revealed that the SMANCS-Lipiodol had infused into the tail of the pancreas. At 2 wk after the procedure, a small amount of SMANCS-Lipiodol remained in the tail, and the margin of the tumor was less clearly defined. However, the body of the pancreas had demonstrated no remarkable change after the 2 wk.

6.3.1. HYPOXIC ABDOMINAL PERFUSION

Isolated hypoxic perfusion is a more invasive technique than celiac trunk infusion. Isolated hypoxic perfusion requires general anesthesia and an average stay of 7 d in hospital. Because of the severe hemodynamic and pathophysiological changes occurring during these therapies a postoperative observation in an intensive care unit is often necessary. The procedure causes severe side effects, primarily affecting the intestine with disorders such as diarrhea and emesis. Isolated hypoxic perfusion therefore has a negative impact on quality of life *(34)*.

Lorenz et al. *(35)* performed isolated hypoxic perfusion with MMC in patients with advanced pancreatic cancer. None of the patients was found to respond to treatment. Furthermore, the median survival was 4.2 mo, similar to that of the untreated patients. This regimen resulted in severe side effects and perioperative complications. Most of the side effects affected the gastrointestinal tract, resulting in nausea, emesis, and diarrhea, with 40% of the patients suffering from severe side-effects. In addition, five patients (29%) suffered deep vein thrombosis following the procedure.

Van IJken et al. *(13)* performed a hypoxic abdominal perfusion with MMC and melphalan followed by a celiac trunk infusion in 12 patients with advanced pancreatic cancer. One patient died after the celiac trunk infusion owing to acute mesenteric ischemia. The study team did not consider any of the patients to be resectable following treatment. Median survival after this chemotherapy was 6 mo. They did not recommend this chemotherapy as a therapeutic option in patients with advanced pancreatic cancer.

6.3.2. INTRAPERITONEAL CHEMOTHERAPY

Oman et al. *(29)* treated nonresectable pancreatic cancer with intraperitoneal 5-FU and leucovorin. All patients had abdominal discomfort and distension during intraperitoneal installation. Median survival time was 7 mo. There was no difference in the survival times between patients with different grading, staging, or tumor size. They concluded that intraperitoneal administration of 5-FU was feasible for patients with nonresectable pancreatic cancer. The study showed that the treatment could induce a temporary stabilization of tumor growth and eventually prolong survival without adverse effects.

6.4. HYPERTHERMIA

Kouloulias et al. *(22)* treated seven patients who had unresectable pancreatic cancer with a combination of cytoreductive surgery and preoperative chemotherapy (5-FU) plus external beam postoperative irradiation and a single session of intraoperative hyperthermia with intraoperative regional chemotherapy. Postoperative recovery was uneventful for all patients. The median overall survival was 18.5 mo.

These clinical results showed both that the treatment was effective at prolonging survival and that patients could tolerate the treatment. This suggests that a combination of cytoreductive resection, preoperative chemotherapy, intraoperative chemohyper-thermia, and external beam postoperative radiotherapy is potentially beneficial for the management of advanced pancreatic cancer.

6.5. Radiation

The Gastrointestinal Tumor Study Group randomized 194 patients with locally unresectable pancreatic cancer into three groups: those who underwent radiotherapy (60 gy) alone; those who underwent 40 gy radiotherapy plus 5-FU; and those who under-went 60 gy radiotherapy plus 5-FU. Median survival time was 17 wk in the radiotherapy-alone group compared with 32 wk for the 40 gy plus 5-FU group and 44 wk for the 60 gy plus 5-FU group. It was recognized that radiation therapy with concurrent 5-FU pro-longed survival in patients with unresectable pancreatic cancer (36,37).

6.5.1. CHEMORADIOTHERAPY

A number of studies have demonstrated how chemoradiotherapy can be used to achieve clinical downstaging of pancreatic cancer by enabling a resection to be performed on previously unresectable cancers.

Pilepich and Miller (38) performed a second-look laparotomy in 11 of the 17 patients in their study, following preoperative irradiation. They were able to resect the tumor in six of the patients and two of the patients, are still alive after 5 yr.

Hoffman et al. (39) reported that, of 34 patients with localized pancreatic cancer who were treated with radiotherapy in combination with 5-FU and MMC, 11 patients were able to undergo a pancreas resection. The median survival time in these 11 patients was 45 mo, with a 5-yr survival rate of 40 %.

Jessup et al. (40) treated 16 patients, who had locally advanced tumors, with external radiation therapy plus continuous infusion of 5-FU. Ten patients underwent a second-look laparotomy that resulted in two resections. These two patients remained free of disease at the time of their report, 20 and 22 mo later.

Wilkowski et al (41) studied the effect that chemoradiotherapy combined with gemcitabine and cisplatin had on locoregional control, in 47 patients with primary inop-erable pancreatic cancer. Following the chemoradiotherapy, 9 patients (19.1%) achieved a complete response and 23 patients (48.9%) a partial response. The overall response rate was 68%. After the chemoradiography, the lesions were considered resectable in 27 patients, and 25 of the 27 patients underwent laparotomy. The other 20 patients under-went a definitive pancreatic resection. The median survival amounted to 10.7 mo for all patients, whereas it was prolonged to 24.2 mo for those who had the R0 resection. They concluded that gemcitabine and cisplatin can safely be combined with external beam radiation.

These studies all indicate that a small number of patients with unresectable pancreatic cancer, who do not have distant metastases, may benefit from palliative chemoradio-therapy in such a way that resection subsequently becomes possible. This prolongs sur-vival and even presents a small chance of cure.

6.6. Gene Therapy

Hoshida et al. *(32)* studied the effects of gene therapy for pancreatic cancer in mice by using an adenovirus vector encoding soluble flt-1 VEGF receptor. They concluded that antiangiogenic gene therapy using soluble flt-1 might be an effective approach for pancreatic cancer treatment in humans.

REFERENCES

1. Lawrence T. Gemcitabine as a radiation sensitizer. Semin Oncol 1995;2:68–71.
2. Lygidakis NJ, Sgourakis G, Georgia D, Vlachos L, Raptis S. Regional targeting chemoimmunotherapy in patients undergoing pancreatic resection in an advanced stage of their disease: a prospective randomized study. Ann Surg 2002;236:806–813.
3. Ensminger WD, Gyves JW, Stetson P, Walker-Andrews S. Phase I study of hepatic arterial degradable starch microspheres and mitomycin. Cancer Res 1985;45:4464–4467.
4. Ikeda K., Saitoh S., Suzuki Y., et al. Effect of arterial administration of a high molecular weight antitumor agent, styrene maleic acid neocarzinostatin, for multiple small liver cancer—a pilot study. J Gastroenterol 1997;32:513–520.
5. Hirashima N., Sakakibara K., Itazu I., et al. Zinostatin stimalamer-transcatheter arterial embolization for hepatocellular carcinoma: a comparison with lipiodol- transcatheter arterial embolization. Sem Oncol 1997;24:S6-91–S6-96.
6. Konno T., Maeda H., Iwai K., et al. Effect of arterial administration of high-molecular-weight anticancer agent SMANCS with lipid lymphographic agent on hepatoma: a preliminary report. Eur J Cancer Clin Oncol 1983;19:1053–1065.
7. Maeda H., Ueda M., Morinaga T., et al. Conjugation of poly (styrene-co-maleic acid) derivatives to the antitumor protein neocarzinostatin: pronounced improvements in pharmacological properties. J Med Chem 1985;28:455–461.
8. Donatini B. A systematic study of the vascularisation of the pancreas. Surg Radiol Anat 1990;12:173–180.
9. Pansky B. Anatomy of the pancreas. Emphasis on blood supply and lymphatic drainage. Int J Pancreatol 1990;7:101–108.
10. Meyer F, Grote R, Lippert H, Ridwelski K. Marginal effects of regional intra-arterial chemotherapy as an alternative treatment option in advanced pancreatic carcinoma. Langenbecks Arch Surg 2004;389:32–39.
11. Aigner KR, Gailhofer S, Kopp S. Regional versus systemic chemotherapy for advanced pancreatic cancer: a randomized study. Hepatogastroenterology 1998;45:1125–1129.
12. Theodors A, Bukowski RM, Hewlett JS, Livingston RB, Weick JK. Intermittent regional infusion of chemotherapy for pancreatic adenocarcinoma. Phase I and II pilot study. Am J Clin Oncol 1982;5:555–558.
13. van IJken MG, van Etten B, Guetens G, et al. Balloon catheter hypoxic abdominal perfusion with mitomycin C and melphalan for locally advanced pancreatic cancer: a phase I-II trial. Eur J Surg Oncol 2004;30:671–680.
14. Maurer CA, Borner MM, Lauffer J, et al. Celiac axis infusion chemotherapy in advanced nonresectable pancreatic cancer. Int J Pancreatol 1998;23:181–186.
15. Muchmore JH, Preslan JE, George WJ. Regional chemotherapy for inoperable pancreatic carcinoma. Cancer. 1996;78:664–673.
16. Gansauge F, Gansauge S, Link KH, Beger HG. p53 in relation to therapeutic outcome of locoregional chemotherapy in pancreatic cancer. Ann N Y Acad Sci 1999;880:281–287.
17. Papachristou E, Link KH, Schoenberg MH. Regional celiac artery infusion in the adjuvant treatment of pancreatic cancer. Anticancer Res 2003;23:831–834.
18. Link KH, Formentini A, Gansauge F, Papachristov E, Beger HG. Regional celiac artery infusion as adjuvant treatment after pancreatic cancer resection. Digestion 1997;58:529–532.
19. Yoshida H, Onda M, Tajiri T, et al. New techniques: Splenic artery embolization followed by intraarterial infusion chemotherapy for the treatment of pancreatic cancer. Hepatogastroenterology 1999;46:2024–2027.

20. Yoshida H, Onda M, Tajiri T, et al. Experience with intraarterial infusion of styrene maleic acid neocarzinostatin (SMANCS)-Lipiodol in pancreatic cancer. Hepatogastroenterology 1999;46: 2612–2615.

21. Bayar S, Unal E, Tez M, Kocaoglu H, Demirci S, Akgul H. Regional chemotherapy for advanced pancreatic carcinoma. Hepatogastroenterology 2003;50:550–552.

22. Kouloulias VE, Nikita KS, Kouvaris JR, et al. Cytoreductive surgery combined with intraoperative chemo-hyperthermia and postoperative radiotherapy in the management of advanced pancreatic adenocarcinoma: feasibility aspects and efficacy. J Hepatobiliary Pancreat Surg 2001;8:564–5670.

23. Lygidakis NJ, Stringaris K. Adjuvant therapy following pancreatic resection for pancreatic duct carcinoma: a prospective randomized study. Hepatogastroenterology 1996;43:671–6780.

24. Ohigashi H, Ishikawa O, Imaoka S, et al. A new method of intra-arterial regional chemotherapy with more selective drug delivery for locally advanced pancreatic cancer. Hepatogastroenterology 1996;43:338–345.

25. Ishikawa O, Ohhigashi H, Sasaki Y, Furukawa H, Imaoka S. Extended pancreatectomy and liver perfusion chemotherapy for resectable adenocarcinoma of the pancreas. Digestion 1999;60:135–128.

26. Ishikawa O, Ohigashi H, Imaoka S, et al. Regional chemotherapy to prevent hepatic metastasis after resection of pancreatic cancer. Hepatogastroenterology 1997;44:1541–1546.

27. Ishikawa O, Ohigashi H, Sasaki Y, et al. Liver perfusion chemotherapy via both the hepatic artery and portal vein to prevent hepatic metastasis after extended pancreatectomy for adenocarcinoma of the pancreas. Am J Surg 1994;168:361–364.

28. Nakayama S, Takeda S, Kawase Y, Inoue S, Kaneko T, Nakao A. Clinical significance of dihydropyrimidine dehydrogenase in adjuvant 5-fluorouracil liver perfusion chemotherapy for pancreatic cancer. Ann Surg 2004;240:840–844.

29. Oman M, Blind PJ, Naredi P, Gustavsson B, Hafstrom LO. Treatment of non-resectable pancreatic cancer with intraperitoneal 5-FU and leucovorin IV. Eur J Surg Oncol 2001;27:477–481.

30. Colacchio TA, Coughlin C, Taylor J, Douple E, Ryan T, Crichlow RW. Intraoperative radiation therapy and hyperthermia. Morbidity and mortality from this combined treatment modality for unresectable intra-abdominal carcinomas. Arch Surg 1990;125:370–375.

31. Ashayeri E, Bonney G, DeWitty RL, Goldson AL, Leffall LD, Thomas JN. Preliminary survivorship report on combined intraoperative radiation and hyperthermia treatments for unresectable pancreatic adenocarcinoma. J Natl Med Assoc 1993;85:36–340.

32. Hoshida T, Sunamura M, Duda DG, et al. Gene therapy for pancreatic cancer using an adenovirus vector encoding soluble flt-1 vascular endothelial growth factor receptor. Pancreas 2002;25:111–21.

33. Tajiri T, Onda M, Yoshida H, Mamada Y, Taniai N, Kumazaki T. Long-term hematological and biochemical effects of partial splenic embolization in hepatic cirrhosis. Hepatogastroenterology 2002;49:1445–1448.

34. Lorenz M, Heinrich S, Staib-Sebler E, et al. Regional chemotherapy in the treatment of advanced pancreatic cancer—is it relevant? Eur J Cancer 2000;36:957–965.

35. Lorenz M, Petrowsky H, Heinrich S, Janshon G, Staib-Sebler E, Poloczek Y, Gog C, Oremek G, Encke A. Isolated hypoxic perfusion with mitomycin C in patients with advanced pancreatic cancer. Eur J Surg Oncol 1998;24:542–547.

36. Moertel CG, Frytak S, Hahn RG, et al. Therapy of locally unresectable pancreatic carcinoma: a randomized comparison of high dose (6000 rads) radiation alone, moderate dose radiation (4000 rads + 5-fluorouracil), and high dose radiation + 5-fluorouracil: The Gastrointestinal Tumor Study Group. Cancer 1981;48:1705–1710.

37. A multi-institutional comparative trial of radiation therapy alone and in combination with 5-fluorouracil for locally unresectable pancreatic carcinoma. The Gastrointestinal Tumor Study Group. Ann Surg 1979;189:205–208.

38. Pilepich MV, Miller HH. Preoperative irradiation in carcinoma of the pancreas. Cancer 1980;46: 1945–1949.

39. Hoffman JP, Weese JL, Solin LJ, et al. A pilot study of preoperative chemoradiation for patients with localized adenocarcinoma of the pancreas. Am J Surg 1995;169:71–77.

40. Jessup JM, Steele G Jr, Mayer RJ, et al. Neoadjuvant therapy for unresectable pancreatic adenocarcinoma. Arch Surg 1993;128:559–564.

41. Wilkowski R, Thoma M, Schauer R, Wagner A, Heinemann V. Effect of chemoradiotherapy with gemcitabine and cisplatin on locoregional control in patients with primary inoperable pancreatic cancer. World J Surg 2004;28:1011–1018.

18 Regional Breast Cancer Treatment

Moshe Z. Papa, MD, and
Siegal Sadetzki, MD, MPH

Contents

Summary

Advances in technology and the increase in screening for breast cancer that identifies tumors at earlier stages have made it possible to destroy tumors in situ without surgery. This can also be used to treat locally advanced tumors. These locoregional ablative techniques include minimally invasive surgical as well as noninvasive ablative modalities, new radiation technologies, and regional chemotherapy. New developments in imaging modalities such as MR make these treatment opportunities more precise and reliable. The regional minimally invasive technologies provide treatment options that are physiologically, cosmetically, and psychologically more acceptable to the patient. Many of these need further investigation before they become an accepted sound practice. This paper reviews and discusses the up-to-date data and feasibility of technologies for locoregional treatment of breast cancer

Key Words: Breast cancer; minimal invasive surgical procedures; radiofrequency; cryoablation; microwave ablation; focused ultrasound ablation; radiation partial; regional chemotherapy.

From: *Cancer Drug Discovery and Development: Regional Cancer Therapy*
Edited by: P. M. Schlag and U. S. Stein © Humana Press Inc., Totowa, NJ

1. INTRODUCTION

Breast cancer is the most common malignant tumor among women; approximately 12.5% of all women in the industrialized countries will develop breast cancer in their lives *(1)*. One of the cornerstones of breast cancer treatment is surgery along with radiation therapy and systemic treatment with chemotherapy, endocrine manipulation, and (recently) biological therapy.

Breast cancer has been treated by surgical intervention under general anesthesia, and the results have revealed a low incidence of local recurrence (5–8%). Adjuvant radiotherapy is important for reducing local recurrence and is associated with inconvenience, increased expense, and possible impairment of cosmesis *(2)*.

The concept that cancer is a systemic disease from its early stages necessitating local control with adjuvant systemic treatment caused a change in the extent of locoregional surgical treatment from radical mastectomy to modified radical mastectomy and later to lumpectomy with axillary sampling. Local recurrence after breast-conserving surgery and radiation for early breast cancer has shown high salvage and survival rates *(3)*. The prognosis of locally recurrent breast cancer after conservation therapy is favorable compared with postmastectomy chest wall recurrence *(4)*. Randomized studies conducted in the United States and Italy have supported the notion of minimizing surgical treatments, having demonstrated no difference in local recurrence between radical and conserving surgery even after 20 yr *(5,6)*. The addition of systemic chemotherapy resulted in increased 5-yr survival, up to >90% in stage 1 *(7)*.

As screening programs of breast cancer are more widely used, breast cancer is being detected at earlier stages. This has resulted in smaller tumors being excised, further strengthening the trend toward local control with breast conservation. While not hampering the outcome, it enables women to keep their breast with good cosmetic results.

A similar trend was observed in treating the axilla by the use of sentinel node excision instead of axillary clearance, thus decreasing the number of unnecessary axillary lymph node dissections and reducing disabling complications such as lymphedema, pain, and limitation of arm movement *(8)* .

Breast preservation is currently offered not only to partients with early-stage tumors but also to partients with more advanced disease when the tumor extent was decreased following neoadjuvant chemotherapy treatment *(9)*.

On the other hand, local procedures are also indicated for patients with primary or recurrent tumors as a palliative procedure.

Locoregional therapy can be subdivided into:

- Surgery:
  — Conventional invasive surgery (mastectomy/lumpectomy)
  — Sterotactic excision (the ABBI system).
- Ablative therapies:
  — Minimal invasive: cryoablation, radiofrequency ablation, interstitial laser ablation,
  — Noninvasive/virtual surgery: microwave thermotherapy and focused ultrasound ablation
- Interstitial radiotherapy.
- Locoregional chemotherapy.

2. SURGICAL METHODS

2.1. Conventional Invasive

A full discussion of the surgical approach to breast cancer is beyond the scope of this review.

The surgical treatment of breast cancer has changed dramatically in the last 100 yr from extended radical mastectomy to breast preservation. Changes in the understanding of the biology of breast cancer, earlier detection by screening, and improvement in radiotherapy technique were crucial in the development of breast-conserving therapy. Equivalent survival between mastectomy and breast-conserving surgery approaches was confirmed in both short- and long-term (20 yr) follow-up *(5,6)*. Studies have also demonstrated high rates of local control with satisfactory cosmetic results.

Since a growing number of tumors are detected in early stages and are therefore small in size and not palpable, needle localization is used to direct the surgeon to the tumor anatomical site. Clear microscopic lumpectomy margins are necessary for optimal local control *(10)*. There is no consensus regarding the width of the clear margins; however, most surgeons agree on at least 2 mm. Since during surgery it is difficult to determine the pathological margin, even an experienced surgeon will have to go back and reexcise some patients to reach clear margins. Consequently, about 30% of patients will need relumpectomy, which means the inconvenience that is associated with an additional surgical procedure. A study published recently demonstrated that the risk of local recurrence after breast-conserving surgery increases progressively with the number of reexcisions needed to achieve clear margins *(11)*.

2.2. Stereotactic Surgical Excision

This procedure uses a biopsy needle directed by mammography to excise repeatedly pieces of tumor. Sterotactic breast surgical excision can be carried out by instruments such as the Advanced Breast Biopsy Instrumentation (ABBI™, US Surgical, Norwalk CT) and vacuum-assisted core biopsy instruments such as the Mammotome (Biopsy Medical, Cincinnati OH) or the MIBB (US Surgical).

This procedure was initially used for diagnostic purposes; however, the increasing number of early detected small tumors increased the potential of these diagnostic modalities: they could also be used for minimally invasive image-guided therapy. The disadvantages are that a small incision is still needed, and it is difficult to assess the margins of the excised specimen. Therefore, this procedure is limited to the excision of benign lesions and very small cancers only *(12)*.

The ABBI technology has been approved for therapeutic purposes, whereas the vacuum-assisted core biopsy instruments have been approved for diagnostic procedures only. Clinical trials are needed to evaluate the role of these minimally invasive technologies as replacement for surgical lumpectomy for the treatment of breast cancer *(12,13)*.

3. ABLATIVE THERAPIES

The idea of this group of procedures is to use thermal energy (heating or cooling) to cause cellular damage and thus tumor destruction. The various technologies differ in the way the energy is generated and applied to the tissue.

The main challenges are to target and destroy the tumor while imaging it in real time, thus ensuring complete ablation of the tumor with negative margins together with minimal damage to normal tissue. Because of tissue destruction one needs to obtain all necessary pathological and biological information such as markers and receptors prior to treatment. Ablative therapies are applied via minimal or non-skin penetration (minimally invasive or virtual).

3.1. Minimally Invasive Techniques

3.1.1. Cryoablation of Breast Lesions

Cryoablation uses cold temperature to freeze and destroy a breast mass. The target temperature is between $-190°C$ and $-160°C$. The efficiency is maximized by multiple freeze-thaw cycles, which result in disruption of the cell membrane. Cryoablation can be done in the physician's office using local anesthesia, since the freezing procedure itself anesthetizes the breast tissue. The patient is awake throughout the procedure. Following application of the local anesthesia, a small incision is made in the skin overlying the lesion to insert the probe. The probe is entirely insulated except for the tip, which is placed into the tumor. Real-time ultrasound is used to guide the probe into the center of the tumor. Argon gas is used as a cooling agent. The ice ball created is observed by the ultrasound, and its diameter is monitored continuously until it reaches the size necessary to encompass all the tumorous area along with a 10-mm margin of healthy tissue to ensure clear margins. Two freeze-thaw cycles are performed, the first lasting 7 to 10 min, followed by a 5-min thaw. The second thaw lasts until the ice ball melts to the point that allows removal of the cryoprobe.

Cell destruction following this procedure is relatively slow; therefore, pathological assessment of tissue damage is difficult for up to a week after the cryoablation. If the destroyed tissue is left *in situ*, the body will reabsorb it within 3 to 6 mo. Normal activity can be resumed by the patient the day after treatment.

Cryoablation has othr potential uses. It can be used to replace wire localization, and the margins created by the ice ball can guide breast-conserving surgery, adding a safety element and decreasing the rate of reexcision.

Limitations and complications are as follows:

- Tumors close to the skin or chest wall may cause thermal burn if the ice ball gets too close.
- Since freezing destroys the tissue, all information relevant for staging and treatment needs to be obtained prior to treatment by core needle biopsy.
- There is no way to ensure complete tumor cell destruction without excision, since no molecular imaging is available following the procedure.
- Malignant cells are more resistant to lethal damage from freezing but more sensitive to hyperthermic damage than normal cells *(14)*.
- Ductal carcinoma *in situ* is more resistant to cryoablation than invasive cancer *(15,16)*.
- Tumor size may affect the success rate of the procedure; tumors less than 2 cm are best treated *(17)*
- Considerable time is taken to form and then throw the ice ball.

Rand et al. were the first to treat breast cancer by cryoablation in 1985 *(18)*. Pfleiderer treated 15 females with 16 breast cancers under ultrasound guidance; the mean tumor diameter was $21 ± 7.8$ mm. Although no severe side effects were noted, they found that only the invasive portions of the tumors were successfully ablated by cryotherapy; the *in situ* components were resistant. This finding is of concern since the existence of ductal carcinoma *in situ* (DCIS) in the tumor may not be detected prior to the treatment *(16)*. The size of the lesion being frozen affects the outcome and effectiveness of this procedure; lesions less than 16 mm are best treated by this modality. Even when this criterion was used, only three of five tumors were completely destroyed *(19)*.

In a multiinstitutional cryoablation study in 29 women, Sable et al. *(17)* reemphasized the importance of tumor size as well as the presence of *in situ* cancer. All tumors <1 cm were fully ablated, tumors between 1 and 1.5 cm without an in situ component were destroyed, whereas tumors over 1.5 cm were not reliably eradicated. The noncalcified type of DCIS caused most treatment failures. They recommended limiting this treatment to tumors smaller than 1.5 cm with a minimal component of *in situ* tumor on core biopsy.

In summary, large tumor size and the presence of DCIS appear to be contraindications. The impact of the destroyed area on imaging studies, recurrence and survival rates, and the impact of freezing on tissue response to adjuvant therapy need to be studied. The major advantages of this modality are the lack of pain and the need for only superficial local anesthesia. Further studies are needed to evaluate the long-term effectiveness of cryoablation.

3.1.3. RADIOFREQUENCY ABLATION THERAPY OF BREAST TUMORS

Radiofrequency ablation (RFA) is a thermal treatment that uses high-frequency (460 kHz) alternating current that flows via the electrode tip into the surrounding tissue and destroys the tumor *in situ*. The alternating current that passes through the tumor heats it to temperatures >55°C, which causes thermal coagulation and protein denaturation. The size of the electrode tip dictates the ablation field. Enlargement of the treated field can be achieved either by increasing the size of the tip to form a star-like array or by infusing saline solution through the tip of the electrode. The tissue surrounding the electrode, rather than the electrode itself, is the source of heat since the ions that compose the tissue attempt to follow the changes in the direction of alternating current, which results in friction that increases the tissue temperature further to 80°C to 110°C. Thus, heat is the main mechanism for tissue injury; heat drives extracellular and intracellular water out of the tissue, resulting in coagulative necrosis *(20,21)*. The treated tissue usually does not show changes for 48 h; thus pathological examination immediately after ablation may not reveal the characteristic pattern. NADH staining is used in addition to hematoxylin and eosin staining to evaluate cell viability *(22)*. This technology has already been used successfully for the treatment of liver tumors and other malignancies *(23,24)*.

Clinical experience with RFA in breast cancer is rather limited. The first feasibility study of RFA in women suffering from breast cancer was described in 1999 by Jeffrey et al. *(25)*. This study, along with a few subsequent ones, evaluated ultrasound-guided RFA in relatively small breast cancers, which was carried out under general anesthesia in the operating room just prior to surgical excision *(26–30)*. Results from these first studies have been encouraging, with complete tumor ablation of 80 to 100%. However, the problem was that they were done immediately prior to the operative lumpectomy or mastectomy, thus making pathological evaluation of tumor destruction somewhat unreliable. Another study has shown a high (23%) rate of complete destruction failure *(31)*. Burak et al. *(32)* found that RFA of small breast malignancies (mean tumor size of 1.2 cm; range 0.8–1.6 cm) can be done with ultrasound guidance under local anesthesia. One of 10 patients failed the treatment and was found to have residual disease. Another study

(28), conducted to evaluate RFA treatment of T1 breast cancer, demonstrated the discrepancy between sonographically confirmed complete ablation and pathologically complete ablation. Thus accurate real-time imaging of complete ablation is needed. A postablation MRI scan appeared to predict the histologic findings *(33)*.

The results from these limited series demonstrate that this is a safe procedure with minimal treatment-related complications. The treatment does not take long, the comfort level is relatively high, and it can be carried out under local anesthesia in the physician's office.

Limitations of RFA treatment include:

- It still is an invasive procedure.
- Dense breast tissue might bend the probe tips.
- Tumor close to the chest wall or the skin cannot be treated owing to heat damage.
- Imaging of the procedure is ultrasound dependent, which limits visualization of the three-dimensional tumor shape and thus accurate positioning of the probe.
- Tumor multifocality may be missed using RFA.
- A pathological consideration is that the presence of extensive DCIS may compromise the efficiency of RFA, since it is relatively resistant to treatment.

There are still no data on long-term morphologic changes of the tumor and surrounding tissue after RFA. It also unknown how quickly the treated tissue is absorbed following RFA; one possibility is that a disturbing hard lump will remain in the area. One study has shown that the scar becomes clinically impalpable as well as invisible by ultrasound in 12 mo *(34)*.

Considering the limitations of ultrasound imaging before and after RFA, magnetic resonance imaging (MRI) may serve as a valuable tool for treatment guidance as well for assessment of tumor response. When MR-compatible probes are available, real-time imaging of thermal changes as well as accurate measurement of the treated zone (with margins of normal tissue) will be possible.

Based on this information, it is possible that in the future RFA will be used as a sole treatment modality for breast cancer and will possibly substitute for breast-conserving surgery. However, to evaluate the natural history of RFA ablation of breast tumors without resection, further studies are needed. Until the results of these trials published, RFA treatment of breast malignancy remains an investigational tool.

3.1.3. INTERSTITIAL LASER ABLATION OF BREAST MALIGNANCY (ILA)

ILA uses heat energy to destroy the breast tumor. The heat source originates from the laser light, which is delivered directly to the tumor via optical fibers inserted into the tissue. Several types of lasers can be used; the most common are the semiconductor diode laser (805 nm) and the argon ion laser (488 and 518 nm). The technique is simple: no general anesthesia is necessary, the skin is locally anesthetized, a small skin incision is made, and a stereotactic 16- to 18-gage laser-omitting optic fiber is inserted. The fiber can be guided by mammogram, ultrasound, or MR. The size of the burn can be increased by using multiple fibers with an optical beam splitter or by using the "pull-back" technique. In this technique the probe is repeatedly inserted deep into the involved tissue and then gradually withdrawn through the tumor. Treatment of >1000 J per fiber produces a burn in the tissue of the size of 10 mm. One centimeter and parallel to the stereotactic needle a multisensing probe is inserted to monitor the temperature of the surrounding tissue. The temperature around the core should reach 80° to 100°C. Throughout the treatment, saline is continuously dripped from the tip of the laser probe to prevent overheating. The best way to monitor this procedure is by MRI, which allows one to observe the ablated area and the temperature reached in real time *(35)*.

The main limitations and complications noted with this procedure are skin and muscle burns. Skin burns can be prevented by cooling the skin either with cold water or ice packs. Other limitations are no different from those that are relevant for heat ablation techniques. Another limitation is the relatively small size of the lesion that is ideally treated (<1.5 cm in diameter) *(19)*.

Bloom et al. *(36)* treated 40 patients with breast cancers measuring >2 cm by interstitial laser therapy. The tumors were excised at a different session 5 to 42 d later. Macroscopically, the treated area consisted of a central charred cavity surrounded by an area of pale tissue with a peripheral hemorrhagic rim. Pathologic evaluation revealed changes in accordance with the distance from the laser tip. The first, around the tip, demonstrated charred tissue, the second coagulation similar to the electrocautery effect, the third histological tumor cells that were not viable, the fourth preserved tumor architecture with changes in cytoplasmatic and nuclear structure, and the fifth a hyperemic, inflammatory zone with fat necrosis. They concluded that it is the outer zone of fat necrosis that delineates the actual area of effective ablation and that may help in guiding the resection *(36)*.

Dowlatshahi et al. *(37)* completed a study on 56 women with breast cancers smaller than 23 mm. Two women were treated out of protocol. Tumors were excised within 2 mo of the ILA treatment; 30% (16 of 54) of the patients still had residual tumor. The authors attempted to explain this high rate of tumor viability by the learning curve, patient compliance, and technical as well as target visualization problems. Two treated patients were observed without excision of primary tumor, and at 2 yr no residual carcinoma was identified.

As mentioned, MRI has been suggested to monitor ILA. Gadolinium may help to locate the lesion, and the T1-weighted gradient echo sequences can be used to monitor therapy. The extent of laser damage is seen as areas of nonenhancement, and these correspond with areas of necrosis seen on histopathological examination. Two studies evaluated MR-guided interstitial laser ablation and concluded that it is an effective and safe alternative to lumpectomy for relatively small tumors *(38,39)*. It should be mentioned that the laser probes are MR-invisible unless specially coated. ILA has also been used by some investigators to treat breast fibroadenomas *(40)*.

In summary, ILA has the potential to ablate *in situ* small breast cancers and fibroadenomas. The combination of ILA with MR is the preferred way to treat these patients since it allows one to monitor the area that was treated as well as observe the temperature generated by the probe in real time. Further studies are needed to evaluate the role for ILA as a replacement to lumpectomy and its long-term local effects.

4. NONINVASIVE/VIRTUAL SURGERY

4.1. Focused Ultrasound

High-energy ultrasound beams can be directed and focused to penetrate the soft tissue and destroy tumors by increasing the local temperature The boundaries of the treatment area are sharply demarcated (focused) without causing damage to the surrounding organs.

Although the idea of using sound waves to ablate tumors was first demonstrated in the 1940s, only ongoing technical developments have enabled the technology to become more feasible. The major breakthrough came when the process was coupled to advanced imaging to guide the sound beams and when an effective way to evaluate the temperature and extent of tissue destruction was developed, thus achieving focal destruction of the lesion with minimal damage to the surrounding breast tissue and other organs. The development of MR as the foundation to guide and evaluate the end results of focused ultrasound (FUS) treatment has pushed this novel technology forward in oncologic practice *(41,42)*.

The patient is positioned on the MR/FUS bed in the prone position. An MR scan to evaluate the breast anatomy and tumor location is performed. If the tumor is identifiable on MR images and accessible by the device for treatment, and if the patient meets all the inclusion criteria, treatment will be carried out. The treating physician than draws the treatment volume using the MR images; this plan includes a minimum boundary of at least 5 mm of healthy tissue beyond the tumor margin. A small area in the center of the tumor is treated with focused ultrasound energy for 5 to 30 s and heats the tissue to between 60 and 90°C to induce thermal coagulation. MR images are taken to provide image quality, a quantitative real-time temperature map, and confirmation of targeting accuracy. Then sonication of the entire tumor is initiated. The duration of each sonication lasts between 16 and 24 s. The ultrasound transducer is automatically moved from one treatment point to the next until the entire volume is treated. The procedure time is dependent on the tumor size. After the treatment is completed, a final MR scan is done including T1- and T2-weighted sequences with contrast to evaluate the treatment effect. MRI is repeated at 72 h for better assessment of treatment success after the posttreatment edema has subsided. The experimental protocol included standard breast cancer surgical treatment by either lumpectomy or mastectomy to evaluate the pathological response to treatment *(43)*.

This technique is not without limitations, as follows:

- Tumor location may limit its application. Currently it is used for tumors smaller than 2 cm located at least 1 cm from the skin and chest wall. The addition of a new cooling system that will protect the skin from heating may minimize the risk of this complication.
- Tumors larger than 3 cm are not treated at this time owing to the treatment time needed. Currently a typical treatment lasts about 2 h, during which the patient must lie still within the enclosed confines of the MR machine.
- Claustrophobia and patient discomfort are important issues. Some patients find lying in the machine psychologically difficult and can become anxious and claustrophobic.
- The effect of this treatment on noncircumscribed, multifocal as well as DCIS tumors is unknown. Since the use of MR can identify this situation, combined with the precision of the FUS, it is conceivable that multifocal DCIS could be eradicated using this technology.

Our initial experience with 10 patients using the ExAblate 2000 (inSightec, Haifa Israel LTD) demonstrated that 2 had complete pathological tumor destruction, 2 had microscopic foci of residual tumor, 3 had 10% residual tumor, and 3 had between 10 and 30% of residual tumor. Procedure-related complications included pain necessitating analgesia and additional sedation during the treatment. In one patient a skin burn developed over the treatment area *(43)*. This system has been used experimentally in Canada, the United States, and Japan.

A Canadian group treated 23 patients successfully, with minimal morbidity. These patients were at increased operative risk or refused conventional surgery *(44)*.

As experience with this technology develops further, it may have the potential to replace surgery for certain breast cancers. At this point, our experience and the results of other centers demonstrate that it is feasible to destroy breast tumors with various degrees of efficacy and with minimal discomfort to the patient. As MR is increasingly becoming a diagnostic tool in breast cancer, it may push forward the use of MR-guided ablation of these tumors by FUS. The precision and three-dimensional image of the tumor, as well as real-time temperature measurements, allows the use of FUS with a remarkable degree of accuracy. In contrast to the other ablative techniques described previously, MR-guided FUS is completely noninvasive, with real-time assessment possible.

The fate of the tumor after FUS ablation needs further investigation. The effect of the ablated tumor on the immune system and the effects on the rest of the body of leaving in nonviable tumor cells (which have an ongoing inflammatory response) deserve further research. Other unsolved questions include the need for radiotherapy following FUS: is there a need to radiate at all? Should the tumor bed only be irradiated or the whole breast with or without a boost to the tumor bed?

The impact of FUS ablation on the ability to identify sentinel nodes deserves further study. It is unclear whether FUS may alter the lymphatic anatomy/physiology to preclude sentinel lymph node identification. In our limited experience with two patients we had no technical problems finding sentinel nodes after ablation.

Tumor heating by FUS may increase the efficacy of chemotherapy when it is applied in the neoadjuvant setting or when the drugs are administered to fixed, nonresectable tumor. Local heating may also be used in the future to target medication to the specific tissue. Another breast disease process that can benefit from FUS ablation is fibroadenoma. This relatively common benign lesion can present in a multifocal fashion. Currently surgery is the only solution; when indicated, however, FUS may enable us to destroy these lesions *in situ* without the need to scar the breast. At our center we have a limited but successful experience in treating fibroadenomas by FUS ablation *(45)*.

In conclusion, the ability to ablate tumors using FUS under MR guidance opens a window to a future in which noninvasive virtual surgery can be safely and repeatedly done with relatively low morbidity. Further clinical studies are needed.

4.2. Microwave Ablation

Microwave ablation is a noninvasive technique that uses heat to destroy the tumor selectively by microwave radiation. Since breast cancer cells have a higher water content than the glandular and fatty tissue that surrounds them, cancer tissue heats more rapidly than the surrounding tissue during microwave treatment.

During the treatment the breast is compressed between two electrodes that generate the microwave energy. To monitor temperature, one electrode is placed in the tumor and the other on the skin. The surface of the breast is cooled by air produced by a special fan. The core/target temperature should reach 43°C *(46)*.

In a pilot study (10 patients) Gardner et al. *(46)* achieved tumor response in 8 patients; significant tumor size reduction as well as tumor necrosis was noted in 4 patients. However, a high complication rate was noted later during the definitive surgery; 3 patients developed full-thickness flap necrosis following mastectomy, probably because of heat trauma to the skin *(46)*. In a study on 25 women with cancers averaging 18 mm,

VargSecond Pagesas et al. concluded that tumor necrosis can be achieved by microwave therapy and that the size of the destruction is a function of the thermal dose *(47)*. A third study *(48)* demonstrated that this is a safe, well-tolerated relatively quick procedure that results in tumor destruction.

One of the problems with microwave breast cancer treatment, as opposed to FUS, is the lack of real-time imaging technology. Another possible advantageous use of microwave heating is thermal enhancement of chemotherapeutic tumoricidal effects *(49)*, particularly in the neoadjuvant setting. Ongoing studies are now examining these effects.

5. REGIONAL RADIOTHERAPY

The standard 5 to 7 wk postoperative radiotherapy after local tumor excision has been one of the reasons for breast conservation underutilization by some patients. Certain patents prefer to undergo mastectomy rather than breast-conserving therapy, even for small breast tumors. Only 60 to 86% of the women who undergo breast-conserving surgery actually receive radiation *(50)*. Partial breast radiation could be an alternative to total breast radiation plus a boost to the area of the lumpectomy. The rationale for this treatment is that most local recurrences occur in the proximity of the tumor bed. Thus it might not be necessary to give whole breast radiation to all patients (especially those with early disease) in order to avoid local failure *(51–53)*.

Until recently brachytherapy was the most common way to apply accelerated partial breast irradiation. Brachytherapy can shorten the treatment course to 4 to 5 d. Early European studies used it mainly for boost irradiation of the primary tumor site. However, results were less than satisfactory because of failure to select the patients appropriately and secondary to suboptimal treatment techniques. Recent studies applying multicatheter brachytherapy as the sole radiation therapy after breast-conserving surgery using strict patient selection criteria have resulted in equivalent recurrence rates *(54,55)*. The North American experience has also been that brachytherapy has a great potential to overcome the barriers that prevented women for choosing breast-conserving therapy *(56)*.

Inserting the brachytherapy catheters requires training and expertise. The surgeon needs to leave clips in the lumpectomy site, at cranial, caudal, left, and right as well at the deepest point of the posterior resection margin. Catheter insertion is done under mammographic or ultrasound guidance using steel needles; this can be painful since multiple punctures are required. Irradiation is performed using an afterloading device either at a high dose rate or at a pulsed dose rate via the catheters. Cosmesis might be affected.

A new brachytherapy device, the MammoSite, was designed to simplify this procedure. It consists of a silicon balloon catheter with an inflation channel and a port for passage of the radiation source. The MammoSite balloon is inflated with saline solution mixed with a small amount of contrast material to allow its visualization. An Iridium-192 source, connected to a computer-controlled high-dose-rate remote afterloader, is inserted into the balloon to deliver the needed radiation dose. The prescription dose is 32 to 35 Gy given in 10 fractions of 3.4 Gy per fraction, b.i.d, with a minimum of 6 h between daily fractions. The iridium source covers a concentric volume within a radius of 10 mm *(52,57)*. The location of the balloon is confirmed by a CT scan. The balloon should be at a minimal distance of 5 mm from the skin. To date there have been no long-term results from clinical trials validating this device. An upcoming National Surgical Adjuvant

Breast and Bowel Project (NSABP) study will randomize patients between partial breast irradiation and external whole breast radiotherapy.

Another possibility for partial breast radiation is interstitial radiotherapy during the operative procedure (IORT). The goal is to apply high single doses of 10 to 22 Gy to a small target volume. Two devices have been developed for this purpose. The first, the Intrabeam technique, was developed by the Middlesex Hospital London. Intrabeam is essentially a miniature low-energy X-ray source (50 kV), which is modulated by spherical applicators of different sizes that provide a uniform dose to the tumor bed. The dose received by the tissue is proportional to the treatment length. The chest wall and skin should be protected to avoid radiation damage. Early pilot study results were encouraging, and a multinational TARGIT trial has been initiated to evaluate the Intrabeam technology (58).

The second intraoperative radiation source, Novac7, was developed by Veronesi's group in Milan. This is a mobile linear electron accelerator with a rotating head that delivers electron beams with energies from 3 to 12 MeV. Special tube applicators collimate the beams to a small target volume. The therapeutic depth is between 13 and 40 mm depending on the energy used. The radiation is applied once tumor resection with negative margins is completed and while protecting the pectoral muscle and the skin. Currently the European Institute of Oncology in Milan is evaluating the sole use of IORT using the Novac7 technology with external beam irradiation of the breast after breast-conserving surgery in a randomized trial (59).

Another possibility for applying partial breast irradiation postoperatively is via the 3D conformal radiation device.

From the preliminary phase I and II results, we believe that partial breast radiation has the potential to control local recurrence adequately and to alleviate the discomfort associated with whole breast external radiation. Future studies along with better breast imaging modalities such as MRI will define the appropriate patients that will benefit from this treatment.

6. REGIONAL CHEMOTHERAPY TREATMENT OF BREAST CANCER

Regional infusion of chemotherapy takes advantage of the first pass effect of the chemotherapeutic drug via the tumor, generating higher local drug concentrations at the tumor cell and thus enhancing its uptake. This infusion is targeted by a catheter placed in the feeding artery of the tumor. The uptake of the drug can be enhanced by producing local hyperthermia. Depending on the tumor location and the richness of the blood supply, when equal chemotherapeutic doses are given systemically or locally, the response may vary greatly. Thus, a better response can be expected with locoregional administration. The development of new drug modalities such as slow release methods may even further increase treatment efficacy.

The blood supply to the breast is variable and must be determined before regional chemotherapy is delivered. The subclavian artery and its tributaries, the internal mammary artery, and the lateral thoracic artery are the target vessels through which the angiographer should place the catheter, which is then used to infuse chemotherapy to treat large nonresectable primary breast cancers or chest wall recurrences (60). Doughty et al. (61) demonstrated that the internal mammary artery perfuses 67% of the breast and the lateral thoracic artery 15%. In 33%, the lateral thoracic artery did not contribute to breast perfusion; which was done from a further branch of the subclavian or axillary artery. A cuff can be placed around the upper arm to avoid leakage into the hand, thus increasing the concentration at the breast region. Injecting blue dye will stain the area treated, thus confirming that the tumor on the chest wall is indeed receiving the drug. Some oncologists have combined regional chemotherapy with transcatheter arterial embolization.

We have treated 13 patients with advanced breast cancer with intraarterial chemotherapy. Adriamycin and 5-FU were administered via the subclavian artery into the internal mammary artery. We obtained an overall 62% clinical response rate. One patient had a complete response, and 7 had partial responses that lasted between 2 and 12 mo. There are no well-controlled studies in the literature; all the reported studies demonstrate local tumor response, feasibility, and tolerability of this procedure *(62–65)*. Thus, intraarterial chemotherapy for locally advanced or recurrent breast cancer is feasible and has relatively low toxicity and significant local tumor response rates. It should be part of the physician's armamentarium to be used either as adjuvant or neoadjuvant treatment for the right indications.

7. OTHER REGIONAL TREATMENTS

Photodynamic laser therapy has been used for advanced breast cancer *(66)*, and local hyperthermia combined with external irradiation for regional recurrent breast carcinoma *(67)*.

8. DISCUSSION

The current trend in treating breast cancer is toward decreasing the extent of surgery of the breast and axilla. Although the gold standard for local disease control in the breast is surgical excision, currently we have not been able to make the leap to a minimally invasive or completely virtual knife. The data available from recent studies demonstrate that the use of a minimally ablative technique it is feasible; nevertheless there are still problems to be solved before this method can be adapted and substitute for the standard surgical procedure. Ablative treatment uses thermal energy; either cooling the tumor by cryosurgery or heating the tumor and causing cell death.

These procedures are minimally or noninvasive, they can be done under sedation in an outpatient setting, and they are attractive to both the patient and the health care system. Becaus of breast cancer screening and the advances in breast imaging, there is a decrease in the size of the tumors detected, making them more suitable for *in situ* ablation. The fact that the extent of local treatment probably does not affect survival may enhance its future use.

A multidisciplinary team approach is necessary to carry out minimally invasive procedures. The surgeon as well as the radiologist, pathologist, oncologist, and radiation oncologist need to work in close collaboration. All tumor data needed from the tumor for future treatment, in addition to tissue diagnosis, need to be acquired prior to tissue ablation. If necessary, core biopsies can be repeated.

Imaging technology has been crucial in the application of ablative therapies. Imaging is necessary for identifying the extent of the disease, targeting, planning, ablative margin planning, real-time monitoring of treatment, and assessing whether complete tumor ablation with free margins was achieved. MRI is currently superior to CT and ultrasonography. MRI can assist in identifying, targeting, and giving a real-time image of the lesion. On the other hand, MRI is limited because of magnetic field interference, the need to have special MR-compatible equipment, and the relative discomfort to the patient. From the pathological point of view, since we are unable to image complete tumor destruction down to the cellular level, repeated core biopsies will be necessary to confirm tumor destruction. Determining margin negativity is also problematic, although accurate treatment planning and observation in real time by MR can give some assurance.

FUS ablation, a completely noninvasive procedure, combined with MRI to produce a 3D image of the tumor as well as real-time temperature readings, can be used with high accuracy, making FUS the most promising ablative tool of the future.

Unfortunately, clinical experience with ablative modalities in comparison with conventional surgery is limited. Such techniques should be considered technically feasible, and the many associated issues (such as the accuracy and completeness of ablation and long term oncologic and aesthetic outcomes) should be further investigated in controlled studies.

Nevertheless, with greater advances in technology, imaging, and scientific knowledge, these less aggressive noninvasive novel treatments should substitute for the standard approach to breast cancer. The future generation of surgeons treating breast cancer will be required to change their classic approach of "surgery with the scalpel" and will have to acquire imaging, technological, molecular biology, and teamwork expertise.

Acknowledgments

The authors would like to thank Dr. D Zipple for his editorial comments, Mrs. Nina Hakak for data acquisition and Drs. Y. Inbar, J. Itscahk, A. Yosipovivch, and U. Kopilovich. for data and assistance with FUS treatment of breast cancer.

REFERENCES

1. Willett WC, Rockhill B, Hankinson SE, Hunter D, Colditz GA. Nongenetic factors in the causation of breast cancer, in Diseases of the Breast, 3rd ed. (Harris JR, Lippman ME, Morrow M, Osborne CK, eds.), Philadelphia, PA: Lippincott Williams & Wilkins, 2004:223–276.
2. Morrow M, Harris JR. Local management of invasive cancer: breast, in Diseases of the Breast, 3rd ed. (Harris JR, Lippman ME, Morrow M, Osborne CK, eds.), Philadelphia, PA: Lippincott Williams & Wilkins, 2004:719–744.
3. Solin LJ, Fourquet A, Vicini FA, et al. Salvage treatment for local recurrence after breast conserving surgery and radiation as initial treatment for mammographically detected ductal carcinoma in situ of the breast. Cancer 2001;91:1090–1097.
4. Huston TL, Simmons RM. Locally recurrent breast cancer after conservation therapy. Am J Surgery 2005;189:229–235.
5. Fisher B, Anderson S, Bryant J, et al. Twenty-year follow-up of a randomized trial comparing total mastectomy,lumpectomy and lumpectomy plus irradiation for the treatment of breast cancer. N Engl J Med 2002:347:1233–1241.
6. Veronesi U, Cascinelli N, Mariana L. Twenty year follow-up of a randomized study comparing breast conserving surgery with radical mastectomy for early breast cancer. N Engl J Med 2002:347: 1227–1232.
7. van der Hage JA, Putter H, Bonnema J, Bartelink H, Therasse P, van der Valde CJH. Impact of locoregional treatment on the early-stage breast cancer patients :a retrospective analysis. Eur J Cancer 2003;39:2192–2199.
8. Krag D, Weaver D, Ashikaga T. The sentinel node in breast cancer –a multicenter validation study. N Engl J Med 1988:339:941–946.
9. Cance WG, Carey LA, Calvo BF. Long term outcome of neoadjuvant therapy for locally advanced breast carcinoma: effective clinical downstaging allows breast preservation and predicts outstanding local control and survival. Ann Surg 2001:236:295–302.

10. Park CC, Mitsumori M, Nixon A, et al. Outcome of 8 years after breast conserving surgery and radiation therapy for invasive breast cancer: influence of margin status and systematic therapy on local recurrence. Clin Oncol 2000;18:1668–1675.

11. Menes TH, Tartter PI, Bleiweiss I, Godbold JH, Estabrook A. The consequence of multiple re-excisions to obtain clear lumpectomy margins in breast cancer patients. Ann Surg Oncol 2005; 12:1–5.

12. Singletary SE. Minimally invasive techniques in breast cancer treatment. Semin Surg Oncol 2001;20:246–250.

13. Noguchi M. Minimally invasive surgery for small breast cancer. J Surg Oncol 2003;84:94–101.

14. Steeves RA. Hyperthermia in cancer therapy: where are we today and where are we going? Bull NY Acad Med 1992;68:341–350.

15. Stocks LH, Chang HR, Kaufman CS, et al. Pilot study of minimally invasive ultrasound-guided cryoablation in breast cancer. Presented at the American Society of Breast Surgeons Meeting, Boston, MA, 2002.

16. Pfleiderer SO, Freesmeyer MG, Marx C, et al. Cryotherapy of breast cancer under ultrasound guidance Initial results and limitations. Eur Radiol 2002;12:3009–3014.

17. Sabel S, Kaufman CS, Whitworth PW, et al. Cryoablation of early stage breast cancer. Work in progress report of a multi-institutional trial. Ann Surg Oncol 2004;11:542–549.

18. Rand W, Rand RP, Eggerding FA, et al. Cryolumpectomy for carcinoma of the breast. Surg gynecol Obstet 1987;165:392–396.

19. Huston TL, Simmons RM. Ablative therapies for the treatment of malignant diseases of the breast. Am J Surg 2005;189:694–701.

20. Hall-Craggs MA, Vaidya JS. Minimally invasive therapy for the treatment of breast tumors. Eur J Radiol 2002;42:52–57.

21. Singletary SE, Fornage BD, Sneige N, et al. Radiofrequency ablation of early-stage invasive breast tumors: an overview. Cancer J 2002;8:177–180.

22. Mirza AN, Fornage BD, Sneige N, et al. Radiofrequency ablation of solid tumors. Cancer J 2001; 7:95–102.

23. Raut CP, Izzo F, Marra P, et al .Significant long-term survival after radiofrequency ablation of unresectable hepatocellular carcinoma in patients with cirrhosis. Ann Surg Oncol 2005;12:616–628.

24. McGahan JP, Prowning PD, Brock JM, Tesluk H. Hepatic ablation using radiofrequency electrocautery. Invest Radiol 19990;25:267–270.

25. Jeffrey SS, Birdwell RJ, Ikeda DM, et al. Radiofrequency ablation of breast cancer. Arch Surg 1999;134:1064–1068.

26. Izzo F, Thomas R, Delrio P, et al. Radiofrequency ablation in patients with primary breast carcinoma. A pilot study in 26 patients. Cancer 2001;92:2036–2044.

27. Singletary SE. New approaches to surgery for breast cancer. Endocr Rel Cancer 2001;8:265–286.

28. Singletary SE. Feasibility of radiofrequency ablation for primary breast cancer. Breast Cancer 2003;10:4–9.

29. Noguchi M. Radiofrequency ablation treatment for breast cancer to meet the next challenge: how to treat primary breast tumor without surgery. Breast Cancer 2003;10:1–3.

30. Elliott RL, Rice PB, Suits JA, et al. Radiofrequency ablation of a stereotactically localized nonpalpable breast carcinoma. Am Surg 2002;68:1–5.

31. Hayasi A, Silver SF, van der Westhuizen NG. Treatment of invasive breast carcinoma with ultrasound-guided radiofrequency ablation. Am J Surg 2003;185:429–435.

32. Burak WE Jr., Povoski SP, Yanssens TL, et al. Radiofrequency ablation of invasive breast cancer followed by delayed surgical excision. Radiofrequency ablation of invasive breast cancer followed by delayed surgical excision. Breast Cancer Res Treat 2002;96:s116.

33. Burak WE, Angese MA, Povoski SP, et al. Radiofrequency ablation of invasive breast carcinoma followed by delayed surgical excision. Cancer 2003;98:1369–1376.

34. Hall-Craggs MA. Interventional MRI of the breast: minimally invasive therapy. Eur Radiol 2000;10:59–62.

35. Harms S. Percutaneous ablation of breast lesions by radiologists and surgeons. Breast Dis 2001;13: 67–75.

36. Bloom KJ, Dowlatshahi K, Assad L. Pathologic changes after interstitial laser therapy of infiltrating breast carcinoma. Am J Surg 2001;182:384–388.

37. Dowlatshahi K, Francescatti D, Bloom KJ. Laser therapy for small breast cancers. Am J Surg 2002;184:359–363.
38. Harms S, Mumtaz H, Hyslop B, et al. RODEO MRI guided laser ablation of breast cancer. Proc Int Soc Opt Eng 1999;3590:484–489.
39. Izzo F, Thomas R, Delrio P, et al. Radiofrequency ablation in patients with primary breast carcinoma—a pilot study of 26 patients. Cancer 2001;92:2036–2044.
40. Lai LM, Hall-Craggs MA, Mumtaz H, et al. Interstitial laser photocoagulation for fibroadenomas of the breast. Breast 1999;8:89–94.
41. Hill CR, ter Haar GR, Review article: high intensity focused ultrasound—potential for cancer treatment. Br J Radiol 1995;68:1296–1303.
42. Gianfelice D, Khiat A, Amara M, Belblidia A, Boulanger Y. MR imaging-guided focused US ablation of breast cancer: histopathologic assessment of effectiveness-initial experience. Radiology 2003;227:849–855.
43. Zippel DB, Papa MZ. The use of MRI imaging guided focused ultrasound in breast cancer patients; a preliminary phase one study and review. Breast Cancer 2005;12:32–38.
44. Gianfelice D, Khiat A, Boulanger Y, Amara M, Belblidia A. Feasibility of magnetic resonance imaging-guided focused ultrasound surgery as an adjunct to tamoxifen therapy in high-risk surgical patients with breast carcinoma. J Vasc Interv Radiol 2003;14:1275–1282.
45. Hynynen K, Pomeroy O, Smith DN, et al. MR imaging-guided focused ultrasound surgery of fibroadenomas in the breast: a feasibility study. Radiology 2001;219:176–185.
46. Gardner RA, Vargas HI, Block JB, et al. Focused microwave phased array thermotherapy for primary breast cancer. Ann Surg Oncol 2002;9:326–332.
47. Vargas HI, Dooley WC, Gardner RA, et al. Focused microwave phases array thermotherapy for ablation of early-stage breast cancer. Results of thermal dose escalation. Ann Surg Oncol 2004;11:139–146.
48. Fujimoto S, Kobayashi K, Takahashi M, et al. Clinical pilot studies on pre-operative hyperthermic tumour ablation for advanced breast carcinoma using an 8 MHz radiofrequency heating device. Int J Hyperthermia 2003;19:13–22.
49. Gardner RA, Heywang-Kobrunner SH, Dooley WC, et al. Phase II clinical studies of focused microwave phased array thermotherapy for primary breast cancer. A progress report. Presented at the American Society of Breast Surgeons Meeting, Boston, MA, 2002.
50. Malin JL, Schuster MA, Kahn KA, et al. Quality of breast cancer care: what do we know? J Clin Oncol 2002;20:4381–4393.
51. Vicini FA, Kestin L, Chen P, Benitez P, Goldstein NS, Martinez A. Limited-field radiation therapy in the management of early-stage breast cancer. J Natl Cancer Inst 2003;95:1205–1211.
52. DiFronzo LA, Tsai PI, Hwang JM, et al. Breast conserving surgery and accelerated partial breast irradiation using the MammoSite system. Arch Surg 2005;140:787–794.
53. Sauer G, Strnad V, Kurzeder C, Kreienberg R, Sauer R. Partial breast irradiation after breast-conserving surgery. Strahlenther Onkol 2005;181:1–8.
54. King TA, Bolton JS, Kuske RR, et al. Long-term results of wide-field brachy- therapy as the sole method of radiation therapy after segmental mastectomy for T(is 1,2) breast cancer. Am J Surg 2000;180:299–304.
55. Strnad V, Otto O, Potter R, et al. Interstitial brachytherapy alone after breast conserving surgery: interim results of a German-Austrian multicenter phase II trial. J Brachyther 2004;3:115–119.
56. Vicini FA, Baglan KL, Kestin LL, et al. Accelerated treatment of breast cancer. J Clin Oncol 2001;19:1993–2001.
57. Dickler A, Kirk MC, Chu J, Nguyen C. The MammoSiteTM breast brachtherapy applicator: a review of technique and outcomes. Brachytherapy 2005;4:130–136.
58. Vaidya JS, Tobias JS, Baum M, et al. Intraoperative radiotherapy for breast cancer. Lancet Oncol 2004;5:165–173.
59. Veronesi U, Orecchia R, Luini A, et al. A preliminary report of intraoperative radiotherapy (IORT) in limited-stage breast cancers that are conservatively treated. Eur J Cancer 2001;37:2178–183.
60. Aigner KR. Intra-arterial infusion: overview and novel approaches. Semin Surg Oncol 1998;14:248–253.
61. Doughty JC, McCarter DH, Kane E, Reid AW, Cooke TG, McArdle CS. Anatomical basis of intra-arterial chemotherapy for patients with locally advanced breast cancer. Br J Surg 1996;83:1128–1130.

62. Cantore M, Fiorentini G, Cavazzini G, et al. Four years experience of primary intra-arterial chemo-therapy (PIAC) for locally advanced and recurrent breast cancer. Minerva Chir 1997;52:1077–1082.
63. Koyama H, Wada T, Takashashi Y, Iwanaga T, Aoki Y. Intra-arterial infusion chemotherapy as preoperative treatment for locally advanced breast cancer. Cancer 1975;36:1603–1612.
64. Gorich J, Hasan I, Sittek H, et al. Superselective intra-arterial chemotherapy in breast cancer. Radiologe 1993;33:308–312.
65. Morandi C, Colopi S, Cantore M, et al. Intra-arterial chemotherapy in locally advanced or recurrent breast neoplasms. Radiol Med 1996;92:101–104.
66. Schmidt S. Photodynamic laser therapy of advanced breast carcinomas. Geburtshilfe Frauenheilkd 1996;56:M153–M156.
67. Gong L, Mitsumori M, Ogura M, et al. Local hyperthermia combined with external irradiation for regional recurrent breast carcinoma. In J Clin Oncol 2004;9:179–183.

19 Regional Therapy in Ovarian Cancer

Marcello Deraco, MD, Francesco Raspagliesi, MD, and Shigeki Kusamura, MD

CONTENTS

SUMMARY

Advanced epithelial ovarian cancer (EOC) is an aggressive disease that remains and progresses inside the peritoneal cavity for most of its natural history. Despite the initial relative sensibility to first-line chemotherapy, most patients relapse and ultimately die of chemoresistant disease. The best second treatment option for recurrent disease has not been defined thus far. Secondary cytoreductive surgery (CRS) associated with hyperthermic intraperitoneal chemotherapy (HIPEC) seems to constitute a possible second-line treatment option based on the results of phase II studies. A prospective randomized study testing the effectiveness of CRS + HIPEC in EOC is ongoing and the future prospects should aim at the refinement of its indications.

Key Words: Advanced epithelial ovarian cancer; regional therapy; HIPEC; CRS.

1. INTRODUCTION

Epithelial ovarian cancer (EOC) is a clinically important health problem in Western countries, ranking fifth highest in incidence and fourth highest in site-specific causes of cancer deaths in women. In spite of progress in surgical techniques and chemotherapy using platinum alone or platinum and paclitaxel in combination, the long-term survival rates remain poor, and median survival is on the order of 36 mo for advanced cases *(1)*.

The conventional clinical approach for advanced (stage III/IV) EOC is based on cytoreductive surgery (CRS) followed by systemic chemotherapy. The initial relative

From: *Cancer Drug Discovery and Development: Regional Cancer Therapy*
Edited by: P. M. Schlag and U. S. Stein © Humana Press Inc., Totowa, NJ

good responsiveness to chemotherapy is well known. Clinical studies have shown that cisplatin and/or paclitaxel-based first-line chemotherapy allows the achievement of response rates of about 70 to 80%, with a significant proportion of complete responses (2). However, negative second-look laparotomy does not necessarily mean the patient is cured. Unfortunately, a considerable percentage of these patients relapse and ultimately die of chemoresistant disease.

2. CYTOREDUCTION

A recent metaanalysis (3) has confirmed that maximal cytoreduction is one of the most powerful determinants of cohort survival in stage III to IV EOC.

However, some authors challenge the independent influence of cytoreduction on final outcome, arguing that complete cytoreduction in most cases is possible thanks to relatively small tumor burdens and presumed diminished tumor aggressiveness rather than to maximal surgical effort (4,5). Some studies have shown differences in survival between patients who are already optimal at the beginning of surgery and patients who are optimal as a result of the first operation (5,6). According to Hoskin et al., at initial CRS, a patient presenting with large-volume tumor would not have the same chance for survival as a patient with small-volume disease (6). On the other hand, Le et al. did not find a significant difference between patients with initial microscopic disease and patients with large-volume disease at the time of exploration and reduction of the tumor to microscopic residuals (7).

Another criticism raised against cytoreduction is that it can only benefit a small proportion of patients. In fact, the rate of optimal cytoreduction has ranged from 25 to 40%, according to the current literature (4,8–11). Thus, an ultraradical procedure has been proposed by some surgeons, who have achieved a rate of optimal cytoreduction as high as 91% (5,12–16). However, there is no consensus on whether the level of intervention can be translated to survival benefit, or that it necessarily results in increased risk of morbidity.

Eisenkop et al. evaluated 213 stage III EOC patients who had to cytoreduction using procedures such as extrapelvic bowel resection, diaphragm stripping, full-thickness diaphragm resection, modified posterior pelvic exenteration, peritoneal implant ablation and/or aspiration, and excision of grossly involved retroperitoneal lymph nodes (17). They verified that survival was independently influenced only by the extent of peritoneal carcinomatosis that required removal. Use of these procedures as well as the type of adjuvant chemotherapy did not impact on the final outcome. The authors concluded that the need to resect a widespread peritoneal carcinomatosis correlates with biological aggressiveness and diminished survival, but not significantly enough to justify abbreviation of the operative effort.

In summary, whether a maximal surgical effort could outweigh the inherent biological aggressiveness of the tumor and produce a favorable impact on the final outcome of patients is a matter of heated debate in the literature, and clarification of the issue will be provided only by a prospective controlled trial.

2.1. Secondary Cytoreduction

About 50% of the patients with EOC have residual disease after first-line chemotherapy due to partial or no response. On the other hand, up to 47% of complete responders to first-line chemotherapy relapse within 5 yr, and the disease-free survival does not generally exceed 18 mo *(18,19)*.

Thus, several alternatives have been proposed as second-line treatment. One of them is the surgical approach. However, the value of secondary cytoreduction has not been clearly defined. When it is performed at the time of second look, most studies, which are not randomized *(20–23)* demonstrate some survival advantage for patients whose tumors can be cytoreduced to microscopic or small macroscopic residual disease. When the second-look operation is performed and residual tumor is detected, it seems advisable to remove all macroscopic disease if technically feasible.

According to a retrospective review of the literature, optimal cytoreduction was achievable in 38 to 87% of the relapsing cases with an acceptable perioperative complication and mortality rate. Unfortunately, there is no randomized evidence supporting the use of secondary CRS as salvage therapy in EOC. Current data suggest that patients left with no gross residual disease after secondary cytoreduction seem to benefit from prolonged survival, in the range of 44 to 60 mo *(24)*. The actual evidence suggests that the removal of all recurrent macroscopic disease should be accomplished if technically feasible, especially in patients with a disease-free interval of more than 12 mo, for platinum-sensitive tumors, and in the absence of ascites *(25)*.

3. SYSTEMIC SECOND-LINE THERAPIES

During the last decade, several new drugs have been shown to have some activity in second-line therapy. Paclitaxel, pegylated liposomal doxorubicin, topotecan, docetaxel, gemcitabine, oxaliplatin, vinorelbine, and ET-743 have joined other, more "classical" drugs like carboplatin, cisplatin, epirubicin, ifosfamide, altretamine, or oral etoposide. Despite the growing number of randomized trials addressing second-line treatments for EOC, no drug, alone or in combination, has been elected as the best. The management of recurrent disease constitutes a complex decision-making process requiring the consideration of several parameters such as platinum sensibility and treatment-free interval. The available data show overall response rates for these drugs chemotherapies ranging from 3.3 to 16%, with a median overall survival (OS) of 35 to 41 wk in the subset of patients with platinum-refractory EOC *(26,27)*.

4. SECONDARY CYTOREDUCTION OR SECOND-LINE CHEMOTHERAPY?

Gungor et al. *(28)* reported on 75 patients with ovarian cancer of whom 44 had salvage surgery and 31 had salvage chemotherapy alone for the treatment of gross recurrent disease. All patients had been clinically free of disease more than 6 mo from the completion of primary treatment. Survival was significantly longer in patients who had salvage surgery compared with those who had salvage chemotherapy alone ($p = 0.03$). The authors concluded that patients with recurrent EOC may benefit in terms of outcome from a salvage surgical cytoreduction specially if macroscopically complete.

The European Organization for the Research and Treatment of Cance (EORTC) (Protocol 55963) is conducting a randomized trial to provide more conclusive data for the management of recurrent EOC. The inclusion criteria are disease recurrence after a minimum of three cycles of primary chemotherapy and a disease-free interval of 12 mo.

Patients are randomized to either six cycles of single-agent platinum (carboplatin or cisplatin) or three cycles of the same chemotherapy, followed by surgical exploration and three more cycles of chemotherapy. They are stratified by initial stage, progression-free survival (<24 vs >24 mo), initial response to primary therapy, and tumor burden. Anticipated accrual is 700 patients, and survival is the primary end point.

To summarize, the standard treatment strategy for patients with relapsing or persistent ovarian cancer after completion of upfront first-line chemotherapy has not yet been clearly defined.

5. REGIONAL TREATMENT APPROACH FOR EOC

The rationale for regional treatment for EOC is based on the natural history of the disease, which remains confined in the peritoneal cavity for most of its course. This pattern of spread would seem to indicate the potential usefulness of selectively increasing drug concentration in the tumor-bearing area direct intraperitoneal chemotherapy instillation (29). A large intergroup trial randomized 546 optimally cytoreduced stage III patients with EOC to intraperitoneal cisplatin plus intravenous cyclophosphamide or intravenous cisplatin plus intravenous cyclophosphamide (30). Intraperitoneal therapy was associated with a significantly improved median survival (49 vs 41 mo) and fewer toxic side effects. In a subsequent Gynecologic Oncology Group trial, 523 patients were randomized to intravenous cisplatin/paclitaxel or high-dose carboplatin followed by intraperitoneal cisplatin plus intravenous paclitaxel. The preliminary results demonstrated a significant increase in recurrence-free interval (28 vs 22 mo), without the same favorable impact on overall survival (31). The results of these trials have, however, not substantially altered clinical practice.

6. CYTOREDUCTIVE SURGERY AND INTRAPERITONEAL HYPERTHERMIC PERFUSION FOR EPITHELIAL OVARIAN CANCER

Intraperitoneal chemotherapy under normothermia was generally judged to create more logistical problems than survival benefit. Poor drug distribution from surgical adhesions, inadequate drug penetration into tumor nodules or tumor entrapped in scar tissue, and repeated failures with long-term peritoneal access have led to this conclusion.

Thus a new multimodality treatment approach comprising CRS and hyperthermic intraperitoneal chemotherapy (HIPEC) was conceived to overcome these drawbacks. Using intraperitoneal chemotherapy as a planned part of a cytoreduction for carcinomatosis, such logistical problems may no longer occur. All adhesions are taken down, scar tissue is resected, and visible cancer nodules are resected. Intraperitoneal chemotherapy is required to eradicate microscopic residual disease; however, it should be performed under hyperthermic perfusion.

The rationale for the use of hyperthermia is multifactorial. Hyperthermia itself has a direct cytotoxic effect caused by denaturation of proteins, induction of heat-shock proteins (which may serve as receptors for natural killer cells), induction of apoptosis, and inhibition of angiogenesis (32–34). The biophysical effects of hyperthermia also include alterations in multimolecular complexes such as the insulin receptor (35) and in the cytoskeleton (36), as well as changes in enzyme complexes for DNA synthesis and repair (37). Moreover, the architecture of the vasculature in solid tumors is chaotic, resulting in regions with low pH, hypoxia, and low glucose levels *(38)*. This susceptible microenvironment renders solid tumors more sensitive to hyperthermia. In addition, hyperthermia also acts in synergy with chemotherapies such as mitomycin C, cisplatin, mitroxantrone, taxanes, and doxorubicin. Increased cell-membrane permeability at higher temperatures can increase drug uptake by tumor tissue *(39)*. The pharmacokinetics of these drugs can also be affected by altered active drug transport and cell metabolism. Furthermore, at 40 to 42°C, neoplastic cells become more chemosensitive owing to an increase in the intracellular concentration of drugs and their activation process, especially for alkylating agents, and to alterations in the DNA repair process *(40,41)*. It has been demonstrated that the formation of platinum-DNA adducts after cisplatin exposure in hyperthermic conditions is enhanced and/or adduct removal is decreased in heated cells, resulting in relatively higher DNA damage *(42,43)*. Besides this synergistic effect, hyperthermia can also diminish the systemic toxicity of some drugs (e.g., doxorubicin and cyclophosphamide) by increasing their alkylation and/or excretion *(44)*.

6.1. Technique of Cytoreductive Surgery

The peritonectomy procedure described by Sugarbaker is used *(45)*. Residual disease after surgery is classified according to Sugarbaker criteria *(46)*: cc-0: no residual disease; cc-1: minimal residual disease, 0 to 2.5 mm; cc-2: residual disease 2.5 mm to 2.5 cm; cc-3: residual disease >2.5 cm.

The surgical procedure starts with a xyphopubic, midline incision; the successive layers of abdominal wall are dissected until the parietal peritoneum is visualized. Then dissection of the parietal peritoneum from the abdominal wall starts without opening of the peritoneal cavity and continues until the identification of major retroperitoneal structures such as the lower segment of the aorta, the vena cava, the iliac arteries/veins, and the ureters. The parietal peritoneum is then incised and full access to the abdominal cavity is achieved through the use of a Thompson self-retaining retractor. A ball-tip electrosurgical handpiece is used to dissect the tumor on peritoneal and visceral surfaces from normal tissue *(47)*. The electrosurgery is used on a pure cut at high voltage.

Each procedure that composes the peritonectomy technique has a definite resection that requires an orderly sequence of surgical maneuvers. One or more of following steps can be performed depending on previously performed surgical procedures or disease extension at the time of laparotomy: (1) infragastric resection of the great omentectum, right parietal peritonectomy, and right colon resection; (2) left upper quadrant peritonectomy, splenectomy, and left parietal peritonectomy; (3) right upper quadrant peritonectomy and Glissonian's capsule resection; (4) lesser omentectomy, cholecystectomy and stripping of omental bursa ± antrectomy; (5) pelvic peritonectomy with sigmoid colon resection ± hysterectomy + bilateral salpingo-oophorectomy if still present; and (6) other intestinal resection and/or abdominal mass resection.

Some considerations are worth discussing. First, the surgical effort should aim at a cytoreduction down to nodules less than 2.5 mm and not the traditional cut-off adopted by gynecologic oncologists of 1 to 2 cm. The rationale for this new concept of oncological radicality is based on the fact that the depth of maximum tumor penetration of the drugs used for HIPEC is no more than 2.5 mm *(48)*.

The second point is that the oncological principle of *en bloc* resection should be followed especially in cases requiring resection of pelvic visceras (rectosigmoid ± genital tract) along with the pelvic peritoneum *(16,49)*. Dissection of the pelvic peritoneum starts on the right and left sides of the bladder. The apex of the bladder is maintained on strong traction with clamps. Broad traction on the entire anterior parietal peritoneal surface and frequent saline irrigation reveal the cleavage plain that is precisely located between the bladder musculature and its adherent fatty tissue. The peritoneum with the underlying fatty tissue is stripped away from the surface of the bladder down to the uterine cervix. The stripping of the peritoneum continues in a centripetal fashion in the rest of the pelvis.

Attention must be paid to the lateral aspects of the bladder near its base, where the ureters can be localized. Sometimes dissection of the ureters from the parametrium is required to ensure better visualization of their entry point into the bladder. The uterine arteries are ligated extraperitoneally, just above the ureter and close to the base of the bladder. The bladder is moved gently off the cervix, and the vagina is entered. The vaginal cuff anterior and posterior to the cervix is transected, and the rectovaginal septum is entered. A linear stapler is used to divide the sigmoid colon at the junction of the sigmoid and descending colon or just above the limits of the pelvic tumor. The vascular supply of the distal portion of the bowel is traced back to its origin on the aorta. The inferior mesenteric artery and vein are ligated, sutured, and divided. Ball-tipped electrosurgery is used to divide the perirectal fat beneath the peritoneal reflection. This ensures that all tumors occupying the cul-de-sac are removed intact with the specimen. The rectal musculature is skeletonized, and the lower half of the rectum is preserved. A reticular stapler is used to close off the rectal stump and the rectum is sharply divided above the stapler.

Surgery extension is usually defined according to macroscopic disease extension. However, some procedures such as resection of the lesser omentum are always indicated, even in the absence of metastatic disease in this structure, because this maneuvre allows better distribution of the perfusate containing the drugs in the upper abdomen region, during HIPEC.

Reconstructive procedures such as bowell anastomosis could be performed after or before the HIPEC, without significant difference in the postoperative complications rate. Protective ostomies could be indicated according to the surgeon's discretion. At the National Cancer Institutie (NCI) of Milan, we adopt a policy of performing protective ostomies only in the presence of extremely high-risk bowel anastomosis*(50)*, and the rate of bowel complications had not increased significantly with respect to data from the literature.

6.3. Hyperthermic Intraperitoneal Chemotherapy

After the CRS, four Tenckhoff catheters are placed in the abdominal cavity. Two inflow catheters are placed in the right subphrenic cavity and at a deep pelvic level, respectively, and two further catheters are placed in the left subphrenic cavity and in the superficial pelvic site.

6.3.1. THE DEVICE

HIPEC requires the use of a lung-heart machine, comprising a roller pump, a thermostat, a heat exchanger, and an extracorporeal circuit. The perfusate flow is controlled (as well as the heat exchanger, which adjusts the temperature of perfusate) by circulating water at a desired temperature in the arterial phase of the circuit. The extracorporeal circuit consists of interconnected tubes that have: (1) an input section (inflow); (2) an output section (outflow); (3) an axis for rapid filling; (4) a central body connected with a filter; (5) a deflow section; and (6) a series of multiperforated catheters in the extremities

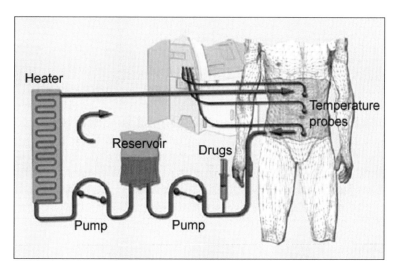

Fig. 1. The device and the extracorporeal circuit for hyperthermic intraperitoneal chemotherapy.

of the tubes (Fig. 1). The device should be approved by CE accreditation. Several centers are using the Performer LRT® (RAND, Medolla, Italy).

6.3.2. THE PERFUSATE

The perfusate, defined as the liquid filling the circuit, could be of various types: a peritoneal dialysis solution *(51)*, a physiologic solution *(52)*, or a Normosol solution R, pH 7.4, mixed with Haemagel (in a 2:1 proportion). The priming volume ought to be abundant enough to achieve homogeneity and constancy of heating, but not excessive, to avoid abdominal distension and bodily thermodilution. For optimal effect, 2 L/m^2 of perfusate for the open technique and 3.5 L/m^2 for closed technique are usually sufficient *(53–55)*.

6.3.3. OPTIMAL DRUG COMBINATION

Various drug combinations for ovarian cancer have been tested by experimental and phase I/II clinical studies: cisplatin alone *(56,57)*, carboplatin alone *(58)*, mitoxantrone alone *(59)*, cisplatin + doxorubicin *(60)*, and docetaxel *(55)*. The criteria for choosing the ideal combination should be based on the pharmacokinetic profile of the drug, tumor chemosensitivity, and toxicity. Ideally, the drug should be water soluble and of high molecular weight, to guarantee a low peritoneal clearance. This, combined with a high systemic clearance, will result in a pharmacological advantage expressed by a higher exposure of tumor to the agent (high AUC_{pe}/AUC_{pl} ratio). For intraperitoneal therapy to be oncologically effective, the drug must have good tumor penetration. The influence of temperature in the cytotoxicity should also be of concern: the higher the cell killing capacity of the drug owing to the hyperthermia the better. Finally, non-cell-cycle-specific drugs are preferred because they are cytotoxic even after a relatively short exposure time.

Since its advent, cisplatin has become the most widely used agent in the systemic treatment of ovarian cancer, with a response rate of 50%. When cisplatin was employed intraperitoneally in the treatment of EOC, a comparable distinctive antiblastic effect was shown. Cisplatin has a high AUC_{pe}/AUC_{pl} ratio, compared with other cytostatic drugs, a deep tumor penetration, and partial response rate of up to 65% in normothermic conditions *(61)*.

Another eligible agent for HIPEC is carboplatin. Despite a better therapeutic index than cisplatin, with substantially less renal toxicity, nausea, and neurotoxicity, carboplatin does not have as favorable pa harmacokinetic profile as cisplatin (58,57). In fact, the AUC_{pe}/AUC_{pl} ratio, tumor penetration, and response rate are markedly lower *(63,64)*.

Doxorubicin has one of the highest AUC_{pe}/AUC_{pl} ratios, about 80 *(65,66)*. Irrespective of its limited tumor diffusion ability (not more than several cell layers), a response rate of 30% was reported when doxorubicin was administered intraperitoneally, under normothermic conditions *(67)*. The dose-limiting toxicity (chemically induced peritonitis) makes doxorubicin feasible for HIPEC only at very low doses.

Oxaliplatin *(68)*, paclitaxel *(69)*, gemcitabine *(70)*, and docetaxel *(55)* are also promising for HIPEC in the treatment of ovarian cancer. However, since they are still under experimental use or have not been tested in phase II clinical investigations, they should be further investigated before being evaluated in a prospective phase III trial.

In summary, the best chemotherapy combination for HIPEC for patients with EOC is still to be defined. Experimental and phase I/II clinical studies suggest a combination of cisplatin and doxorubicin as the currently most advisable regimen. The drug doses are: cisplatin (CDDP; 43.0 mg/L of perfusate) and Adriamycin (Dx; 15.25 mg/L of perfusate) *(71,72)*.

6.3.4. MODALITIES OF EXECUTION: OPEN, CLOSED ABDOMINAL, OR SEMICLOSED TECHNIQUES *(72–74)*

In the closed technique the skin of abdominal wall is temporarily closed with a running suture, and the Tenckhoff catheters are connected to the circuit, to initiate the HIPEC. In the open modality, also known as the Coliseum technique *(74)*, the abdomen is covered with a plastic sheet and drug vapor is evacuated to protect the operating room personnel.

The catheters are connected to the extracorporeal circuit, and the preheated polysaline perfusate containing cisplatin and Adriamycin is instilled in the peritoneal cavity using the heart-lung pump at a mean flow of 600 to 1000 mL/min for 90 min. To achieve an intrabdominal temperature of 42.5°C, we maintain an inflow temperature of approx 44°C. Throughout the perfusion, if the open technique is adopted, the surgeon will continuously manipulate the viscera to distribute both heat and chemotherapy. Following perfusion, the perfusate is quickly drained, and the abdomen is closed after careful intracavitary inspection.

7. LITERATURE DATA

Many centers worldwide have initiated regional therapy programs for carcinomatosis secondary to ovarian cancer (Table 1) after seeing the promising results obtained by phase II and III trials testing the combined approach of CRS + HIPEC in other types of cancer.

At the NCI of Milan, 40 patients *(75)* with histologically confirmed advanced EOC were treated by CRS and HIPEC *(75)*. Median follow-up was 26.1 mo (range: 0.3–117.6 mo). Thirteen patients were treated in a second-look setting and 27 in a salvage setting. The median number of systemic chemotherapy lines was two (range: 1-5) which consisted of cisplatin-based, paclitaxel-based or paclitaxel/platinum-containing regimens. HIPEC

Table 1

Phase II studies on cytoreductive surgery and hyperthermic intraperitoneal chemotherapy in ovarian cancer.

Author/year	Disease No.	Setting	Drug schedule	OS	Median OS (mo)	Median PFS (mo)	Median DFS (mo)	Toxicity/complications/mortality
Raspagliesi et al., 2005 (75)	40	Recurrent or partially responsive to first line CHT	CDDP (25 mg/m^2/L) + MMC (3.3 mg/m^2/L) or CDDP (43.0 mg/L) + Dx (15.25 mg/L)	5-yr = 15%	41.4 (mean)	23.9 (mean)	—	Morbidity rate = 5% Toxicity (mild) rate = 15% No treatment-related mortality
Hager et al., 2001 (76)	36	—	CDDP 100 mg/ CBDCA 450 mg	5-yr = 16 ± 7%	19 ± 4 mo	—	—	Mild nausea, vomiting, subileus, peritoneal irritation
Piso et al., 2004 (77)	19	Primary/recurrent	CDDP 75 mg or mitoxantrone 15 mg/m^2	5-yr = 15%	33(± 6)	18	—	Anastomotic leak, bleeding No toxicity One postoperative death;
Zanon et al., 2004 (78)	30	Completion of at least a first line CDDP based CHT	CDDP 100 mg/m^2– 150 mg/m^2	2-yr = 60%	28.1 95%: CI 21.4–34.7	—	—	Major complications: 16.7% intestinal perforation, acaleculus cholecystitis, anastomotic leak, and massive pleural effusion Mortality 3.3%
Ryu et al., 2004 (79)	57	Mainly recurrent	CBDCA 350 mg/m^2 + INF-α 5.000,000 UI/m^2	5-yr = 63.4%	—	—	48.7	Intestinal rupture/obstruction, sepsis, renal failure, hernia
Gori et al., 2005 (53)	29	Consolidation therapy	CDDP 100 mg/m^2	—	64.4	—	—	No intraoperative complication; postop eventration

Abbreviations: OS, overall survival; PFS, progression free survival; DFS, disease-free survival; RD, residual disease; CDDP, cisplatin; MMC, mitomycin-C; CBDCA, carboplatin; CHT, chemotherapy.

was performed with the closed abdomen technique, with cisplatin (25 mg/m^2/L) + mito-mycin-C (3.3 mg/m^2/L) or cisplatin (43.0 mg/L of perfusate) and Adriamycin (15.25 mg/L of perfusate). After the CRS, 33 (83%) patients presented no macroscopic residual disease. Five-year OS was 15%; the mean overall and progression-free survivals were 41.4 and 23.9 mo, respectively. Three variables were shown to be of prognostic significance: completeness of cytoreduction, World Health Organization (WHO) performance status, and extent of carcinomatosis. The treatment-related morbidity was 5%. Six (15%) patients had mild acute toxicity. There was no treatment-related mortality.

In 2001 Hager et al. *(76)* conducted a prospective clinical trial on 36 patients with ovarian cancer treated by CRS + HIPEC . Median OS time from the first HIPEC chemotherapy treatment was 19 ± 4 months. The 5-yr OS rate of all patients from the start of the first HIPEC was 16 ± 7%. The complications were mild especially compared with systemic chemotherapy. In 3 of 162 treatments, clinical ileus was observed.

Piso et al. *(77)* reported on 19 patients with ovarian cancers (11 recurrent and 8 primary). Intraperitoneal chemotherapy consisted of either cisplatin or mitoxantrone. Complete cytoreduction <2 mm was achieved in nine patients. A 5-yr survival rate of 15% was reported even though nine patients had concomitant liver metastases. Survival was the same for both primary and recurrent cases.

Zanon et al. treated 30 patients affected with a relapsing EOC *(78)*. Patients underwent CRS followed by intraoperative HIPEC with cisplatin. Complete cytoreduction down to no or minimal residual disease (cc0-cc1) was obtained in 23 patients (77%). One patient died postoperatively from a pulmonary embolism. Major postoperative morbidity occurred in 5 of the 30 patients (16.7%). Complications were as follows: one case of anastomotic leakage, a spontaneous ileum perforation, a postoperative cholecystitis, a hydrothorax, and one patient with bone marrow toxicity. Median locoregional relapse-free survival and median overall survival were 17.1 mo and 28.1 mo, respectively.

Ryu et al. *(79)* published a retrospective series on ovarian cancer patients treated by CRS with or without HIPEC consisting of carboplatin and interferon-α. All patients had previously undergone the primary standard staging procedure for ovarian cancer. A total of 117 patients were reviewed, and 74 of them had stage III disease. For this subgroup, the median survival was 60.9 mo for the 35 patients receiving both CRS and HIPEC compared with only 22.3 mo for patients in the CRS-only group ($p = 0.0015$). Five-year OS was 53.8% for the former and 33.3% for the latter. The 5-yr disease-free survival reached 26.9% for the former and 10.3% for the latter ($p = 0.0070$). The use of IPHP was shown to be a positive independent prognostic factor along with residual disease <1 cm. The originality of this report relates to the intraperitoneal administration of interferon-α. This immunotherapy was not associated with a higher complication rate than after conventional chemotherapy administered intraperitoneally.

Gori et al. (53) investigated the effect of HIPEC as consolidation therapy in stage III ovarian cancer, following CRS and systemic chemotherapy (cisplatin-cyclophospha-mide). In a multicenter prospective trial, 29 patients with complete or optimal CRS and systemic treatment were included in the consolidation group and received HIPEC, which was performed with the open-abdomen technique, using cisplatin 100 mg/m^2 for 60 min. Disease-free survival, overall survival, and side effects were compared with a control group of patients who refused a second-look surgery and intraperitoneal chemotherapy. The consolidation therapy group showed a better 5-yr survival rate and lower recurrent disease rate, but differences were not statistically significant.

It is hard to ascertain to what extent this apparently longer survival time (OS ranging from 16 to 64%) reported by clinical studies resulted from individual physician selection bias. In addition, most of the studies were retrospective, without a randomized control group and some authors have reported on heterogeneous study populations with the inclusion of histological subtypes other than epithelial and different stage distributions at different time settings in disease evolution (primary disease vs recurrent). Furthermore, the HIPEC modality , drug schedules, and duration of perfusion were not uniform. Finally, most of the studies did not provide information on the percentage of platinum resistant cases in their series.

7.1. Phase III Protocol

To confirm the apparently encouraging results provided by the growing number of phase II studies, the Italian Society of integrated locoregional therapy (SITILO) is conducting a prospective multicenter randomized study to test the effectiveness of secondary CRS associated with HIPEC in patients with cisplatin-resistant advanced EOC *(81)*. Patients with EOC stage III/IV who have had to surgical staging and six courses of first-line platinum-based chemotherapy, and with persistent but clinically resectable disease, or early relapsing tumors (<6 mo after the completion of first-line chemotherapy), will be randomly allocated to one of two treatment groups: (1) study group: secondary CRS and HIPEC followed by second-line chemotherapy; or (2) control group: second-line chemotherapy. Patients will be stratified according to the participating centers. Anticipated accrual is 100 patients per arm, and the primary end point is overall and progression-free survival.

8. FINAL CONSIDERATIONS

The outcome results provided by phase II studies on CRS and HIPEC to treat EOC warrant confirmation by prospective randomized trials. Currently CRS + HIPEC is under investigation as a second-line treatment option. Future efforts should pursue the identification of subsets of patients who would best benefit the most. We need studies testing CRS + HIPEC in other circumstances of disease evolution and also investigations on prognostic factors. For example, CRS + HIPEC could be proposed in the context of a clinical trial in patients with complete response to first-line chemotherapy as a consolidation approach. Studies on clinical and/or biological markers with prognostic significance and predictive value for treatment response would be of utmost importance. The high cost and the considerable morbidity rate point out the need for a judicious choice of patients, a highly skilled surgical team with expertise in peritonectomy procedures, and a well-structured multidisciplinary unit devoted exclusively to the management of peritoneal surface malignancy.

REFERENCES

1. McGuire WP, Hoskin WJ, Brady MF, et al. Cyclophosphamide and cisplatin compared with paclitaxel and cisplatin in patients with stage III and IV ovarian cancer. N Engl J Med 1996;334:1–6.
2. Conte PF, Gadducci A, Cianci C. Second-line treatment and consolidation therapies in advanced ovarian cancer. Int J Gynecol Cancer 2001;11(Suppl 1):52–56.
3. Bristow RE, Tomacruz RS, Armstrong DK, Trimble EL, Montz FJ. Survival effect of maximal cytoreductive surgery for advanced ovarian carcinoma during the platinum era: a meta-analysis. J Clin Oncol 2002;20:1248–1259.

4.   Hoskins WJ, Bundy BN, Thigpen JT, Omura GA. The influence of cytoreductive surgery on recurrence-free interval and survival in small-volume stage III epithelial ovarian cancer: a Gynecologic Oncology Group study. Gynecol Oncol 1992;47:159–166.
5.   Eisenkop SM, Friedman RL, Wang HJ. Complete cytoreductive surgery Is feasible and maximizes survival in patients with advanced epithelial ovarian cancer: prospective study. Gynecol Oncol 1998;69:103–108.
6.   Heintz APM, van Oostrom AT, Trimbos JBMC, et al. The treatment of advanced ovarian carcinoma. I. Clinical variables associated with prognosis. Gynecol Oncol 1988;30:348–358.
7.   Le T, Krepart GV, Lotocki RJ, Heywood MS. Does debulking surgery improve survival in biologically aggressive ovarian carcinoma. Gynecol Oncol 1997;67:208–214.
8.   Bertelson K. Tumor reduction surgery and long-term survival in advanced ovarian cancer: a DACOVA study. Gynecol Oncol 1990;38:203–209.
9.   Eisenkop SM, Spirtos NM, Montag TW, Nalick RH Wang HW. The impact of subspecialty training on the management of advanced ovarian cancer. Gynecol Oncol 1992;47:203–209.
10. LoCoco S, Covens A, Carney M, et al. Does aggressive therapy improve survival in suboptimal stage IIIc/IV ovarian cancer? A Canadian-American comparative study. Gynecol Oncol 1995;59:194–199.
11. Neijt JP, ten Bokkel Huinink WW, et al. Randomised trial comparing two combination chemotherapy regimens (Hexa-CAF vs CHAP-5) in advanced ovarian carcinoma. Lancet 1984;2:594–600.
12. Michel G, De Iaco P, Castaigne D, El-Hassan MJ, et al. Extensive cytoreductive surgery in advanced ovarian carcinoma. Eur J Gynecol Oncol 1997;18:9–15.
13. Brand E, Pearlman N. Electrosurgical debulking of ovarian cancer: a new technique using the argon beam coagulator. Gynecol Oncol 1990;39:115–118.
14. Deppe G, Malviya VK, Boike G, Malone JM Jr. Use of Cavitron surgical aspirator for debulking of diaphragmatic metastases in patients with advanced carcinoma of the ovaries. Surg Gynecol Obstet 1989;168:455–456.
15. Rose PG.The cavitational ultrasonic surgical aspirator for cytoreduction in advanced ovarian cancer. Am J Obstet Gynecol 1992;166:843–846.
16. Benedetti-Panici P, Maneschi F, Scambia G, Cutillo G, Greggi S, Mancuso S. The pelvic retroperitoneal approach in the treatment of advanced ovarian carcinoma. Obstet Gynecol 1996;87:532–538.
17. Eisenkop SM, Spirtos NM. Procedures required to accomplish complete cytoreduction of ovarian cancer: is there a correlation with "biological aggressiveness" and survival? Gynecol Oncol 2001;82:435–441.
18. De Gramont A, Drolet Y, Varette C, et al. Survival after second-look laparotomy in advanced ovarian epithelial cancer. Study of 86 patients. Eur J Cancer Clin Oncol 1989;25:451–457.
19. Gershenson DM, Copeland LJ, Wharton JT, Atkinson EN, Sneige N, Edwards C.L, Rutledge FN. Prognosis of surgically determined complete responders in advanced ovarian cancer. Cancer 1985;5:1129–1135.
20. Podratz KC, Schray MF, Wieand HS, et al. Evaluation of treatment and survival after positive second-look laparotomy. Gynecol Oncol 1988;31:9–24.
21. Hoskins WJ, Rubin SC, Dulaney E, et al. Influence of secondary cytoreduction at the time of second-look laparotomy on the survival of patients with epithelial ovarian carcinoma. Gynecol Oncol 1989;34:365–371.
22. Williams L, Brunetto VL, Yordan E, DiSaia PJ, Creasman WT. Secondary cytoreductive surgery at second-look laparotomy in advanced ovarian cancer: a Gynecologic Oncology Group Study. Gynecol Oncol 1997;66: 171–178.
23. Obermaier A, Sevelda P. Impact of second look laparotomy and secondary cytoreductive surgery at second-look laparotomy in ovarian cancer patients. Acta Obstet Gynecol Scand 2001;80:432–436.
24. Munkarah AR, Coleman RL. Critical evaluation of secondary cytoreduction in recurrent ovarian cancer. Gynecol Oncol 2004;95:273–280. Review.
 5. Salom E, Almeida Z, Mirhashemi R. Management of recurrent ovarian cancer: evidence-based decisions. Curr Opin Oncol 2002;14:519–527. Review.
26. ten Bokkel Huinink WW, Gore M, Carmichael J, et al. Topotecan versus paclitaxel for the treatment of recurrent epithelial ovarian cancer. J Clin Oncol 1997;15:2183–2193.
27. Gordon AN, Fleagle JT, Guthrie D, Parkin DE, Gore ME, Lacave AJ. Recurrent epithelial ovarian carcinoma: a randomized phase III study of pegylated liposomal doxorubicin versus topotecan. J Clin Oncol 2001;19:3312–3322.
28. Gungor M, Ortac F, Arvas M, Kosebay D, Sonmezer M, Kose K. The role of secondary cytoreductive surgery for recurrent ovarian cancer. Gynecol Oncol 2005;97:74–79.
29. Markman M, Kelsen D. Efficacy of cisplatin-based intraperitoneal chemotherapy as treatment of malignant peritoneal mesothelioma. J Cancer Res Clin Oncol 1992;118:547–555.
30. Alberts DS, Liu PY, Hannigan EV, et al. Intraperitoneal cisplatin plus intravenous cyclophosphamide versus intravenous cisplatin plus intravenous cyclophosphamide for stage III ovarian cancer. N Engl J Med 1996;335:1950–1955.
31. Markman M, Bundy BN, Alberts DS, et al. Phase III trial of standard-dose intravenous cisplatin plus paclitaxel versus moderately high-dose carboplatin followed by intravenous paclitaxel and intraperitoneal cisplatin in small-volume stage III ovarian carcinoma: an intergroup study of the Gynecologic Oncology Group, Southwestern Oncology Group, and Eastern Cooperative Oncology Group. J Clin Oncol 2001;19:1001–1007.
32. Christophi C, Winkworth A, Muralihdaran V, Evans P. The treatment of malignancy by hyperthermia. Surg Oncol 1999;7:83–90.

33. Dahl O, Dalene R, Schem BC, Mella O. Status of clinical hyperthermia. Acta Oncol 1999;38:863–873.
34. Roca C, Primo L, Valdembri D, et al. Hyperthermia inhibits angiogenesis by a plasminogen activator inhibitor 1-dependent mechanism. Cancer Res. 2003;63:1500–1507. Erratum in: Cancer Res. 2003;63:2345.
35. Calderwood SK, Hahn GM Thermal sensitivity and resistance of insulin-receptor binding. Biochim Biophys Acta 1983;756:1–8.
36. DuBose DA, Hinkle JR, Morehouse DH, Ogle PL. Model for environmental heat damage of the blood vessel barrier. Wilderness Environ Med 1998;9:130–136.
37. Xu M, Myerson RJ, Straube WL, et al. Radiosensitization of heat resistant human tumor cells by 1 hour at 41.1 degrees C and its effect on DNA repair. Int J Hyperthermia 2002;18:385–403.
38. Vaupel PW. The influence of tumor blood flow and microenvironmental factors on the efficacy of radiation, drugs and localized hyperthermia. Klin Padiatr 1997;209:243–249.
39. Storm FK. Clinical hyperthermia and chemotherapy. Radiol Clin North Am 1989;27:621–627.
40. Engelhardt R. Hyperthermia and drugs. Recent Results Cancer Res 1987;104:136–203.
41. Teicher BA, Kowal CD, Kennedy KA, Sartorelli AC. Enhancement by hyperthermia of the in vitro cytotoxicity of mitomycin C toward hypoxic tumor cells. Cancer Res 1981;41:1096–1099.
42. Vaart PJM, Vange N, Zoetmulder FAN, et al. intraperitoneal cisplatin with regional hyperthermia in advanced ovarian cancer: pharmacokinetics and cisplatin-DNA adduct formation in patients and ovarian cancer cell lines. Eur J Cancer 1998;34:148–154.
43. Hettinga JVE, Lemstra W, Meijer C, et al. Mechanism of hyperthermic potentiation of cisplatin action in cisplatin-sensitive and -resistant tumor cells. Br J Cancer 1997;75:1735–1743.
44. Bull JMC. An update on the anticancer effects of a combination of chemotherapy and hyperthermia. Cancer Res 1984;44:4853s–4856s.
45. Sugarbaker P.H. Peritonectomy procedures. Ann Surg 1995;221:29–42.
46. Jacquet P, Sugarbaker PH. Current methodologies for clinical assessment of patients with peritoneal carcinomatosis. J Exp Clin Cancer Res 1996;15:49–58.
47. Sugarbaker PH. Laser-mode electrosurgery. Cancer Treat Res 1996;82:375–385.
48. Deraco M, Raspagliesi F, Kusamura S. Management of peritoneal surface component of ovarian cancer. Surg Oncol Clin North Am 2003;12:561–583.
49. Paul H. Sugarbaker PH. Complete parietal and visceral peritonectomy of the pelvis for advanced primary and recurrent ovarian cancer, in Peritoneal Carcinomatosis: Drugs and Diseases (Sugarbaker PH, ed.), Kluwer. Boston: 1996:75–87.
50. Younan R, Kusamura S, Baratti D, et al. Bowel complications in 203 cases of peritoneal surface malignancies treated with peritonectomy and closed-technique intraperitoneal hyperthermic perfusion. In press Ann Surg Oncol 2005;12:910–918.
51. Stephens AD, Alderman R, Chang D, et al. Morbidity and mortality analysis of 200 treatments with cytoreductive surgery and hyperthermic intraoperative intraperitoneal chemotherapy using the coliseum technique. Ann Surg Oncol 1999;6:790–796.
52. Salle B., Gilly F.N., Carry P.Y., Sayag A., Brachet A., Braillon G. Intraperitoneal chemo-hyperthermia in the treatment of peritoneal carcinomatosis of ovarian origin. Initial cases, physiopathologic data. J Gynecol Obstet Biol Reprod (Paris) 1993;22:369–371.
53. Elias D, Matsuhisa T, Sideris L, et al. Heated intra-operative intraperitoneal oxaliplatin plus irinotecan after complete resection of peritoneal carcinomatosis: pharmacokinetics, tissue distribution and tolerance. Ann Oncol 2004;15:1558–1565.
54. Deraco M, Raspagliesi F, Kusamura S. Management of peritoneal surface component of ovarian cancer. Surg Oncol Clin N Am. 2003;12:561–583.
55. de Bree E, Rosing H, Beijnen JH, et al. Pharmacokinetic study of docetaxel in intraoperative hyperthermic i.p. chemotherapy for ovarian cancer. Anticancer Drugs. 2003;14:103–110.
56. Vaart P.J.M., Vange N., Zoetmulder F.A.N., et al. intraperitoneal cisplatin with regional hyperthermia in advanced ovarian cancer: pharmacokinetics and cisplatin-DNA adduct formation in patients and ovarian cancer cell lines. Eur J Cancer 1998;34:148–154.
57. van der Vange N, van Goethem AR, Zoetmulder FA, et al. Extensive cytoreductive surgery combined with intra-operative intraperitoneal perfusion with cisplatin under hyperthermic conditions (OVHIPEC) in patients with recurrent ovarian cancer: a feasibility pilot. Eur J Surg Oncol 2000;26:663–668.
58. Steller M.A., Egorin M.J., Trimble E.L., et al. A pilot phase I trial of continuous hyperthermic peritoneal perfusion with high-dose carboplatin as primary treatment of patients with small-volume residual ovarian cancer. Cancer Chemother. Pharmacol 1999;43:106–114.
59. Nicoletto MO, Padrini R, Galcotti F, et al. Pharmacokinetics of intraperitoneal hyperthermic perfusion with mitoxantrone in ovarian cancer. Cancer Chemother Pharmacol 2000;45:457–462.
60. Deraco M., Rossi C.R., Pennacchioli E., et al. Cytoreductive surgery followed by intraperitoneal hyperthermic perfusion in the treatment of recurrent epithelial ovarian cancer: a phase II clinical study. Tumori 2001;87:120–126.
61. Cohen CJ. Surgical considerations in ovarian cancer. Semin Oncol 1985;12:53–56.
62. Los G, van Vugt MJ, Pinedo HM. Response of peritoneal solid tumors after intraperitoneal chemohyperthermia treatment with cisplatin or carboplatin. Br J Cancer 1994;69:235–241.

20

Regional Therapy of Bladder Tumors

Ingo Kausch, MD and Dieter Jocham, MD

CONTENTS

SUMMARY

The urinary bladder is an ideal organ for local topical treament. Numerous agents have been instilled intravesically during the last century to decrease bladder tumor recurrence and prevent progression and subsequent patient mortality. Today, intravesical immunotherapy with BCG and chemotherapy are routinely used as an adjunct to surgical resection of superficial bladder tumors. Photodynamic therapy with different photosensitizers and thermotherapy in combination with intravesical chemotherapy or percutaneous radiotherapy have been evaluated in phase III studies and may soon be widely available tools for the clinical treatment of bladder cancer. The first clinical phase I trials demonstrating safe application have been reported for intravesical gene therapy and antisense therapy approaches. Despite initial promising results of HIFU therapy and interventional radiotherapy, it cannot be anticipated that these two techniques will enter the clinical routine in the near future. Although the bladder is an easily accessible organ for regional treatment, a glycosaminoglycan (GAG) layer on the bladder mucosa can prevent the sufficient uptake and integration of many intravesically applied therapeutical compounds. Iontophoresis has shown clinical success in enhancing the uptake of, for instance, chemotherapeutic agents. Furthermore, magnetically targeted carriers, microspheres, and nanocarriers have been tested preclinically.

Key Words: Bladder cancer; intravesical therapy; novel therapeutics; regional therapy; chemotherapy; immunotherapy.

From: *Cancer Drug Discovery and Development: Regional Cancer Therapy*
Edited by: P. M. Schlag and U. S. Stein © Humana Press Inc., Totowa, NJ

1. INTRODUCTION

More than 90% of bladder cancers are transitional cell carcinomas; the remainder are squamous cell or adenocarcinomas. Bladder cancers are the second most common urologic malignancy in the Western world. Seventy percent of patients present with their cancers at a superficial stage (e.g., confined to the mucosa = Ta, T1, carcinoma *in situ* [CIS]). The mainstay of treatment for superficial bladder cancer has always been complete transurethral resection and close cystoscopic surveillance. However, approximately two-thirds of patients diagnosed with superficial bladder cancer experience a recurrence of their tumor, and 10 to 20% of recurring cancers demonstrate progression to muscle-invasive disease. As an adjunct to tumor resection, chemotherapeutic and immunotherapeutic agents are routinely used to reduce the frequency of tumor recurrence and possibly delay or inhibit tumor progression to muscle-invasive disease. The gold standard treatment for muscle-invasive bladder cancer remains radical cystectomy. Alternatively, radiotherapy with or without chemosensitizing can be performed. For metastatic disease, polychemotherapy is usually recommended. Although the exact cause of bladder cancer is not known, smokers are twice as likely to get the disease as nonsmokers. Hence, smoking is considered the greatest risk factor for bladder cancer. Workers who are exposed to certain chemicals used in the dye industry and in the rubber, leather, textile, and paint industries are believed to be at a higher risk for bladder cancer. The disease is also three times more common in men than in women; Caucasians also are at an increased risk. The risk of bladder cancer increases with age. Most cases are found in people who are 50 to 70 yr old.

2. SURGICAL STRATEGIES

2.1. Superficial Bladder Cancer

The diagnosis of bladder cancer ultimately depends on cystoscopic examination. If a bladder tumor has been visualized, a transurethral resection (TUR) is performed under general or spinal anesthesia. A small wire loop on the end of the cystoscopically introduced resectoscope is used to remove the cancerous area and to coagulate the deep layer with an electric bipolar or monopolar current. Depending on the current, different fluids are necessary for continuous irrigation of the bladder during TUR. In addition or alternatively to TUR, high-energy lasers may be used for fulguration of tumors. Superficial tumors can be safely treated with TUR. Disease-specific survival of patients with superficial tumors has been correlated with tumor grade and after 15 yr ranged between 62 and 100% *(1)*. Since approximately two-thirds of patients experience tumor recurrence, in most cases additional intravesical treatment with intravesical chemotherapy or immunotherapy (*see* **Subheading 3**) is recommended.

2.2. Muscle-Invasive Bladder Cancer

Although muscle-invasive tumors may in principal be treated with deep TUR and subsequent immuno- or chemotherapy, it is well accepted and confirmed by clinical studies that invasive tumors need more aggressive treatment. Generally, radical cystectomy is the gold standard treatment in most countries. However, radiotherapy and/or chemotherapy as the first choice may be performed, especially in older patients (>70 yr) with concomitant diseases. The 10-yr-recurrence-free survival in patients with muscle-

Table 1
Prognostic Risk Profile of Superficial Bladder Tumors
According to the Guidelines of the European Association of Urology

Risk	Characteristics
Low	Monofocal, Ta, G1, <3 cm diameter
High	T1, G3, multifocal or highly recurrent, CIS
Intermediate	All other tumors, Ta-1, G1–2, multifocal, >3 cm diameter

invasive tumors ranged after radical cystectomy from 87% (T2) to 45% (T4) and 34% in lymph node-positive patients *(2)*.

Radical cystectomy consists of removal of the bladder and neighboring organs, such as the prostate and seminal vesicles in men and the uterus and adnexa in women. Furthermore, regional lymph nodes are removed. Additional urethrectomy is performed depending on the tumor localization and the form of urinary diversion. Depending on life quality, patient compliance, and tumor characteristics, an orthotopic neobladder, continent pouches, and incontinent stomas using part of the bowel can be considered for urinary diversion as well as ureterosigmoidostomy (rarely performed today owing to long-term complications) or ureterocutaneostomy. Bladder-sparing surgery (partial cystectomy) together with neoadjuvant or adjuvant chemotherapy and/or radiation may be a reasonable alternative to radical cystectomy in selected cases.

3. Local Immuno- and Chemotherapy

Since the urinary bladder is an ideal organ for local topical treatment, numerous agents have been instilled intravesically during the last century in order to decrease recurrence and eventually progression of superficial tumors. Today, intravesical chemotherapy with agents such as mitomycin C (20–40 mg), epirubicin (50–80 mg), or doxorubicin (50 mg) as well as immunotherapy with bacillus Calmette-Guérin (BCG; 2×10^8 to 3×10^9 colony forming units) is routinely recommended as an adjuvant treatment after TUR depending on the recurrence and progression risk (Table 1).

The mechanism of BCG activity is not completely understood. It has been found that immunomodulation is mainly mediated by local activation of urothelial antigen-presenting cells, granulocytes and mononuclear cells, and natural killer cells with a predominat Th1 immune response, which results in elevated interleukin-2 (IL-2), IL-12, and interferon-γ (IFN-γ) concentrations, as well as mainly perforin-mediated tumor cell killing.

A single instillation of chemotherapeutic agents within 6 h of TUR is able to reduce the disease recurrence rate by about 50% *(3)* and is therefore advocated in all superficial bladder tumors. Monofocal low-risk tumors need no further treatment as the recurrence rate is very low (<0.2/yr). In intermediate- and high-risk tumors, a single early chemotherapy instillation is not sufficient *(4)*, and subsequent induction instillations have been recommended. The application of intravesical agents is quiet well standardized. Chemotherapeutic agents or BCG are dissolved in 30 to 50 mL of physiological solution or water and are kept in the bladder for 1 to 2 h. Usually four to six weekly treatments are given as an induction cycle. In higher risk patients, maintenance therapy can be recommended for up to 3 yr.

The side effects of intravesical BCG and chemotherapy are mostly local irritation and flu-like symptoms. Although the ideal doses and application protocols are not optimized and as yet rather empirical, numerous clinical trials and metanalyses have shown the following facts:

- Intravesical BCG and chemotherapy result overall in a 30 to 80% reduction of tumor recurrence compared to TUR alone *(5–7)*.
- BCG is not superiour to chemotherapy in low-risk tumors *(8,9)*.
- BCG induces more severe and more pronounced side effects than chemotherapy *(8,10)*.
- BCG is more effective than chemotherapy in CIS *(11)*.
- BCG can reduce tumor progression (overall 9.8% (BCG) vs 13.8% [untreated]) when maintenance is given *(3)*.
- There is as yet no proof that intravesical BCG or chemotherapy has an impact on survival

The local effectiveness of further chemotherapeutic agents such as alimta and Gemcitabine is currently being evaluated in phase III studies. Other immunomodulating agents that have proved successful in the prevention of disease recurrence, that are as active as chemotherapeutic agents, and that are currently being evaluated in phase III studies include IFN-α and keyhole limpet hemocyanin (KLH).

4. PHOTODYNAMIC THERAPY

Almost 30 yr ago, the use of photosensizing drugs for the diagnosis and treatment of bladder cancer was advocated. Initially, photodynamic therapy (PDT) for the treatment and prevention of bladder tumor recurrence was mainly performed with hematoporphyrin derivate (HPD) or dihematoporphyrin ether given systemically. Despite clinical effectiveness, considerable morbidity and toxicity occurred. Frequent side effects have been skin photosensitivity and inflammation. A major drawback of the synthetic porphyrin mixtures is the risk of damaging the bladder muscle and causing bladder shrinkage. Permanent bladder contraction owing to fibrosis has been reported in up to 40% of treated patients *(12)*. Radioprotective substances and dose modifications have been used with limited success. An alternative method to increase the selectivity of photosensitizers is to attach the photosensitizer to tumor-specific substances *(13)*. In our own as yet unpublished randomized clinical phase III study, the effectiveness of PDT with Photofrin® was compared with BCG in 124 patients with superficial bladder tumors. After a follow-up of 2 yr, the overall recurrence-free survival was significantly higher in the BCG group.

More recent approaches have used PDT with topical application of newer photosensitizers, such as PpIX induced by 5-aminolevulinic acid (ALA) or ALA derivates. Clinical experience has shown that HPD instilled intravesically did not demonstrate tumor specificity, whereas ALA instilled into the bladder showed increased tumor levels of endogenous protoporphyrin IX *(14)*. Although ALA is today frequently used for photodynamic diagnosis of bladder tumors as an adjunct to normal cystoscopy, PDT approaches with successful clinical results have only been described in small series *(14,15)*. Kriegmair's group *(16)* has described four complete remissions and (interestingly) no photodermatosis or bladder shrinkage after PDT with ALA in 10 bladder cancer patients. It has been suggested that ALA-PDT is more suitable for patients with flat lesions than for patients with papillary tumors *(16)*. According to in vitro data, the uptake of ALA may be further increased by electromotive diffusion (EMD) *(14)*. ALA derivates such as hexylester aminolevulinate (HAL) or new photosensitizers such as hypericin, a constituent of the plant *Hypericum perforatum*, have shown excellent fluorescence intensity as well as sensitivity and specificity (up to 98.5 and 93%, respectively, for CIS) in bladder cancer *(17,18)* and may improve clinical effectiveness in the future.

5. GENE THERAPY

Advances in genetic and molecular biology have led to numerous novel approaches for gene therapeutic cancer treatment. Several clinical trials have been approved worldwide.

Intralesional injection and intravesical instillation of transgenes may achieve successful gene transfer, especially in locally advanced or superficial bladder tumors. The most important obstacle for clinical application is the method for sufficient delivery and expression of the transferred genes. Although the bladder is an easily accessible organ, a glycosaminoglycan (GAG) layer on the bladder mucosa prevents the integration of intravesically applied genetic vectors.

The various strategies for inhibiting cancer growth by gene therapy include the reversion of the malignant phenotype by correcting abberrant gene expression, induction of genes that inhibit tumor growth, immune gene concepts, cytoreductive approaches, and modulation of multidrug resistance. Inhibition of overexpressed critical factors such as oncogenic genes is a property of antisense compounds (*see* **Subheading 5.1.**).

The induction of genes that inhibit tumor growth or the restoration of tumor suppressor genes have been examined for several genes (*p53*, *Rb*, *p21*, and *p16*). Clinical studies have already been performed for *p53* and *Rb*. *p53* mutations are the most common genetic defect in human tumors. The major role of *p53* are induction of apoptosis, cell cycle regulation, and DNA repair. In a phase I study, adenovirus-mediated *p53* gene transfer by intravesical instillation was safe and feasible in 13 patients with advanced bladder cancer. However, no local increase in *p53* and only one case of tumor response was noted *(19)*.

Immunogene therapy strategies involve the administration of genetically modified cancer cell vaccines, vaccination with tumor antigen nucleic acids, or the direct induction of cytokines. Several studies have shown the feasibility of immune gene approaches in bladder cancer. Studies with intravesical application of irradiated autologous mouse bladder tumor cells or cytokine gene-modified tumor cells have demonstrated only modest antitumor activity in mouse models. In addition, several preclinical systemic vaccination studies have been published *(20)*.

Most intravesical immune gene studies have been performed with direct induction of cytokines. Various cytokines, such as IL-2, IL-12, granulocyte/macrophage colony-stimulating factor (GM-CSF), and IFNs, have been used. The main purpose of the transfer of cytokine genes is to enhance local cytokine production and possibly to reduce the systemic side effects of systemic cytokine application. Furthermore, continuous expression may result in steady concentrations at the site of action. Although several studies have demonstrated the feasibility of intravesical and intralesional cytokine gene transfer preclinically *(20)*, it has still to be proved that local production of these cytokines yields an advantage over local administration.

Cytoreduction therapy by induction of suicide genes implies the selective destruction of cancer cells when prodrugs are selectively activated within targeted cells previously transduced by suicide genes. The effectiveness of this approach (herpes simplex virus thymidine kinase plus ganciclovir) was demonstrated in bladder cancer mouse models.

Replication-competent oncolytic viruses (ONYX-015, G207) have also shown antitumor activity in bladder cancer cell culture *(21)*.

Regional gene therapeutic modulation of multidrug resistance has not yet been evaluated in bladder cancer.

To improve the delivery of therapeutic genes, a broad range of techniques involved with nonviral delivery systems such as lipofection, liposomes, electrotransfection, and others has been investigated. Efficient transduction to deeper tissue layers was accomplished with a particle gun and electrotransfection *(22)*. Strategies attempting to increase transfer efficacy by disruption of the GAG layer in bladder cancer have already shown safety and usefulness *(23)*. Sufficient gene transfer seems to be dependent on the volume and the intravesical pressure *(24)*, as well as, at least for adenoviral transfer, certain receptors such as the CAR receptor *(25)*.

5.1. Antisense Therapy

Antisense oligonucleotides are short DNA sequences (10–25 nucleotides) designed to modulate the information transfer from gene to protein. Sequence-related hybridization with the mRNA of a specific protein results in selective inhibition of gene expression and downregulation of protein expression, which allows the study of gene function and the application of therapy on a molecular level. Antisense oligonucleotide inhibitors can be designed directly from genomic sequence information by simply making the reversed complement of the desired sequence. However, active compounds are more effectively generated by computer-based approaches. One antiviral antisense drug (fomivirsene) has already been approved by the Food and Drug Administration (FDA). Phase III studies with several antisense constructs in cancer patients are under way or have been finished. Some results have been particularly encouraging, although antitumoral effects have to a certain extent been attributed to nonspecific immunostimulatory mechanisms. Inhibition of individual gene expression with antisense oligonucleotides has shown promising activity in bladder cancer cell culture. Targeting of different critical genes (*bcl-2, Ki-67, ras, raf, PKC-α,* transforming growth factor-β, telomerase, clusterin, survivin, insulin-like growth factor, basic fibroblast growth factor) resulted in inhibition of cell proliferation, induction of apoptosis, and/or inhibition of tumor growth *(26)*. Furthermore, different combinations of antisense constructs and chemotherapy have demonstrated promising preclinical results.

Pharmacokinetic and toxicity data have shown the relative safety of therapeutic doses of systemic and intravesical oligonucleotides as well as the ability to downregulate the target gene mRNA and protein. Our own as yet unpublished studies have shown high local uptake and low systemic concentrations of intravesically applied oligonucleotides. The results of a first clinical trial with intravesical oligonucleotides (against the target gene Ki-67) are expected.

In bladder cancer, antisense oligonucleotides have the potential as both systemic and intravesical therapy. However, for most medical applications, several obstacles (related to toxicity, stability, affinity, cellular delivery, and specificity) remain to be clarified and may be overcome by new chemical modifications. Further antisense constructs such as interfering RNA or ribozymes have not yet reached clinical application.

6. INTERVENTIONAL RADIOTHERAPY

Brachytherapy for bladder cancer is only performed in a few specialized centers, mainly in Europe (France, the Netherlands, and Belgium). Only a few studies on a small number of patients have been published in the United States. Today, there is general agreement about the potential indications for brachytherapy: a solitary tumor smaller than 5 cm and stages T1 to T3a *(27)*. A short course of prebrachytherapy external beam radiotherapy (EBRT) prevents iatrogenic scar implants caused by tumor manipulation. Although there is general agreement on the use of preoperative EBRT, the dose and fractionation schedule have varied widely (1–25 fractions with 2–8.5 gy). In most of the published studies, brachytherapy was combined with regional lymphadenectomy and partial cystectomy. Until the end of the last century, the dose of brachytherapy treatment was delivered at a continuous low-dose rate (LDR). The treatment was hand loaded until the 1990s, when afterloading techniques became widely available. More recently, pulsed dose rate (PDR) and high-dose rate (HDR) brachytherapy machines with a single iridium source have been introduced to allow dose distribution optimization and reduction in treatment time.

Different brachytherapy series for bladder cancer are not comparable, since the radioactive source and the implantation technique have changed. Local control rates after radium and cesium-137 brachytherapy ranged from 74 to 91% for T1 to T3 tumors. More recent reports with iridium-192 showed 5-yr survival rates of 70 to 80% (T1G3), 50 to 76% (T2), and 61 to 72% (T3a) *(28)*. The total delivered dose rates have ranged from 30 to 65 gy.

Some reports have shown excellent local control rates of between 70 and 90% and 5-yr survival rates (47–86%) that were comparable to cystectomy series. The late toxicity was in general low, with 90 to 95% functioning bladders in long-term survivors *(27)*. However, owing to patient selection in studies (often monofocal smaller tumors) and frequently performed additional partial cystectomy and EBRT, the true value of brachytherapy in bladder cancer is not clear.

7. THERMOTHERAPY

The benefit of combined treatment modalities has been described in bladder cancer for radiofrequency or microwave hyperthermia together with chemotherapy or radiotherapy. The combination of thermal energy and chemotherapy has demonstrated increased effectiveness in preclinical studies mediated by different mechanisms (e.g., increased cellular permeability and increased reaction with DNA or inhibition of DNA repair) depending on the chemotherapeutic agent. Clinical data have been published for mitomycin C treatment of superficial bladder cancer. Van der Heijden et al. *(29)* treated 90 patients with intermediate- and high-risk tumors with mitomycin C (20 mg) and microwave (SB-TS 101) hyperthermia. The treatment regimen included six to eight weekly sessions followed by six to eight monthly sessions, each lasting 60 min. Mitomycin C was instilled in a volume of 50 mL via the SB-TS 101 system, which is a specially designed transurethral catheter containing a 915-MHz microwave applicator that directly heats the bladder wall and five thermocouples that control the temperature. The results were quite promising, with 14.3% and 24.6% recurrence rates after 1 and 2 yr of follow-up, respectively. One case of severe and prolonged thermal reaction was noted. Comparable data were reported by Colombo et al. from 83 patients with intermediate- and high-risk tumors after appplication with the same hyperthermia device *(30)*. Subjective intolerance and clinical complications were significantly higher but were transient and moderate in the combined treatment group.

Results from radiotherapy plus hyperthermia have been presented by the Dutch Deep Hyperthermia Group *(31)*: 358 cancer patients including 101 patients with bladder cancer (stage T2-T4) were randomly assigned to radiotherapy alone or radiotherapy plus hyperthermia. Then 66 to 70 gy were administered in fractions of 2 gy to the bladder, with regional pelvic lymph nodes included in the field to a total dose of 40 gy. Hyperthermia (BSD-2000 system) was given once weekly during the period of external radiotherapy, to a total of five treatments. Hyperthermia was generally well tolerated. A statistically significant higher rate of complete responses was seen in bladder cancer patients in the radiotherapy plus hyperthermia group (26%) compared with the radiotherapy group (22%). There was a trend toward duration of local control after 3 yr (42% vs 33%) and of overall survival (28% vs 22%) for the combined treatment groups. Although these results were not statistically significant, it was shown that the addition of hyperthermia to radiotherapy may improve local tumor control in patients with advanced bladder cancer.

8. ULTRASOUND-GUIDED THERAPY

The therapeutic application of high-intensity focused ultrasound (HIFU) has been frequently described in prostate disease, but only a few reports for the treatment of bladder cancer exist. A feasibility study in pigs with 1.7 MHz of extracorporeal focused-bowl ultrasonic transducers has shown that focused ultrasound can successfully destroy regions of the bladder wall *(32)*. Further preclinical data described a synergism of HIFU and mitomycin chemotherapy *(33)*. Clinical results from a phase II study have been presented after ablation of superficial bladder tumors in 25 patients *(34)*. With focused extracorporeal pyrotherapy (300 shots), tumors were undetectable after 1 mo in 15 patients. The effect was most likely owing to mechanical damage induced by shock waves. Despite initial feasibility studies of HIFU in bladder cancer, no recent clinical data have been published.

9. MICROSPHERES, NANOCARRIERS, AND DRUG DELIVERY

The use of magnetically targeted carriers (MTCs) to aggregate doxorubicin to specific regions of the bladder has been examined by Leakakos et al. *(35)*. After instillation of MTCs in swine bladders and placement of external magnet guides, MTCs indeed localized to targeted sites.

Bioadhesive paclitaxel microspheres were shown to optimize paclitaxel release and adhesion at the urothelial surface in mice *(36)*. Compared with free paclitaxel, which is poorly soluble and of which 85% was washed out of mice bladders within the first void, a significant amount of paclitaxel microspheres were still adherent to the bladder mucosa 48 h after instillation. This better availability correlated with lower incidence of tumors in an orthotopic mouse bladder tumor model. Lu et al. *(37)* found 2.6 times increased drug concentrations in the urothelium and lamina propria tissue layers in dogs when an intravesical dose of paclitaxel-loaded gelatin nanoparticles (600–1000 nm) was given, compared with a dose of normal paclitaxel *(37)*. Several further approaches with immunoliposomes, immunonanospheres, or nanoparticle-adsorbed antisense oligonucleotides have been tested in bladder cancer cell culture with mostly promising results but without existing in vivo data.

10. ELECTROMOTIVE DRUG APPLICATION (EMDA)

EMDA, or iontophoresis of therapeutic substances, is frequently used for treatment of cystitis and chronic pain conditions. In 1988 Thiel et al. reported on intravesical iontophoresis of the positively charged drug proflavine for recurrence prophylaxis of superficial bladder cancer without local or systemic toxicity *(38)*. Recent data support the concept that EMDA enhances drug transport through the urothelium into deeper layers of the bladder. Riedl et al. have performed treatment with EMDA and 40 mg mitomycin C in 22 patients with high-risk bladder cancer *(39)*. Following insertion of a small indwelling catheter containing a spiral silver electrode, the bladder was drained and washed and subsequently filled with 150 mL of the nonionized mitomycin C solution. This volume is supposed to result in an ideal spherical bladder configuration. Two electrode pads were placed at the abdomen, and the current generator was connected to the electrodes. Maximum current was 23 mA. Treatment was well tolerated. Only one patient presented with severe bladder pain and an ulcer of the bladder wall. Colombo et al. treated low/intermediate-risk patients ($n = 80$) with mitomycin C as a standard procedure or in combination with local microwave-induced hyperthermia or with EMDA *(40)*. The EMDA technique was comparable in effectiveness to the other methods. Local toxicity induced by thermochemotherapy was more severe than that registered for EMDA and standard instillation. The number of patients is as yet too small to draw conclusions on effectiveness.

REFERENCES

1. Herr HW. Tumor progression and survival of patients with high grade, noninvasive papillary (TaG3) bladder tumors: 15-year outcome. J Urol 2000;163:60–61.
2. Stein JP, Lieskovsky G, Cote R, et al. Radical cystectomy in the treatment of invasive bladder cancer: long-term results in 1,054 patients. J Clin Oncol 2001;19:666–675.
3. Sylvester RJ, van der Meijden AP, Lamm DL. Intravesical bacillus Calmette-Guérin reduces the risk of progression in patients with superficial bladder cancer: a meta-analysis of the published results of randomized clinical trials. J Urol 2002;168:1964–1970.
4. Sylvester RJ, Oosterlinck W, van der Meijden AP. A single immediate postoperative instillation of chemotherapy decreases the risk of recurrence in patients with stage Ta T1 bladder cancer: a meta-analysis of published results of randomized clinical trials. J Urol 2004;171:2186–2190
5. Shelley MD, Kynaston H, Court J, et al. A systematic review of intravesical bacillus Calmette-Guérin plus transurethral resection vs transurethral resection alone in Ta and T1 bladder cancer. BJU Int 2001;88:209–216.
6. Huncharek M, Geschwind JF, Witherspoon B, McGarry R, Adcock D. Intravesical chemotherapy prophylaxis in primary superficial bladder cancer: a meta-analysis of 3703 patients from 11 randomized trials. J Clin Epidemiol 2000;53:676–680
7. Huncharek M, McGarry R, Kupelnick B. Impact of intravesical chemotherapy on recurrence rate of recurrent superficial transitional cell carcinoma of the bladder: results of a meta-analysis. Anticancer Res 2001;21:765–769
8. Shelley MD, Court JB, Kynaston H, Wilt TJ, Coles B, Mason MD. Intravesical bacillus Calmette-Guérin versus mitomycin C for Ta and T1 bladder cancer. Cochrane Database Syst Rev 2003;3: CD003231.
9. Malmstrom PU, Wijkstrom H, Lundholm C, Wester K, Busch C, Norlen BJ. 5-Year followup of a randomized prospective study comparing mitomycin C and bacillus Calmette-Guérin in patients with superficial bladder carcinoma. Swedish-Norwegian Bladder Cancer Study Group. J Urol 1999; 161:1124–1127.
10. Böhle A, Jocham D, Bock PR. Intravesical bacillus Calmette-Guérin versus mitomycin C for superficial bladder cancer: a formal meta-analysis of comparative studies on recurrence and toxicity. J Urol 2003;169:90–95.
11. de Reijke TM, Kurth KH, Sylvester RJ, et al. European Organization for the Research and Treatment of Cancer-Genito-Urinary Group Bacillus Calmette-Guérin versus epirubicin for primary, secondary or concurrent carcinoma in situ of the bladder: results of a European Organization for the Research and Treatment of Cancer-Genito-Urinary Group Phase III Trial (30906). J Urol 2005;173:405–409.

12. Nseyo UO, DeHaven J, Dougherty TJ, et al. Photodynamic therapy (PDT) in the treatment of patients with resistant superficial bladder cancer: a long-term experience. J Clin Laser Med Surg 1998; 16:61–68.

13. Morgan J, Lottman H, Abbou CC, Chopin DK. A comparison of direct and liposomal antibody conjugates of sulfonated aluminum phthalocyanines for selective photoimmunotherapy of human bladder carcinoma. Photochem Photobiol 1994; 60:486–496.

14. Stenzl A, Eder I, Kostron H, Klocker H, Bartsch G. Electromotive diffusion (EMD) and photodynamic therapy with delta-aminolaevulinic acid (delta-ALA) for superficial bladder cancer. J Photochem Photobiol B 1996;36:233–236.

15. Kriegmair M, Baumgartner R, Lumper W, Waidelich R, Hofstetter A. Early clinical experience with 5-aminolevulinic acid for the photodynamic therapy of superficial bladder cancer. Br J Urol 1996;77:667–671

16. Waidelich R, Beyer W, Knuchel R, et al. Whole bladder photodynamic therapy with 5-aminolevulinic acid using a white light source. Urology 2003;61:332–337

17. Marti A, Jichlinski P, Lange N, et al. Comparison of aminolevulinic acid and hexylester aminolevulinate induced protoporphyrin IX distribution in human bladder cancer. J Urol 2003; 170:428–432.

18. Kamuhabwa A, Agostinis P, Ahmed B, et al. Hypericin as a potential phototherapeutic agent in superficial transitional cell carcinoma of the bladder. Photochem Photobiol Sci 2004;3:772–780.

19. Pagliaro LC, Keyhani A, Williams D, et al. Repeated intravesical instillations of an adenoviral vector in patients with locally advanced bladder cancer: a phase I study of p53 gene therapy. J Clin Oncol 2003;21:2247–2253.

20. Ardelt P, Kausch I, Böhle A. Gene and antisense therapy of bladder cancer. Adv Exp Med Biol 2003;539:155–158.

21. Irie A. Advances in gene therapy for bladder cancer. Curr Gene Ther 2003;3:1–11.

22. Harimoto K, Sugimura K, Lee CR, Kuratsukuri K, Kishimoto T. In vivo gene transfer methods in the bladder without viral vectors. Br J Urol 1998;81:870–874

23. Kuball J, Wen SF, Leissner J, et al. Successful adenovirus-mediated wild-type p53 gene transfer in patients with bladder cancer by intravesical vector instillation. J Clin Oncol 2002;20:957–965.

24. Siemens DR, Austin JC, See WA, Tartaglia J, Ratliff TL. Evaluation of gene transfer efficiency by viral vectors to murine bladder epithelium. J Urol 2001;165:667–671.

25. Loskog A, Hedlund T, Wester K, et al. Human urinary bladder carcinomas express adenovirus attachment and internalization receptors. Gene Ther 2002;9:547–553.

26. Glackin AJ, Gray SB, Johnston SR, Duggan BJ, Williamson KE. Antisense oligonucleotides in the treatment of bladder cancer. Expert Opin Biol Ther 2005;5:67–77.

27. Pos F, Moonen L. Brachytherapy in the treatment of invasive bladder cancer. Semin Radiat Oncol 2005;15:49–54.

28. Van Poppel H, Lievens Y, Van Limbergen E, Baert L. Brachytherapy with iridium-192 for bladder cancer. Eur Urol 2000;37:605–608

29. van der Heijden AG, Kiemeney LA, Gofrit ON, et al. Preliminary European results of local microwave hyperthermia and chemotherapy treatment in intermediate or high risk superficial transitional cell carcinoma of the bladder. Eur Urol 2004;46:65–71.

30. Colombo R, Da Pozzo LF, Salonia A, et al. Multicentric study comparing intravesical chemotherapy alone and with local microwave hyperthermia for prophylaxis of recurrence of superficial transitional cell carcinoma. J Clin Oncol 2003;21:4270–4276.

31. van der Zee J, Gonzalez Gonzalez D, van Rhoon GC, van Dijk JD, van Putten WL, Hart AA. Comparison of radiotherapy alone with radiotherapy plus hyperthermia in locally advanced pelvic tumours: a prospective, randomised, multicentre trial. Dutch Deep Hyperthermia Group. Lancet 2000; 355:1119–1125

32. Watkin NA, Morris SB, Rivens IH, Woodhouse CR, ter Haar GR. A feasibility study for the non-invasive treatment of superficial bladder tumours with focused ultrasound. Br J Urol 1996;78: 715–721.

33. Wang GM, Yang YF, Sun LA, Xu ZB, Xu YQ. An experimental study on high intensity focused ultrasound combined with mitomycin treatment of bladder tumor. Zhonghua Wai Ke Za Zhi 2003;41:897–900.

34. Vallancien G, Harouni M, Guillonneau B, Veillon B, Bougaran J. Ablation of superficial bladder tumors with focused extracorporeal pyrotherapy. Urology 1996;47:204–207.
35. Leakakos T, Ji C, Lawson G, Peterson C, Goodwin S. Intravesical administration of doxorubicin to swine bladder using magnetically targeted carriers. Cancer Chemother Pharmacol 2003; 51:445–450.
36. Le Visage C, Rioux-Leclercq N, Haller M, Breton P, Malavaud B, Leong K. Efficacy of paclitaxel released from bio-adhesive polymer microspheres on model superficial bladder cancer. J Urol 2004;171:1324–1329.
37. Lu Z, Yeh TK, Tsai M, Au JL, Wientjes MG. Paclitaxel-loaded gelatin nanoparticles for intravesical bladder cancer therapy. Clin Cancer Res 2004; 10:7677–7684.
38. Thiel, KH. Die intravesikale antineoplastische Iontophorese. Ein unblutiges Verfahren zur Therapie und Rezidivprophylaxe des Blasenkarzinoms, in Verhandlungsbericht der Deutschen Gesellschaft für Urologie, 40. Tagung: Springer-Verlag, 1988.
39. Riedl CR, Knoll M, Plas E, Pfluger H. Electromotive drug administration and hydrodistention for the treatment of interstitial cystitis. J Endourol 1998;12:269–272.
40. Colombo R, Brausi M, Da Pozzo L, et al. Thermo-chemotherapy and electromotive drug administration of mitomycin C in superficial bladder cancer eradication. A pilot study on marker lesion. Eur Urol 2001;39:95–100.

21 Regional Therapy of Rectal Cancer

*Stefano Guadagni, MD, Mario Schietroma, MD,
Giammaria Fiorentini, MD,
Maurizio Cantore, MD, Claudio Lely,
Cristina Ruscitti, MD, Marco Clementi, MD,
Evangelos Kanavos, MD, and
Gianfranco Amicucci, MD*

CONTENTS

SUMMARY

Histopathologic examinations of resected specimens have revealed that the development of local recurrence after rectal surgery for cancer is related to the resection margin of the mesorectum. The incidence rate of local pelvic recurrence after standard "curative" surgery for rectal cancer varies widely. The treatment of local recurrence remains a challenge. Extensive resection (abdominal sacral resection with or without pelvic exenteration) gives the best chance of survival. For patients with unresectable recurrent rectal cancer, neither intravenous systemic chemotherapy nor intraarterial chemotherapy achieve desirable results in terms of pain control and tumor response. To improve clinical response, several methods of regional chemotherapy delivery have been suggested. One of these is regional pelvic perfusion. In our study, hypoxic pelvic perfusion has been proposed as palliative treatment in patients with unresectable locally recurrent rectal cancer who are nonresponders or who have disease progression after the standard modalities. The median survival time (12.2 mo) registered after one course of hypoxic pelvic perfusion is comparable to that obtained by irradiation or reirradiation

From: *Cancer Drug Discovery and Development: Regional Cancer Therapy*
Edited by: P. M. Schlag and U. S. Stein © Humana Press Inc., Totowa, NJ

355

in non-pretreated patients. Considering the vascular damage following radiotherapy, a different sequence in the multimodular treatment of unresectable recurrent rectal cancer could be more useful. Further studies are necessary to establish whether hypoxic pelvic perfusion improves the quality of life and survival of these patients if administered before radiotherapy with or without concomitant systemic chemotherapy. In conclusion, hypoxic pelvic perfusion is a good palliative treatment for patients with unresectable locally recurrent rectal cancer, but it should be considered as a link of a chain in a multimodular approach.

Key Words: Regional perfusion; stop-flow; rectal cancer; pharmacokinetics; mitomycin c; chemofiltration; mesorectal excision; pelvic exenteration; adjuvant therapy.

1. INTRODUCTION

Histopathologic examination of resected specimens have revealed that the development of local recurrence after rectal surgery for cancer is related to the resection margin of the mesorectum *(1)*. An analysis of pelvic recurrences after resection of rectal cancer supports this conclusion *(2)*. Furthermore, nearly 75% of the recurrences were detected in the perirectal tissue with the vast majority near the rectal anastomosis. Distal resection margins of less than 1 cm and resection of fewer than 14 lymph nodes have been identified as independent prognostic factors for developing locally recurrent disease *(3)*. The incidence rate of local pelvic recurrence after standard "curative" surgery for rectal cancer varies widely according to the definition employed, accuracy of diagnosis, completeness of follow-up, and whether and how often postmortem examinations were performed *(4,5)*. In control groups included in prospective randomized trials or in epidemiological studies, the 5-yr local recurrence rates vary from 20 to 30% *(6)*. A retrospective review of preoperative radiotherapy followed by resection of tethered or fixed rectal cancers demonstrated a local recurrence rate of 16% *(7)*. In contrast, a local recurrence rate of 35% was observed in patients with mobile cancers treated with surgery alone. Two prospective randomized trials comparing preoperative radiotherapy and surgery vs surgery alone for tethered or fixed tumors reported a significant decrease in the local recurrence rate with the use of preoperative radiotherapy *(8,9)*. The value of adding radiotherapy to surgery in the treatment of patients with resectable primary rectal cancer has been demonstrated in trials using postoperative and especially preoperative irradiation *(10)*.

2. TREATMENT FOR LOCAL RECURRENCE

The use of total mesorectal excision (TME) has been associated with a dramatic reduction in local recurrence without the use of adjuvant therapy *(11)*. Bokey et al. reported their experience with wide anatomical resection without the use of adjuvant therapy *(12)*. A total of 596 patients were analyzed with nearly 40% having lymph node metastases. The overall 5-yr actuarial local recurrence rate was 11%. Multivariate analysis identified positive nodes and venous invasion as pathological features that were independent predictive factors for local recurrence. Merchant et al. reviewed their experience of TME without adjuvant treatment in 95 patients with T3 N0 M0 (stage II). The overall local recurrence rate was 9%, and the only histopathologic feature significant for predicting local failure was lymphatic invasion *(13)*.

However, treatment for local recurrence remains a challenge since, without surgical intervention, the reported survival rate of patients with local recurrence of rectal cancer is less than 4% at 5 yr, and the median life expectancy is 7 mo (6). Although 50% of recurrences are associated with disseminated disease (14), most patients die of local and/ or regional progression of disease rather than systemic metastases (15). Extensive resection (abdominal sacral resection with or without pelvic exenteration) gives the best chance of survival (16–18). Operative mortality varies from 0 to 10%, the 5-yr survival rate varies from 20 to 30%, and the median life expectancy varies from 39 to 44 mo (16–18). Results from such radical surgery seem to be optimized by applying multimodality approaches, including external beam radiotherapy, sensitizing chemotherapy, and intraoperative radiation therapy (19–21). The actuarial 2-yr overall survival is approximately 50%, and the actuarial 5-yr disease-free survival is approximately 35% (19–21). However, if the resected recurrent cancer does not have margins free on histopathologic examination, the actuarial 2-yr survival rate is significantly lower (approximately 35%). Unfortunately, extensive surgery is not feasible in almost two-thirds of patients with recurrent rectal cancer (22). In general, the demonstration of pelvic side wall involvement, growth into the sciatic notch, involvement of the first and/or second sacral vertebra, and/or encasement of the bladder or iliac vessels, contraindicates surgery (19).

Although occasional cases of complete remission have been reported (23), radiotherapy alone or in conjunction with chemotherapy provides palliative benefit and extension of mean or median survival, but long-term survival (>2 yr) is rare (24–27). Recent studies using radiotherapy alone have reported a median survival time of 17.9 mo in a group of patients able to receive a dose of 50 to 60 gy (28); on the other hand, after a mean dose of 30 gy, a median survival time of 14 mo has been observed in chemotherapy- and radiotherapy-naïve patients (29), whereas a median survival time of 12 mo has been reported for palliative reirradiation (30).

3. REGIONAL CHEMOTHERAPY DELIVERY

For patients with unresectable recurrent rectal cancer, neither intravenous systemic chemotherapy nor intraarterial chemotherapy achieve desirable results in terms of pain control and tumor response (31–38). To improve clinical response, several methods of regional chemotherapy delivery have been suggested. One of these methods is regional pelvic perfusion. In 1958, Creech et al. (39) proposed the technique of isolated perfusion, in which the blood supply of a body region was isolated: the aorta and the vena cava are occluded with vessel clamps and perfused by means of cannulae with thigh tourniquet application to reduce collateral circulation. Actually, the perfused compartment was not fully isolated. Pharmacokinetic evaluations of 5-fluorouracil (5-FU) in patients with pelvic recurrence of colorectal cancer (40) showed that isolation perfusion was advantageous compared with intraarterial or intravenous administration. This technique is still in use (41).

Isolated perfusion incorporating laparotomic aortic and caval cannulation was modified by the use of femoral cannulation (42–47). In 1960, Watkins et al. (48) described a technique using balloon catheters to achieve blockage of the aorta and inferior vena cava. In 1963, Lawrence et al. (49) reported a technique using balloon occlusion catheters and a large abdominal external tourniquet. In a 1987 study of hyperthermic pelvic infusion with 5-FU, Wile and Smolin (45) reported the occlusion of the great vessels by means of balloon catheters and femoral cannulation in 11 of 27 patients with refractory pelvic cancer. In 1993, a similar technique was reported by Turk et al. (50) in six patients with recurrent unresectable rectal cancer who underwent perfusion with 5-FU, cisplatin, and mitomycin C (MMC). In 1996, Wanebo et al. *(51)* published the results of normothermic pelvic perfusion with the same regimen in 14 patients with unresectable and 5 with resectable recurrent rectal cancer. In 1994, Aigner and Kaevel *(52)* presented the results of pelvic perfusion with MMC and melphalan in 41 patients with recurrent unresectable rectal cancer. Both occlusion of the great vessels and perfusion were done with only two catheters, which were surgically introduced through the femoral vessels. The 2-yr survival rate in the group of patients pretreated with radiotherapy and/or chemotherapy was 35%. A similar technique using percutaneous catheters was later performed by Thompson et al. *(53)* in seven patients with recurrent rectal cancer who underwent perfusion with MMC and 5-FU or cisplatin.

Microenviromental alterations, including tissue hypoxia and low cellular pH, occur during isolated pelvic perfusion. MMC is 10 times more toxic to tumor cells in hypoxic conditions *(54,55)*. The pharmacokinetics of MMC in peripheral and inferior vena cava blood were studied by our group *(56)* in four patients with unresectable recurrent rectal cancer under different types of major vessel occlusion. For the type of pelvic perfusion corresponding to the method used by Aigner and Kaevel *(52)*, the area under the plasma concentration-time curve (AUC) ratio for inferior caval vein blood vs systemic circulation was 11.7:1.

4. HYPOXIC PELVIC PERFUSION (STOP-FLOW) TECHNIQUE

4.1. Positioning of Catheters

The femoral artery and vein were exposed through a short longitudinal incision in the groin. After systemic heparinization (150 U/kg), a three-lumen balloon catheter (PfM, Cologne, Germany) was introduced into the inferior vena cava via the saphenous vein and a second one into the aorta via the femoral artery; these were positioned under fluoroscopic control below the renal vessels and above the aortic and venous bifurcation using a guidewire.

4.2. Occlusion of Circulation

Both balloons were filled with isotonic sodium chloride solution, containing the radiopaque dye diatrizoate, and blocked. For isolation of the pelvis, two large-cuff orthopedic tourniquets, placed around each of the upper thighs just below the lower level of the femoral triangle, were inflated just before starting the perfusion.

4.3. Drug Perfusion

The infusion channels of the arterial and venous stop-flow catheters were connected to a hypoxic perfusion set on a roller pump. The set was primed with an isotonic sodium chloride solution containing heparin (10,000 U/L). Once flow was established (approx 200 mL/min), drug therapy was started. The drug, diluted in 250 mL of isotonic sodium chloride solution also containing 16 mg of dexamethasone sodium phosphate, was administered over 3 min. The extracorporeal circuit (Fig. 1) also included both a hemofiltration system and a heater-cooler unit. The hypoxic perfusion circuit was maintained over 20 min (mean 22 ± 4 min). The temperature of the perfusate was 38.5°C.

PELVIC PERFUSION

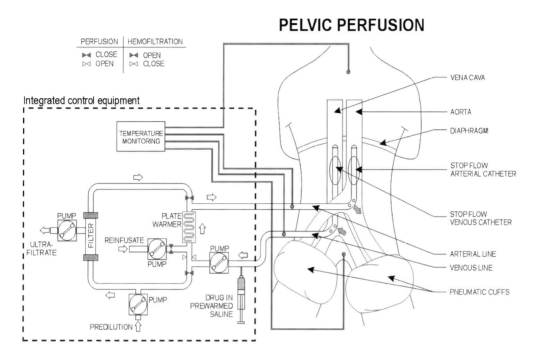

Fig. 1. Scheme of hypoxic pelvic perfusion and extracorporeal circuit incorporating both a hemofiltration system and a heater-cooler unit.

4.4. Reestablishment of Normal Circulation

After perfusion, both catheter balloons and pneumatic cuffs were deflated and the circulation restored. The extracorporal circuit also was used in the hemofiltration section for 80 ± 20 min. A polyamide hemofilter (Hemoflux 20, Gambro, Lund, Sweden) with a surface area of 2 m² was used. Thereafter, the catheters were withdrawn and the vessels repaired.

5. DISCUSSION

For patients with unresectable recurrent rectal cancer, particularly when the surgeon is unable to accomplish a gross total surgical resection of the recurrent cancer, preoperative external irradiation plus continous infusion chemotherapy, intraoperative irradiation, maximal surgical resection, and systemic chemotherapy are currently being studied in clinical trials (19–21,57). When comorbid conditions contraindicate extensive palliative surgery, when intraoperative irradiation is not available, or when external irradiation is not practical, hypoxic pelvis perfusion has been an effective alternative (53).

The relative advantage of intraarterial over intravenous chemotherapy (R_D) is proportional to the increase of drug concentration in the target organ or compartment (R_T) and to the reduction of drug concentration in the systemic circulation (R_S), as can be seen in the following equation:

$$R_D = [(R_T/R_S)] = 1 + [Cl_T/Q(1 - E)]$$

where Cl_T represents the overall amount of blood detoxified in the whole body per minute (drug clearance in the whole body), Q represents the blood flow in the artery in which the drug is infused, and E represents the amount of drug cleared by or held by the organ or compartment in which the drug has been infused *(58)*. The relative advantage of intraarterial over intravenous chemotherapy (R_D) can be increased by reducing Q and increasing Cl_T and E. Hypoxic perfusion with the balloon-occlusion technique can be an effective method for reducing Q. Hemofiltration of venous blood from the infused organ or compartment can increase Cl_T.

Hypoxic pelvic perfusion has potential therapeutic advantages over intraarterial infusion of chemotherapy, as recently demonstrated by a pilot study in which an approximately 10-fold superior MMC pelvic-systemic exposure ratio was measured for hypoxic pelvic perfusion in comparison with intraaortic infusion in patients with unresectable locally recurrent rectal cancer *(56)*. After intravenous push injection of 20 mg/m² of MMC, Door *(59)* reported that the peripheral C_{max} was 6.0 µg/mL with an AUC of 73.3 µg/mL × minutes. In our study *(60)*, after intra-aortic administration of 25 mg/m² of MMC during the hypoxic pelvic perfusion, the mean C_{max} in the pelvic compartment was 54.8 µg/mL, the mean peripheral C_{max} was 25 µg/mL, and the mean peripheral AUC was 50.2 µg/mL × minutes.

The efficiency of the simplified balloon occlusion technique used in our study *(60)* to perform hypoxic pelvic perfusion has been demonstrated by the good mean pelvic-systemic MMC-AUC ratio (13.3:1) measured in our series of 11 treatments, this being higher than both the value of 9.0:1 reported by Wanebo et al. *(51)*, and the value of 4.4:1 reported by Turk et al. *(50)*. The high variability in the range of MMC-AUC ratio values (4.3:1–25.7:1), which is attributable in our opinion to the variability of conditions in different individuals (i.e., anastomotic venous leak from the pelvic circulation to the systemic circulation), explains why both the type of tumor response and the extent of toxic effects in this kind of patient are not accurately predictable.

5.2. Choice of Drug

Several different chemotherapeutic regimens have been used in pelvic perfusion, often as part of a single study. In the treatments performed for recurrent rectal cancer, the agents more frequently used have been 5-FU *(45,50,51)*, and cisplatin *(45,50, 51)* in monochemotherapy or in polychemotherapy. Less frequently and often in small series, the use of nitrogen mustard *(42,43,49)*, cyclophosphamide *(49)*, 2-deoxy-5-fluorouridine *(49)*, melphalan *(52)*, and mitoxantrone *(41)* have been reported. The real value of pelvic perfusion in terms of tumor response is consequently difficult to ascertain. After a pilot study on hypoxic pelvic perfusion *(56)*, we planned a phase II trial based on the use of single-agent MMC, which has been shown to be increasingly cytotoxic in a hypoxic enviroment *(53,54)*. Although 5-FU has been considered more effective than MMC against adenocarcinoma of the rectum, also when administered by pelvic perfusion *(50)*, 5-FU was not selected for this study mainly because most patients had disease progression after systemic chemotherapy with this agent.

In our selected series of patients, one course of hypoxic pelvic perfusion with 25 mg/m² of MMC resulted in an overall response rate of 36.3%. These results are comparable to those reported by Turk et al. *(50)*, which were approx 30% using 5-FU (3000 mg/m²), cisplatin (25–75 mg/m²), and MMC (10 mg/m²). Aigner and Keavel *(52)* reported an overall response rate of 32% in a series of 41 patients treated with MMC (12.5 mg/m²) and melphalan (12.5 mg/m²). Wile and Smolin *(45)* reported an overall response rate of 40% in 17 patients treated with 5-FU (750–1500 mg/m²) by hyperthermic perfusion.

Based on these data, the response rate does not seem to be significantly higher in patients treated with polychemotherapy than in those receiving monochemotherapy. Further studies are necessary to evaluate other drugs that are active in hypoxic conditions (i.e., doxorubicin, tirapazamine), the role of hyperthermia and oxygenation with prolonged isolated perfusion *(45)*, or the use of agents modulating multiple-drug resistance *(50)*.

Strocchi et al. (61) reported an overall response rate of 30% in a series of 10 patients with unresectable pelvic recurrence from colonrectal cancer, treated with a combination of MMC(20 mg/m^2) plus doxorubicin (75 mg/m^2; 8 patients), or epirubicin (75 mg/m^2; 2 patients) infused into the isolated pelvic compartment. Pain remission was observed in 8/10 patients.

5.3. Comparative Response and Survival Rates

In our study the 45.4% response rate of pain relief (not only from tumor shrinkage but mainly from neurotoxic effects) represents good palliation in patients with severe local symptoms. This result, together with the local control of tumor growth (6 mo of median time to disease progression), promotes an improved quality of life for these patients. Further studies are necessary to evaluate whether the median time to disease progression can be improved by long-term administration of heparin *(62)*. If responding patients can become candidates for pelvic surgery, they might have prolonged survival and improved quality of life. Radical removal of the colorectal pelvic relapse gives the patient a chance of survival almost equal to that of a patient with a C2 tumor subjected to primary surgery.

The response and survival rates obtained with the stop-flow technique and schedule are at least comparable to those observed with the other second-line therapies employed in FU-refractory metastatic colorectal cancer such as irinotecan or oxaliplatin *(63,64)*, whereas systemic toxicities are significantly lower.

As reported by Pilati et al. in a review *(65)*, the stop-flow technique is a safe and encouraging procedure in terms of cure and palliation when conventional treatment are no longer possible or have failed.

5.4. Limitations

Since its first description, despite several innovations and significant response rates *(39)*, regional pelvic perfusion has not seen widespread use, first owing to its inherent complexity and second owing to serious adverse effects from local and systemic toxicities. In 1963 Lawrence et al. *(49)* reported a 70% occurrence of local toxic effects (30% of them major) after pelvic perfusion with MMC at a dose of 1 mg/kg. With a dose of 25 mg/m^2 and regional administration of dexamethasone sodium phosphate, no local toxic effects were registered in our series. To reduce systemic exposure, low pressure and flow in the extracorporal circuit with the aim of reducing leakage *(51)* as well as hemofiltration *(66)* were adopted in our study. It has been reported that chemofiltration reduces immediate cytotoxic effects and postpones cumulative toxic effects in patients treated with abdominal stop-flow infusion *(67)*. Strocchi et al. *(61)* provide data showing that a temporary arterio-venous block in the tumor area can actually lead to selective exposition of the tumor to cytostatic drugs, but that hemofiltration is not able to remove MMC and doxorubicin to a significant extent before the circuit from the systemic circulation is removed. For this reason, sample peripheral blood drug concentrations in their patients are similar to those achieved by conventional intravenous chemotherapy. We previously demonstrated that the bioavailability of MMC in the peripheral venous blood can be reduced using safe hemofiltration for 60 min *(56)*. Based on results of our study *(60)*, at the end of the procedure, approx 10% of the total MMC dose administered can be detected in urine and ultrafiltrate. However, the minor clinical consequences of the MMC systemic bioavailability are mainly related, in our opinion, to the use of granulocyte colony-stimulating factor, unfortunately not available in the 1960s.

6. CONCLUSIONS

In our study *(60)*, hypoxic pelvic perfusion has been proposed as palliative treatment in patients with unresectable locally recurrent rectal cancer who are nonresponders or who have disease progression after the standard modalities. The median survival time (12.2 mo) registered after one course of hypoxic pelvic perfusion is comparable to that obtained by irradiation or reirradiation in non-pretreated patients *(29,30)*. Considering the vascular damage following radiotherapy, a different sequence in the multimodular treatment of unresectable recurrent rectal cancer could be more useful. Further studies are necessary to establish whether hypoxic pelvic perfusion improves the quality of life and survival of these patients if administered before radiotherapy with or without concomitant systemic chemotherapy. In conclusion, hypoxic pelvic perfusion is a good palliative treatment for patients with unresectable locally recurrent rectal cancer, but it should be considered as a link of a chain in a multimodular approach.

ACKNOWLEDGMENTS

All the authors contributed equally to the realization of this work.

REFERENCES

1. Quirke P, Durdey P, Dixon MF, Williams NS. Local recurrence of rectal adenocarcinoma due to inadequate surgical resection. Histopathological study of lateral tumor spread and surgical excision. Lancet 1986;2:996–999.
2. Wiig JN, Wolff PA, Tveit KM, Giercksky KE. Location of pelvic recurrence after curative low anterior resection for rectal cancer. Eur J Surg Oncol 1999;25:590–594.
3. Bufalari A, Boselli C, Giustozzi G, Moggi L. Locally advanced rectal cancer: multivariate analysis of outcome risk factors. J Surg Oncol 2000;74:2–10.
4. Holm T, Cedermark B, Rutqvist LE. Local recurrence of rectal adenocarcinoma after "curative" surgery with and without preoperative radiotherapy. Br J Surg 1994;81:452–455.
5. Marsh PJ, James RD, Schofield PF. Definition of local recurrence after surgery for rectal carcinoma. Br J Surg 1995;82:465–468.
6. Sagar PM, Pemberton JH. Surgical management of locally recurrent rectal cancer. Br J Surg 1996;83:293–304.
7. Luna-Perez P, Trejo-Valdivia B, Labastida S, Garcia-Alvarado S, Rodriguez DF, Delgado S. Prognostic factors in patients with locally advanced rectal adenocarcinoma treated with preoperative radiotherapy and surgery. World J Surg 1999;23:1069–1064.
8. Medical Research Council Rectal Cancer Working Party. Randomised trial of surgery alone versus radiotherapy followed by surgery for potentially operable locally advanced rectal cancer. Lancet 1996;348:1605–1610.
9. Marsh PJ, James RD, Schofield PF. Adjuvant preoperative radiotherapy for locally advanced rectal carcinoma. Results of a prospective, randomised trial. Dis Colon Rectum 1994;37:1205–1214.
10. Swedish Rectal Cancer Trial. Improved survival with preoperative radiotherapy in resectable rectal cancer. N Engl J Med 1997;336:980–987.
11. Heald RJ, Husband EM, Ryall RD. The mesorectum in rectal cancer surgery—the clue to pelvic recurrence? Br J Surg 1982;69:613–616.

12. Bokey EL, Ojerskog B, Chapuis PH, Dent OF, Newland RC, Sinclair G. Local recurrence after curative excision of the rectum for cancer without adjuvant therapy: role of total anatomical dissection. Br J Surg 1999;86:1164–1170.

13. Merchant NB, Guillem JG, Paty PB, et al. T3N0 rectal cancer: results following sharp mesorectal excision and no adjuvant therapy. J Gastrointest Surg 1999;3:642–647.

14. Huguier M, Houry S. Treatment of local recurrence of rectal cancer. Am J Surg 1998;175:288–292.

15. Pilipshen SJ, Heilweil M, Quan SHQ, Sternberg SS, Enker WE. Patterns of pelvic recurrence following definitive resections of rectal cancer. Cancer 1984;53:1354–1362.

16. Wanebo HJ, Koness RJ, Vezeridis MP, Cohen SI, Wrobleski DE. Pelvic resection of recurrent rectal cancer. Ann Surg 1994;220:586–597.

17. Suzuki K, Dozois RR, Devine RM, et al. Curative reoperations for locally recurrent rectal cancer. Dis Colon Rectum 1996;39:730–736.

18. Maetani S, Onodera H, Nishikawa T, et al. Significance of local recurrence of rectal cancer as a local or disseminated disease. Br J Surg 1998;85:521–525.

19. Magrini S, Nelson H, Gunderson LL, Sim FH. Sacropelvic resection and intraoperative electron irradiation in the management of recurrent anorectal cancer. Dis Colon Rectum 1996;39:1–9.

20. Lowy AM, Rich TA, Skibber JM, Dubrow RA, Curley SA. Preoperative infusional chemoradiation, selective intaoperative radiation, and resection for locally advanced pelvic recurrence of colorectal adenocarcinoma. Ann Surg 1996;223:1612–1613.

21. Harrison LB, Minsky BD, Henker WE, et al. High dose rate intraoperative radiation therapy (HDR-IORT) as part of the management strategy for locally advanced primary and recurrent rectal cancer. Int J Radiat Oncol Biol Phys 1998;42:325–330.

22. Hoffman JP, Riley L, Litwin S. Isolated locally recurrent rectal cancer: a review of incidence, presentation, and management. Semin Oncol 1993;20:506–519.

23. Hayashi I, Shirai Y, Hatakeyama. Complete remission after radiotherapy for recurrent rectal cancer. Hepatogastroenterology 1997;44:1612–1613.

24. Rominger CJ, Gelber R, Gunderson LL. Radiation therapy alone or in combination with chemotherapy in the treatment of residual or inoperable carcinoma of the rectum and rectosigmoid or pelvic recurrents following colorectal surgery. Am J Clin Oncol 1985;8:118–127.

25. Wong CS, Cummings BJ, Keane TJ, O'Sullivan B, Catton CN. Results of external beam irradiation for rectal carcinoma locally recurrent after local excision or electrocoagulation. Radiother Oncol 1991;22:145–148.

26. Minsky BD, Cohen AM, Enker WE, Sigurdson E, Harrison LB. Radiation therapy for unresectable rectal cancer. Int J Radiat Oncol Biol Phys 1991;21:1283–1289.

27. Dobrowsky W. Mitomycin C, 5-fluorouracil and radiation in advanced, locally recurrent rectal cancer. Br J Radiol 1992;65:143–147.

28. Guiney MJ, Smith JG, Worotniuk V, Ngan S, Blakey D. Radiotherapy treatment for isolated locoregional recurrents of rectosigmoid cancer following definitive surgery: Peter McCallum Cancer Institute experience, 1981–1990. Int J Radiat Oncol Biol Phys 1997;38:1019–1025.

29. Wong CS, Cummings BJ, Brierley JD, et al. Treatment of locally recurrent rectal carcinoma: results and prognostic factors. Int J Radiat Oncol Biol Phys 1998;40:427–435.

30. Lingareddy V, Ahmad NR, Mohiuddin M. Palliative reirradiation for recurrent rectal cancer. Int J Radiat Oncol Biol Phys 1997;38:785–790.

31. Bayer JR, von Heyden HW, Bartsch HH, et al. Intra-arterial perfusion therapy with 5-fluorouracil in patients with metastatic colorectal carcinoma and intractable pelvic pain. Recent Results Cancer Res 1983;86:33–36.

32. Patt YZ, Peters RE, Chuang VP, Wallace S, Claghorn L, Mavligit G. Palliation of pelvic recurrence of colorectal cancer with intraarterial 5-fluorouracil and mitomycin. Cancer 1985;56: 2175–2180.

33. Estes NC, Morphis JG, Hornback NB, Jewell WR. Intraarterial chemotherapy and hyperthermia for pain control in patients with recurrent rectal cancer. Am J Surg 1986;152:597–601.

34. Percivale P, Nobile MT, Vidili MG, et al. Treatment of colorectal cancer pelvic recurrences with hypogastric intraarterial 5-fluorouracil by means of totally implantable port systems. Reg Cancer Treat 1990;3:143–146.

35. Muller H, Aigner KR. Pallation of recurrent rectal cancer with intrarterial mitomycin C/5-fluorouracil via Jet Port aortic bifurcation catheter. Reg Cancer Treat 1990;3:147–151.

36. Tseng MH, Park HC. Pelvic intrarterial mitomycin C infusion in previously treated patients with metastatic, unresectable pelvic colorectal cancer and angiographic determination of tumor vascularity. J Clin Oncol 1985;3:1093–1098.

37. Hafstorm L, Jonsson PE, Landberg T, Owman T, Sundkvist K. Intraarterial infusion chemotherapy (5-fluorouracil) in patients with inextirpable or locally recurrent rectal cancer. Am J Surg 1979;137:757–762.

38. Carlsson C, Hafstrom L, Jonsson PE, Ask A, Kallum B, Lunderquist A. Unresectable and locally recurrent rectal cancer treated with radiotherapy or bilateral internal iliac artery infusion of 5-FU. Cancer 1986;58:336–340.

39. Creech O, Krementz ET, Ryan RF, Winbald JN. Chemotherapy of cancer: regional perfusion utilizing an extracorporeal circuit. Ann Surg 1958;148:616–632.

40. Wile AG, Stemmer EA, Andrews PA, Murphy MP, Abramson IS, Howell SB. Pharmacokinetics of 5-fluorouracil during hypotermic pelvic isolation-perfusion. J Clin Oncol 1985;3:849–852.

41. Vaglini M, Cascinelli F, Chiti A, et al. Isolated pelvic perfusion for the treatment of unresectable primary or recurrent rectal cancer. Tumori 1996;82:459–462.

42. Asten WA, Monaco AP, Richardson GS, Baker WH, Shaw RS, Raker JW. Treatment of malignant pelvic tumors by extracorporeal perfusion with chemotherapeutic agents. N Engl J Med 1959;261: 1037–1045.

43. Ryan RF, Schramel RJ, Creech O Jr. Value of perfusion in pelvic surgery. Dis Colon Rectum 1963;6: 297–300.

44. Shingleton WW, Parker RT, Mahaley S. Abdominal perfusion for cancer chemotherapy with hypothermia and hyperthermia. Surgery 1961;50:260–265.

45. Wile A, Smolin M. Hypertermic pelvic isolation-perfusion in the treatment of refractory pelvic cancer. Arch Surg 1987;122:1321–1325.

46. Lawrence W, Kuehn P, Mori S, Poppel JW, Clarkson B. Regional perfusion of the pelvis: consideration of the "leakage" problem. Surgery 1961;50:248–259.

47. Lathrop JC, Leone LA, Sodeberg CH, Colbert MP, Vargas LL. Perfusion chemotherapy for gynaecological malignancy. Trans N Engl Obstet gynecol Soc 1963;17:47–56.

48. Watkins E, Hering AC, Luna R, Adams HD. The use of intravascolar balloon catheters for isolation of the pelvic vascular bed during pump-oxygenator perfusion of cancer chemotherapeutic agents. Surg gynecol Obstet 1960;111:464–468.

49. Lawrence W, Clarkson B, Kim M, Clapp P, Randall HT. Regional perfusion of pelvis and abdomen by an indirect technique. Cancer 1963;16:567–582.

50. Turk PS, Belliveau JF, Darnowsky JW, Weinberg MC, Leenen L, Wanebo HJ. Isolated pelvic perfusion for unrectable cancer using a balloon occlusion tecnique. Arch Surg 1993;128:533–539.

51. Wanebo HJ, Chung MA, Levy AI, Turk PS, Vezeridis MP, Belliveau JP. Preoperative therapy for advanced pelvic malignancy by isolated pelvic perfusion with the balloo-occlusion tecnique. Ann Surg Oncol 1996, 3:295–303.

52. Aigner KR, Kaevel K. Pelvic stopflow infusion (PSI) and hypoxic pelvic perfusion (HPP) with mitomycin and melphalan for recurrent rectal cancer. Reg Cancer Treat 1994;7:6–11.

53. Thompson JF, Liu M, Waugh RC, et al. A percutaneous aortic "stop-flow" infusion tecnique for regional cytotoxic therapy of the abdomen and pelvis. Reg Cancer Treat 1994;7:202–207.

54. Teicher BA, Lazo JS, Sartorelli AC. Classification of antineoplastic agents by their selective toxicities toward oxigenated and hypoxic tumor cells. Cancer Res 1981;41:73–81.

55. Rockwell S. Effect of some proliferative and environmental factors on the toxicity of mitomycine to tumor cells in vitro. Int J Cancer 1986;38:229–235.

56. Guadagni S, Aigner KR, Palumbo G, et al. Pharmacokinetics of mitomycine C in pelvic stopflow infusion and hypoxic pelvic perfusion with and without hemofiltration: a pilot study of patients with recurrent unresectable rectal cancer. J Clin Pharmacol 1998;38:936–944.

57. Suzuki K, Gunderson LL, Devine RM, et al. Intraoperative irradiation after palliative surgery for locally recurrent rectal cancer. Cancer 1995;75:939–952.

58. Graham RA, Siddik ZH, Hohn DC. Extrcorporeal hemofiltration: a model for digreasing systemic drug exposure with intraarterial chemotherapy. Cancer Chemother Pharmacol 1990;26:210–214.

59. Door RT. New findings in the pharmacokinetic metabolic and drug resistance aspects of mitomycine C. Semin Oncol 1998;15:32–41.

60. Guadagni S, Fiorentini G, Palumbo G, et al. Hypoxic pelvic perfusion with mitomycin C using a simplified balloon-occlusion tecnique in the treatment of patients with unresectable locally recurrent rectal cancer. Arch Surg 2001;136:105–112.

61. Strocchi E, Iaffaioli RV, Facchini G, et al. Stop-flow tecnique for loco-regional delivery of high dose chemotherapy in the treatment of advanced pelvic cancers. EJSO 2004;30:663–670.

62. Hengelberg H. Actions of heparine that may affect the malignant process. Cancer 1999;85:257–272.

63. Fuchs CS, Moore MR, Harker G, Villa L, Rinaldi D, Hecht JR. Phase III comparison of two irinotecan dosing regimens in second-line therapy of metastatic colorectal cancer. J Clin Oncol 2003;21:807–814.

64. Carrato A, Gallego J, Diaz-Rubio E. Oxaliplatin: results in colorectal carcinoma. Crit Rev Oncol Hematol 2002;44:29–44.

65. Pilati P, Mocellin D, Miotto D, et al. Stop-flow tecnique for loco-regional delivery of antiblastic agents: literature review and personal experience. Eur J Surg Oncol 2002;28:544–553.

66. Guadagni S, Fiorentini G, D'Alessandro V, et al. Intrahepatic artery high-dose chemotherapy with concomitant post-hepatic venous blood detoxification: comparison between drug removal systems. Reg Cancer Treat 1995;8:140–150.

67. Aigner KR, Gaihofer S. High dose MMC: aortic stopflow infusion (ASI) with versus without chemofiltration: a comparison of toxic side effects (abstract). Reg Cancer Treat 1993;6(Suppl 1):3.

22 Percutaneous Laser Ablation of Lung Metastases

Christiane Weigel, MD,
Claus-Dieter Heidecke, MD,
and Norbert Hosten, MD

CONTENTS

SUMMARY

CT guidance allows for placement of a laser applicator into a pulmonary metastasis while the patient is under conscious sedation. The metastasis may thus be thermally destroyed. We describe how a laser applicator used in pulmonary lesions is designed; how complications from laser ablation compare to diagnostic biopsies; and how the technique may supplement traditional surgical therapy. It should be mentioned that following laser ablation, lesions enlarge, and it may take weeks or months before scar formation is reached. The technique is compared with other modalities and the necessity to combine it with local pharmaceutical approaches is discussed.

Key Words: Lung, metastases; lung, laser ablation; intervention, pulmonary.

1. INTRODUCTION

Lung metastases develop in 15% of patients with colorectal carcinoma and in 30 to 50% of all cancer patients *(1)*. Surgical studies have long shown that removal of pulmonary metastases improves survival. Over the last decades surgical techniques have been continuously improved, with a trend toward minimally invasive techniques *(2–14)*.

From: *Cancer Drug Discovery and Development: Regional Cancer Therapy*
Edited by: P. M. Schlag and U. S. Stein © Humana Press Inc., Totowa, NJ

Thoracotomy has now been supplemented by video-assisted thoracic surgery (VATS), although this technique is not yet generally accepted to remove metastases. Depending on the primary tumor as well as other factors, 5-yr survival rates after surgical removal of lung metastases may approach 50%. Despite these advances, an image-guided, minimally invasive procedure such as thermoablation may be useful in patients who are (1) primarily not candidates for surgery for different reasons or who are (2) no longer operable following repeated resections. In addition (3), an approach whereby central lesions are laser ablated and peripheral lesions surgically removed in one session also seems feasible.

The capabilities of diagnostic imaging modalities have steadily progressed in the last decades. Current diagnostic imaging is able to visualize pathologic lesions noninvasively. Development of computed tomography (CT) has especially favored image-guided therapies. Resolution today is very good in the spatial as well as temporal domains. CT-fluoroscopy is now available and allows fast and accurate placement of applicators for percutaneous ablative therapies.

The topographic relationship of a lesion to surrounding tissue is easily delineated. This kind of visualization allows for a transcutaneous therapeutic approach in some patients and for selected pathologies. Lesions located within the depth of the body may thus be accessed with needles, catheters, or other instruments, preferably of small caliber. A simple means of treatment is destruction of the lesions; metastastic disease is a main target of these ablative therapies. Different ways of ablating tissue have been described. Ablation of tissue has been successful because tissue within the depth of the body tends to be of limited susceptibility to pain and even large volumes of necrotic tissue can be resorbed by the body without infection or abscess formation. It should be stressed that ablative therapies are not substitutes for surgery. They are generally restricted, because they destroy tissue in a defined diameter, not along anatomic boundaries; on the other hand, interventional therapy may be still performed when a patient's clinical state makes surgery unsuitable. As most ablative therapies can be performed with conscious sedation, patients may be treated with minimal hospitalization. The incidence of most cancers increases with age. With an ageing population, the requirement for tumor therapies that can be applied to older multimorbid patients increases *(15)*.

2. CONDITIONS FOR PERCUTANEOUS, IMAGE-GUIDED THERAPY OF LUNG TUMORS

Ideally, complications after therapeutic pulmonary procedures should not significantly exceed those of percutaneous biopsies of lung nodules *(16)*. A thin caliber of the applicator seems especially important to avoid complications like pneumothorax, hemorrhage, and air embolism *(17)*, or at least to reduce their frequency. As pneumothorax is the most frequent complication to be expected, a modality that adequately visualizes pneumothorax should be chosen for image guidance. CT is the modality of choice. The applicator therefore must be visible on CT.

Experience from tumor ablation indicates that recurrent tumor is a problem with most ablative therapies. Current research therefore aims at a therapy combining thermal ablation and application of ablative pharmaceuticals. The applicator used for thermal ablation should allow for instillation of liquid agents.

3. COMPLICATIONS AFTER DIAGNOSTIC
BIOPSY OF PULMONARY NODULES

The percentages of pneumothoraces after biopsy vary in different publications, the range being between 5 and 61%; the necessity for chest tubes range between 0 and 20% (18–28). Different authors judge factors that favor pneumothorax differently; there seems to be a trend toward fewer pneumothoraces in deeper lesions. Hemorrhage is the most dangerous complication after diagnostic biopsy of pulmonary lesions. Few data have been published recently, but it seems that 3 to 10% of all pulmonary biopsies lead to some degree of hemorrhage, usually along the needle path. Hemoptysis is at the lower end of the range of complications, i.e., it is seen in about 3% of all biopsies. Air embolism is a life-threatening but extremely rare complication; it seems to be favored by air-cooled laser fibers or by abrupt changes in intrathoracal pressure.

Of 51 patients biopsied in our institution, 27 had malignant lung nodules. Pneumothorax was seen in 35%, hemorrhage on CT scans in 33%, and hemoptysis in 4%. In 8% of patients pneumothorax had to be treated. We did not see any cases of air embolism.

4. DEVELOPMENT OF A LASER APPLICATOR

Laser ablation destroys tissue by heating (29). Exposure to a temperature of over 60°C for more than 10 min is supposed to destroy cells completely. Denaturation of proteins is one mechanism of action. Applicators for laser ablation have to be small enough to ensure nearly atraumatic introduction into tissue (30). Carbonization would severely limit heat propagation into the surrounding tissue and must therefore be prevented by permitting the passage of cooling fluid along the laser fiber. Magnetic resonance (MR)-thermometry is another way of controlling heat application (31); it is, however, not yet feasible in the lung. The ablation of larger volumes is thus facilitated.

Introducing a laser fiber into tissue requires a light-transparent guiding structure (applicator), which may be a needle or a catheter. The use of a guiding structure minimizes the risk of damage to both the tissue and the light guide with the diffuser tip. The applicator we developed for thoracic use had to fulfill two requirements. First, the applicator must be introduced into the tumor tissue like a biopsy needle, without additional manipulation that would increase the risk of pneumothorax. Surprisingly, a thin Teflon tube stabilized by a solid needle made from titanium (= mandrin) proved perfectly suitable to penetrate the thoracic wall and reach any position within the lung. Second, the cooling fluid need not be removed. The second canal can thus be dispensed with and the diameter of the applicator kept small.

The main feature of the applicator (Monocath®, Trumpf Medizinsysteme, Umkirch, Germany, [32]) is the Teflon tube, with a diameter of 5.5 French (Fig. 1). The inner diameter of the Teflon tube is large enough to allow for easy passage of a standard laser fiber. The space between the laser fiber and the inner wall of the Teflon tube is large enough to allow the minimal fluid flow required for cooling the diffuser tip. When the Teflon tube is positioned, the mandrin is exchanged for the laser fiber. A headpiece with a thread is attached to one end of the Teflon tube. When the mandrin is removed, a Y-shaped distributor with a hemostatic valve at the straight opening is connected to the Teflon tube. The hemostatic valve holds the laser fiber, which must end within the Teflon tube just before its distal end. The second opening of the Y-shaped distributor receives

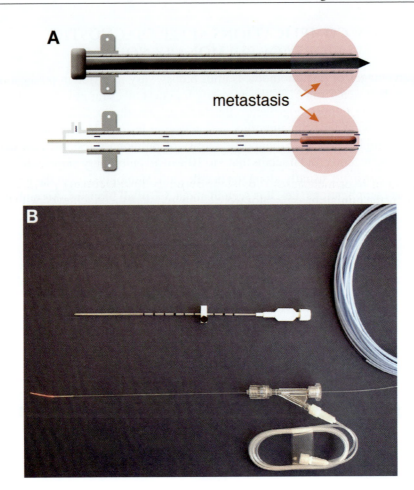

metastasis

Fig. 1. (A) Construction of the applicator. The drawing illustrates how the tube part of the appli-cator is fitted on the titanium mandrin and its position in a metastasis (top); after the titanium mandrin is removed and the Y-shaped distributor is connected, the laser fiber and the infusion line for the cooling fluid are connected to the hemostatic valve (bottom). Note that the scattering dome of the laser fiber is now inside the metastasis. **(B)** Photograph of the applicator. The upper part of the photo shows the applicator ready for introduction: the Teflon tube is mounted on a titanium mandrin. After placement of the applicator, the mandrin is removed and the premounted laser fiber (bottom) is placed inside the Teflon tube instead. The hemostatic valve is connected to the laser fiber and the cooling medium. Exchange of laser fiber for mandrin after placement allows for a small-diameter applicator.

the line supplying the cooling fluid. In short, after the Teflon tube is introduced into the metastasis and the titanium mandrin is removed, the Y-shaped distributor with the fitted laser fiber is connected to the Teflon tube. Ideally the diffuser tip of the laser fiber is positioned inside the metastasis. The length of the dome is chosen in such a way that it reaches 5 mm beyond the margins of the metastasis at both ends. Alternatively, it may be repositioned within the tube during the ablation process to first treat the distal and then the proximal part of the tumor.

For treatment, two Nd:Yag lasers are used (1064 nm, Dornier Medilas 5100 Fibertom, Dornier Medtech Europe, Wessling, Germany). Each laser is fitted with a beam splitter

TT-Switch 3 (Trumpf Medizinsysteme). Up to six fibers can be used simultaneously. Laser fibers (Microdome and Microflexx, Trumpf) are available in lengths of 1, 2, 2.5, and 3 cm. We use the 3- and 2-cm fibers in most cases. The diameters of the laser fiber at the dome are 1.1 mm (Microflexx) and 0.9 mm (Microdome). The flexible diffuser tip is preferred *(33)*. Between one and four laser fibers are used per treatment. The power deposited ranges from 3.0 to 35.0 kW (mean 19.0 kW). The total duration of energy application ranges from 9 to 25 min (mean 15 min). When several fibers are used, they are supplied simultaneously.

The miniature applicator was calibrated against a commercially available applicator for treatment of liver metastases (Somatex, Berlin Teltow, Germany [34]). The areas necrotized by the miniature applicator were compared with those achieved with the liver applicator system. The area of necrosis was 6.0×4.5 cm for the power applicator with standard operating characteristics (20 min, 30 W, 60 mL/min). To achieve a necrosis of that size, the microcatheter had to be powered by 15 W for 20 min with a flow of the cooling fluid of 0.75 mL/min. An area of 6.0×4.0 cm was thus necrotized. We used the aforementioned operating parameters as a starting point for patient therapy.

5. CT-GUIDED LASER ABLATION (LITT) OF LUNG METASTASES

5.1. Technique

In our opinion, the following criteria have to be met for indication of LITT of lung metastases: *(1)* histological proof of a primary tumor known to metastasize to the lung; *(2)* imaging proof of development of a lung lesion, i.e., follow-up studies (contrast-enhanced CT) have to show a new nodule; *(3)* approval of percutaneous laser ablation given by the institution's interdisciplinary tumor board; *(4)* absence of coagulation disorders; and *(5)* informed consent of the patient *(35)*.

The procedure is performed in the CT scanner room. The physician performing the treatment, a nurse, and two technicians operating the CT scanner and the laser are present. Vital signs are monitored during the session. Patients receive an infusion of haloperidol (Haloperidol-GRY®, TEVA, Kirchzarten, Germany), metoclopramide (Cerucal®, TemmLer, Marburg, Germany), and pethidin (Dolantin®, Aventis, Frankfurt, Germany) in 500 mL saline 0.9%. Under this regimen, the procedure is tolerated while patients are conscious and able to respond to breathing instructions.

Applicators and laser fibers are premounted. At the beginning of each session, the infusion pumps (IVAC Medizintechnik, Giessen, Germany) are started and kept running until cooling fluid emerges at the applicators' tips. These preparations were found to be necessary as they reduce table time for the patients. For most patients, lying on the CT table with their arms raised is the most arduous part of the treatment. Functioning of the laser system is controlled for each fiber using the pilot light. After the patient is positioned, the skin is disinfected and the surroundings of the entry site are covered with sterile drapes. The skin at the entry site is anesthetized with local anesthetic (1% lidocaine), and after a few seconds the thoracic wall is infiltrated at the site where the pleura is to be transversed. Contact with the pleura, however, is avoided. The needle is left in place at an angle deemed suitable for positioning of the applicator and the plane of the needle imaged under fluoroscopy. Ideally, the needle and metastases are seen on this image with the needle pointing precisely at the center of the metastasis. If this is not the case, the needle is cautiously repositioned.

A small incision is made after the correct angle for applicator placement is determined and the applicator is introduced. Contact with the pleura is again avoided at this stage while the applicator is introduced as far as necessary to secure a stable position. The distance between the tip of the applicator and the distal margin of the metastasis is then measured and marked with an adjustable stop on the Teflon tube. Another image is obtained under fluoroscopic guidance, and the position of the applicator relative to the metastasis is ascertained. If a single applicator is to be used, the applicator is aimed at the center of the metastasis; if two applicators are deemed necessary, they are aimed at the tumor's periphery. A distance of 10 to 20 mm between applicators is considered ideal, depending on the size of the metastasis. The patients are then instructed to hold their breath in either inspiration or expiration.

The choice of inspiration or expiration is made depending on which better moves the ribs away for accessibility of the metastasis. The applicator is then pushed forward without fluoroscopic control for the distance measured immediately prior to the maneuver (until the clip touches the skin). Fluoroscopy is used to control the position. If the position is considered correct, the applicator is fixed with adhesive tape to the patient's skin. After all applicators are in place, the metal mandrins are removed one by one and immediately replaced by the Y-shaped hemostatic valve holding the laser fiber. Application of energy is then started without further delay. Fluoroscopy is used at various points to monitor treatment, especially to exclude progressive pneumothorax, hemorrhage, changes within the metastasis, and cooling fluid distribution in the lung. After energy application is terminated, the laser fibers and applicators are removed. The canal is not sealed. Fluoroscopy is used to check for pneumothorax below or above the level of the applicators at this point.

The whole process naturally involved learning curve. Placement of the applicators was not more complicated or time consuming than placement of a biopsy gun. Ablation of a single metastasis with two applicators typically took around 60 min.

5.2. Complications

For the miniature applicator the pneumothorax rate was 48%, hemorrhage was seen on CT scans in 21%, and hemoptysis in 9%. Varying complication rates are reported in the literature *(36–39)*. Lee and co-workers *(38)* describe major and minor complications they encountered. Major complications like severe pneumothorax and acute respiratory distress syndrome were seen only in central lesions. Major complications occurred in 3/30 patients. Minor complications were seen in a larger percentage, covering a span of 36% for small pneumothorax in central lesions to pleural effusion in 2/39 cases and hemoptysis in 1/30. Steinke and coworkers *(40,41)* treated 20 patients with pulmonary metastases from colorectal carcinoma with radiofrequency ablation; pneumothorax resulted in 10. Four of these and one patient with a hydropneumothorax required chest tube placement. Spontaneously resolving smaller pleural effusions were seen more often. Steinke et al. *(40,41)* mention cavitations among their complications. Although its precise nature remains to be determined (possibly a valve mechanism or gas development during therapy), in our opinion cavitation is rather a favorable sign. Patients who developed cavitations in our series (8/64) showed complete regression of both cavitations and metastasis in a further course. Steinke and coworkers *(40,41)* observed intraparenchymal hemorrhage in 7.5%, which proved harmless in their series as well as in ours and led to only one case of hemoptysis in each. Both cases resolved spontaneously. All in all, pneumothorax, pleural effusion, and hemoptysis are the complications most often described. For comparison, it must be borne in mind that in our experience emphysema, which makes patients more susceptible to pneumothorax, is more frequent in patients with lung cancer than in patients with metastases.

5.3. Results

Our own work showed the following results. Forty-two patients with 64 lung tumors were treated (39 patients with metastases and 3 with primary tumors). Mean follow-up was 7.6 mo (range 6 wk to 39 mo). Eighty percent of the treatments were technically successful in the first session. Pneumothorax was the main complication and occurred in 50% of the first 20 patients and in 35% of the rest. Two patients required a chest tube. Fourteen lesions were central, and 50 were peripheral. It took several weeks for the effect of therapy to become apparent on follow-up CT. Thirty-nine percent of all lesions increased in size immediately after treatment. Gross reduction in size with scar formation was seen in 50% of the lesions and cavitation in 13%. Local tumor control was achieved in 51 lesions. Progression after therapy was seen in 9% of lesions <1.5 cm but in more than 11% of larger lesions. Progression was also more frequent in lesions located in the basal parts of the lung (47%). Sixteen patients died from systemic progression.

A few approaches to percutaneous ablation of lung nodules have recently been published. Several groups *(36,37)* described successful ablation of a single case. Rose et al. reported that the possibility of microembolization to the brain during radiofrequency ablation of pulmonary nodules requires special attention. Lee and Jin *(38)* have recently published a larger series of non-small cell lung cancer ($n = 27$) and lung metastases ($n = 4$). They used radiofrequency ablation and reached complete necrosis in 38% of lesions. Necrosis proved more difficult to achieve in larger nodules. Our own results with 43% complete ablation did not differ significantly. However, it is not clear at this point whether ablation of lung cancer and of lung metastases is the same.

5.4. Imaging Findings

Imaging findings after thermal ablation are strongly time dependent. In our series we found enlargement of the lesion itself immediately after ablation. It took months before shrinkage and scar formation were observed (Fig. 2). These findings correspond to those reported by other groups. Various authors report volumetric measurements with some metastases increasing and some decreasing after 3 mo. Our experience suggests that some decrease in volume is to be expected in successfully treated lesions at 3-mo follow-up. Jin and co-workers *(39)* devoted a whole paper to the description of CT follow-up after ablation of (mostly primary) lung lesions. The decrease seen after 3 mo was 5.7% in nine completely ablated lesions vs 40% at 15 mo. In our study, completely ablated metastases showed even more pronounced shrinkage with only some scarring remaining. These authors *(39)* found increased volumes in completely ablated lesions. Jin and coworkers describe contrast enhancement as a sign of viable tumor, given that it was already present before ablation. Animal studies *(42–44)* suggest that normal lung tissue is destroyed by heat as well, but little attention has been paid to damage caused by ablation in normal lung tissue. Contrary to the appearance of ablated liver metastases, a successfully ablated lung lesion is not characterized by a rim of overtly damaged normal lung tissue. Neither our data nor those of other groups suggest such a phenomenon. Instead, a completely ablated lung lesion seems to be characterized by the absence of contrast enhancement that was

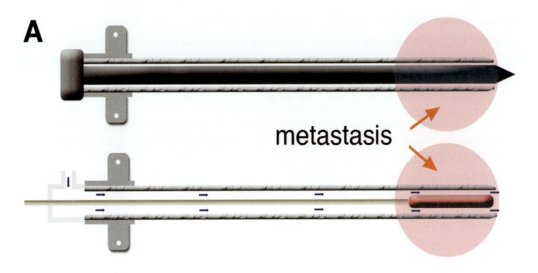

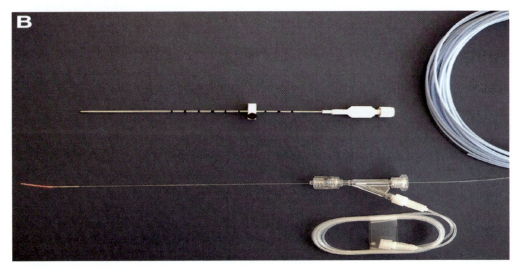

Fig. 2. Follow-up of pulmonary metastases after laser ablation. Soft-tissue (**A**) and lung window CT (**B**) demonstrate lesions located centrally in the right lung before (left) and at 3 (middle) and 6 (right) mo after laser ablation. There is some shrinkage at 3 mo, but regression of the metastasis is slow.

seen before treatment. However, we saw cavitations in nine lesions, and all of them showed complete regression in the further course. The significance of cavernation still has to be determined.

For better delineation of the amount of necrosis achieved, perfusion CT studies may be obtained and perfusion maps calculated from these images (contrast medium bolus, 80 mL, 320 mg iodine/mL, flow 7.2 mL/s, >50 consecutive scans, breath hold, no table movement). The slice should be positioned at the level of the applicator or in the middle of the applicators. Parameter images can then be calculated for blood flow, blood volume, mean transit time, and time to peak.

5.5. *Advantages of LITT of Lung Metastases*

Although radiofrequency has the advantage of being marketed as a complete set ready for therapy, laser ablation has other definite advantages:

1. The laser fiber does not have to be positioned inside a nodule to allow for ablation of lung lesions. The laser light is easily transmitted through air-filled spaces and thermal ablation may be achieved without actual contact.
2. Multiple applicators with multiple fibers may be introduced into a larger metastasis. The applicator described here has the additional advantage of allowing for tissue access.

Suzuki and coworkers *(46)* have demonstrated the feasibility of using ethanol for ablation in the lung. This might be a way to improve ablation results. Chemotherapeutic agents, which may be applied locally in high concentrations, may prove to be a better tolerated agent for local therapy. Immunological phenomena have been described.

5.6. INDICATIONS

Current results indicate that thermal laser ablation of lung metastases is an additional therapeutic option. Its indication appears more successful for nodules that are (1) located centrally and in the upper parts of the lungs and (2) are between 15 and 40 mm. Lesions with contact to the pleura are difficult to treat, because adequate anesthesia is hard to achieve, and applicators have to be placed rather awkwardly parallel to the inner side of the thoracic wall. These lesions, however, are ideal candidates for removal with surgical minimally invasive techniques. Likewise, lesions close to the diaphragm are also difficult to treat with laser ablation, as respiratory movements make placement difficult.

Another modality, which might be used in combination with laser ablation, is local chemotherapy. Chemotherapeutic agents may be introduced via the applicator. Research is ongoing to determine properties of chemotherapeutic agents that allow for optimal contact with the wall of the necrotic cave after laser ablation.

6. CONCLUSIONS

In conclusion, percutaneous laser ablation is a suitable tool for the thermal destruction of lung metastases. Results are best in medium-size lesions (between 2 and 3 cm) and in lesions located more centrally and in the upper parts of the lungs. Complications do not differ significantly from those observed in diagnostic lung biopsy under CT guidance. The applicator used in our study allows for instillation of tumoricidal substances *(46)* after completion of thermal ablation and removal of the laser fiber. In our opinion, this may show potential in treating larger metastases or those not completely ablated by heat alone.

REFERENCES

1. Baron, O, Amimi M, Duveau D, Despins S, Sagan CA, Michaud JL. Surgical resection of pulmonary metastases from colorectal carcinoma. Eur J Cardiothorac Surg 1979;10:347–351.
2. Zanella A, Marchet A, Mainente P, Nitti D, Lise M. Resection of pulmonary metastases from colorectal carcinoma. Eur J Surg Oncol 1997; 23:424–427.
3. Saito Y, Omiya H, Kohno K, et al. Pulmonary metastasectomy for 165 patients with colorectal carcinoma: a prognostic assessment. J Thorac Cardiovasc Surg 2002;124:1007–1013
4. Davidson RS, Nwogu CE, Brentjens MJ, Anderson TM. The surgical management of pulmonary metastasis: current concepts. Surg Oncol 2001;10:35–42.

5. Inoue M, Kotake Y, Nakagawa K, Fujiwara K, Fukuhara K, Yasumitsu T. Surgery for pulmonary metastases from colorectal carcinoma. Ann Thorac Surg 2000;70:380–383.

6. Leo F, Cagini L, Rocmans P, et al. Lung metastases from melanoma: when is surgical treatment warranted? Br J Cancer 2000;83:569–572.

7. Groeger AM, Kandioler D, Mueller MR, End A, Eckersberger F, Wolner E. Survival after surgical treatment of recurrent pulmonary metastases. Eur J Cardiothorac Surg 1997;12:703–705

8. Maniwa, Y, Kanki M, Okita Y. Importance of the control of lung recurrence soon after surgery of pulmonary metastases. Am J Surg 2000;179:122–125.

9. McCormack PM, Attizeh FF. Resected pulmonary metastases from colorectal cancer. Dis Colon Rectum 1979;22:553–556.

10. McCormack PM, Bains MS, Begg CB, Burt ME. Role of VATS in the treatment of pulmonary metastases; results of a prospective trial. Ann Thorac Surg 1996;68:795–796.

11. McCormack PM, Burt ME, Bains MS, Martini N, Rusch VW, Ginsburg RJ. Lung resection for colorectal metastases. 10-year results. Arch Surg 1992;127:1403–1406.

12. Putnam JB. New and evolving treatment. Methods for pulmonary metastases. Semin Thorac Cardiovasc Surg 2002;14:49–56.

13. Okumura S, Kondo H, Tsuboi M, et al. Pulmonary resection for metastatic colorectal cancer: experiences with 159 patients. J Thorac Cardiovasc Surg 1996;112:867–874.

14. The International Registry of Lung Metastases. Long-term results of lung metastasectomy: prognostic analyses based on 5206 cases. J Thorac Cardiovasc Surg 1997;113:37–49.

15. Busemann C, Schmidt CA, Fendrich K, Hoffmann W. [Lung metastases of colorectal tumors: clinical background and development of care supply.] Radiologe 2004;7:711–714.

16. Diederich S, Hosten N. [Percutaneous ablation of pulmonary tumours: state-of-the-art 2004.] Radiologe 2004;7:658–662.

17. Rose SC, Fotooki M, Lewin DL, Harrell JH. Cerebral microembolization during radiofrequency ablation of lung malignancies. J Vasc Interv Radiol 2002;13:1051–1054.

18. Garcia-Rio F, Pino JM, Casadevall J, et al. Use of spirometry to predict risk of pneumothorax in CT-guided needle biopsy of the lung. J Comput Assisted Tomogr 1996;20:20–23.

19. Shaham D. Semi-invasive and invasive procedures for the diagnosis and staging of lung cancer I: Percutaneous transthoracic needle biopsy. Radiol Clin North Am 2000;38:525–534.

20. Huanqi L, Boiselle PM, McLoud TC, Troman-Dickenson B, Shepard AO. Diagnostic accuracy and safety of CT-guided percutaneous needle aspiration biopsy of the lung: comparison of small and large pulmonary nodules. AJR 1996;167:105–109.

21. Gouliamos AD, Giannopoulos DH, Panagi GM, FletoridisNK, Deligeorgie-Polititi HA, Vlahos LJ. Computed tomography-guided fine needle aspiration of peripheral lung opacities. An initial diagnostic procedure? Acta Cytol 2000;44:344–348.

22. Haramati LB, Austin JHM. Complications after CT-guided needle biopsy through aerated versus nonaerated lung. Radiology 1991;181:778.

23. Klein JS, Zarka MA. Transthoracic needle biopsy. Radiol Clin North Am 2000;38:235–266.

24. Laurent F, Michel P, Latrabe V, Tuno de Lara M, Marthan R. Pneumothoraces and chest tube placement after CT-guided transthoracic lung biopsy using a coaxial tehnique: incidence and risk factors. AJR 1999;172:1049–1053.

25. Moore E, Shepard JAO, McLoud TC, Templeton PA, Kosiuk JP. Positional precautions in needle aspiration lung biopsy. Radiology 1990;175:733–735.

26. Westcott JL. Percutaneous transthoracic needle biopsy. Radiology 1988;169:593–601.

27. Westcott JL. Direct percutaneous needle aspiration of localized pulmonary lesions: results in 422 patients. Radiology 1980;137:31–35.

28. Bergquist TH, Bailey PB, Cortese DA, Miller WE. Transthoracic needle biopsy accurcy and complications in relation to location and type of lesion. Mayo Clin Proc 1980;55:475–481.

29. Brooks JAS, Lees WR, Brown SD. Interstitial laser photocoagulation for treatment of lung cancer. AJR 1997;168:357–358.

30. Speck U, Stroszczynski, Puls P, Gaffke G, Hosten N, Felix R. [A miniaturized tissue applicator: in-vitro characterization for laser-induced thermotherapy] ROFO 2002;174:S 303.

31. Hosten N, Puls R, Kreißig R, et al. In vivo temperature measurements and MR-thermometry during laser-induced interstitial thermotherapy (LITT) of liver metastases. Eur Radiol 2000;10:C7–C8.

32. Hosten N, Stier A, Weigel C, et al. [Laser-induced thermotherapy (LITT) of lung metastases: description of a miniaturized applicator, optimization, and initial treatment of patients.] ROFO 2003;175: 393–400.

33. Pech M, Werk M, Beck A, Stohlmann A, Ricke J. [System continuity and energy distribution in laser-induced thermo therapy (LITT).] ROFO 2002;174:754–760.

34. Puls R, Hosten N, Stroszczynski, Kreissig R, Gaffke G, Felix R. [Laser-induced thermotherapy (LITT). Use of round and pointed laser applicator systems—initial results.] ROFO 2001;173:263–265.

35. Weigel C, Kirsch M, Schuchmann S, Speck U, Hosten N. Laser ablation of lung metastases: technique and results after 21 treatments. Med Laser Appl 2004;19:83–90.

36. Highland AM, Mack P, Breen DJ. Radiofrequency thermal ablation of metastatic lung nodule. Eur Radiol 2002:12:5166–5170.

37. Breen MS, Lazebnik RS, Fitzmaurice M, Nour SG, Lewin JS, Wilson DL. Radiofrequency thermal ablation: correlation of hyperacute MR lesion images with tissue response. J Magn Reson Imaging 2004;20:475–486.

38. Lee JM, Jin Gy. Percutaneous radiofrequency ablation for inoperable non-small cell lung cancer and metastases: preliminary report. Radiology 2004;230:125–134.

39. Jin GY, Lee JM, Lee YC, Han YM, Lim YS. Primary and secondary lung malignancies treated with percutaneous radiofrequency ablation: evaluation with follow-up helical CT. AJR 2004;183:1013–1020

40. Steinke K, Glenn D, King J, Morris DL. Percutaneous pulmonary radiofrequency ablation: difficulty achieving complete ablations in big lesions. Br J Radiol 2003;76:742–745.

41. Steinke K, King J, Glenn D, Morris DL. Radiologic appearance and complications of percutaneous computed tomography-guided radiofrequency-ablated pulmonary metastases from colorectal carcinoma. J Comput Assist Tomogr 2003;27:750–757.

42. Glenn DW, Clark W, Morris DL, King J, Zhao J. Percutaneous radiofrequency ablation of colorectal pulmonary metastases. Radiology 2001;201:315.

43. Miao Y, Ni Y, Bosmans H, et al. Radiofrequency ablation for eradication of pulmonary tumor in rabbits. J Surg Res 2001;99:265–271.

44. Morrison PR, van Sonnenberg E, Shankar S, et al. Radiofrequency ablation of thoracic lesions: part 1, experiments in the normal porcine thorax. AJR Am J Roentgenol 2005;184:375–380.

45. Oshima F, Yamakado K, Akeboshi M, et al. Lung radiofrequency ablation with and without bronchial occlusion: experimental study in porcine lungs. J Vasc Intervent Radiol 2004;15:1451–1456.

46. Suzuki K, Moriyama N, Yokose T, et al. Preliminary study of percutaneous alcohol injection into the lung. Jpn J Cancer Res 1998;89:89–95.

1. The treatment of small targets (diameter <4 cm).
2. The application of a stereotactic head frame or similar image-guided techniques for target localization.
3. Convergence of multiple beams on the isocenter with a steep dose gradient.
4. Use of a single fraction of irradiation.

The two most common delivery systems for radiosurgery are dedicated linear accelerator systems and the gamma knife (cobalt-60 sources) *(17–19)*. Linear accelerator units are the most common devices employed. The maximum tolerated doses (enclosing the lesion) of single-fraction radiosurgery are 15 to 24 gy for tumors <20 to 40 mm in maximum diameter *(20)*.

Acute side effects and complications associated with SRS like edema and worsening of preexisting symptoms (seizure, aphasia, or motor deficits) are rare, owing to the small, well-circumscribed target volumes. The potential for acute toxicity increases substantially for larger lesions. Radiosurgery can be applied as a technique for boosting external beam radiotherapy for newly diagnosed malignant gliomas or for the control of recurrences *(21–24)*.

Many studies and retrospective analyses, designed to evaluate the role of radiosurgery as a component of initial management (surgery and external beam radiotherapy), have reported on improved survival of patients *(25–29)*; however, any apparent improvement in outcome seen in these trials may have been attributable to patient selection. Curran et al. *(30)* and Larson et al. *(31)* determined the factors associated with survival differences after radiosurgery and concluded that survival was strongly related to patient selection variables, e.g., pathologic grade, age, Karnofsky performance score (KPS), tumor volume, and radicalism of resection.

To clarify this discussion, the Radiation Therapy Oncology Group (RTOG) conducted a prospective phase III trial evaluating SRS boost in patients treated for glioblastoma multiforme. No survival benefit or changes in general quality of life or cognitive functioning could be demonstrated *(32)*.

2.2. Brachytherapy

Interstitial brachytherapy, where either multiple radioactive sources are placed or one high-activity source is moved within the tumor being treated, is another technique to deliver a boost dose to malignant brain tumors while limiting radiation to the surrounding brain. The common isotopes used are iodine-125 (low dose rate [LDR]) and iridium-192 (high dose rate [HDR]). For intracavitary brachytherapy, phosphorus-32 and yttrium-90 are often used.

Total dose delivered depends on the duration of the implants and the total activity of the isotopes used. ^{125}I is an isotope with lower energy (mean 30 keV) emitting X-rays, compared with the gamma irradiation of ^{192}Ir (approx 300 keV). The sources are generally implanted as seeds either temporarily or permanently and either directly during surgery (^{125}I) or by stereotactic techniques. Remote afterloading devices are used for HDR irradiation or pulsed dose rate (PDR) irradiation.

For more than 20 yr, interstitial brachytherapy has been used as additional treatment modality for malignant brain tumors, and most phase I and II trials have suggested a survival benefit for newly diagnosed patients and reasonable tumor control for recurrent patients *(33–40)*. Studies on the use of low-activity permanent brachytherapy implants, which received attention because of lower toxicity *(41,42)*, revealed comparable survival to that of similar groups of patients who received temporary brachytherapy *(43,44)*.

To clarify the criticism that patient selection alone was responsible for the improved survival *(45,46)*, two phase III trials on interstitial brachytherapy were conducted. The results did not reveal any survival benefit *(47,48)*, which consequently led to a strong decrease in the practice of brachytherapy for primary malignant gliomas. However, we should note that in one particular randomized trial *(49)*, the addition of interstitial hyperthermia to a brachytherapy boost resulted in improved overall survival. Nevertheless, this successful treatment concept was, nevertheless, not further evaluated because of its tremendous demands. However, it confirms the principal rationale and requirement to intensify local effectiveness in the treatment of gliomas.

For patients with recurrent malignant gliomas, there is so far no phase III trial of interstitial brachytherapy.

2.3. GliaSite® Radiation Therapy System (RTS)

Dempsey et al. *(50)* and Tatter et al. *(51)* have described a delivery device that utilizes a liquid ^{125}I isotope as a new approach in intracavitary brachytherapy. The Gliasite radiation therapy system (Proxima Therapeutics, Alpharetta, GA) comprises an inflatable silicon balloon reservoir attached to a positionable catheter, which is intraoperatively implanted into the resection cavity and postoperatively filled with the radionuclide solution. In a phase I trial with 21 patients with recurrent high-grade astrocytomas, the liquid radiation source delivered a total dose of 40 to 60 Gy to all tissues within the target volume *(51)*. The authors concluded that the delivery system was safe and delivered the prescribed dose of radiation efficiently to the tissue at highest risk for tumor recurrence.

The method is basically a special approach of intraoperative radiotherapy (IORT). Future studies in both the newly diagnosed and recurrent settings are planned.

2.4. Radioimmunotherapy

Locoregionally applied radioiodinated monoclonal antibodies are a possible therapeutic option for the treatment of malignant gliomas. Intracavitary implantation of ^{131}I-labeled murine antitenascin monoclonal antibodies into the surgically created resection cavity is in the early stages of clinical evaluation *(52–54)*. Tenascin is an extracellular matrix hexabrachion glycoprotein that is abundantly expressed in gliomas *(55,56)*.

Goetz et al. *(57)* compared side effects and survival after surgery and radioimmunotherapy with yttrium-90 and ^{131}I-labeled antibodies in patients with malignant gliomas and found prolonged survival in a selected group of patients. Patients with anaplastic astrocytomas seemed to benefit more than patients with glioblastoma multiforme *(57)*. In another phase II trial on patients with newly diagnosed malignant gliomas, Reardon et al. found prolonged survival associated with a significantly lower rate of radionecrosis and suggested a randomized phase III study on this subject *(58)*.

3. CHEMOTHERAPY

Even the most intensive combinations of radio- and chemotherapy in treating malignant gliomas are not curative and yield only a modest impact on survival for most patients *(59–61)*. There is a major need for new chemotherapeutic drugs and alternative therapeutic modalities.

The development of temozolomide improved the efficacy for chemotherapy on high-grade gliomas. A European Organization for Research and Treatment of Cancer (EORTC) phase III trial on the addition of temozolomide to radiotherapy for newly diagnosed glioblastoma resulted in a clinically meaningful and statistically significant survival benefit with only minimal additional toxicity. The median survival was 14.6 mo with radiotherapy plus temozolomide and 12.1 mo with radiotherapy alone (5). In general, brain tumor treatment lacks therapeutic strategies capable of overcoming barriers for effective delivery of drugs. Clinical failure of many potentially effective therapeutics often occurs because of shortcomings in the methods by which drugs are delivered to brain tumors. Extensive efforts have been made to develop novel strategies to overcome these obstacles and to deliver drugs to brain tumors in a safe and effective manner.

Gliomas are at least partially shielded from systemic chemotherapeutic agents by the blood-brain barrier. This barrier restricts the entry of agents of high molecular weight or that are hydrophilic or that possess an ionic charge from systemic circulation into the brain, with the result that only a few chemotherapy drugs are capable of reaching cytotoxic concentrations at the tumor target when delivered intravenously (61–64).

Although the blood-brain barrier is largely disrupted within the tumor core (65), allowing some systemic chemotherapeutic agents access to the tumor, it is mostly intact at the margins, where tumors often recur within centimeters of the original location (66,67). Systemic exposure to chemotherapy can result in a variety of toxicities, such as bone marrow suppression, stomatitis, nausea, and vomiting. To minimize the exposure of normal tissues, chemotherapeutic drugs are directly delivered to the tumor area, which bypasses the blood-brain barrier and improves drug concentration compared with systemic delivery.

The methods for administering intratumoral chemotherapy to maintain elevated drug concentrations for extended periods range from intratumoral injection through a catheter (68,69) and convection-enhanced delivery (70) to the use of controlled delivery systems, such as programmable subcutaneous pumps (71,72) and biodegradable polymer matrices.

3.1. Ommaya Reservoir

The Ommaya reservoir is a device surgically implanted beneath the scalp to deliver intermittent bolus injections of anticancer drugs directly into the tumor bed. Agents can be injected percutaneously into the reservoir and then delivered to the tumor by manual compression of the reservoir through the scalp. Thus, the Ommaya reservoir reduces the risk of infection but it does not allow continuous drug delivery. The Ommaya reservoir has been extensively used for local brain tumor chemotherapy in many phase I and II trials (73–76), in which it appeared to be a safe and effective device for intralesional administration; further exploration was recommended in the management of gliomas resistant to conventional forms of treatment.

3.2. Gliadel Wafer

Surgically implantable biodegradable polymer matrices loaded with chemotherapeutic agents provide another approach in regional drug delivery. The drug load is released from the polymer over a certain time period determined by the characteristics of the polymer. In 1996, the carmustine implant (Gliadel® wafer) was approved by the U.S. Food and Drug Administration. Gliadel wafers are designed to slowly release carmustine

(BCNU) over a period of about 2 wk after placement into the resection cavity, thus resulting in locally elevated high concentrations of the chemotherapeutic drug.

Several clinical trials have demonstrated tolerability and effective treatment of malignant gliomas; local delivery of high doses avoided the systemic toxicities encountered with other methods of administration *(77–82)*.

In a phase III trial Westphal et al. *(83)* demonstrated that local chemotherapy with BCNU wafers offers a survival benefit and prolongs time to relapse in patients with initial resective surgery for malignant gliomas. Median survival was 13.9 mo after BCNU wafer treatment compared with 11.6 mo after placebo implant *(83)*.

To encounter the problem of a limited number of chemosensitive tumor cells, phase I trials on combination approaches with Gliadel wafers and intravenous temozolomide *(84)* or carboplatin *(85)* in patients with malignant gliomas have been conducted.

3.3. 5-FU Microspheres

A major restriction to the placement of wafers in resection cavities is that they cannot be implanted intratumorally or intraparenchymally, nor can they be administered stereo-tactically owing to their size (several centimeters).

To achieve larger volumes of tissue penetration, Menei et al. have developed micro-particulate implants as microspheres, which can be stereotactically injected *(86–88)*. The microspheres contain 5-fluorouracil (5-FU), an antimetabolic drug with a powerful radiosensitizing activity *(89)* that does not efficiently cross the blood-brain barrier. The viscid polymer is injected into the walls of the cavity after tumor resection. The drug is then slowly released over more than 1 mo owing to a combination of diffusion and degradation phenomena, thus allowing an optimal radiosensitizing effect.

In a multicenter phase II trial, Menei et al. investigated the effect of perioperative implantation of 5-FU-releasing microspheres and concluded an increase in overall survival *(90)*. A phase III trial is under preparation to confirm their results. Because of the promising results, the authors conducted a phase I trial on stereotactic implantation of 5-FU-releasing microspheres for deep and nonresectable malignant gliomas *(91)*.

4. IMMUNOTOXIN THERAPY

Targeted toxins or immunotoxins represent a new approach for treating malignant gliomas. They comprise two components, a carrier molecule with high specificity for tumor-associated antigens and a potent protein toxin. The optimal technique for administering these agents appears to be regional intracerebral drug delivery via microinfusion, utilizing stereotactically placed catheters. This method, also known as convection-enhanced delivery (CED), administers therapeutic agents directly to brain parenchyma, thus achieving high drug concentrations by circumventing the blood-brain barrier and minimizing systemic toxicity *(92,93)*. In contrast to drug-impregnated polymer implants, in which diffusion is limited to a few millimeters off the implantation site *(94)*, pressure gradient-dependent CED has the potential to distribute even large molecules homogeneously over much greater distances.

Different chimeric fusion proteins are currently under investigation in clinical phase I and II trials on patients with malignant gliomas. Some of these are:

- Interleukin-13 (IL-13) plus *Pseudomonas* exotoxin: chimeric fusion protein composed of human IL-13 and *Pseudomonas* exotoxin, termed IL-13 cytotoxin (IL13-PE38) *(95–97)*

- Transforming growth factor-α (TGF-α) plus *Pseudomonas* exotoxin: TP-38 is a recombinant chimeric protein containing a genetically engineered form of the cytotoxic *Pseudomonas* exotoxin PE-38 and the epidermal growth factor receptor (EGFR) binding ligand TGF-α. TGF-α binds with high affinity to EGFR, which is expressed at very low levels in normal human glia cells but uniformly overexpressed in malignant gliomas, often because of gene amplification *(98)*.
- Transferrin plus diphtheria toxin: transferrin-CRM107 is a conjugate protein of human transferrin (Tf) and a mutant of diphtheria toxin (CRM107) that lacks native toxin binding *(99,100)*.

Promising results of the clinical trials performed so far warrant further studies as well as continued research in the field of targeted toxin therapy.

5. GENE THERAPY

Several clinical gene therapy trials on brain tumors have been performed during the last few years *(101)*, but none of them has advanced to an established adjuvant therapy. Nevertheless, there have been enduring efforts to improve gene therapy. Herpes simplex virus thymidine kinase (HSV-tk) gene therapy combined with ganciclovir medication is a major approach in gene therapy of malignant gliomas *(102,103)*. Using this strategy, eligible patients undergo surgical resection of the tumor followed by injection of the vector-producing cells containing the HSV-tk gene into the brain adjacent to the resection cavity and subsequent ganciclovir treatment.

A phase III trial on HSV-tk/ganciclovir gene therapy for patients with glioblastoma multiforme failed to demonstrate any significant benefit in median survival *(104)*. However, it is assumed that failure of this specific protocol was most likely owing to insufficient transgene delivery to the tumor cells. The principle of this approach is therefore being reinvestigated in another phase III trial with oncolytic adenovirus that began in 2005.

Immonen et al. found a significant increase in mean survival after adenovirus HSV-tk treatment for patients with primary or recurrent malignant gliomas *(105)*. Clinical trials with an oncolytic herpesvirus reported by Rainov et al. also demonstrated encouraging antitumor activity *(106)*.

5.1. Antisense Oligonucleotide Therapy

Malignant gliomas are characterized by a massive overexpression of transforming growth-factor-β2 (TGF-β2). High TGF-β concentrations promote vascularization as well as tumor growth and spreading of tumor cells. Thus, blocking of TGF-β2 expression seems to be an interesting approach in local therapy of malignant gliomas. Preliminary analysis of a phase I/II trial of a new TGF-β2 antisense compound (termed AP 12009), administered intratumorally via high-flow microperfusion, showed safety and tolerability in patients with malignant gliomas *(106a)*. The method has now entered a phase II/III trial.

6. THERMOTHERAPY WITH MAGNETIC NANOPARTICLES (MAGFORCE® NANO CANCER THERAPY)

Although the biological effectiveness and molecular mechanisms of heat in treating cancer is well known and has been partially understood for decades, hyperthermia is not

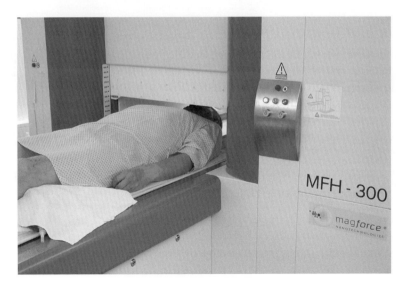

Fig. 1. Thermotherapy treatment of a glioblastoma multiforme patient in the magnetic field applicator MFH® 300F (MagForce Nanotechnologies, Berlin, Germany).

yet well established in clinical routine *(49)*. It seems likely that this discrepancy derives rather from technical limitations that prevent effective temperature distributions in the depth of the human body than from a general lack of biological effectiveness *(107)*.

The major problem with all conventional thermotherapy methods used these days is to achieve an effective temperature distribution in the treated tumor tissue (e.g., minimum temperatures >42°C or any other threshold value). Until now, technically intricate, complex, and costly heating methods with limited effectiveness and without biological specificity have prevented thermotherapy from becoming a routine application for treating cancer.

For lesions of limited size, the utilization of nanofluids might overcome these problems (*see* Chapter 6). This method has been developed over the last 15 yr of basic research at the Charité-University Medicine, Berlin, Germany, as one of the first applications of nanotechnology in medicine *(108–111)*. The new technique, in which a magnetic fluid is injected directly into the tumor and heated by an alternating magnetic field, allows precise heating of almost every part of the body.

The magnetic fluid manufactured by MagForce Nanotechnologies (Berlin, Germany) consists of aminosilane-coated superparamagnetic iron-oxide nanoparticles (core diameter 15 nm) in aqueous solution with an iron concentration of 2 mol/L. The particles generate heat by Brownian and Néel relaxation processes.

Thermotherapy is performed in the alternating magnetic field applicator (MFH® 300F, MagForce Nanotechnologies), operating at a frequency of 100 kHz and a variable field strength of 2.5 to 18 kA/m, especially developed for this type of therapy (Fig. 1). This therapy system for hyperthermia (42–45°C) and thermoablation (≥46°C) for the first time allows the physician to select between treatment temperatures. Depending on clinical indications for different tumor entities, either hyperthermia can be applied to locally enhance the effects of conventional radio- or chemotherapy, or thermoablation alone with temperatures of up to 70°C for direct destruction of tumor cells.

The new method offers several advantages over conventional heating techniques. The magnetic fluid can be distributed in very small portions (0.1 mL) and therefore almost continuously within the targeted area. Owing to their special surface (aminosilane-type shell), the nanoparticles form stable deposits within the tumor thus allowing repeated treatments following a single injection of the magnetic fluid. A collapse of tissue barriers during repeated heatings leads to improved diffusion of the magnetic fluid, resulting in a spreading of the nanoparticles within the target area (109).

In a rat model of glioblastoma multiforme, high efficacy of the new technique with stereotactically applied nanoparticles could be demonstrated, resulting in an up to 4.5-fold prolongation of survival in relation to the applied intratumoral temperatures (112). Because of the very promising results of preclinical studies, a phase I trial on patients with recurrences or inoperable glioblastoma multiforme was started. Fourteen patients received stereotactic injection of the magnetic fluid into the tumor area. Before thermo-therapy was started, the position of the instilled nanoparticles was determined by computed tomography. These data were then matched to presurgical magnetic resonance (MR) images by specially designed software (MagForce NanoPlan®, not commercially available), thus allowing calculation of the expected heat distribution within the treatment area in relation to the magnetic field strength (113).

Patients received 4 to 10 thermotherapy sessions following external beam radiation. Mean maximum intratumoral temperatures reached 45°C (range 42–49°C).

The authors concluded from their data that deep regional thermotherapy using magnetic nanoparticles can be safely applied on glioblastoma multiforme patients with therapeutic temperatures and without side effects (114). A phase II study is in progress to evaluate the efficacy of the new method.

7. CONCLUSIONS

Surgical and radiotherapeutic approaches may have reached their limits in the treatment of malignant gliomas, although interstitial temporary brachytherapy is still being used to treat recurrent malignant gliomas and meningiomas, as well as newly diagnosed and recurrent brain metastases. Two phase III trials on temporary brachytherapy and one on radiosurgery have failed to show a benefit for newly diagnosed glioblastoma. Radiosurgery for recurrent gliomas may offer reasonable palliation compared with other therapies, but further studies are needed to define its exact role. Other promising new approaches in the field of regional therapies for brain tumors have been described over the last decade. Intracavitary chemotherapy using Gliadel wafers has clearly demonstrated its potential value, but also its limitations (limited number of chemosensitive cells, necessity for sealed resection cavities to prohibit ventricular entry, and unknown distance of diffusion). Pericavitary chemotherapy using local injections of 5-FU microspheres is another interesting approach. This technique is still in the early stages of development but has shown encouraging results so far. Its potential lies in the use of other compounds, e.g., with direct cytotoxic or higher radiosensitizing efficacy. There are also promising opportunities in the field of gene therapy, e.g., blocking DNA replication in cancer cells, blocking RNA translation by antisense oligonucleotides, and use of vector-enhanced delivery techniques.

The delivery of chemotherapeutic agents, toxins, or radionuclides to tumor-associated antigens via monoclonal antibodies or other carrier molecules are other approaches with promising outlooks. Future directions of research in the field of targeted therapy include optimizing delivery to targeted brain regions, as well as improvement of treatment efficacy by combining agents targeted to different epitopes.

Thermotherapy using magnetic nanoparticles has demonstrated its feasibility and clinical tolerability and can be regarded as a promising approach in regional cancer therapy. It can be used as monotherapy or in combination to enhance the efficacy of radio- and chemotherapy. It is hoped that new treatment regimens in regional chemo-, immuno-, thermo-, and gene therapy combined with surgery and radiotherapy will lead to significant prolongation of survival together with good quality of life.

REFERENCES

1. Counsell CE, Grant R. Incidence studies of primary and secondary intracranial tumors: a systematic review of their methodology and results. J Neurooncol 1998;37:241–250.
2. Landis SH, Murray T, Bolden S, Wingo PA. Cancer statistics, 1998. CA Cancer J Clin 1998;48:6–29.
3. Cairncross JG, Kim JH, Posner JB. Radiation therapy for brain metastases. Ann Neurol 1980;7: 529–541.
4. Lohr F, Pirzkall A, Hof H, Fleckenstein K, Debus J. Adjuvant treatment of brain metastases. Semin Surg Oncol 2001;20:50–56.
5. Stupp R, Mason WP, van den Bent MJ, et al. Radiotherapy plus concomitant and adjuvant temozolomide for glioblastoma. N Engl J Med 2005;352:987–996.
6. Bashir R, Hochberg F, Oot R. Regrowth patterns of glioblastoma multiforme related to planning of interstitial brachytherapy radiation fields. Neurosurgery 1988;23:27–30.
7. Gaspar LE, Fisher BJ, Macdonald DR, et al. Supratentorial malignant glioma: patterns of recurrence and implications for external beam local treatment. Int J Radiat Oncol Biol Phys 1992;24: 55–57.
8. Davis FG, Freels S, Grutsch J, Barlas S, Brem S. Survival rates in patients with primary malignant brain tumors stratified by patient age and tumor histological type: an analysis based on Surveillance, Epidemiology, and End Results (SEER) data, 1973–1991. J Neurosurg 1998;88:1–10.
9. Prados MD, Levin V. Biology and treatment of malignant glioma. Semin Oncol 2000;27(3 Suppl 6):1–10.
10. Brandes AA, Fiorentino MV. The role of chemotherapy in recurrent malignant gliomas: an overview. Cancer Invest 1996;14:551–559.
11. Wong ET, Hess KR, Gleason MJ, et al. Outcomes and prognostic factors in recurrent glioma patients enrolled onto phase II clinical trials. J Clin Oncol 1999;17:2572–2578.
12. Hau P, Baumgart U, Pfeifer K, et al. Salvage therapy in patients with glioblastoma: is there any benefit? Cancer 2003;98:2678–2686.
13. Walker MD, Strike TA, Sheline GE. An analysis of dose-effect relationship in the radiotherapy of malignant gliomas. Int J Radiat Oncol Biol Phys 1979;5:1725–1731.
14. Bleehen NM, Stenning SP. A Medical Research Council trial of two radiotherapy doses in the treatment of grades 3 and 4 astrocytoma. The Medical Research Council Brain Tumour Working Party. Br J Cancer 1991;64:769–774.
15. Chan JL, Lee SW, Fraass BA, et al. Survival and failure patterns of high-grade gliomas after three-dimensional conformal radiotherapy. J Clin Oncol 2002;20:1635–1642.
16. Leksell L. The stereotaxic method and radiosurgery of the brain. Acta Chir Scand 1951;102:316–319.
17. Kondziolka D, Lunsford LD, Witt TC, Flickinger JC. The future of radiosurgery: radiobiology, technology, and applications. Surg Neurol 2000;54:406–414.
18. Loeffler JS, Siddon RL, Wen PY, Nedzi LA, Alexander E 3rd. Stereotactic radiosurgery of the brain using a standard linear accelerator: a study of early and late effects. Radiother Oncol 1990;17:311–321.
19. Yamamoto M. Gamma knife radiosurgery: technology, applications, and future directions. Neurosurg Clin North Am 1999;10:181–202.
20. Shaw E, Scott C, Souhami L, et al. Single dose radiosurgical treatment of recurrent previously irradiated primary brain tumors and brain metastases: final report of RTOG protocol 90–05. Int J Radiat Oncol Biol Phys 2000;47:291–298.
21. Chamberlain MC, Barba D, Kormanik P, Shea WM. Stereotactic radiosurgery for recurrent gliomas. Cancer 1994;74:1342–1347.

22. Hall WA, Djalilian HR, Sperduto PW, et al. Stereotactic radiosurgery for recurrent malignant gliomas. J Clin Oncol 1995;13:1642–1648.

23. Shaw E, Scott C, Souhami L, et al. Radiosurgery for the treatment of previously irradiated recurrent primary brain tumors and brain metastases: initial report of radiation therapy oncology group protocol *(90–05)*. Int J Radiat Oncol Biol Phys 1996;34:647–654.

24. Shrieve DC, Alexander E 3rd, Wen PY, et al. Comparison of stereotactic radiosurgery and brachytherapy in the treatment of recurrent glioblastoma multiforme. Neurosurgery 1995;36: 275–282; discussion 282–284.

25. Loeffler JS, Alexander E 3rd, Shea WM, et al. Radiosurgery as part of the initial management of patients with malignant gliomas. J Clin Oncol 1992;10:1379–1385.

26. Masciopinto JE, Levin AB, Mehta MP, Rhode BS. Stereotactic radiosurgery for glioblastoma: a final report of 31 patients. J Neurosurg 1995;82:530–535.

27. Sarkaria JN, Mehta MP, Loeffler JS, et al. Radiosurgery in the initial management of malignant gliomas: survival comparison with the RTOG recursive partitioning analysis. Radiation Therapy Oncology Group. Int J Radiat Oncol Biol Phys 1995;32:931–941.

28. Mehta MP, Masciopinto J, Rozental J, et al. Stereotactic radiosurgery for glioblastoma multiforme: report of a prospective study evaluating prognostic factors and analyzing long-term survival advantage. Int J Radiat Oncol Biol Phys 1994;30:541–549.

29. Alexander E 3rd, Loeffler JS. Radiosurgery for primary malignant brain tumors. Semin Surg Oncol 1998;14:43–452.

30. Curran WJ Jr, Scott CB, Weinstein AS, et al. Survival comparison of radiosurgery-eligible and -ineligible malignant glioma patients treated with hyperfractionated radiation therapy and carmustine: a report of Radiation Therapy Oncology Group 83–02. J Clin Oncol 1993;11:857–862.

31. Larson DA, Gutin PH, McDermott M, et al. Gamma knife for glioma: selection factors and survival. Int J Radiat Oncol Biol Phys 1996;36:1045–1053.

32. Souhami L, Seiferheld W, Brachman D, et al. Randomized comparison of stereotactic radiosurgery followed by conventional radiotherapy with carmustine to conventional radiotherapy with carmustine for patients with glioblastoma multiforme: report of Radiation Therapy Oncology Group 93–05 protocol. Int J Radiat Oncol Biol Phys 2004;60:853–860.

33. Scharfen CO, Sneed PK, Wara WM, et al. High activity iodine-125 interstitial implant for gliomas. Int J Radiat Oncol Biol Phys 1992;24:583–591.

34. McDermott MW, Sneed PK, Gutin PH. Interstitial brachytherapy for malignant brain tumors. Semin Surg Oncol 1998;14:79–87.

35. Sneed PK, Lamborn KR, Larson DA, et al. Demonstration of brachytherapy boost dose-response relationships in glioblastoma multiforme. Int J Radiat Oncol Biol Phys 1996;35:37–44.

36. Gutin PH, Bernstein M. Stereotactic interstitial brachytherapy for malignant brain tumors. Prog Exp Tumor Res 1984;28:166–182.

37. Loeffler JS, Alexander E 3rd, Hochberg FH, et al. Clinical patterns of failure following stereotactic interstitial irradiation for malignant gliomas. Int J Radiat Oncol Biol Phys 1990;19:1455–1462.

38. Sneed PK, Russo C, Scharfen CO, et al. Long-term follow-up after high-activity ^{125}I brachytherapy for pediatric brain tumors. Pediatr Neurosurg 1996;24:314–322.

39. Leibel SA, Gutin PH, Wara WM, et al. Survival and quality of life after interstitial implantation of removable high-activity iodine-125 sources for the treatment of patients with recurrent malignant gliomas. Int J Radiat Oncol Biol Phys 1989;17:1129–1139.

40. Bernstein M, Laperriere N, Glen J, Leung P, Thomason C, Landon AE. Brachytherapy for recurrent malignant astrocytoma. Int J Radiat Oncol Biol Phys 1994;30:1213–1217.

41. Halligan JB, Stelzer KJ, Rostomily RC, Spence AM, Griffin TW, Berger MS. Operation and permanent low activity ^{125}I brachytherphy for recurrent high-grade astrocytomas. Int J Radiat Oncol Biol Phys 1996;35:541–547.

42. Patel S, Breneman JC, Warnick RE, et al. Permanent iodine-125 interstitial implants for the treatment of recurrent glioblastoma multiforme. Neurosurgery 2000;46:1123–1128; discussion 1128–1130.

43. Larson DA, Suplica JM, Chang SM, et al. Permanent iodine 125 brachytherapy in patients with progressive or recurrent glioblastoma multiforme. Neurooncology 2004;6:119–126.

44. Gaspar LE, Zamorano LJ, Shamsa F, Fontanesi J, Ezzell GE, Yakar DA. Permanent [125]iodine implants for recurrent malignant gliomas. Int J Radiat Oncol Biol Phys 1999;43:977–982.

45. Florell RC, Macdonald DR, Irish WD, et al. Selection bias, survival, and brachytherapy for glioma. J Neurosurg 1992;76:179–183.

46. Haines SJ. Moving targets and ghosts of the past: outcome measurement in brain tumour therapy. J Clin Neurosci 2002;9:109–112.

47. Laperriere NJ, Leung PM, McKenzie S, et al. Randomized study of brachytherapy in the initial management of patients with malignant astrocytoma. Int J Radiat Oncol Biol Phys 1998;41: 1005–1011.

48. Selker RG, Shapiro WR, Burger P, et al. The Brain Tumor Cooperative Group NIH Trial 87–01: a randomized comparison of surgery, external radiotherapy, and carmustine versus surgery, interstitial radiotherapy boost, external radiation therapy, and carmustine. Neurosurgery 2002;51:343–355; discussion 355–357.

49. Sneed PK, Stauffer PR, McDermott MW, et al. Survival benefit of hyperthermia in a prospective randomized trial of brachytherapy boost +/- hyperthermia for glioblastoma multiforme. Int J Radiat Oncol Biol Phys 1998;40:287–295.

50. Dempsey JF, Williams JA, Stubbs JB, Patrick TJ, Williamson JF. Dosimetric properties of a novel brachytherapy balloon applicator for the treatment of malignant brain-tumor resection-cavity margins. Int J Radiat Oncol Biol Phys 1998;42:421–429.

51. Tatter SB, Shaw EG, Rosenblum ML, et al. An inflatable balloon catheter and liquid ^{125}I radiation source (GliaSite Radiation Therapy System) for treatment of recurrent malignant glioma: multicenter safety and feasibility trial. J Neurosurg 2003;99:297–303.

52. Bigner DD, Brown MT, Friedman AH, et al. Iodine-131-labeled antitenascin monoclonal antibody 81C6 treatment of patients with recurrent malignant gliomas: phase I trial results. J Clin Oncol 1998;16:2202–2212.

53. Riva P, Franceschi G, Frattarelli M, et al. [131]I radioconjugated antibodies for the locoregional radioimmunotherapy of high-grade malignant glioma—phase I and II study. Acta Oncol 1999;38: 351–359.

54. Akabani G, Cokgor I, Coleman RE, et al. Dosimetry and dose-response relationships in newly diagnosed patients with malignant gliomas treated with iodine-131-labeled anti-tenascin monoclonal antibody 81C6 therapy. Int J Radiat Oncol Biol Phys 2000;46:947–958.

55. Zalutsky MR, Moseley RP, Coakham HB, Coleman RE, Bigner DD. Pharmacokinetics and tumor localization of ^{131}I-labeled anti-tenascin monoclonal antibody 81C6 in patients with gliomas and other intracranial malignancies. Cancer Res 1989;49:2807–2813.

56. Ventimiglia JB, Wikstrand CJ, Ostrowski LE, Bourdon MA, Lightner VA, Bigner DD. Tenascin expression in human glioma cell lines and normal tissues. J Neuroimmunol 1992;36:41–55.

57. Goetz C, Riva P, Poepperl G, et al. Locoregional radioimmunotherapy in selected patients with malignant glioma: experiences, side effects and survival times. J Neurooncol 2003;62:321–328.

58. Reardon DA, Akabani G, Coleman RE, et al. Phase II trial of murine (131)I-labeled antitenascin monoclonal antibody 81C6 administered into surgically created resection cavities of patients with newly diagnosed malignant gliomas. J Clin Oncol 2002;20:1389–1397.

59. Green SB, Byar DP, Walker MD, et al. Comparisons of carmustine, procarbazine, and high-dose methylprednisolone as additions to surgery and radiotherapy for the treatment of malignant glioma. Cancer Treat Rep 1983;67:121–132.

60. Walker MD, Green SB, Byar DP, et al. Randomized comparisons of radiotherapy and nitrosoureas for the treatment of malignant glioma after surgery. N Engl J Med 1980;303:1323–1329.

61. Stewart LA. Chemotherapy in adult high-grade glioma: a systematic review and meta-analysis of individual patient data from 12 randomised trials. Lancet 2002;359:1011–1108.

62. Azizi SA, Miyamoto C. Principles of treatment of malignant gliomas in adults: an overview. J Neurovirol 1998;4:204–216.

63. Chang CH, Horton J, Schoenfeld D, et al. Comparison of postoperative radiotherapy and combined postoperative radiotherapy and chemotherapy in the multidisciplinary management of malignant gliomas. A joint Radiation Therapy Oncology Group and Eastern Cooperative Oncology Group study. Cancer 1983;52:997–1007.

64. Shapiro WR, Green SB, Burger PC, et al. Randomized trial of three chemotherapy regimens and two radiotherapy regimens and two radiotherapy regimens in postoperative treatment of malignant glioma. Brain Tumor Cooperative Group Trial 8001. J Neurosurg 1989;71:1–9.

65. Vick NA, Khandekar JD, Bigner DD. Chemotherapy of brain tumors. Arch Neurol 1977;34:523–526.

66. Forsting M, Albert FK, Kunze S, Adams HP, Zenner D, Sartor K. Extirpation of glioblastomas: MR and CT follow-up of residual tumor and regrowth patterns. AJNR Am J Neuroradiol 1993;14:77–87.
67. Giese A, Westphal M. Glioma invasion in the central nervous system. Neurosurgery 1996;39: 235–250; discussion 250–252.
68. Garfield J, Dayan AD, Weller RO. Postoperative intracavitary chemotherapy of malignant supratentorial astrocytomas using BCNU. Clin Oncol 1975;1:213–222.
69. Bosch DA, Hindmarsch T, Larsson S, Backlund EO. Intraneoplastic administration of bleomycin in intracerebral gliomas: a pilot study. Acta Neurochir Suppl (Wien) 1980;30:441–444.
70. Lidar Z, Mardor Y, Jonas T, et al. Convection-enhanced delivery of paclitaxel for the treatment of recurrent malignant glioma: a phase I/II clinical study. J Neurosurg 2004;100:472–479.
71. Nierenberg D, Harbaugh R, Maurer LH, et al. Continuous intratumoral infusion of methotrexate for recurrent glioblastoma: a pilot study. Neurosurgery 1991;28:752–761.
72. Chandler WF, Greenberg HS, Ensminger WD, et al. Use of implantable pump systems for intraarterial, intraventricular and intratumoral treatment of malignant brain tumors. Ann N Y Acad Sci 1988;531:206–212.
73. Jacobs A, Clifford P, Kay HE. The Ommaya reservoir in chemotherapy for malignant disease in the CNS. Clin Oncol 1981;7:123–129.
74. Voulgaris S, Partheni M, Karamouzis M, Dimopoulos P, Papadakis N, Kalofonos HP. Intratumoral doxorubicin in patients with malignant brain gliomas. Am J Clin Oncol 2002;25:60–64.
75. Boiardi A, Eoli M, Salmaggi A, et al. Efficacy of intratumoral delivery of mitoxantrone in recurrent malignant glial tumours. J Neurooncol 2001;54:39–47.
76. Patchell RA, Regine WF, Ashton P, et al. A phase I trial of continuously infused intratumoral bleomycin for the treatment of recurrent glioblastoma multiforme. J Neurooncol 2002;60:37–42.
77. Brem H, Piantadosi S, Burger PC, et al. Placebo-controlled trial of safety and efficacy of intraoperative controlled delivery by biodegradable polymers of chemotherapy for recurrent gliomas. The Polymer-Brain Tumor Treatment Group. Lancet 1995;345:1008–1012.
78. Brem H, Mahaley MS Jr, Vick NA, et al. Interstitial chemotherapy with drug polymer implants for the treatment of recurrent gliomas. J Neurosurg 1991;74:441–446.
79. Walter KA, Tamargo RJ, Olivi A, Burger PC, Brem H. Intratumoral chemotherapy. Neurosurgery 1995;37:1128–1245.
80. Engelhard HH. The role of interstitial BCNU chemotherapy in the treatment of malignant glioma. Surg Neurol 2000;53:458–464.
81. Subach BR, Witham TF, Kondziolka D, Lunsford LD, Bozik M, Schiff D. Morbidity and survival after 1,3-bis(2-chloroethyl)-1-nitrosourea wafer implantation for recurrent glioblastoma: a retrospective case-matched cohort series. Neurosurgery 1999;45:17–22; discussion 23.
82. McGovern PC, Lautenbach E, Brennan PJ, Lustig RA, Fishman NO. Risk factors for postcraniotomy surgical site infection after 1,3-bis (2-chloroethyl)-1-nitrosourea (Gliadel) wafer placement. Clin Infect Dis 2003;36:759–765.
83. Westphal M, Hilt DC, Bortey E, et al. A phase 3 trial of local chemotherapy with biodegradable carmustine (BCNU) wafers (Gliadel wafers) in patients with primary malignant glioma. Neurooncology 2003;5:79–88.
84. Gururangan S, Cokgor L, Rich JN, et al. Phase I study of Gliadel wafers plus temozolomide in adults with recurrent supratentorial high-grade gliomas. Neurooncology 2001;3:246–250.
85. Limentani SA, Asher A, Heafner M, Kim JW, Fraser R. A phase I trial of surgery, Gliadel wafer implantation, and immediate postoperative carboplatin in combination with radiation therapy for primary anaplastic astrocytoma or glioblastoma multiforme. J Neurooncol 2005;72:241–244.
86. Menei P, Benoit JP, Boisdron-Celle M, Fournier D, Mercier P, Guy G. Drug targeting into the central nervous system by stereotactic implantation of biodegradable microspheres. Neurosurgery 1994;34:1058–1064; discussion 1064.
87. Menei P, Venier MC, Gamelin E, et al. Local and sustained delivery of 5-fluorouracil from biodegradable microspheres for the radiosensitization of glioblastoma: a pilot study. Cancer 1999;86:325–330.
88. Benoit JP, Faisant N, Venier-Julienne MC, Menei P. Development of microspheres for neurological disorders: from basics to clinical applications. J Control Release 2000;65:285–296.
89. Koutcher JA, Alfieri AA, Thaler H, Matei C, Martin DS. Radiation enhancement by biochemical modulation and 5-fluorouracil. Int J Radiat Oncol Biol Phys 1997;39:1145–1152.

90. Menei P, Capelle L, Guyotat J, et al. Local and sustained delivery of 5-fluorouracil from biodegradable microspheres for the radiosensitization of malignant glioma: a randomized phase II trial. Neurosurgery 2005;56:242–248; discussion 248.

91. Menei P, Jadaud E, Faisant N, et al. Stereotaxic implantation of 5-fluorouracil-releasing microspheres in malignant glioma. Cancer 2004;100:405–410.

92. Lieberman DM, Laske DW, Morrison PF, Bankiewicz KS, Oldfield EH. Convection-enhanced distribution of large molecules in gray matter during interstitial drug infusion. J Neurosurg 1995;82: 1021–1029.

93. Groothuis DR, Ward S, Itskovich AC, et al. Comparison of ^{14}C-sucrose delivery to the brain by intravenous, intraventricular, and convection-enhanced intracerebral infusion. J Neurosurg 1999;90:321–331.

94. Merlo A, Mueller-Brand J, Maecke HR. Comparing monoclonal antibodies and small peptidic hormones for local targeting of malignant gliomas. Acta Neurochir Suppl 2003;88:83–91.

95. Debinski W, Obiri NI, Powers SK, Pastan I, Puri RK. Human glioma cells overexpress receptors for interleukin 13 and are extremely sensitive to a novel chimeric protein composed of interleukin 13 and pseudomonas exotoxin. Clin Cancer Res 1995;1:1253–1258.

96. Kunwar S. Convection enhanced delivery of IL13-PE38QQR for treatment of recurrent malignant glioma: presentation of interim findings from ongoing phase 1 studies. Acta Neurochir Suppl 2003;88:105–111.

97. Parney IF, Kunwar S, McDermott M, et al. Neuroradiographic changes following convection-enhanced delivery of the recombinant cytotoxin interleukin 13-PE38QQR for recurrent malignant glioma. J Neurosurg 2005;102:267–275.

98. Sampson JH, Akabani G, Archer GE, et al. Progress report of a Phase I study of the intracerebral microinfusion of a recombinant chimeric protein composed of transforming growth factor (TGF)-alpha and a mutated form of the *Pseudomonas exotoxin* termed PE-38 (TP-38) for the treatment of malignant brain tumors. J Neurooncol 2003;65:27–35.

99. Laske DW, Youle RJ, Oldfield EH. Tumor regression with regional distribution of the targeted toxin TF-CRM107 in patients with malignant brain tumors. Nat Med 1997;3:1362–1368.

100. Weaver M, Laske DW. Transferrin receptor ligand-targeted toxin conjugate (Tf-CRM107) for therapy of malignant gliomas. J Neurooncol 2003;65:3–13.

101. Engelhard HH. Gene therapy for brain tumors: the fundamentals. Surg Neurol 2000;54:3–9.

102. Sandmair AM, Loimas S, Puranen P, et al. Thymidine kinase gene therapy for human malignant glioma, using replication-deficient retroviruses or adenoviruses. Hum Gene Ther 2000;11: 2197–2205.

103. Prados MD, McDermott M, Chang SM, et al. Treatment of progressive or recurrent glioblastoma multiforme in adults with herpes simplex virus thymidine kinase gene vector-producer cells followed by intravenous ganciclovir administration: a phase I/II multi-institutional trial. J Neurooncol 2003;65:269–278.

104. Rainov NG. A phase III clinical evaluation of herpes simplex virus type 1 thymidine kinase and ganciclovir gene therapy as an adjuvant to surgical resection and radiation in adults with previously untreated glioblastoma multiforme. Hum Gene Ther 2000;11:2389–2401.

105. Immonen A, Vapalahti M, Tyynela K, et al. AdvHSV-tk gene therapy with intravenous ganciclovir improves survival in human malignant glioma: a randomised, controlled study. Mol Ther 2004;10:967–972.

106. Rainov NG, Ren H. Oncolytic viruses for treatment of malignant brain tumours. Acta Neurochir Suppl 2003;88:113–123.

106a. Hau. Presented at the Meeting of the American Society of Clinical Oncologists, Orlando, FL, 2002.

107. Wust P, Hildebrandt B, Sreenivasa G, et al. Hyperthermia in combined treatment of cancer. Lancet Oncology 2002; 3:487–497.

108. Jordan A, Wust P, Fahling H, John W, Hinz A, Felix R. Inductive heating of ferrimagnetic particles and magnetic fluids: physical evaluation of their potential for hyperthermia. Int J Hyperthermia 1993;9:51–68.

109. Jordan A, Scholz R, Wust P, et al. Effects of magnetic fluid hyperthermia (MFH) on C3H mammary carcinoma in vivo. Int J Hyperthermia 1997;13:587–605.

110. Jordan A, Scholz R, Maier-Hauff K, et al. Presentation of a new magnetic field therapy system for the treatment of human solid tumors with magnetic fluid hyperthermia. J Magnetism Magn Mater 2001;225:118–126.

111. Jordan A, Wust P, Scholz R, et al. Cellular uptake of magnetic fluid particles and their effects on human adenocarcinoma cells exposed to AC magnetic fields in vitro. Int J Hyperthermia 1996;12:705–722.

112. Jordan A, Scholz R, Maier-Hauff K, et al. The effect of thermotherapy using magnetic nanoparticles on rat malignant glioma. J Neurooncl 2006;78:7–14.

113. Gneveckow U, Jordan A, Scholz R, et al. Description and characterization of the novel hyperthermia- and thermoablation-system MFH 300F for clinical magnetic fluid hyperthermia. Med Phys 2004;31:1444–1451.

114. Maier-Hauff K, Rothe R, Scholz R, et al. Deep regional thermotherapy using magnetic nanoparticles: results of a feasibility study with 14 glioblastoma multiforme patients. J Neurooncol 2007;81:53–60.

24 Hyperthermic Intrapleural Chemotherapy in Pleural Malignancy

Frans A.N. Zoetmulder MD, PhD, *and*
Serge van Ruth MD, PhD

CONTENTS

SUMMARY

Hyperthermic intrapleural chemotherapy for malignant pleural disease aims to increase the exposure of malignant cells at the pleural surface to chemotherapeutic agents. Evidence is presented that indeed intrapleural perfusion can result in local exposure for cisplatin and doxorubicin of 60 to 100 times the systemic exposure. Combining chemotherapeutic perfusion of the pleural cavity with mild hyperthermia of 40°–42°C can probably further increase effective tumor cell kill. Effective penetration of the drugs is limited, however. This type of therapy can therefore only work in cases of microscopic residual disease, after complete surgical resection of all malignant pleural disease. A review is presented of studies using this approach in malignant pleural mesothelioma and in pleural involvement in non-small cell lung cancer. In neither disease is there any solid evidence to prove effectivness of hyperthermic pleural chemotherapy. Only in patients with pleural metastases of malignant tymoma has this approach resulted in some unexpected long-term survivors.

Key Words: Mesothelioma; pleural carcinomatosis; thymoma; intrapleural chemotherapy.

From: *Cancer Drug Discovery and Development: Regional Cancer Therapy*
Edited by: P. M. Schlag and U. S. Stein © Humana Press Inc., Totowa, NJ

1. INTRODUCTION

Primary and secondary malignancy of the pleural cavity is a common event. Asbestos-induced mesothelioma is at present reaching its peak, with an incidence of around 4 per 100.000 inhabitants in western Europe. Secondary involvement of the pleural cavity is, however, far more frequent, with lung and breast cancer the most common primaries. Both tumorous pleural growth and effusion can cause significant complaints and can contribute to early death. In a series of 417 patients with malignant pleural effusions, Heffner et al. found a median survival of only 4 mo *(1)*. Better control of pleural disease can thus have an important impact on quality of life and survival in these patients. Treatment by systemic chemotherapy has in general been disappointing, both in primary mesothelioma and in metastatic pleural disease. Although responses do occur, the duration is usually short, with the exception of some breast cancer cases. The main factor limiting the effect of systemic chemotherapy is the relative insensitivity of most of these malignancies to chemotherapeutic agents. In the laboratory, this relative resistance can be overcome by increased exposure. In addition, the cell killing capacity of a number of cytostatic agents can be improved by an increase in temperature, so-called mild hyperthermia. The aim of regional chemotherapeutic treatments is to translate these laboratory findings into practical and effective treatment strategies.

2. PATHOPHYSIOLOGY OF MALIGNANCIES OF THE PLEURAL CAVITY

The pleural cavity is the virtual space between the visceral pleural covering of the lung and the parietal pleura, covering the inside of the chest wall, the mediastinum, and the diaphragm. The parietal pleura consists of a single layer of mesothelial cells, covering loose irregular connective tissue. Deep to the parietal pleura is the endothoracic fascia. The parietal pleura contains lymphatic stomata, corresponding to an extensive lymphatic network. These stomata are thought to be the main passage for drainage of pleural fluid and corpuscular material. The corresponding lymphatic network drains anteriorly to the parasternal lymph node chain and posteriorly to the mediastinal nodes.

The visceral pleura in humans is relatively thick and consists of a mesothelial surface and a connective tissue layer. The visceral pleura contains no lymphatic stomata. There is an extensive lymphatic network in the connective tissue layer, which drains ultimately to mediastinal lymph glands. The visceral pleura is vascularized from the bronchial artery, whereas its venous outflow goes to the pulmonary vein.

The pleural cavity contains a few milliliters of fluid, which is thought to have the function of lubricating the movement between the lung and the chest wall. The visceral pleura is considered to be the main production site for this pleural fluid, at a rate of 1 to 2 ml per hour. The drainage capacity through the lymphatic lacunae is, by contrast, about 10 times as much. This system maintains the normal situation with only a very limited amount of pleural fluid.

Pleural effusion will develop when either the amount of fluid production at the visceral pleura exceeds the capacity of the lymphatic drainage, or the lymphatic drainage gets blocked. In malignant pleural disease, both events usually play a role. Tumor growth will disrupt the normal membrane characteristics of the pleura, increasing fluid production, whereas blockage of the lymphatic stomata by tumor cells will limit drainage.

In pleural mesothelioma, the primary event is thought to take place in the parietal pleura, where asbestos fibers tend to accumulate in milky spots, first described by Kampmeyer's group *(2)*. From there malignant cells spread via the pleural cavity to both parietal and visceral pleural surfaces, often accompanied by massive pleural effusion. Ultimately the whole lung will be encased in tumor.

Metastatic pleural disease is thought to originate most often at the visceral pleura, by tumor emboli reaching the pleura via the pulmonary artery *(3)*. In primary lung cancer, direct tumor penetration through the visceral pleura is of course an alternative route. Involvement of the parietal pleura appears to be secondary in these cases. Lymphatic spread from the pleural cavity toward parasternal and mediastinal lymph nodes appears to be common. In case of pleural metastases based on hematogenic spread, extrapleural metastases will almost always be present as well.

3. PRINCIPLES OF INTRAPLEURAL CHEMOTHERAPY

3.1. Principles

Intrapleural chemotherapy has the advantage of very high local concentrations of cytostatic drugs, while drug concentrations in the systemic compartment will remain below toxic levels. Because of practical constraints, the time the pleural surface can be exposed is limited. This means that only directly cytotoxic drugs can be used in this setting, such as cisplatin, mitomycin C, and doxorubicin. Van Ruth et al. have shown convincingly for doxorubicin that effective infiltration will only reach a few cell layers deep below the surface of the pleural cavity *(4)*. The consequence is that only very limited microscopic tumor residue on the surface of the chest cavity can be exposed to effective doses during intracavitary delivery of drugs. In almost all patients this means that extensive surgery is needed to remove all macroscopic cancer, before the start of intrapleural chemotherapy. This is in accordance with the experience in intraperitoneal chemotherapy, in which the only long-term survivors are those in whom all macroscopic disease can be removed *(5)*.

Combining hyperthermia with regional chemotherapy is an attractive idea. Many cytostatic drugs exhibit enhanced activity once the temperature exceeds 39°C. The temperature in intracavitary delivery systems can be manipulated very easily. It is important that the increased temperature in fluid in the cavity only penetrates 1 or 2 mm deep *(6)*. This means that the enhanced therapeutic action is limited to the surface of the cavity and the tissue directly below. It also means that no additional systemic toxicity has to be feared. Despite its theoretical advantages, clinical evidence of the synergism of cytotoxic drugs and heat is limited to just one randomized study, showing a significant benefit for the combination of intraperitoneal chemotherapy plus hyperthermia over intraperitoneal chemotherapy alone in operable gastric cancer *(7)* To maintain the temperature at a constant level in the pleural cavity, or in the abdominal cavity it is important to perfuse the cavity with fluid at an adjustable inflow temperature. The system should employ intracavitary temperature probes, registering the temperature at the target area. The inflow temperature is then adjusted until the target tissue is at the chosen temperature. Most studies in this field have used a temperature between 40 and 42°C. Such a perfusion apparatus can be rather simple, consisting of a roller pump, a reservoir, a heat exchanger, and connecting tubing (Fig. 1). Commercial systems are also available.

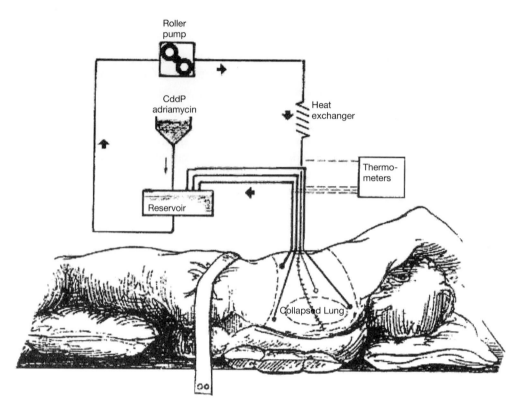

Fig. 1. Schematic overview of the intraoperative hyperthermic intrathoracic perfusion circuit.

3.2. Pharmacokinetics

Both doxorubicin and cisplatin have been widely used for intrapleural application. This choice has been based on the recorded sensitivity of both mesothelioma and non-small cell lung cancer after intravenous application and on the directly cytotoxic action pattern of both drugs. van Ruth et al. studied the combination of cisplatin with doxorubicin at a temperature of 40 to 41°C and a perfusion time of 90 min *(4)*. Cisplatin was given at a fixed dose of 80 mg/m^2, and the doxorubicin dose was slowly increased in a dose-finding study that reached a maximum dose of 25 mg/m^2. This dosing method proved to be problematic. To ensure complete exposure of the pleural cavity surface, the whole cavity has to be filled with fluid. In practice, they found a wide variation in the volume needed to fill the cavity completely, forcing them to add extra volume in many patients, and thus reducing the drug concentration. As drug delivery and movement of drug over the pleural membrane is thought to be influenced by concentration, this is undesirable. So, to the end of the study, they changed toward dosing per liter of perfusate.

The maximum dosage reached was 40 mg of cisplatin/L and 21 mg doxorubicin/L, corresponding to a total dose of 160 to 200 mg of cisplatin and 80 to 100 mg of doxorubicin. Drug concentrations were measured at regular intervals in the perfusate and in plasma. The plasma measurements were continued until 20 h after perfusion (Fig. 2 and Fig. 3). The concentrations of both doxorubicin and cisplatin were decreased gradually in the perfusate, essentially according to first-order elimination kinetics, with a half-life

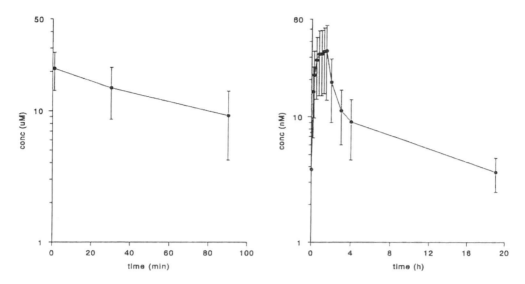

Fig. 2. Course of doxorubicin concentration (mean ± SD) on a logarithmic scale in relation to time measured in perfusate (left) and plasma (right).

of 74 min for doxorubicin and 138 min for cisplatin. At the end of the 90-min perfusion time, 35% of the original dose of doxorubicin and 52% of the cisplatin was recovered from the perfusate. The plasma concentration was gradually increased during perfusion, reaching a steady state at 90 min. After cessation of the perfusion, the plasma concentration decreased according to two-compartmental decay kinetics. The dose advantage expressed as the ratio between the area under the curve (AUC) in perfusate (0–90 min) and the AUC in plasma (0–20 h), was almost 100 for doxorubicin and 60 for cisplatin. Also important was that the AUC in plasma remained about 10 times below the AUC at commonly used systemic doses. Yellin et al. *(21)* published a dose-finding study on hyperthermic intrapleural cisplatin, in which they reached a total dose of 200 mg, without systemic toxicity.

3.3. Toxicity

As the systemic exposure after intrapleural perfusion with doxorubicin and cisplatin remains well below that reached after the usual intravenous application, it is not surprising that little toxicity is reported. In their 20 patients, van Ruth et al. *(4)* reports 1 patient with transient grade 2 renal toxicity, most likely related to low blood pressure during surgery. None of their patients developed alopecia. Local toxicity owing to exposure to doxorubicin was not an important feature. Although it remains difficult to distinguish mild doxorubicin toxicity in the postoperative wound, no case of important soft tissue necrosis was reported. It is also of interest that no cardiac toxicity was observed, even though the chest was perfused with an open pericardium in eight patients, exposing the epicardium to heated doxorubicin. It can be concluded that at these dose levels, both local and systemic toxicity has been very limited. This probably means that dose levels can be further increased safely. Whether that would add effectiveness is of course to be studied.

The combination treatment of cytoreduction with hyperthermic intrapleural chemotherapy is not without complications. Attempts at complete resection of malignant

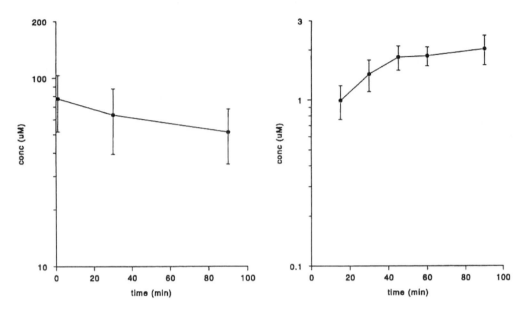

Fig. 3. Course of cisplatin concentration (mean ± SD) on a logarithmic scale in relation to time measured in perfusate (left) and plasma (right).

mesothelioma involve major surgery, with all the associated risks. Even in the most experienced hands, a pleuropneumonectomy carries a risk for major complications of at least 20% and a risk for therapy-related death of 5% *(23)*.

4. PATIENT STUDIES AND CLINICAL RESULTS

Most studies on intrapleural chemotherapy are phase I type feasibility studies or small phase II studies. There are no randomized studies on this topic. Studies concentrating on pleural mesothelioma, non-small cell lung cancer, and pleural metastases of thymoma have survival as the end point. Studies that have looked at intrapleural chemotherapy as a palliative measure in malignant effusion have considered time to recurrent effusion as end point.

4.1. Studies on Malignant Pleural Mesothelioma

All studies on locoregional therapy in mesothelioma are faced with the difficulty of selection. Entry to most studies has been restricted to patients with unilateral disease, without signs of lymph node involvement (Butchart stage I, Sugarbaker stage I, IMIG stage I) with good performance status and adequate pulmonary function *(8–10)*. Although the three staging systems have a considerable overlap, there are also some important differences that may have important prognostic significance, making the comparison of study results difficult.

All studies in this field have combined intrapleural chemotherapy with some kind of surgery, either extrapleural pneumonectomy, or pleurectomy/decortication (Table 1). The acceptance of both surgical strategies in intrapleural chemotherapy studies has been defended by the observation that the type of surgery did not influence survival in surgery-

Table 1
Surgery with Adjuvant Intrapleural Chemotherapy

Study	Treatment	Year	No. of patients	Median survival (mo)	2-yr survival (%)	Mortality (%)
Lee et al. *(12)*	S, IPC	1995	15	12	16	0
Rice et al. *(16)*	S, IPC, C	1994	19	13	25	5
Rusch et al. *(13)*	S, IPC, C	1994	27	18	40	4
Sauter et al. *(15)*	S, IPC, C	1995	13	9	15	8
Colleoni et al. *(14)*	S, IPC, C	1996	20	12	34	0
van Ruth et al. *(17)*	S, IPC, RT	2003	20	11	15	0

Abbreviations: C, chemotherapy; IPC, intrapleural chemotherapy; RT, radiotherapy; S, surgery.

alone studies *(11)*. Lee et al. *(12)* gave intrapleural cisplatin and cytosine arabinoside to patients who had had incomplete surgery. Rusch et al. *(13)*, Colleoni et al. *(14)*, Sauter et al. *(15)*, and Rice et al. *(16)* all report on intrapleural chemotherapy after complete cytoreduction but do not define exactly what they mean. All patients in these studies also received systemic adjuvant chemotherapy. van Ruth et al. *(17)* published a series of 20 patients who after surgery and hyperthermic intrapleural chemotherapy also received radiotherapy on the surgical wound. In all studies survival was disappointing and probably not significantly different from untreated controls, if the patients were selected for similar stage and performance. Important observations are that in all studies local recurrence dominated and that patients after truly complete resection did significantly better than those with macroscopic residue, even if it was very small.

4.2. Studies on Pleural Metastases of Non Small Cell Lung Cancer

Theoretically, pleural involvement in non-small cell lung cancer (NSCLC) can still be considered regional cancer spread. This is the rationale that has prompted investigators, especially from Japan, to study the addition of intrapleural chemotherapy to resection in patients with NSCLC and tumor-positive pleural effusion.

Shigemura et al. *(18)* reported on a series of 19 patients who underwent video assisted thoracoscopic resection of their lung tumor, combined with a 1- or 2-h perfusion of the pleural cavity at 42°C with cisplatin 200 mg/m^2. They observed local lung damage attributed to the perfusion in four cases. The median survival was 18 mo; it was not significantly influenced by the duration of perfusion. Matsuzaki et al. *(19)* treated 11 patients using primary adenocarcinoma of the lung and pleural metastases with resection and intrapleural perfusion with 200 cisplatin mg/m^2 at 42°C for 2 h and saw a median survival of 20 mo, compared with 6 mo for a nonrandomized control group.

Ichinose et al. *(20)* reported the results of a randomized study that was prematurely stopped because of recruitment problems. Patients with NSCLC and tumor-positive pleural fluid after resection either were treated by intrapleural infusion of cisplatin or received no adjuvant therapy. Forty-nine patients were randomized. There was no significant difference in survival, but the recurrence in the pleura was reduced from 42 to 8%.

4.3. Pleural Metastases of Thymoma

Thymoma has a well-known tendency to present with unilateral or bilateral pleural metastases or to recur in that fashion after resection of the mediastinal primary. Small studies have now been published reporting on the outcome after cytoreduction combined with hyperthermic intrapleural chemotherapy. In his publication on hyperthermic intrapleural chemotherapy from the Netherlands Cancer Institute, De Bree included three patients with pleural metastases of thymoma. At present this series has grown to seven cases (unpublished data). Five patients are alive, of whom three are without evidence of disease, after a median follow up of 40 mo, and two are alive for longer than 5 yr. The experience published by Yellin et al. *(21)* and Refaely et al. *(22)* gives a similar impression. In their 15 patients, they achieved an R0 resection in 10. Nine patients were alive at the time of writing, four of them for longer than 5 yr. All long-term survivors were among the R0 resection group.

So, although the numbers are small, the combination therapy seems to produce interesting results in pleural metastases of thymoma.

4.4. Studies on Palliative Intrapleural Chemotherapy to Treat Malignant Effusion

Hyperthermic intrapleural chemotherapy is an aggressive therapy. All groups interested in this modality have limited its use to patients with good performance status who are treated with curative intent. On the other hand, there is quite an extensive literature on the use of instillation chemotherapy to palliate malignant pleural effusion. Mitoxantrone in particular has been widely studied as a means of treating malignant effusion; it has some very enthusiastic supporters *(24–26)*. In a randomized comparison, however, Groth et al. *(26)* did not find any advantage of intrapleural mitoxantrone over simple drainage. The idea was that mitoxantrone would kill the malignant cells in the pleural effusion, thus limiting overproduction of pleural fluid. With a better understanding of the physiology underlying malignant pleural effusion, it seems more likely that intrapleural cytostatic drugs simply act as another sclerosing agent, comparable to the action of tetracycline derivates.

5. DISCUSSION

The theoretical advantages of hyperthermic intrapleural chemotherapy remain very attractive. On the other hand, it must be admitted that despite 20 yr of research we still do not have any solid evidence that it is of any practical value. There are a number of reasons for this. In the first place, the types of cancer that have been most extensively studied are of a highly malignant nature. This means that even if the treatment succeeded in controlling regional disease, it would still be unlikely that these patients could be cured by regional therapies alone. Another factor is that both mesothelioma and NSCLC belong to the most chemotherapy-resistant cancer types. It is questionable whether dose intensification can really overcome the resistance of these cells.

Mesothelioma is a disease characterized by dominance of the locoregional problem. True metastases are rare, and late, strongly suggesting an aggressive locoregional treatment policy. Surgical cytoreduction combined with hyperthermic intrapleural chemotherapy is such an approach and is worth investigating.

A dominant problem in mesothelioma is proper patient selection. Closely related to selection is the question of whether the tumor can be resected completely. Any surgeon who has ventured into the surgical treatment of mesothelioma has experienced the unpredictability of these operations. Our present-day computed tomography (CT) and MRI scans can inform us perfectly on the place and the size of the tumor, but they do not give reliable information on the ease by which a tumor can be separated from nontumorous tissue. The same CT picture of thickened parietal pleura can indicate an easy, blunt extrapleural dissection, but this can also mean dense tumorous fixations to the chest wall that necessitate sharp dissection, leaving cancer cells all over the thoracic wall. The observation that such a growth pattern corresponds to reduced lung volume and reduced respiratory movements is useful but remains difficult to quantify in the selection of patients for surgery.

Another unsettled point is the best approach to the diaphragm. In most cases of diffuse mesothelioma tumor deposits are present on the diaphragm. For the tendinous part in particular, complete resection is only possible by resection of the diaphragm, or at least the central part. Thus the abdomen is opened, also opening the way for the spread of tumor cells from the chest to the abdomen. In a disease with such a well-documented tendency for implantation metastases, this is a risky situation. On the other hand, leaving macroscopic tumor on the diaphragm is also a certain route to recurrence. Abdominal recurrences are usually considered distant metastases, obscuring the fact that they are probably better understood as regional recurrences, on the same line as incisional or drain tract recurrences. There is also no consensus as to what to do if the diaphragm has been removed. Should a graft be put in place to allow the perfusion to be limited to the pleural cavity? Or should the perfusion be done with an open diaphragm, thus including the abdominal cavity? This would make sense in the prevention of peritoneal implants but could potentially change the pharmacokinetics of intrapleural perfusion, as it would increase the membrane size between the intracavitary compartment and the systemic compartment by a factor 10. From experience with hyperthermic intracavitary chemotherapy in the abdomen it is clear that complete cytoreduction is a prerequisite for long-term success. Although the data are limited, they suggest that the same holds true in the chest.

6. CONCLUSIONS

Summarizing the experience in mesothelioma, it seems obvious that at present no evidence is available to support the use of hyperthermic intrapleural chemotherapy. Future studies with this treatment modality will have to pay special attention to the selection of patients who can undergo complete cytoreduction and to the surgical techniques involved. Obvious lines of research would be to increase the dose of well-studied drugs like cisplatin and doxorubicin, up to the maximum tolerated dose, and the study of newer drugs in this setting. Sugarbaker is at present studying the effects of higher doses in intrapleural cisplatin therapy *(24)*.

The use of hyperthermic intrapleural chemotherapy in NSCLC with tumor-positive pleural effusion remains a difficult concept. NSCLC is characterized by early distant dissemination and a dominance of distant metastases. It is difficult to see how this will be influenced by more aggressive locoregional therapy. It is also questionable whether pleural involvement represents true regional spread or just a form of distant metastases, as is suggested by postmortem studies on this subject *(3)*. If hyperthermic intrapleural chemotherapy has a place in the treatment of these NSCLC patients, it should be restricted to those with direct infiltration of the visceral pleura by the primary tumor. In general, it would appear that the future for these patients is to be found in better systemic drugs, rather then in more intensive regional use of known drugs.

Patients with pleural metastases of thymoma are a small but interesting group. As these tumors are usually slow growing, with little tendency to true distant metastases, intensifying locoregional therapy is an obvious choice. Although the numbers are small, the published results are encouraging, both in treatment morbidity and toxicity and in middle to long-term survival. The observation that pleural metastases of thymoma are usually quite easily removed from the parietal pleura, only rarely needing pneumonectomy to reach a complete cytoreduction is of use. Pleural metastases of thymoma are thought to be implants from the primary mediastinal tumor that occur either when the primary infiltrates the mediastinal pleura or during surgical removal of the primary, when the pleura is opened in the presence of free tumor cells. During resection of pleural metastases, the circumstances for new implantations seem ideal. Possibly the observed effect of hyperthermic intrapleural chemotherapy in this situation is mainly the prevention of new implants. Whatever the explanation, cytoreduction and hyperthermic intrapleural chemotherapy in pleural metastases of thymoma is at present the only hopeful spark in the otherwise gloomy picture of malignant pleural disease.

REFERENCES

1. Heffner JE, Nietert PJ, Barbieri C. Pleural fluid pH as a predictor of survival in patients with malignant pleural effusions. Chest 2000;117:79–86.
2. Boutin C, Dumortier P, Rey F, et al. Black spots concentrate oncogenic asbestos fibers in the parietal pleura. Thoracosopic and mineralogic study. Am J Respir Crit Care Med 1996;153:444–449.
3. Rodrigues-Panadero F, Borderas Naranjo F, Lopez Meijas J. Pleural metastatic tumours and effusions. Frequency and pathogenic mechanisms in a post-mortem series. Eur Respir J 1989;2:366–399.
4. van Ruth S, Tellingen O van, Korse CM, et al. Pharmacokinetics of doxorubicin and cisplatin used in intra-operative hyperthermic chemotherapy after cytoreductive surgery for malignant pleural mesothelioma and pleural thymoma. Anticancer Drugs 2003;14:57–65.
5. Verwaal V, van Ruth S, de Bree E, et al. Randomized trial of cytoreduction and hyperthermic intraperitoneal chemotherapy versus systemic chemotherapy and palliative surgery in patients with peritoneal carcinomatosis of colorectal cancer. J Clin Oncol 2003;21:3737–3743.
6. Ruth S van, Verwaal VJ, Hart AAM, et al. Heat penetration in locally applied hyperthermia in the abdomen during intra-operative intraperitoneal chemotherapy. Anticancer Res 2003;23:1501–1508.
7. Yonemura Y, de Aretetxabala X, Fujimura T, et al. Intraoperative chemohyperthermic perfusion as an adjunct to gastric cancer: final results of a randomized controlled study. Hepatogastroenterology 2001;48:1776–1782.
8. Butchart EG, Ashcroft T, Barnsley WC, et al. Pleuropneumonectomy in the management of diffuse malignant mesthelioma of the pleura. Experience with 29 patients. Thorax 1976;31:15–24.
9. Sugarbaker DJ, Strauss GM, Lynch TJ, et al. Node status has prognostic significance in the multimodality therpy of diffuse malignant mesothelioma. J Clin Oncol 1993;11:1172–1178.
10. Rusch VW. A proposed new international TNM staging system for malignant pleural mesothelioma. From the International Mesothelioma Interest Group. Chest 1995;108:1122–1128.
11. Rusch VW, Piantadosi S, Holmes EC. The role of extra pleural pneumonectomy in malignant pleural mesothelioma. A Lung Cancer Study Group Trial. J Thorac Cardiovasc Surg 1991;102:1–9.
12. Lee DJ, Perez S, Wang HJ, et al. Intrapleural chemotherapy for patients with incompletely resected malignant mesothelioma: the UCLA experience. J Surg Oncol 1995;60:262–267.
13. Rusch VW, Saltz L, Venkatraman E, et al. A phase II trial of pleurectomy/decortication followed by intrapleural and systemic chemotherapy for malignant pleural mesothelioma. J Clin Oncol 1994;12:1156–1163.

14. Colleoni M, Sartori F, Calabro F, et al. Surgery followed by intracavitary plus systemic chemotherapy in malignant pleural mesothelioma. Tumori 1996; 82: 53–56.

15. Sauter ER, Langer C, Coia IR, et al. Optimal management of malignant mesothelioma after subtotal pleurectomy: revisiting the role of intrapleural chemotherapy and post-operative radiation. J Surg Oncol 1995;60:100–105.

16. Rice TW, Adelstein DJ, Kirby TJ, et al. Aggressive multimodality therapy for malignant pleural mesothelioma. Ann Thorac Surg 1994;58:24–29.

17. van Ruth S, Baas P, Haas RLM et al, Cytoreductive surgery combined with intra-operative hyperthermic intrathoracic chemotherapy for stage I malignant pleural mesothelioma. Ann Surg Oncol 2003;10:176–182.

18. Shigemura N, Akashi A, Nakagiri T et al, Pleural perfusion thermo-chemotherapy under VATS: a new less invasive modality for advanced lung cancer with pleural spread. Ann Thorac Surg 2004;77: 1016–1021.

19. Matsuzaki Y, Edagawa M, Shimizu T, et al. Intrapleural hyperthermic perfusion with chemotherapy increases apoptosis in malignant pleuritis. Ann Thorac Surg 2004;78:1769–1772.

20. Ichinose Y, Tsichiya R, Koike T, et al. A prematurely terminated phase III trial of intrapleural hypotonic cisplatin treatment in patients with resected non small cell lung cancer with positive pleural lavage cytology: the incidence of carcinomatous pleuritis after surgical intervention. J Thorac Cardiovasc Surg 2002;123:695–699.

21. Yellin A, Simansky DA, Paley M, et al. Hyperthermic pleural perfusion with cisplatin: early experience. Cancer 2001;92:2197–2203.

22. Refaely Y, Simansky DA, Paley M et al, Resection and perfusion thermochemotherapy: a new approach for the treatment of thymic malignancies with pleural spread. Ann Thorac Surg 2001;72: 366–370.

23. Sugarbaker DJ, Garcia JP, Richards WG, et al. Extrapleural pneumonectomy in the multimodality therapy of malignant pleural mesothelioma. Results in 120 consecutive patients. Ann Surg 1996;224:288–294.

24. Janne PA, Baldini EH. Patterns of failure following surgical resection for malignant pleural mesothelioma. Thorac Surg Clin 2004;14:567–573.

25. Morales M, Exposito MC. Intrapleural mitoxantrone for palliative treatment of malignant pleural effusions. Support Care Cancer 1995;3:147–149.

26. Aasebo U, Norum J, Sager G, et al. Intrapleurally installed mitoxantrone in metastatic pleural effusions: a phase II study. J Chemother 1997;9:106–111.

27. Groth G, Gatzemeier U, Haussingen K, et al. Intrapleural palliative treatment of malignant pleural effusions with mitoxantrone versus placebo (pleural tube alone). Ann Oncol 1991;2:213–215.

25 Isolated Limb Perfusion in Advanced Soft Tissue Sarcomas

*Peter M. Schlag, MD, PhD, and
Per-Ulf Tunn, MD*

CONTENTS

INTRODUCTION
CLINICAL MANAGEMENT OF STS
ISOLATED LIMB PERFUSION WITH TNF-α AND MELPHALAN
CONCLUSIONS
REFERENCES

SUMMARY

Management of locally advanced soft tissue sarcomas (STS) of the extremities that leads to an increase in preservation of functional limb continues to be a challenge. Isolated limb perfusion (ILP) with TNF-α and melphalan is a locoregional approach for advanced soft tissue sarcomas that has proved to be very effective to achieve this goal. The most prominent antineoplastic effect of TNF-α involves tumor vascularization, owing to early and selective alterations in tumor-associated endothelial cells, resulting in destruction of the tumor vessels. ILP may render a nonresectable tumor resectable and may reduce the local recurrence rate; in cases with widespread metastases, it can be used palliatively to avoid ablative surgery. ILP with TNF-α and melphalan has been shown to result in excellent response rates over 75% and to achieve long-term limb salvage rates in approx 80% of patients.

Key Words: Soft tissue sarcoma; isolated limb perfusion; surgery; limb salvage; prognosis; interdisciplinary therapy.

1. INTRODUCTION

Soft tissue sarcomas (STS) form a heterogeneous group of malignant tumors stemming from mesenchymal connective tissue. They are rare and, together, account for 1 to 2% of all malignancies. The overall incidence is about 1.8 cases per 100,000 population per annum *(1,2)*. Although they can develop at any anatomic site, about 60% of these tumors occur in the extremities, most of them in the lower limb. The tumor typically appears as a painless swelling and is often large at the time of initial diagnosis.

From: *Cancer Drug Discovery and Development: Regional Cancer Therapy*
Edited by: P. M. Schlag and U. S. Stein © Humana Press Inc., Totowa, NJ

Sarcomas exhibit a striking tendency towards local recurrence following a marginal excision. In order to achieve local control in patients with a nonmetastatic stage of STS, a wide or compartmental resection of the tumor to achieve an R0 resection is essential. A radical surgical treatment for locally advanced, non-R0-resectable STS may therefore consist in amputation or exarticulation of the affected limb. Preservation of the extremity as well as a good limb function has become increasingly important in light of evidence that amputations do not improve survival rates in patients with large (>5 cm), deep-seated high-grade sarcomas, as even with local tumor control, more than half of the patients die of disseminated disease *(3)*. Distant metastases of STS are usually localized in the lungs (>80%) and rarely in the liver (<10%) or other organs. Lymphogenic metastases of STS are uncommon. An adjuvant chemotherapy does not influence the number of distant failures but may reduce the local failure rate after an adequate local surgical treatment *(4)*.

In most cases a combined modality approach including preoperative or postoperative radiation therapy is used. The management of locally advanced STS of the extremities that leads to an increase in preservation of a functional limb is complex and continues to be a challenge. Isolated limb perfusion (ILP) with tumor necrosis factor-α (TNF-α) and melphalan as a neoadjuvant locoregional therapeutic approach for primarily nonresectable STS was recently introduced and has improved the prognosis dramatically. In the last few years, this method has been intensively studied in settings of advanced and irresectable STS of the extremities. This novel treatment led to impressive clinical outcomes, with an overall response rate of approximately 70 to 80% and a limb salvage rate of 75 to 80% *(5–7)*. This chapter summarizes the current status of the ILP in the treatment of advanced STS.

2. CLINICAL MANAGEMENT OF STS

2.1. Diagnosis

Current diagnostic tools have improved the diagnosis and staging of STS. Magnetic resonance imaging (MRI) and positron emission tomography (PET) provide more accurate radiologic images of the extent of the disease than heretofore and allow the use of a targeted biopsy. In addition, modern diagnostics are enhanced by immune histology and genetic profiling to assess the typical genetic changes that occur in different sarcoma entities. Complete staging and treatment planning by a multidisciplinary team of cancer specialists is required to determine the optimal treatment for patients with this disease.

2.2. Prognosis

The prognosis depends on several factors, including the patient's age and the size, histological grade, and type of the tumor. Factors associated with a poorer prognosis include age over 60 yr, tumor >5 cm, or high-grade histology. The 5-yr survival rate reported for extremity STS varies from 40 to 60%, which can be attributed to an aggressive local growth and a propensity for hematogenic dissemination *(8)*. Surgery is the primary treatment of choice, and adjuvant high-dose external beam radiotherapy is imperative after narrow or positive surgical margins (R1 resection). With this approach, the local recurrence rate of extremity STS is approx 15% *(9)*.

2.3. Current Treatment Options

The treatment has been improved in the last several years with advances in radiation oncology techniques and with development of new chemotherapeutic and molecular targeting agents. Multimodal therapy, planned at the time of diagnosis by an experienced team, is the key to success. Less radical surgery is often possible for these patients, thus maintaining and maximizing limb function with no increase in the rates of recurrence or development of a metastatic disease.

Locally advanced STS of the extremities can be particularly difficult to treat successfully with standard surgical and radiotherapy techniques. If the tumor is large or involves a major nerve, blood vessel, or joint, it may be impossible to achieve surgical clearance, especially in cases of extracompartmental localizations. About 10% of STS in the extremities are nonresectable. Surgery for locally advanced and nonresectable extremity STS may consist in an amputation or exarticulation.

Limb-sparing surgical procedures, if at all possible, are extensive and usually followed by high-dose radiation therapy. This combination may compromise and mutilate limb function considerably. Therefore, preoperative therapeutic concepts to improve limb salvage have been developed to avoid amputation and improve local control. Various locoregional approaches have been proposed and investigated. A major breakthrough was achieved in 1992 when Lejeune et al. introduced TNF-α in the ILP procedure *(10)*. Over the last 15 yr the technique of hyperthermic ILP with TNF-α and melphalan has been shown to be an effective limb-salving treatment modality for locally advanced STS.

3. ISOLATED LIMB PERFUSION WITH TNF-α AND MELPHALAN

3.1. History

The technique of ILP using an extracorporal circuit was first described by Creech et al. in 1958 *(11)*. The advantage of this treatment modality is that a high dose of a cytostatic drug can be administered to the tumor-bearing extremity without inducing systemic side effects. ILP permits regional cytostatic concentrations 15 to 20 times higher than those reached after a systemic administration. Various attempts to improve tumor responses to ILP using methods such as hyperthermia have increased its efficacy. ILP is most commonly used in the treatment of melanoma patients with a local recurrent satellitosis, and in transit metastasis of the extremity. Because of its efficacy and low regional toxicity profile, melphalan is the standard agent for ILP. In patients with multiple melanoma in transit metastases, hyperthermic ILP with melphalan results in a complete remission rate of about 50% and an overall response rate of 75 to 80% *(7,12,13)*. The technique had also been applied in the treatment of locally advanced STS of the extremities with a variety of chemotherapeutic agents but rather poor results *(14,15)*.

In 1992, Lejeune et al. pioneered the use of TNF-α in combination with ILP and reported high rates of complete response not only in patients with stage III melanoma but (remarkably) also in four patients with advanced extremity STS *(10)*. This led to a European multicenter study that showed to favorable results of this treatment modality for primarily local nonresectable STS of the extremities *(5)*. Despite theoretical possibilities, the addition of interferon-γ (IFN-γ) to TNF/melphalan seems to provide no further advantage. The efficacy of TNF-based ILP against drug-resistant STS has led to the approval of recombinant human (rh)TNF-α (Tasonermin) by the EMEA for use in combination with melphalan.

3.2. Surgical Technique

Isolation of the blood circuit of a limb is achieved by clamping the major artery and vein, ligating the collateral vessels, and applying a tourniquet around the base of the limb to compress remaining minor vessels in the muscles, subcutaneous tissue, and skin. Isolated perfusion of the legs may be conducted at four levels (external iliac, high femoral, femoropopliteal, or popliteal) whereas of the arm at two levels (axilliary or brachial). After the cannulation of the vessels, the isolated extremity is provided with artificial circulation by means of an oxygenated extracorporeal circuit, into which the cytostatic agent is injected.

The dose of melphalan is calculated according to the limb volume to be perfused. This volume can easily be determined by immersion of the limb in water *(16)*. The maximal dose of melphalan tolerated by normal tissues at an acceptable risk of toxicity is 10 mg/L perfused tissue for lower limb perfusions, and 13 mg/L perfused tissue for upper limb perfusion. The general recommended dose of TNF-α to be administered during an ILP in our clinic is 1 mg.

Tissue temperature in the subcutaneous and intramuscular compartments is continuously monitored by temperature probes inserted into the respective compartments. Leakage monitoring is performed by using a precordial scintillation probe to detect the leakage of radiolabeled albumin or autologous erythrocytes injected into the perfusion circuit. The adjustment of the flow rate (35–40 mL/L limb volume/min) and the tourniquet are required to ensure that leakage from the perfusion circuit to the systemic circulation is prevented or minimized. TNF-α should only be administered if leakage is less than the 5% over 90 min.

ILP consists of a 90-min-long perfusion at mild hyperthermia (39–40°C). TNF-α should be injected as a bolus into the arterial line provided the limb tissue temperature is >38°C. Melphalan should be administered 30 min later at limb temperature between 39 and 40°C. At the end of the procedure, the perfusate is washed out and the limb is rinsed with an electrolyte solution until the perfusate is clear.

Toxicity and postoperative management after ILP with TNF-α does not differ significantly from those after ILP with melphalan alone. Currently, most patients remain 2 or 3 d in the ICU before they are transferred to the surgical ward. Resection of the residual tumor mass is performed no earlier than 6 to 8 wk after ILP.

3.3. Mechanism of Action of TNF-α

In the regional ILP system, TNF-α is administered at a 10-fold higher dose compared with the maximum tolerable dose in a systemic administration. The systemic use of TNF-α has been limited by its toxicity, in particular causing severe hypotension. The maximum tolerated dose of TNF-α in a systemic administration is approximately 350 µg/m², a dose associated with plasma concentrations far below those necessary for antitumor effects *(18)*.

TNF-α is a highly potent antineoplastic agent which acts via multiple direct and indirect mechanisms that contribute to the antitumor activity. It exerts its effect mainly by affecting the tumor vasculature *(17)*. Namely it has been shown that, beside direct antiproliferative and cytotoxic effects on tumor cells, TNF-α activates adhesion mol-

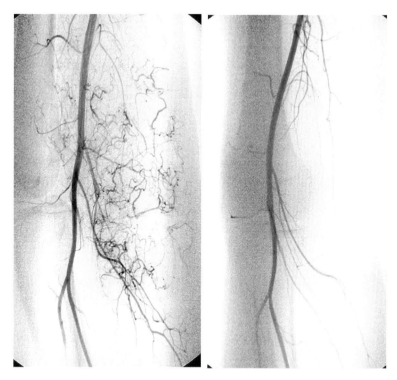

Fig. 1. Angiography pre-ILP (left) and post-ILP (right) of the fossa poplitea showing complete selective destruction of tumor vascular bed in a 42-yr-old male patient with pleomorph sarcoma (NOS).

ecules on the surface of endothelial cells within the tumor, as well as membrane receptors on macrophages and leukocytes. Adhesion of these cells to the endothelial surface of the tumor's capillary bed, followed by release of oxygen free radicals and cytokines, leads to exclusive destruction of the tumor vasculature, which is accompanied by thrombus formation and hemorrhagic necrosis of the tumor *(18)*.

The selective destructive effects of TNF-ILP on tumor-associated vessels are demonstrated by pre- and post-ILP angiographies, regardless of whether a good histological response is expected or not *(22)* (Fig. 1). Complete disappearance of all tumor-associated vessels has been described within 7 to 14 d after hyperthermic ILP, whereas other vessels remained uneffected. The efficacy of the technique can be shown by MRI before and after ILP (Fig. 2).

The addition of high-dose TNF-α to the perfusate results in four- to sixfold increased uptake of the cytostatic agent by the tumor. de Wilt et al. found an increased accumulation of melphalan in tumor tissue after ILP with TNF-α and melphalan compared with melphalan alone *(19)*. Melphalan uptake was tumor specific, no increased uptake was noted in normal tissues, thus emphasizing the relative selective effect of TNF-α on the tumor-associated vasculature. This increased melphalan accumulation correlates well with the observed tumor response, suggesting that higher melphalan concentrations may be an additional mechanism by which TNF-α enhances the antitumor response. The effect correlates with the vascularity of the tumor. The more vascular the tumor, the better the synergistic effect between TNF-α and the chemotherapeutic agent.

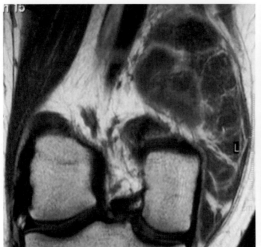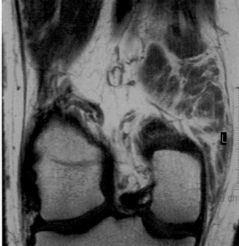

Fig. 2. Magnetic resonance images of a 23-yr-old patient with a liposarcoma of the lower leg and an infiltration of the knee joint before (left) and after ILP (right). A decrease in tumor mass can be seen.

3.4. Regional and Systemic Toxicity

The toxicity attributed to systemic leakage of TNF-α from the perfusion circuit is severe. The incidence of adverse events, such as septic shock and hypotension, has been decreased with increasing experience of the technique, and systemic toxicity should be minimal in the absence of leakage (20). From our experience >90% of the patients exhibited no detectable leak and no severe systemic toxicity was encountered. Moderate systemic toxicity such as fever, sometimes with chills is easily treatable. Optimal hydration of the patient before, during, and after ILP is recommended and may help to maintain high fluid pressure in the systemic compartment.

The regional toxicity of hyperthermic ILP today generally classified in accordance with a system proposed by Wieberdink et al. (16). Epidermal inflammatory reactions and neurological symptoms determine the various grades of toxicity. Almost all patients have a perfusion reaction grade II and III that commonly develops within 48 h after ILP and usually resolves within 14 d. This is similar to the toxicity observed after ILP with melphalan alone.

3.5. Clinical Outcome and Results

The key parameters that define treatment outcome are the clinical and histological response, the final treatment outcome, the local recurrence rate, the limb salvage, and the systemic metastasis rate. The efficacy of TNF combined with a cytostatic agent in the setting of ILP in patients with locally advanced STS has been well established. Ever since the first report, response rates over 75% have been noted in expanding multicenter experiences (5,6,21).

The efficacy and safety of ILP with TNF-α were initially assessed in three open-label, uncontrolled, multicenter clinical trials and in an Investigator's Own Responsibility program. More than 400 STS patients have been recruited for these trials. The overall

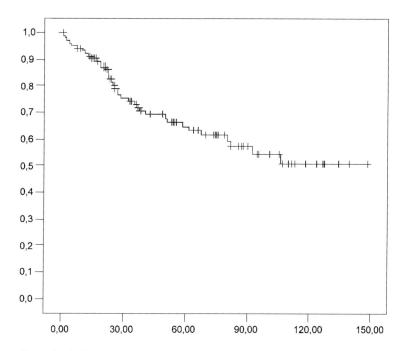

Fig. 3. Overall survival of patients treated with ILP in advanced soft tissue sarcomas between 1993 and 2004 (*n* = 125)

response rate was approximately 80%, with a 20 to 30% complete remission rate. Limb salvage has been achieved in 74 to 87% of the patients *(5,6)*.

TNF-based ILP was introduced in our department in 1993. During the period 1993 to 2004, 125 patients, 54% men and 46% women, with a mean age of 51 yr (range 11–76 yr), and locally advanced extremity STS were treated by ILP with melphalan and TNF according to the method described previously. The tumor was localized in the lower limbs in 109 patients (87%) and in the upper extremity in 16 patients (13%). The histological types included synovial sarcoma (23%), malignant fibrous histiocytoma (19%), liposarcoma (17%), malignant peripheral nerve sheath tumor (7%), pleomorph sarcoma, not otherwise specified NOS (7%), leiomyosarcoma (5%), and other sarcoma types (23%). Because of the tumor extent and localization, an amputation or exarticulation of the extremity would have been considered for all patients. Two patients had metastases at the time of the procedure.

The resection of the residual tumor mass was performed six to eight weeks after ILP with TNF and melphalan (81% R0, 12% R1, 7% R2). Limb salvage has been achieved in 81% of the patients. The 5-yr overall survival rate was 63% (Fig. 3), and the 5-yr disease-free survival rate was 46%. The 5-yr recurrence-free survival of all patients was 76%. Systemic and local toxicities of TNF-ILP are listed in Table 1.

Our data are in accord with the results of several studies in which patients with advanced STS were treated with TNF-based ILP *(5,6)*. Recently, 246 patients with locally advanced STS, enrolled in a European multicenter study, were reviewed by an independent review committee and the results were compared with those of patients treated conventionally. According to the classification of the review committee, 80% of these patients would

Table 1
Systemic and Local Toxicity After ILP[a]

Reaction grade	% of patients	Reaction
I	26.4	No reaction
II	45.9	Slight erythema and/or edema
III	22.3	Substantial erythema and/or edema with some blistering, slightly disturbed motility permissible
IV	5.4	Extensive epidermolysis and/or obvious damage to the deep tissue, causing definite functional disturbances; threatening or manifested compartmental syndrome
V	1.4	Reaction that may necessitate amputation

[a] Classification of Acute Tissue Reactions According to Wieberdink et al. *(24)*.

normally have been managed with an amputation or a functionally debilitating resection and radiotherapy. After TNF-based ILP, a major response was observed in 82% of the patients, rendering these large sarcomas respectable in most cases. In a median follow-up of almost 2 yr, limb salvage was achieved in 82% *(23)*. The local recurrence rate depended greatly on whether the tumor resection was performed after ILP and whether one or multiple tumors were present in the extremity.

4. CONCLUSIONS

TNF-based ILP provides an excellent tool to achieve local control and avoid amputation in patients with advanced nonresectable STS of the extremities. The technique of ILP with TNF-α and melphalan is well established but not yet as widely practiced for sarcomas of the limb as it could be. There is an improved indication for ILP with TNF-α as an adjunct to surgery for subsequent resection of the tumor in order to prevent or delay amputation. TNF-based ILP may render a nonresectable tumor resectable and may reduce the local recurrence rate; in cases with widespread metastases, it can be used palliatively to avoid ablative surgery. ILP with TNF-α and melphalan results in excellent response rates and has been shown to achieve limb salvage rates of approximately 80%. Our experience shows that the procedure is safe, associated with only moderate regional and systemic toxicity. In patients with advanced STS of the extremities, no other available treatment or combination of treatment has been able to produce comparable results. The local management of advanced STS of the extremities should be identical whether the intent is curative or palliative, as local control improves the quality of life.

REFERENCES

1. Gustafson P. Soft tissue sarcoma. Epidemiology and prognosis in 508 patients. Acta Orthop Scand 1994;259:1–31.
2. Greenlee RT, Hill-Harmon MB, Murray T, Thun M. Cancer statistics. Cancer J Clin 2001;51:15–36.
3. Hoekstra HJ, Schraffordt, Koops H, Oldhoff J. Soft tissue sarcoma of the extremity. Eur J Surg Oncol 1994;20:3–6.

4. Bramwell V, Rouesse J, Steward W, et al. Adjuvant CYVADIC chemotherapy for adult soft tissue sarcoma—reduced local recurrence but no improvement in survival: a study of the European Organization for Research and Treatment of Cancer Soft Tissue and Bone Sarcoma Group. J Clin Oncol 1994;12:1137–1149.

5. Eggermont AMM, Schraffordt Koops H, Lienard D, et al. Isolated limb perfusion with high-dose tumor necrosis factor-α in combination with interferon-γ and melphalan for nonresectable extremity soft tissue extremity sarcomas: a muliticenter trial. Ann Surg 1996;224:756–765.

6. Eggermont AMM, Schraffordt Koops H, Klausner JM, et al. Isolated limb perfusion with tumor necrosis factor and melphalan for limb salvage in 186 patients with locally advanced soft tissue extremity sarcomas. The cumulative multicenter European experience. Ann Surg 1996;224:756–765.

7. Eggermont AMM, de Wilt JHW, ten Hagen TLM. Current uses of isolated limb perfusion in the clinic and a model system for new strategies. Lancet Oncol 2003;4:429–437.

8. Chang AE, Sondak VK. Clinical evaluation and treatment of soft tissue tumors, in Soft Tissue Tumors, 3rd ed. (Enzinger FM, Weiss SW, eds.), Mosby, St. Louis 1995;17–31.

9. Potter DA, Glenn J, Kinsella T, et al. Patterns of recurrence in patients with high-grade soft-tissue sarcomas. J Clin Oncol 1985;3:353–366.

10. Lienard D, Delmotte JJ, Renard N, Ewalenko P, Lejeune FJ. High-dose recombinant tumor necrosis factor-alpha in combination with interferon gamma and melphalan in isolation perfusion of the limbs for melanoma and sarcoma. J Clin Oncol 1992;10:52–60.

11. Creech O Jr, Krementz ET, Ryan RF, Winblad JN. Chemotherapy of cancer: regional perfusion utilizing an extracorporeal circuit. Ann Surg 1959;148:616–632.

12. Lienard D, Eggermont AMM, Schraffordt Koops H, et al. Isolated limb perfusion with tumor necrosis factor-alpha and melphalan with or without interferon-gamma for the treatment of in-transit melanoma metastases: a multicentre randomized phase II study. Melanoma Res 1999;9:491–502.

13. Grünhagen DJ, Brunstein F, Graveland WJ, van Geel AN, de Wilt JHW, Eggermont AMM. One hundred consecutive isolated limb perfusions with TNF-α and melphalan in melanoma patients with multiple in-transit metastases. Ann Surg 2004;240:939–948.

14. Klaase JM, Kroon BBR, Benckhuysen C, van Geel AN, Albus-Lutter CE, Wieberdink J. Results of regional isolation perfusion with cytostatics in patients with soft tissue tumors of the extremities. Cancer 1989;64:616–621.

15. Rossi CR, Vecchiato A, Foletto M, et al. Phase II study on neoadjuvant hyperthermic-antiblastic perfusion with doxorubicin in patients with intermediate of high grade limb sarcomas. Cancer 1994;73:2140–2146.

16. Wieberdink J, Benckhuijsen C, Braat RP, van Slooten EA, Olthuis GA. Dosimetry in isolation perfusion of the limbs by assessment of perfused tissue volume and grading of toxic tissue reactions. Eur J Cancer Clin Oncol 1982;18:905–910.

17. Carswell EA, Old LJ, Kassel RL. An endotoxin induced serum factor that causes necrosis of tumors. Proc Natl Acad Sci U S A 1975;72:3666–3370.

18. Sidhu RS, Bollon AP. Tumor necrosis factor activities and cancer therapy—a perspective. Pharmacol Ther 1993;57:79–128.

19. de Wilt JHW, ten Hagen TLM, de Boeck G, van Tiel ST, de Bruijn EA, Eggermont AMM. Tumour necrosis factor alpha increases melphalan concentration in tumor tissue after isolated limb perfusion. Br J Cancer 2000;82:1000–1003.

20. Vrouenraets BC, Kroon BBR, Ogilvie AC, et al. Absence of severe systemic toxicity after leakage-controlled isolated limb perfusion with tumor necrosis factor-α and melphalan. Ann Surg Oncol 1999;6:405–412.

21. Olieman AFT, van Ginkel RJ, Molenaar WM, Schraffordt Koops H, Hoekstra HJ. Hyperthermic isolated limb perfusion with tumor necrosis factor-α and melphalan as palliative limb-saving treatment in patients with locally advanced soft-tissue sarcomas of the extremities with regional or distant metastases. Is it worthwhile? Arch Orthop Trauma Surg 1998;118:70–74.

22. Olieman AFT, van Ginkel RJ, Hoekstra HJ, Mooyaart EL, Lejeune F. The angiographic response of locally advanced soft tissue sarcomas following hyperthermic isolated limb perfusion with tumor necrosis factor. Ann Surg Oncol 1997;4:64–69.

23. Eggermont AMM, ten Hagen TLM. Isolated limb perfusion for extremity soft-tissue sarcomas, in-transit metastases, and other unresectable tumors: credits, debits, and future perspectives. Curr Oncol Rep 2001;3:359–367.

26 Isolated Limb Perfusion for Melanoma In Transit Metastases

Flavia Brunstein, MD, Dirk J. Grünhagen, MD,
Timo ten Hagen, PhD, and
Alexander M. M. Eggermont, MD, PhD

Contents

Summary

The treatment of melanoma in transit metastases can vary widely and is dependent on the size and number of lesions. When many, large lesions exist, isolated limb perfusion (ILP) can be used as an attractive treatment option with high response rates. We review here the various methods of treatment for melanoma in transit metastases, with a focus on ILP. Indications and results are discussed, and the extra value of tumour necrosis factor (TNF) is evaluated. ILP with melphalan results in complete response rates of 40 to 82% (54% in a large retrospective metaanalysis). The addition of TNF can improve these complete response rates (59–85%), and although no data from randomized controlled trials are available, TNF seems of particular value in large, bulky lesions or in patients with recurrent disease after previous ILP. TNF-based ILP has earned a permanent place in the treatment of patients with melanoma it transit metastases. In patients with a high tumor burden, TNF-based ILP is the most efficacious procedure to obtain local control and achieve limb salvage.

Key Words: TNF, ILP, melanoma, in transit metastasis, limb salvage.

1. INTRODUCTION

The occurrence of multiple melanoma in transit metastases in the extremities has led to a search for a surgical treatment that could deal with all metastases by one procedure.

From: *Cancer Drug Discovery and Development: Regional Cancer Therapy*
Edited by: P. M. Schlag and U. S. Stein © Humana Press Inc., Totowa, NJ

This prompted the development of isolated limb perfusion (ILP). In transit metastases develop in 5 to 8% of melanoma patients with a high-risk primary melanoma (>1.5 mm). They present as single or multiple cutaneous and/or subcutaneous tumors in the viscinity of the primary or scattered throughout the extremity. The prognosis of patients presenting with both in transit metastases and regional lymph node involvement is even worse. The management of regionally recurrent melanoma is complex in the sense that one can choose from many options according to the size and number of lesions and the general condition of the patient (1).

Obviously one or a few lesions can easily be treated by excision, and some oncologists have advocated carbon-dioxide laser for multiple small lesions (2). Other groups have studied intralesional administration of immunostimulants such as bacillus Calmette-Guérin, or cytokines such as interferon, usually with limited success and reponses of short duration (1). It is clear from the literature that ILP has superior response rates. The method is described here.

2. ISOLATED LIMB PERFUSION: METHODOLOGY

The ILP technique was pioneered by Creech, Krementz, and co-workers at Tulane University in New Orleans (3). Regional concentrations of chemotherapeutic agents 15 to 25 times higher than those possible with systemic administration can be achieved by ILP in the tumor-bearing extremity without systemic side effects (4). Isolation of the blood circuit of a limb is achieved by clamping and cannulation of the major artery and vein, connection to an oxygenated extracorporeal circuit, ligation of collateral vessels, and application of a tourniquet. Once isolation is secured, drugs can be injected into the perfusion circuit. Because of its efficacy and low regional toxicity profile, melphalan (L-phenyl-alanine mustard) is the standard drug, most commonly used at a dose of 10 mg/L perfused tissue for a leg and at 13 mg/L for an arm (5). Tissue temperatures in the limbs are monitored, and radiolabeled albumin or erythrocytes are injected into the extracorporeal circuit so leakage into the systemic circulation can be detected with a precordial scintillation probe (6). Leakage monitoring is mandatory, especially now that high doses of tumor necrosis factor-α (TNF-α) are used in the treatment of soft tissue sarcomas.

After 1 to 1.5 h of perfusion, the limb is rinsed with an electrolyte solution, cannulas are removed, and the vessels are repaired. Classification of acute tissue reactions after perfusion is done according to Wieberdink et al. (7): grade I, No reaction; grade II, slight erythema and/or edema; grade IIII, considerable erythema and/or edema with some blistering (slightly disturbed motility permissible); grade IV, extensive epidermolysis and/or obvious damage to the deep tissues, causing definite functional disturbances; threatening or manifest compartmental syndrome; and grade V, reaction that may necessitate amputation.

3. ILP FOR IN TRANSIT MELANOMA METASTASIS

Various attempts to improve tumor responses to ILP by using methods such as hyperthermia or by adding drugs such as TNF-α, have increased the efficacy of ILP for in transit melanoma metastases over the years. These developments are summarized in Table 1.

Table 1
Treatments for Melanoma In Transit Metastases)

ILP Strategy	No. of patients	CR %	PR %	Overall RR	TTLP median mets	Study
Melphalan alone)						
Normothermia						
37–38°C	58	41	24	65	6	Klaase et al., 1994 (20)
2X ILP[a]	42	76	14	90	6	Klaase et al, 1993 (21)
Mild hyperthermia						
39–40°C	80	26	36	62	ns	Rosin et al, 1980 (22)
	23	65	26	91	ns	Lejeune et al, 1983 (23)
	67	ns	ns	78	ns	Skene et al, 1990 (24)
	35	60	34	94	ns	Kettelhack et al, 1990 (25)
	111	73	13	86	9.5	Thompson et al, 1997 (26)
	103	52	25	77	14	Lienard et al, 1999 (44)[a]
Borderline/true hyperthermia)						
40–41°C	32	56	25	ns	85	Vaglini et al, 1981 (28)
	85	40	42	82	ns	Bryant et al., 1995 (29)
41.5–43°C	72	36	60	ns	87	Cavaliere et al, 1996 (39)
	46	48	39	87	ns	Di Filippo et al, 1989 (31)
	11	64	27	91	6+	Kroon et al, 1992 (32)
Repeat ILP	19	74	5	79	6+	Klop et al., 1996 (33)
Isolated limb infusion (= hypoxic isolated limb perfusion)						
37–38°C	128	41	44	85	ns	Lindner et al, 2002 (34)
2X ILI	47	41	47	88	18	Lindner et al, 2004 (35)
TNF–based ILP						
(39–40°C)	19	89	11	100[b]	8+	Lienard et al, 1992 (38)
	44	90	10	100[b]	18+	Lejeune et al, 1993 (39)
	4	100	0	100	ns	Hill et al, 1993 (40)
	11	64	0	64[b]	ns	Vaglini et al, 1994 (41)
	58	88	12	100[b]	26	Eggermont et al, 1994 (42)
	26	76	16	92[b]	ns	Fraker et al, 1996 (43)
	32	78	22	100[b]	14	Lienard et al, 1999 (44)
	32	69	22	91	14	Lienard et al, 1999 (44)
	100	69	26	95	16+	Grünhagen et al, 2004 (45)
Bulky disease only	39	16	75	ns	02	Fraker et al, 1959 (46)
	20	70	25	95	ns	Rossi et al, 2004 (47)
	50	58	34	83	8	Grünhagen et al, 2004 (45)
Repeat ILP	17	65	29	94	6+	Bartlett et al, 1997 (48)
	26	75	25	100	14	Grünhagen et al, 2005 (49)

[a] Abbreviations: CR, complete resonse; ILI, isolated limit infusion; ILP, isolated limb perfusion; PR, partial response; Overall RR, overall response rate (CR +- PR); TNF, tumor necrosis factor .

[b] TNF + interferon-γ.

3.1. Hyperthermia

Prevention of vasoconstriction in cutis and subcutis by using a warm water mattress is advocated in the treatment of superficial in transit melanoma metastases. In vivo drug uptake by in transit metastases is two times higher at 39.5°C than at 37°C *(8)*. Moreover, tumor cells *per se* are sensitive to heat, and hyperthermia also improves uptake of drug by the tumor cells, especially at temperatures >41°C *(9,10)*. In the normothermia to true hyperthermia temperature (range from 37 to 43°C) we distinguish the following states:

1. Normothermia (37–38,C): normothermic ILP with melphalan has been reported to result in a complete response (CR) rate of about 40%, a partial response (PR) rate of about 35%, and a median duration of local tumor control of about 6 mo *(11)*. Two perfusions at a 4-wk interval improves the the CR-response rate (77%) but does not improve duration of local control *(12)*.
2. Mild hyperthermia (39–40°C): several reports have claimed improved response rates *(13–17)*, but a comparative study did not show a significant benefit for mild hyperthermia over normothermia *(18)*.
3. Borderline true hyperthermia (40–41°C): this seems to be associated with higher CR rates but may also be associated with increased regional toxicity *(19–21)*.
4. True hyperthermia (41–43°C): this yields high CR rates *(22,23)* but is associated with unacceptable regional toxicity and even amputations in some reports *(24)*.

It is interesting that patients with local recurrence after a response to ILP have a similar response rate when treated again by ILP *(25)*. Overall, ILP with melphalan alone is associated with about a 50% CR rate and a 25 to 30% PR rate. Response rates improve somewhat with hyperthermia, but so does toxicity.

3.2. Percutaneous Hypoxic ILP

Isolated limb infusion with application of a tourniquet, which was developed by Thompson and co-workers in 1993, is essentially a low-flow, normothermic, hypoxic ILP with melphalan, but it has been called isolated limb "infusion" (ILI) to differentiate it from ILP *(9)*. The ILI procedure is technically less complex than ILP, as small-caliber catheters are inserted percutaneously into the vessels of the limb via the common femoral artery and vein in the contralateral groin. After 30 min the limb is flushed with saline, the tourniquet is deflated, and the catheters are removed.

With a CR rate of 41% and a PR rate of 44% in 207 cases, the results of ILI seem similar to those obtained with classical ILP *(26)*. However, these results are usually obtained in patients with only lesions in the distal two-thirds of the legs, where ILP easily achieves CR rates of 60 to 70%. Two ILI procedures at a 6-wk interval did not yield better results than a single perfusion *(27)*. However, ILI offers an effective, simple, and cheap alternative to the technically (heart-lung machine) more complicated and more expensive ILP procedure. Response rates are superior with ILP.

4. TUMOR NECROSIS FACTOR-A IN MELANOMA

ILP with melphalan or doxorubicin alone is not effective in the treatment of large tumors such as soft tissue sarcomas (STS). This has been demonstrated in the past and also recently by a trial at the M.D. Anderson Cancer Center, where Feig and collegues reported a 0% response rate and a 75% amputation rate in patients with locally advanced STS *(28,29)*. This situation changed dramatically with the advent of TNF *(30)*. TNF-based ILP has been established as a highly effective new method of induction biochemotherapy in extremity soft tissue sarcoma,s with a 20 to 30% CR rate and about a 50% PR rate *(31–34)*. On the basis of results in multicenter trials in Europe, TNF was approved and registered for sarcoma in 1998 *(34)*. The European TNF/ILP assessment group evaluated 246 patients with nonresectable STS enrolled over 10 years in four studies. All cases were reviewed by an independent review committee and compared with conventionally treated patients (often by amputation) from a population-based Scandinavian STS database. Major responses were seen in 56.5 to 82.6% of the patients, after which resection of the sarcoma usually became possible. Limb salvage was achieved in 74 to 87% in these four studies. It was concluded that TNF in combination with melphalan in the ILP setting represents a new and succesful option in the management of nonresectable locally advanced extremity STS *(34)*.

These results have now been confirmed by large single-institution studies reporting response rates varying from 63 to 91% and limb salvage rates from 58 to 94% *(35–44)*. Two reports on the combination of TNF with doxorubicin show very similar response rates of 62 to 90% and limb salvage rates of 71 to 85%, with more regional toxicity after doxorubicin than with melphalan *(37,41)*. Thus, we consider melphalan therefore still the drug of choice.

5. TNF-BASED ILP FOR MELANOMA IN TRANSIT METASTASES

ILP with melphalan alone for melanoma in transit metastases (IT-mets) has been reported the literature to result in a CR rate of about 50% and an overall response rate of 80% *(1)*. The introduction of TNF in this setting was reported to increase CR rates to 70 to 90% and overall response rates to 95 to 100% *(30,45–55)*. These results are summarized in the lower part of Table 1. Early on, however, it was observed that ILP with TNF + melphalan (TM-ILP) was especially effective against bulky tumors such as STS, whereas ILP with melphalan alone (M-ILP) fails, as was explained previously. We also used TM-ILP in melanoma patients, especially in those with bulky disease or those who had failed prior ILP. In Rotterdam we performed 100 consecutive TM-ILPs in 87 melanoma patients *(47)*, 45 for stage IIIA (IT-mets without positive lymph nodes), 39 for stage IIIAB (IT-mets with positive nodes), and 16 for stage IV (IT-mets + distant mets) disease. Most patients had bulky disease (0–10 lesions in 45 patients, 11–50 in 32 patients, and >50 in 25 patients) and/or had failed multiple prior treatments. In 21 patients we performed a second or third TM-ILP because the patient failed a prior M-ILP or TM-ILP.

The overall response rate was 95%, with 69 CRs (68%), 26 PRs (27%), and 5 incidences of stable disease (5%). CR rates differed significantly by stage: 82% in stage IIIA, 64% in stage IIIAB, and 38% in stage IV. Local recurrences in CR patients were seen in 50%. Mean time to recurrence/progression in CR patients was 11 mo (range 3–129+ mo); in PR patients it was 5 mo, with overall time to progression being 10 mo. With the 75% of stage IV patients at or after ILP, the mean time to distant metastases was 14 mo. At a median follow-up of 21.7 mo (range 1–132+ mo) overall 5-yr survival was 33% and 10-yr survival 17%. Repeat TM-ILPs had a 71% CR rate, indicating that repeat TM-ILPs are just as effective as first TM-ILPs. Local toxicity was mild: Wieberdink toxicity grades of I (15%), II (54%), III (27%), IV (4%), and V (1%). Median leakage was 0%, and no grade 3/4 systemic toxicity was observed, not even in five patients with high leakage

(10–21%). The CR rate up to 1996 (52 ILPs) was 77% compared with 58% in 48 ILPs since 1996 ($p = 0.048$).

This difference reflects a change in policy to offer TM-ILP only to patients with bulky disease and or multiple recurrences after multiple surgical interventions and/or after vaccine therapy trials, which many patients had entered. We managed patients with small tumors and a small number of tumors increasingly by repeated excisions and vaccine protocols and offered TNF-based ILP more and more exclusively to patients with a high tumor burden. This patient category, with highly unfavorable characteristics, was analyzed separately as the second 50 ILPs in our series; the CR rate was still 58%. This is still superior to the response rate in the historical group of patients treated with melphalan alone without such unfavorable patient selection, and it is similar to observations in the United States (52). In a interim analysis of a randomized trial by Fraker et al., TNF-based ILP was of significant benefit in patients with a high tumor load; the CR rate increased from 19% for MILP to 58% for TM-ILP (52). Moreover, Rossi and co-workers recently reported a CR rate of 70% after TNF-based ILP in a series of 20 melanoma patients with a high tumor burden (53)

Our experience demonstrates the extraordinary efficacy of TNF-based ILP in melanoma patients: as it results in a very high overall response rate (95%) was seen in patients with multiple IT-mets in a patient population dominated by those with high tumor burden and multiple prior treatments. Limb salvage was achieved in 99%.

A second indication for TM-ILP is failure after previous ILP therapy. The results of our study are similar to the response rates observed for repeat ILPs by Bartlett et al. (54). We performed 26 ILPs for recurrences in the limb after previous ILP treatment. The overall response rate of repeat ILP was 96% (CR 73%, PR 23%, no charge 3%). This did not differ from rates of the primary ILPs in our series, and no increased toxicity was observed (55). This observation underscores the efficacy of TNF-based ILP in the repeat ILP setting (55).

6. OBSERVATIONS IN THE LABORATORY AND FUTURE PERSPECTIVES

6.1. TNF Enhances Selective Drug Uptake in Tumor

We have recently demonstrated that the addition of high-dose TNF to the perfusate results in a four- to sixfold increased uptake by the tumor of the cytostatic drug. For melphalan and for doxorubicin it was demonstrated that this uptake was tumor specific and that no increased uptake was noted in normal tissue, thus emphasizing the relatively selective action of TNF on the tumor-associated vasculature (56,57). Moreover, we have demonstrated that the effect correlates with the vascularity of the tumor: the more vascular the tumor, the better the synergistic effect between TNF and the chemotherapeutic agent (58). We also demonstrated that 10-µg of TNF (a fivefold reduction in the "standard" dose of 50 µg) was the threshold dose for activity of TNF in our rat tumor extremity perfusion model. At 2 µg, all TNF effects were lost (59). Our tumor models predict a threshhold activity for 1 mg TNF in the clinical situation and we recommend not going below that dose. We demonstrated that hyperthermia, when combined with TNF and melphalan, leads to amputations because of normal tissue damage, and we do not recommend it in the clinic (59). Furthermore, we showed that actinomycin D, commonly used in the clinical setting, led to idiosyncratic toxicity in our models to both tumor and normal tissues resulting in amputation in all cases. We strongly caution not to use TNF in combination with actinomycin D *(60)*.

6.2. New Vasoactive Drugs

Various vasoactive drugs have been and are being studied in our laboratory models. We have recently noted that histamine can enhance selective drug uptake in tumors and can lead to intratumoral hemorrhage within 24 h, followed by massive tumor necrosis *(61)*. Similarly, but without causing intratumoral hemorrhage, interleukin-2 can enhance selective intratumoral drug uptake and act synergistically in the ILP setting *(62)*.

6.3. Potential Systemic Utility

Based on the findings of selective drug uptake enhancement of chemotherapeutics, we studied TNF in the systemic setting. Here we found that repeated administration of nontoxic low doses of TNF could enhance the intrumoral uptake of liposomal doxorubicin, but not free doxorubicin. We demonstrated this in various tumor models and thus identified a potential development for TNF in the systemic setting in the clinic *(63,64)*.

7. CONCLUSIONS AND FUTURE DIRECTIONS

ILP provides us with an excellent clinical tool to obtain local control and avoid limb amputations in patients with limb-threatening tumors and patients with multiple melanoma in transit metastases. This has been largely achieved by the success of the antivascular TNF-based biochemotherapy in this setting. TNF, for the first time, has given us an effective treatment against large, bulky tumors. TNF-based ILP is a highly successful treatment option to achieve limb salvage in the management of advanced, multiple, or drug-resistant extremity tumors. TNF-based ILPs are now performed in some 35 cancer centers in Europe with referral programs for limb salvage. TNF-based antivascular therapy of cancer is here to stay and its potential needs to be studied further, including its use in the systemic setting. In the Isolated perfusion field, newly discovered vasoactive drugs await evaluation in clinical trials *(65)*.

REFERENCES

1. Eggermont AMM. Treatment of melanoma in transit metastases confined to the limb. Cancer Surv 1996;26:335–349.
2. Hill S, Thomas JM. Treatment of cutaneous metastases from malignant melanoma using the carbon-dioxide laser. Eur J Surg Oncol 1993;19:173–177.
3. Creech O, Krementz E, Ryan E, Winblad J. Chemotherapy of cancer: regional perfusion utilising an extracorporeal circuit. Ann Surg 1958;148:616–632.
4. Benckhuijsen C, Kroon BB, van Geel AN, et al. Regional perfusion treatment with melphalan for melanoma in a limb: an evaluation of drug kinetics. Eur J Surg Oncol 1988;14:157–163.
5. Thompson JF, Gianoutsos MP. Isolated limb perfusion for melanoma—effectiveness and toxicity of cisplatin compared with that of melphalan and other drugs. World J Surg 1992;16:227–233.
6. Klaase JM, Kroon BBR, Van Geel AN, Eggermont AMM, Franklin HR. Systemic leakage during isolated limb perfusion for melanoma. Br J Surg 1993;80:1124–1126.
7. Wieberdink K, Benckhuijsen C, Braat RP, Van Slooten EA, Olthuis GAA. Dosimetry in isolation perfusion of the limbs by assessment of perfused tissue volume and grading of toxic tissue reactions. Eur J Cancer Clin Oncol 1982;18:905–910.
8. Omlor G, Gross G, Ecker KW, Burger I, Feifel G. Optimization of isolated hyperthermic limb perfusion. World J Surg 1993;16:1117–1119.

9. Cavaliere R, Ciocatto RC, Giovanella BC, et al. Selective heat sensitivity of cancer cells: biochemical and clinical studies. Cancer 1967;20:1351–1381.

10. Clark J, Grabs AJ, Parsosn PG, Smithers BM, Addison RS, Roberts MS. Melphalan uptake, hyperthermic synergism and drug resistance in a human cell culture model for the isolated limb perfusions of melanoma. Melanoma Res 1994;4:365–370.

11. Klaase JM, Kroon BBR, Van Wijk J, et al. Limb recurrence-free interval and survival in patients with recurrent melanoma of the extremities treated with normothermic isolated perfusion. J Am Coll Surg 1994;178:564–572.

12. Klaase JM, Kroon BBR, Van Geel AN, Eggermont AMM, Franklin HR, Van Dongen JA. A retrospective comparative study evaluating the results of a single perfusion versus a double perfusion schedule with melphalan in patients with recurrent melanoma of the lower limb. Cancer 1993;71:2990–2994.

13. Rosin RD, Westbury G: Isolated limb perfusion for malignant melanoma. Practitioner 1980;224: 1031–1036.

14. Lejeune FJ, Deloof T, Ewalenko P. Objective regression of unexcised melanoma in transit metastases after hyperthermic isolation perfusion of the limbs with melphalan. Recent Results Cancer Res 1983;86:268–276.

15. Skene AI, Bulman AS, Williams TR, Meirion Thomas J, Westbury G. Hyperthermic isolated perfusion with melphalan in the treatment of advanced malignant melanoma of the lower limb. Br J Surg 1990;77:765–767.

16. Kettelhack C, Kraus T, Hupp T, Manner M, Schlag P. Hyperthermic limb perfusion for malignant melanoma and soft tissue sarcoma. Eur J Surg Oncol 1990;16:370–375.

17. Thompson JF, Hunt JA, Shannon KF, Kam PC. Frequency and duration of remission after isolated limb perfusion for melanoma. Arch Surg 1997;132:903–907.

18. Lejeune F, Lienard D, Eggermont A, et al. Rationale for using TNF alpha and chemotherapy in regional therapy of melanoma. J Cell Biochem 1994; 56:52–61.

19. Klaase JM, Kroon BBR, Eggermont AMM, et al. A retrospective comparative study evaluating the results of "mild" hyperthermic versus "controlled" normothermic perfusion for recurrent melanoma of the extremities. Eur J Cancer 1995; 31:73–81.

20. Vaglini M, Andreola S, Attili A, et al. Hyperthermic antiblastic perfusion in the treatment of cancer of the extremities. Tumori 1985;71:355–359.

21. Bryant PJ, Balderson GA, Mead P, Egerton WS. Hyperthermic isolated limb perfusion for malignant melanoma: response and survival. World J Surg 1995;363–368.

22. Cavaliere R, Calabro A, Di Filippo F, Carlini S, Giannarelli D. Prognosic parameters in limb recurrent melanoma treated with hyperthermic antiblastic perfusion. Proceedings of the International Conference on Regional Cancer Treatment, 1987, Ulm G7:163.

23. Di Filippo F, Calabro A, Giannarelli D, et al. Prognostic variables in recurrent limb melanoma treated with hyperthermic antiblastic perfusion Cancer 1989;63:2551–2561.

24. Kroon BBR, Klaase JM, Van Geel AN, Eggermont AMM. Application of hyperthtmermia in regional isolated perfusion for melanoma of the limbs. Reg Cancer Treat 1992;4:223–226.

25. Klop WM, Vrouenraets BC, van Geel BN, et al. Repeat isolated limb perfusion with melphalan for recurrent melanoma of the limbs. J Am Coll Surg 1996;182:467–472.

26. Lindner P, Doubrovsky A, Kam PCA, Thompson JF. Prognostic factors after isolated limb infusion with cytotoxic agents for melanoma. Ann Surg Oncol 2002;9:127–136.

27. Lindner P, Thompson JF, De Wilt JH, Colman M, Kam PC. Double isolated limb infusion with cytotoxic agents for recurrent and metastatic limb melanoma. Eur J Surg Oncol 2004 May;30: 433–9.

28. Klaase JM, Kroon BBR, Benckhuysen C, Van Geel AN, Albus-Lutter ChE, Wieberdink J. Results of regional isolation perfusion with cytostatics in patients with soft tissue tumors of the extremities. Cancer 1989;64:616–621.

29. Feig BW, Ross MI, Hunt J, et al. A prospective evaluation of isolated limb perfusion with doxorubicin in patients with unresectable extremity sarcomas. Ann Surg Oncol 2004;11:S80.

30. Lienard D, Ewalenko, Delmotte JJ, Renard N, Lejeune FJ. High-dose recombinant tumor necrosis factor alpha in combination with interferon gamma and melphalan in isolation perfusion of the limbs for melanoma and sarcoma. J Clin Oncol 1992;10:50–62.

31. Eggermont AMM, Liénard D, Schraffordt Koops H, Rosenkaimer F, Lejeune FJ. Treatment of irresectable soft tissue sarcomas of the limbs by isolation perfusion with high dose TNF-α in combi-

nation with gamma-interferon and melphalan, in Tumor Necrosis Factor: Molecular and Cellular Biology and Clinical Relevance (Fiers W, Buurman WA, eds.), Basel: Karger Verlag, 1993:239–243.

32. Eggermont AMM, Schraffordt Koops H, Lienard D, et al. Isolated limb perfusion with high-dose tumor necrosis factor-alpha in combination with interferon-gamma and melphalan for nonresectable extremity soft tissue sarcomas: a multicenter trial [see comments]. J Clin Oncol 1996;14:2653–2665.

33. Eggermont AMM, Schraffordt Koops H, Klausner JM, et al. Isolated limb perfusion with tumor necrosis factor and melphalan for limb salvage in 186 patients with locally advanced soft tissue extremity sarcomas. The cumulative multicenter European experience. Ann Surg 224:756–764; discussion 1996:764–765.

34. Eggermont AMM, Schraffordt Koops H, Klausner JM, et al. Limb salvage by isolation limb perfusion with tumor necrosis factor alpha and melphalan for locally advanced extremity soft tissue sarcomas: results of 270 perfusions in 246 patients. Proc ASCO 1999;11:497.

35. Gutman M, Inbar M, Lev-Shlush D, et al. High dose tumor necrosis factor-α and melphalan administered via isolated limb perfusion for advanced limb soft tissue sarcoma results in a >90% response rate and limb preservation. Cancer 1997;79:1129–1123.

36. Olieman AF, Pras E, van Ginkel RJ, Molenaar WM, Schraffordt Koops H, Hoekstra HJ. Feasibility and efficacy of external beam radiotherapy after hyperthermic isolated limb perfusion with TNF-alpha and melphalan for limb-saving treatment in locally advanced extremity soft-tissue sarcoma. Int J Radiat Oncol Biol Phys 1998;40:807–814.

37. Rossi CR, Foletto M, Di Filippo F, et al. Soft tissue limb sarcomas: Italian clinical trials with hyperthermic antiblastic perfusion. Cancer 1999;86:1742–1749.

38. Lejeune FJ, Pujol N, Lienard D, et al. Limb salvage by neoadjuvant isolated perfusion with TNF-alpha and melphalan for non-resectable soft tissue sarcoma of the extremities. Eur J Surg Oncol 2000;26:669–678.

39. Hohenberger P, Kettelhack C, Hermann A, Schlag PM. Functional outcome after preoperative isolated limb perfusion with rhTNF-alpha/melphalan for high-grade extremity sarcoma. Eur J Cancer 2001;37:S34–S35.

40. Noorda EM, Vrouwenraets BC, Nieweg OE, Slooten GW, Kroon BBR. Isolated limb perfusion with TNFα and melphalan for irresectable soft tissue sarcoma of the extremities. Ann Surg Oncol 2003;10;1:S36.

41. Rossi CR, Mocellin S, Pilati P, et al. Hyperthermic isolated perfusion with low-dose tumor necrosis factor alpha and doxorubicin for the treatment of limb-threatening soft tissue sarcomas. Ann Surg Oncol 2005;12:398–405.

42. Grünhagen DJ, de Wilt JH, Graveland WJ, et al. Outcome and prognostic factor analysis of 217 consecutive isolated limb perfusions with tumor necrosis factor-α and melphalan for limb-threatening soft tissue sarcoma. Cancer 2005;106(8):1776–1784.

43. Bonvalot S, Laplanche A, Lejeune F, et al. Limb salvage with isolated perfusion for soft tissue sarcoma: could less TNF-alpha be better? Ann Oncol 2005;16:1061–1068.

44. Grünhagen DJ, de Wilt JHW, Verhoef C, Graveland WJ, van Geel AN et al. TNF Dose Reduction in Isolated Limb Perfusion. Eur J Surg Oncol 2005;21:1011–1019.

45. Lejeune FJ, Lienard D, Leyvraz S, Mirimanoff RO. Regional therapy of melanoma. Eur J Cancer 1993;29A:606–612.

46. Hill S, Fawcett WJ, Sheldon J, Soni N, Williams T, Thomas JM. Low dose tumor necrosis factor-alpha and melphalan in hyperthermic isolated limb perfusion. Br J Surg 1993;80:995–997.

47. Vaglini M, Belli F, Ammatuna M, et al. Treatment of primary or relapsing limb cancer by isolation perfusion with high-dose TNF, gamma-IFN and melphalan. Cancer 1994;73:483–492.

48. Eggermont AMM, Liénard D, Schraffordt Koops H, et al. High dose tumor necrosis factor-alpha in isolation perfusion of the limb: highly effective treatment for melanoma in transit metastases or unresectable sarcoma. Reg Cancer Treat 1995;7:32–36.

49. Fraker DL, Alexander HR, Andrich M, Rosenberg SA. Treatment of patients with melanoma of the extremity using hyperthermic isolated limb perfusion with melphalan, tumor necrosis factor, and interferon gamma: results of a tumor necrosis factor dose-escalation study. J Clin Oncol 1996;14:479–489.

50. Lienard D, Eggermont AMM, Schraffordt Koops H, et al. Isolated limb perfusion with tumor necrosis factor-alpha and melphalan with or without interferon-gamma for the treatment of in transit melanoma metastases: a multicentre randomized phase II study. Melanoma Res 1999;9:491–502.

51. Grünhagen DJ, Brunstein F, Graveland WJ, van Geel AN, de Wilt JH, Eggermont AM. One hundred consecutive isolated limb perfusions with TNF-alpha and melphalan in melanoma patients with multiple in transit metastases. Ann Surg 2004;240:939–947; discussion 947–948.

52. Fraker DL, Alexander HR, Ross M, et al. A phase III trial of isolated limb perfusion for extremity melanoma comparing melphalan alone versus melphalan plus tumor necrosis factor (TNF) plus interferon gamma (IFN). Ann Surg Oncol 2002;9:S8.

53. Rossi CR, Foletto M, Mocellin S, et al. Hyperthermic isolated limb perfusion with low-dose tumor necrosis factor-alpha and melphalan for bulky in transit melanoma metastases. Ann Surg Oncol 2004;11:173–177.

54. Bartlett DL, Grace M, Alexander HR, Libutti SK, Fraker DL. Isolated limb perfusion with tumor necrosis factor and melphalan in patients with extremity melanoma after failure of isolated limb perfusion with chemotherapeutics. Cancer 1997;80:2084–2090.

55. Grünhagen DJ, van Etten B, Brunstein F, et al. Efficacy of repeat isolated limb perfusions with tumor necrosis factor alpha and melphalan for multiple in transit metastases in patients with prior isolated limb perfusion failure.Ann Surg Oncol 2005;12:609–615.

56. De Wilt JHW, ten Hagen TLM, de Boeck G, van Tiel ST, de Bruijn EA, Eggermont AMM. Tumour necrosis factor alpha increases melphalan concentration in tumor tissue after isolated limb perfusion. Br J Cancer 2000;82:1000–1003.

57. Veen vd AH, Wilt de JHW, Eggermont AMM, van Tiel ST, ten Hagen TLM. TNF-α augments intratumoral concentration of doxorubicin in TNF-α-based isolated limb perfusion in rat sarcoma models and enhances antitumor effects. Br J Cancer 2000;82:973–980.

58. van Etten B, de Vries M, van IJken M, et al. Degree of tumor vascularity correlates with drug accumulation and tumor response upon TNF-based isolated hepatic perfusion. Br J Cancer 2003;87:314–319.

59. DeWilt JHW, Manusama ER, van Tiel ST, van IJken MGA, ten Hagen TLM, Eggermont AMM. Prerequisites for effective isolated limb perfusion using tumor necrosis factor-alpha and melphalan in rats. Br J Cancer 1999;80:161–166.

60. Seynhaeve ALB, de Wilt JHW, vanTiel SA, Eggermont AMM, ten Hagen TLM. Combination of actinomycin D with TNF-α in isolated limb perfusion results in improved tumor response in soft tissue sarcoma-bearing rats but is accompanied by severe dose limiting local toxicity. Br J Cancer 2002;86:1174–1179.

61. Brunstein F, Hoving S, Seynhaeve AL, et al. Synergistic antitumor activity of histamine plus melphalan in isolated limb perfusion: preclinical studies. J Natl Cancer Inst 2004;96:1603–1610.

62. Hoving S, Brunstein F, aan de Wiel-Ambagtsheer G, et al. Synergistic antitumor response of interleukin 2 with melphalan in isolated limb perfusion in soft tissue sarcoma-bearing rats. Cancer Res 2005;65:4300–4308.

63. Ten Hagen TL, Van Der Veen AH, Nooijen PT, et al. Low-dose tumor necrosis factor-alpha augments antitumor activity of stealth liposomal doxorubicin (DOXIL) in soft tissue sarcoma-bearing rats. Int J Cancer 2000;87:829–837.

64. Brouckaert P, Takahashi N, van Tiel ST, et al. Tumor necrosis factor-alpha augmented tumor response in B16BL6 melanoma-bearing mice treated with stealth liposomal doxorubicin (Doxil) correlates with altered Doxil pharmacokinetics. Int J Cancer 2004;109:442–448.

65. Ten Hagen TLM, FJ Lejeune, Eggermont AMM. TNF is here to stay—revisited. Trends Immunol 2001;22:127–129.

27 Outpatient Brachytherapy with Seeds

Alternative Treatment Option for Patients with Localized Prostate Cancer

Frank Kahmann, MD and Thomas Oliver Henkel, MD

CONTENTS

SUMMARY

Prostate cancer and lung carcinoma are the most common cancers in the western world. Better screening methods especially the introduction of prostate specific antigen (PSA) screening in the beginning of the 1990s, have increased the early detection rate. In the United States only 30% of prostate tumors discovered were at an early stage before the introduction of PSA screening, compared with >60% nowadays. Early detection also increased the number of younger men among these patients. Patient demands have increased with respect to incontinence and impotence, especially among those young patients. Radical prostatectomy is still the gold standard for therapy of localized prostate cancer. Better operating techniques have decreased the side effects of this operation, but many patients still do not undergo this operation because they fear the side effects. Low dose rate (LDR) brachytherapy using permanent seeds originated in the United States and has had a renaissance in recent years. In 2004 alone, more than 50,000 patients were successfully treated using this technique. Ten-year data published as early as 1998 showed similar results compared with a multitude of radical prostatectomy studies and superior results to most of the published external beam studies, with significantly fewer side effects. Recently published 15-yr follow-up data support these findings. In Germany and Western Europe, more and more centers began with LDR

From: *Cancer Drug Discovery and Development: Regional Cancer Therapy*
Edited by: P. M. Schlag and U. S. Stein © Humana Press Inc., Totowa, NJ

brachytherapy. In contrast to the United States, where brachytherapy is mostly performed as an outpatient procedure, many European centers do only inpatient brachytherapy, with only a few centers performing outpatient procedures. Among them is the Ambulantes Operationszentrum im Ullsteinhaus in Berlin. The results from this center are very encouraging: few complications, high-quality treatment, and high patient acceptance.

Key Words: Prostate carcinoma; brachytherapy; seeds; iodine-125; Pd-103.

1. INTRODUCTION

Prostate cancer and lung cancer are the most common male malignant diseases in Western European countries. The European health authorities have estimated an incidence of 280,000 new prostate cancer patients in 2003. More than 100,000 of these patients have localized disease and can be treated curatively. In Europe, radical prostatectomy is still the gold standard treatment. Prostate brachytherapy has enjoyed increasing popularity, beginning in the early 1990s. During the 1970s, prostate brachytherapy was performed intraoperatively with a freehand technique popularized by Whitmore and Hilaris. Brachytherapy seemed to be the perfect solution to deliver high doses within the target organ under maximal protection of the surrounding organs. However, long-term results with the freehand retropubic approach were discouraging, partly because of poor patient selection (since prognostic parameters such as prostate-specific antigen [PSA] were not available during that time) and partly owing to limited technical resources such as dose planning programs or needle guiding templates. The retropubic, freehand approach required an open laparotomy, dissection of the prostate, and implantation of the seeds under digital rectal guidance without any preplanning of the dose delivered to the prostate (Fig. 1). As anticipated, this technique showed poor seed distribution, thus leading to a very inhomogenous implant with unsatisfactory dose delivery within the prostate.

Nowadays, doctors have much better tools to calculate the likelihood of extraprostatic disease, lymph node involvement, or bone metastases. PSA screening has helped us to diagnose tumors earlier. The seed implant procedure has totally changed: modern, powerful, and user-friendly computer systems allow fast and precise dose planning, the transperineal template-guided seed implant allows us to implant the radioactive seeds precisely, and quality control can be performed using computed tomography (CT)-based postplanning. All of these improvements have led to very good long term results.

2. INDICATION FOR LOW DOSE RATE BRACHYTHERAPY

The typical indication for interstitial low dose rate (LDR) brachytherapy is localized cancer of the prostate. LDR brachytherapy, therefore, is in direct competition to other treatment options such as radical prostatectomy. The American Brachytherapy Society (ABS) first published guidelines describing patient selection for prostate seed brachytherapy in 1999. Patients were divided into two different risk groups (low and high risk) according to their clinical results (biopsy Gleason score, rectal exam, clinical staging). Clinical results are often divided into three profile groups: low, intermediate, and high risk. Therapy options are decided according to the specific risk assesment of each patient. Patients with a low risk of extracapsular extension of the tumor can be treated with interstitial LDR brachytherapy implementing seeds as a monotherapy, whereas patients with a higher risk for extracapsular extension should be treated with a combina-

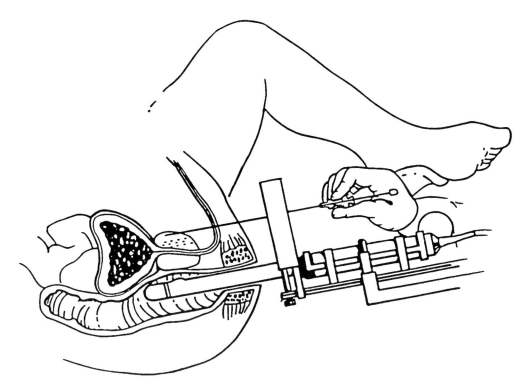

Fig. 1. Retropubic technique: impregnating the seeds via an open approach.

tion therapy. For this combined treatment option, the external beam radiation (EBRT) dose of 45 gy is boosted with a reduced seed implant dose. According to the American Association of Physicists in Medicine Task Group 43 (AAPM TG 43). When one is using ^{125}I-seeds, the dose of 145 gy for monotherapy will be reduced to 110 gy for the combined treatment. When one is using ^{103}P-seeds, the planned dose will be 125 gy (for monotherapy) and 100 gy (for combination therapy).

All seed implant patients should have a minimal life expectancy of 5 yr, and metastatic disease should, if necessary, be excluded using CT and a bone scan. Table 1 shows the indications according to the ABS guidelines for prostate brachytherapy for both monotherapy and combination therapy.

Patients will be considered at a higher risk if only one of the parameters is elevated. The ABS did not give specific recommendations for Gleason scores of 7 and PSA between 10 and 20 ng/mL. For these patients, individual treatment decisions are to be discussed with the patient.

European and German guidelines were published in December 2000. These guidelines only recommend monotherapy treatment for low-risk tumors. Additional clinical parameters were included, such as micturition measurements (see Table 2).

A possible contraindication for prostate seed brachytherapy is a transurethral resection or the prostate (TURP) prior to the implant since the risk of postoperative incontinence is significantly increased. Results from a very experienced group in Seattle revealed an increase in the postoperative incontinence rate up to 40% after TURP compared with 1% without prior TURP. The latest implant techniques, using peripheral loading, have

Table 1
Indications for Monotherapy/Combined Therapy
According to American Brachytherapy Society (ABS) Guidelines

Parameter	Monotherapy	Combined therapy	No recommendation
PSA	<10 ng/mL	>20 ng/mL	10–20 ng/mL
Gleason Score	≤6	≥8	7
Prostate volume	<60 cm^3	<60 cm^3	
Clinical stage	≤cT2a	cT2b	

Abbreviation: PSA, prostate-specific antigen.

Table 2
Indications for Seed Brachytherapy
According to European (EAU/ESTRO) Guidelines

Parameter	Monotherapy
PSA	<10 ng/mL
Gleason score	≤6
Prostate volume	<60 cm^3
Clinical stage	≤cT2a
IPSS	≤8
Flow Q_{max}	>15 mL/s

Abbreviations: IPSS, international prostate symptom score;
PSA, prostate-specific antigen.

reduced the risk to 9%. Our own data using high-activity seeds (0.729 mCi) and the peripheral loading technique only showed a slight increase in postoperative incontinence compared with non-TURP patients as long as an interval of at least 6 mo had passed between TURP and the seed implant. High international prostate symptom scores (IPSS) also led to an increased risk of postoperative voiding problems or possible urinary retention.

If the biopsy shows perineural invasion, the risk of capsular penetration is increased to 50%. It recommended that patients with such a biopsy result receive combination therapy. Multifocal tumors with more than four positive biopsy cores and bilateral disease also have a higher risk for extracapsular disease and may show better results when treated with combination therapy.

3. TECHNIQUE OF PERMANENT SEED BRACHYTHERAPY

Many brachytherapy centers in the United States are still performing preplan dosimetry studies 3 to 4 wk prior to the implant. The prostate is examined using transrectal ultrasound (TRUS), 5 mm cross-sectional slices of the prostatic anatomy as well as of the rectum, bladder, and urethra are registered. These ultrasound images are transfered to the dose planning system. The dose planning computer reconstructs the 3D anatomy of

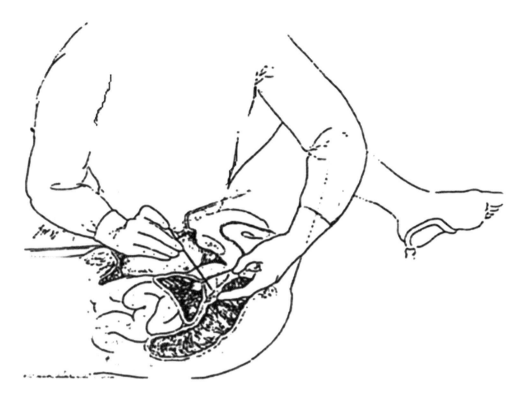

Fig. 2. Transperineal technique.

the prostate and the surrounding tissues. The number, activity, and position of the seeds within the prostate are calculated, and an implant protocol is printed.

On the day of operation, the patient must be placed in the exact same position in the preplan. Inaccuracies are still possible. To eliminate such innaccuracies, more and more centers are using intraoperative dose planning systems. In contrast to the preplan 3 to 4 wk before, the complete dose plan is calculated intraoperatively while the patient is anesthetized. Optimal accuracy between the plan and the actual intraoperative situation can be achieved. To perform the intraoperative plan, the patient will be placed in the dorsal lithotomy position, anesthetized and catheterized (Fig. 2).

After intraprostatic insertion of the fixation needles (Fig. 3), the prostate is registered using planimetric ultrasound measurements. The 3D reconstruction of the prostatic, urethral, and rectal anatomy permits dose calculation and creates the implant protocol printout. There is no patient movement between the dose planning and the actual implant. Other variables such as filling of the bladder and the rectum, which can influence the dose plan significantly, are kept constant. A further improvement for dose planning and implant quality was the introduction of *dynamic dosimetry*, whereby the dose plan is re-evaluated after every implanted needle. If any needle/seed displacement can be detected under ultrasound and fluoroscopy control, the dose plan is recalculated and adjusted to the actual situation by changing the position of the remaining seeds. Thus, optimal dose distribution within the prostate can be achieved, and the quality of the implant can be documented.

Table 3
Dose Recommendations for Iodine-125 and Palladium-103[a] (AAPM TG 43)

Seed type	Monotherapy dose (gy)	Combination therapy dose (gy)[b]
[125]I (before TG 43)	160	110–120
[125]I (after TG 43)	144	100–110
[103]Pd	125	100

[a] According to guidelines of the American Association of Physicists in Medicine Task Group 43 (AAPM TG 43).
[b] Plus 40–50 gy of external beam radiotherapy (EBRT).

The first PSA test should be performed after 3 or 6 mo; a PSA nadir will usually be attained within 12 to 18 mo. The criteria for biochemical monitoring are being reexamined. Some centers use the American Society for Therapeutic Radiology and Oncology (ASTRO) definition of three consecutive rises in PSA as an indicator for biochemical recurrence, whereas others prefer to use a nadir of 0.5 or 1.0 ng/mL.

4. DOSE PLANNING FOR SEED IMPLANTS

In 1995, the AAPM TG 43 changed the calculation algorithm for implants using ^{125}I seeds. They adjusted the dose from 160 to 144 gy. The task group changed the calculation and therefore the amount in gy, but not the total implanted activity. The dose calculation for [103]Pd was not changed significantly. The current recommendation from the AAPM for [103]Pd is 125 gy. Table 3 gives an overview of the currently used doses for brachytherapy using ^{125}I or [103]Pd.

The introduction of [103]Pd in 1986 meant that a second isotope was available. [103]Pd emits photons with a lower energy than those emitted by ^{125}I, which leads to a steeper decrease of the dose within the tissue. Therefore the geometric position of the seeds within the prostate is more critical than with iodine. Ling et al. compared the biological effectiveness of palladium vs iodine using theoretical radiobiological models. They postulated that rapidly proliferating tumors with high Gleason grades would be treated more effectively with palladium, whereas slowly growing tumors would react better when treated with iodine. On the basis of these considerations, several centers in the United States treated patients with Gleason scores above 7 using palladium only. Comparative studies in the last few years showed no differences in clinical effectiveness between the two isotopes within the first 5 yr after treatment. The ABS guidelines do not give any recommendation as to which isotope to use at the present moment. Owing to higher costs and more complicated logistics (17-d half life of palladium vs 60 d with iodine), palladium is not commonly used in Europe.

The dose planning computers are equipped with planning algorithms that can vary in particular details; the main planning parameters are specified by the AAPM and the ABS.

The main planning parameter is coverage of the prostate with the prescription isodose (V_{100}). Nowadays, the V_{100} in a preplan should be 99% minimum. A safety margin of the 100% isodose around the prostate would be 3 to 5 mm. An additional planning parameter is the D_{90} (dose that covers 90% of the prostate volume). In our center, we try to have a preimplant D_{90} of 185 gy or higher. We limit the maximum dose at the urethra to 160% of the prescription dose (232 gy), and only 2% of the contoured rectum surface will receive 145 gy. The dose parameters for the urethra and the rectum vary significantly between the different centers within Europe. A further dose parameter that should be monitored is the D_{50} (dose that covers 50% of the prostate volume). Our own data have revealed that the D_{50} directly correlates with toxicity, especially at the urethra. Urethral toxicity will be significantly lower if the D_{50} is below 240 gy. If combined therapy is administered (110 gy seeds) or if [103]Pd is being used, the dose parameters will be lowered accordingly.

5. POSTOPERATIVE QUALITY SURVEILLANCE

Every patient should receive a postoperative quality surveillance using either CT or MRI scans. Postplans permit monitoring of the actual dose truly received by the patient. Not only is the postplan the sole way to monitor the dose to the patient, it is also the one and only means for the implant team to control the quality of their own work. This is considered mandatory in order to overcome the initial learning curve and later on to keep track of the implant parameters. The ABS guidelines demand a postplan for every patient.

Until the beginning of the 1990s, postplans were performed using anteroposterior and lateral X-ray scans; the seed number could be detected easily, but the 3D reconstruction of the seed position within the prostate was very complicated. Furthermore, anatomical structures such as the prostate, bladder, rectum, and urethra could not be depicted. Dose-volume histograms were insufficient, at times only rough estimates. Nowadays, the CT or MRI scans used are either directly imported into the planning computer via DICOM 3 files or digitized using a digitizer (Fig. 6). Both image modalities have their advantages and disadvantages. CT gives very good seed recognition but has limitations with the specific definition of the prostate boundaries; MRI demonstrates the prostate quite accurately, but the intraprostatic seed position can be hard to define. Comparisons between CT and TRUS imaging of the prostate showed a discrepancy of up to 30% in prostate size because definition of the prostate on CT scans are imprecise. This leads to a significant error in dose calculation for the prostate in the postplan. Some centers use image fusion technologies (fusing CT and MRI pictures) to gain the advantages of both imaging modalities (Fig. 7).

New developments in seed technology such as the use of plastic seeds or seeds with MRI contrast dye can help to overcome these limitations of the postplan and will lead to better means of critical judgment for postplans. Another crucial parameter for postplan dosimetry is the actual timing of the imaging. If the calculation is performed too early, the prostate could still be significantly swollen owing to intraprostatic hematoma and edema, making the calculated dose within the prostate possibly 10 to 30% too low. Studies have demonstrated that the optimal interval for postplans following ^{125}I implants is 3 to 5 wk and for [103]Pd implants 2 to 3 wk postoperatively. Nevertheless, because of logistical reasons, many centers perform the postplan on the first postoperative day.

As mentioned above in Subheading 4., the following parameters should be calculated and documented on a proper postplan (according to the AAPM):

D_{100}: Dose that covers 100% of the prostate (also called *minimal peripheral dose* or *minimal dose to the prostate*)

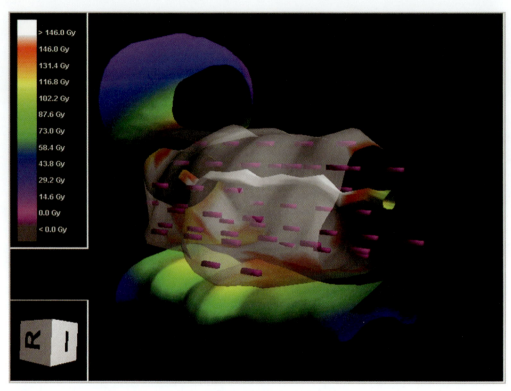

Fig. 6. Postplan 3D reconstruction.

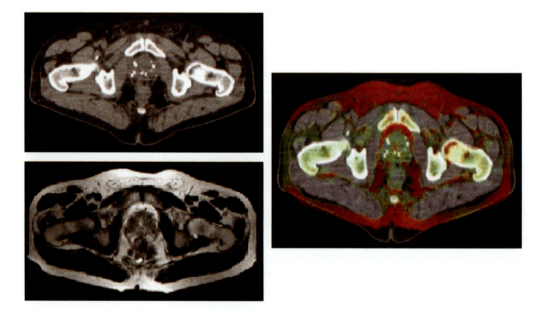

Fig. 7. Image fusion postplan with CT and MRI.

Table 4
Parameters for Postplan Dosimetry

Therapy type	D_{100} (gy)	D_{90} (gy)	V_{100} (%)
[125]I Monotherapy	>110	>144	>80
[125]I Combined therapy	>80	>100	>80
[103]Pd Monotherapy	>100	>115	>80
[103]Pd Combined therapy	>70	>90	>80

Abbreviations: D_{100}, dose that covers 100% of the prostate; D_{90}, dose that covers 90% of the prostate; V_{100}, volume of the prostate covere by 100% of the prescription dose.

D_{90}:   Dose that covers 90% of the prostate
V_{100}:   Volume of the prostate that is covered by 100% of the prescription dose

Further parameters that should be calculated for documentation of postoperative quality surveillance are the D_{50}, D_{80}, V_{80}, V_{90}; V_{150}, and V_{200}. The 50, 80, 90, 100, 150, and 200% isodose lines should be recognized during therapy visualization.

Table 4 shows the different dose parameters for postimplant quality surveillance.

The only statistically proven prognostic parameter for biochemical control (no PSA relapse) defined by the postplan is the D_{90}. A cutoff point was calculated at 140 gy. Patients with a D_{90} on the postplan below 140 gy were biochemically relapse free in 68% after 6 yr, in comparison to 92% without biochemical relapse if the D_{90} was above 140 gy ($p = 0,02$).

Wallner has described correlations between dosimetric parameters and the rate of side effects for LDR prostate brachytherapy. Patients who reported Radiation Therapy Oncology Group (RTOG) grade 0 to 1 genitourinary side effects had an average of 10 mm of the prostatic urethra irradiated with more than 400 gy, in comparison to 20 mm in patients with RTOG grade 2 to 3 genitourinary side effects. Similar correlations could be proved for rectal side effects with RTOG defined grade 1 to 2 gastrointestinal side effects if more than 17 mm^2 of the rectum were treated with more than 100 gy. Patients did not report rectal side effects if less than 11 mm^2 of the rectal surface received 100 gy. Our own results have shown that rectal toxicicty is significantly lower if the volume that receives the prescription dose is below 1 cm^3.

6. RESULTS OF PROSTATE BRACHYTHERAPY FOR LOCALIZED TUMORS

In 1998, Ragde, Blasko, and Grimm from Seattle reported the first 10-yr results for LDR prostatc brachytherapy using a transperineal approach under image guidance for ^{125}I seeds as monotherapy or combined therapy with EBRT. One hundred fifty-two patients with T1 to T3 tumors were treated with brachytherapy between January 1987 and June 1988.

Ninety-eight patients were considered at low risk for extracapsular extension of the tumor and were consequently treated with monotherapy using iodine (group 1). The other 54 patients had a higher risk for tumor spread beyond the capsule and were treated with a combination consisting of 100-gy seeds followed by 45 gy EBRT (group 2).

The average preoperative parameters were PSA of 11 ng/mL, T2 tumors, and a Gleason score of 5. Median follow-up was 119 mo. Overall survival after 10 years was 65%. Only 2% of the patients died because of the tumor, which means a disease-specific survival of 98%. After a follow-up of 10 yr, 64% of the patients were free from biochemical failure; the average PSA was 0.18 ng/mL. Surprisingly, no significantly statistical differences in survival were seen after 10 yr between group 1 and group 2, even though group 2 had significantly worse tumor parameters than group 1.

Ragde and his colleagues postulated that the results after 10 yr of follow-up were comparable with most studies after radical prostatectomy and better than most series done with EBRT for low-risk prostate cancers.

Similar data were published after a 12- and 14-yr follow-up comprising a slightly larger number of patients that had already been reported on by Ragde et al. They presented similar survival data as seen in recent radical prostatectomy data; the average PSA was still 0.18 ng/mL.

In 1998, Patrick Walsh and his colleagues from Baltimore published a retrospective comparison of brachytherapy patients treated by the Seattle group with patients treated with radical prostatectomy by his own group. A matched pair analysis with single matching was calculated.

The patient data from Seattle were acquired from a publication by Ragde et al. in 1997, who reported a 79% survival rate after 7 yr. The Baltimore group reported a 97% 7-yr survival after radical prostatectomy. The parameter for biochemical progress was a PSA of above 0.5 ng/mL for the brachytherapy group and 0.2 ng/mL for the radical prostatectomy group. The Baltimore group recommended caution with the use of prostate LDR brachytherapy for localized prostate cancer.

A similar retrospective study was performed in 1999 by Catalona and colleagues from St. Louis. They reported on a 5-point match comparison between the same patient group reported by Ragde et al. and a patient group from St. Louis.

The criterion for biochemical progress was again defined to be 0.5 ng/mL PSA for the LDR brachytherapy group; for the radical prostatectomy patients, an even more generous margin (of 0.3 ng/mL) was permitted. In contrast to the results from Baltimore, the St. Louis study could not show any statistically significant difference in patient survival. Patients treated by radical prostatectomy showed a 7-yr biochemically free survival of 84% compared with 79% in the Seattle group.

A further study, published by d'Amico, also compared patients after radical prostatectomy restrospectively with brachytherapy patients. Patients were classified into 3 risk goups according to preoperative clinical data: low, intermediate, and high risk. No differences in survival after 5 yr were seen in the low-risk group. Patients with an intermediate or high risk did better after receiving a radical prostatectomy.

In summary, none of the three retrospective studies showed clear results, owing to inhomogeneities between the groups of patients compared. All authors concluded that prospective studies were necessary to obtain proper data about the safety and effectiveness of prostate LDR brachytherapy for localized prostate cancer.

To overcome the lack of prospective randomized data, the SPIRIT study was introduced, with the goal of prospectively comparing radical prostatectomy and brachytherapy patients. Unfortunately, the study had to be closed because of the low number of enrolled patients who were willing to have their treatment modality randomly chosen.

Nowadays, most centers use Partin tables and a Kattan nomogram when counseling patients for the treatment of localized prostate cancer. The Partin tables reveal the pre-operative likelihood of organ-confined disease and extracapsular extension as well lymph node and seminal vesical involvement. PSA, biopsy Gleason score, and clinical stage are the necessary parameters for the Partin tables. The Kattan nomogram uses the same data and can estimate 5-yr biochemical freedom of recurrence for the different treatment modalities. Using those tools, the patient can be properly guided and informed about his treatment options.

7. OUTPATIENT BRACHYTHERAPY IN EUROPE AND GERMANY

During the last 5 yr, Europe has experienced an LDR prostate brachytherapy boom. Many new centers have established their own brachytherapy programs. In Germany, more than 50 hospitals and outpatient practices have begun to implant seeds into cancer-ous prostates. Unfortunately, many of these centers only perform a limited number of implants per year. Since the learning curve is considered to be as high as 40 to 60 patients, it is feared that the results from centers with limited patient numbers will not meet the standards defining good implants. In contrast to the United States, where implants are mostly performed as outpatient treatments, brachytherapy in Europe is predominantly done as an inpatient procedure. The major reason for this preference is the reimbursement situation in most European countries. In Germany, brachytherapy is generally reim-bursed in an inpatient setting, whereas a case-by-case reimbursement has to be negotiated for each outpatient treatment with the respective health insurance companies. The first outpatient procedure was performed in Germany in 1999. Since then only a few brachytherapy programs have treated a large number of patients. In Germany, approx 2000 patients are treated per year, which is less than 10% of the potential curative treat-ment for localized prostate cancer. In the United States approx 35% of curative treatments are brachytherapy.

We have treated more than 800 patients on an outpatient basis in our brachytherapy center in Berlin. The patients tolerated the outpatient procedure very well. Because of the outpatient situation, seed implantation was performed under general anesthesia. Average time of anesthesia was 76 min and the average length of stay was 250 min. Eighty percent of our patients were considered low risk according to ABS guidelines and were treated with 145 gy iodine monotherapy. The remaining 20% were considered intermediate or high risk and were treated with combination therapy consisting of 110-gy seeds followed by 45 gy EBRT. Over 90% of the patients received intraoperative dosimetry planning, which did not significantly prolong the duration of anesthesia (+10 min). Since 2003, we have introduced dynamic dosimetry, which has increased the accuracy of the dose plan-ning even more.

Acute toxicity has been limited; approx 4% of the patients required postoperative catheterization. Half of these patients, however, were in need of long-term catheteriza-tion and required a TURP afterward. Nearly all patients reported urethral toxicity grade 1 to 2. This consists of an increase in dysuria, frequency, urge, and nocturia. Patients with a high preoperative AUA symptom score reported more problems than patients with good voiding function prior to the implant. Urethral toxicity reaches its peak after 4 to 6 wk and slowly subsides to 8 to 12 wk after implantation. No patients experienced grade 3 or 4 rectal toxicity. The low side effect rate of our implant patients could only be achieved with intraoperative dosimetry planning and a stringent quality surveillance program enforcing strict limitations on urethral and rectal doses during the implant.

Patient acceptance was very high. Patients were sent questionnaires about their general health and brachytherapy-related problems as well as their postimplant PSA. Patients were also asked whether they felt safe in the outpatient setting, whether they would still choose the same form of treatment, and whether they would recommend this treatment option to other patients. All patients reported that they felt safe in the outpatient setting. Eighty-one percent would choose again brachytherapy as their preferred treatment option and would recommend it to another patient. Sixty-nine percent returned to their daily routine or went back to work immediately, 25% after 1 wk, and only one patient reported that he required 4 wk of recovery before returning to his normal activities. Also, toxicity parameters for acute as well as long-term side effects were questioned. The most important factor for patient satisfaction in the long run is continence. Almost no high-grade incontinence was seen after prostate brachytherapy. This could only be achieved through a strict limitation of the dose to the urethra using intraoperative and dynamic dose planning. Especially for the younger patients, preservation of potency, leading to a better quality of life, was also a major factor influencing their preference toward LDR brachytherapy as a treatment option.

8. CONCLUSIONS

LDR brachytherapy is a valid treatment alternative to radical prostatectomy for localized prostate cancer. The minimal side effects, with hardly any incontinence and a lower impotence rate compared with radical prostatectomy, is a particularly important decision-making criterion for younger patients. LDR brachytherapy requires close cooperation between urology and radiooncology. It is a team effort also involving physicists, anesthetists, and a highly motivated nursing staff. Long-term analysis shows similar results for progression-free survival compared with studies on radical prostectomy and better results compared with EBRT or HDR-brachytherapy for T1 and T2 tumors.

Technical improvements in the last few years involving not only dose planning but also the implant technique give hope for even better results. In comparison with the United States, where most treatments are done on an outpatient basis, most patients in Europe are still treated as inpatients in larger hospitals. However, results from specialized centers in Germany demonstrate that the outpatient mode is safe and leads to good postoperative results. Patient acceptance of outpatient treatment has been high.

More and more urologists and radiation oncologists are becoming interested in LDR prostate brachytherapy. The patient numbers are largest in the United States. Whether Europe will follow suit is not yet clear and will largely depend on the reimbursement situation in the different European countries.

REFERENCES

1. Ling CC. Permanent implants using Au-198, Pd-103 and I-125: radiobiological considerations based on the linear quadratic model. Int J Radiat Oncol Biol Phys 1992;23:81–87.
2. Ling CC, Roy J, Sahoo N, et al. Quantifying the effect of dose inhomogeneity in brachytherapy: application to permanent prostatic implant with ^{125}I seeds. Int J Radiat Oncol Biol Phys 1994;28: 971–978.
3. Blasko JC, Wallner K, Grimm PD, Ragde H. Prostate specific antigen based disease control following ultrasound guided [125]iodine implantation for stage T1/T2 prostatic carcinoma. J Urol 1995;154:1096–1099.

4. Porter AT, Blasko JC, Grimm PD, et al. Brachytherapy for prostate cancer. CA Cancer J Clin 1995; 45:165–178.

5. Dattoli M, Wallner K, Sorace R, et al. ^{103}Pd brachytherapy and external beam irradiation for clinically localized, high-risk prostatic carcinoma. Int J Radiat Oncol Biol Phys 1996;35:875–879.

6. Grimm PD, Blasko JC, Ragde H, et al. Does brachytherapy have a role in the treatment of prostate cancer? Hematol Oncol Clin North Am 1996;10:653–673.

7. Stock RG, Stone NN, DeWyngaert JK, et al. Prostate specific antigen findings and biopsy results following interactive ultrasound guided transperineal brachytherapy for early stage prostate carcinoma. Cancer 1996;77:2386–2392.

8. Beyer DC, Priestley JB Jr. Biochemical disease-free survival following ^{125}I prostate implantation. Int J Radiat Oncol Biol Phys 1997;37:559–563.

9. Critz FA, Levinson K, Williams WH, et al. Prostate-specific antigen nadir of 0.5 ng/mL or less defines disease freedom for surgically staged men irradiated for prostate cancer. Urology 1997;49:668–672.

10. Luse RW, Blasko J, Grimm P. A method for implementing the American Association of Physicists in Medicine Task Group-43 dosimetry recommendations for ^{125}I transperineal prostate seed implants on commercial treatment planning systems. Int J Radiat Oncol Biol Phys 1997;37:737–741.

11. Merrick GS, Butler WM, Dorsey AT, et al. Prostatic conformal brachytherapy: ^{125}I/^{103}Pd postoperative dosimetric analysis. Radiat Oncol Invest 1997;5:305–313.

12. Ragde H, Blasko JC, Grimm PD, et al. Interstitial iodine-125 radiation without adjuvant therapy in the treatment of clinically localized prostate carcinoma. Cancer 1997;80:442–453.

13. Ragde H, Blasko JC, Grimm PD, et al. Brachytherapy for clinically localized prostate cancer: results at 7-and 8-year follow-up. Semin Surg Oncol 1997;13:438–443.

14. Willins J, Wallner K. CT-based dosimetry for transperineal I-125 prostate brachytherapy. Int J Radiat Oncol Biol Phys 1997;39:347–353.

15. Bice WS Jr, Prestidge BR, Prete JJ, et al. Clinical impact of implementing the recommendations of AAPM Task Group 43 on permanent prostate brachytherapy using ^{125}I. American Association of Physicists in Medicine. Int J Radiat Oncol Biol Phys 1998;40:1237–1241.

16. Bice WS Jr, Prestidge BR, Grimm PD, et al. Centralized multiinstitutional postimplant analysis for interstitial prostate brachytherapy. Int J Radiat Oncol Biol Phys 1998;41:921–927.

17. D'Amico AV, Whittington R, Malkowicz SB, et al. Biochemical outcome after radical prostatectomy, external beam radiation therapy, or interstitial radiation therapy for clinically localized prostate cancer. JAMA 1998;280:969–974.

18. Kirkpatrick J. Biochemical outcome after radical prostatectomy, external beam radiation therapy, or interstitial radiation therapy for clinically localized prostate cancer. J Insur Med 1998;30:204–205.

19. Polascik TJ, Pound CR, DeWeese TL, Walsh PC. Comparison of radical prostatectomy and iodine 125 interstitial radiotherapy for the treatment of clinically localized prostate cancer: a 7-year biochemical (PSA) progression analysis. Urology 1998;51:884–889; discussion 889–890.

20. Polascik TJ, Pound CR, DeWeese TL, Walsh PC. Comparison of radical prostatectomy and iodine 125 interstitial radiotherapy for the treatment of clinically localized prostate cancer: a 7 year biochemical (PSA) progression analysis. Urology 1998;51:884–889.

21. Prestidge BR, Bice WS, Kiefer EJ, et al. Timing of computed tomography-based postimplant assessment following permanent transperineal prostate brachytherapy. Int J Radiat Oncol Biol Phys 1998;40:1111–1115.

22. Prete JJ, Prestidge BR, Bice WS, et al. Comparison of MRI- and CT-based post-implant dosimetric analysis of transperineal interstitial permanent prostate brachytherapy. Radiat Oncol Invest 1998;6: 90–96.

23. Prete JJ, Prestidge BR, Bice WS, et al. A survey of physics and dosimetry practice of permanent prostate brachytherapy in the United States. Int J Radiat Oncol Biol Phys 1998;40:1001–1005.

24. Ragde H, Elgamal AA, Snow PB, et al. Ten-year disease free survival after transperineal sonography-guided iodine-125 brachytherapy with or without. 45-gray external beam irradiation in the treatment of patients with clinically localized, low to high Gleason grade prostate carcinoma. Cancer 1998;83:989–1001.

25. Willins J, Wallner K. Time-dependent changes in CT-based dosimetry of I-125 prostate brachytherapy. Radiat Oncol Invest 1998;6:157–160.

26. Cha CM, Potters L, Ashley R, et al. Isotope selection for patients undergoing prostate brachytherapy. Int J Radiat Oncol Biol Phys 1999;45:391–395.

27. Davis BJ, Pisansky TM, Wilson TM, et al. The radial distance of extraprostatic extension of prostate carcinoma: implications for prostate brachytherapy. Cancer 1999;85:2630–2637.
28. Grado GL, Collins JM, Kriegshauser JS, et al. Salvage brachytherapy for localized prostate cancer after radiotherapy failure. Urology 1999;53:2–10.
29. Lee WR, McQuellon RP, Case LD, et al. Early quality of life assessment in men treated with permanent source interstitial brachytherapy for clinically localized prostate cancer. J Urol 1999;162:403–406.
30. Merrick GS, Butler WM, Dorsey AT, et al. Potential role of various dosimetric quality indicators in prostate brachytherapy. Int J Radiat Oncol Biol Phys 1999;44:717–724.
31. Merrick GS, Butler WM, Dorsey AT, et al. The dependence of prostate postimplant dosimetric quality on CT volume determination. Int J Radiat Oncol Biol Phys 1999;44:1111–1117.
32. Nag S, Beyer D, Friedland J, et al. American Brachytherapy Society (ABS) recommendations for transperineal permanent brachytherapy of prostate cancer. Int J Radiat Oncol Biol Phys 1999;44:789–99.
33. Ramos CG, Carvalhal GF, Smith DS, et al. Retrospective comparison of radical retropubic prostatectomy and 125-iodine brachytherapy for localized prostate cancer. J Urol 1999;161:1212–1215.
34. Vicini FA, Kini VR, Edmundson G, et al. A comprehensive review of prostate cancer brachytherapy: defining an optimal technique. Int J Radiat Oncol Biol Phys 1999;44:483–491.
35. Walsh PC. Ten-year disease free survival after transperineal sonography-guided iodine-125 brachytherapy with or without 45-gray external beam irradiation in the treatment of patients with clinically localized, low to high gleason grade prostate carcinoma. J Urol 1999;161:357–358.
36. Yu Y, Anderson LL, Li Z, et al. Permanent prostate seed implant brachytherapy: report of the American Association of Physicists in Medicine Task Group No. 64. Med Phys 1999;26:2054–2076.
37. Potters L. Permanent prostate brachytherapy: lessons learned, lessons to learn. Oncology (Williston Park) 2000;14:981–991; discussion 991–982, 997–989.
38. Ragde H, Grado GL, Nadir B, et al. Modern prostate brachytherapy. CA Cancer J Clin 2000;50:380–393.
39. Ragde H, Korb L. Brachytherapy for clinically localized prostate cancer. Semin Surg Oncol 2000;18:45–51.
40. Sharkey J, Chovnick SD, Behar RJ, et al. Minimally invasive treatment for localized adenocarcinoma of the prostate: review of 1048 patients treated with ultrasound-guided palladium-103 brachytherapy. J Endourol 2000;14:343–350.
41. Singh A, Zelefsky MJ, Raben A, et al. Combined 3-dimensional conformal radiotherapy and transperineal Pd-103 permanent implantation for patients with intermediate and unfavorable risk prostate cancer. Int J Cancer 2000;90:275–280.
42. Stock RG, Stone NN, Lo YC, et al. Postimplant dosimetry for (125)I prostate implants: definitions and factors affecting outcome. Int J Radiat Oncol Biol Phys 2000;48:899–906.
43. Stock RG, Stone NN, Lo YC. Intraoperative dosimetric representation of the real-time ultrasound-guided prostate implant. Tech Urol 2000;6:95–98.
44. Nag S, Bice W, DeWyngaert K, et al. The American Brachytherapy Society recommendations for permanent prostate brachytherapy postimplant dosimetric analysis. Int J Radiat Oncol Biol Phys 2000..
45. Bice WS, Prestidge BR, Sarosdy MF. Calibration, calculation, and prescription issues in permanent prostate brachytherapy with (103)Pd. Int J Radiat Oncol Biol Phys 2001;49:289–291.
46. Deger S, Bohmer D, Roigas J, et al. [Brachytherapy of local prostatic carcinoma]. Urologe A 2001;40:181–184.
47. Merrick GS, Butler WM, Dorsey AT, et al. Effect of prostate size and isotope selection on dosimetric quality following permanent seed implantation. Tech Urol 2001;7:233–240.
48. Nag S, Ciezki JP, Cormack R, et al. Intraoperative planning and evaluation of permanent prostate brachytherapy: report of the American Brachytherapy Society. Int J Radiat Oncol Biol Phys 2001;51:1422–1430.
49. Pommier P, Villers A, Bataillard A, et al. [Standards, Options, and Recommendations for brachytherapy in patients with prostate cancer: efficacy and toxicity]. Cancer Radiother 2001;5:770–786.
50. Ragde H, Grado GL, Nadir BS. Brachytherapy for clinically localized prostate cancer: thirteen-year disease-free survival of 769 consecutive prostate cancer patients treated with permanent implants alone. Arch Esp Urol 2001;54:739–747.

51. Beaulieu L, Aubin S, Taschereau R, et al. Dosimetric impact of the variation of the prostate volume and shape between pretreatment planning and treatment procedure. Int J Radiat Oncol Biol Phys 2002;53:215–221.

52. Blasko JC, Mate T, Sylvester JE, et al. Brachytherapy for carcinoma of the prostate: techniques, patient selection, and clinical outcomes. Semin Radiat Oncol 2002;12:81–94.

53. Crook J, Milosevic M, Catton P, et al. Interobserver variation in postimplant computed tomography contouring affects quality assessment of prostate brachytherapy. Brachytherapy 2002;1:66–73.

54. Kaulich TW, Lamprecht U, Paulsen F, et al. [Physical basics and clinical realization of interstitial brachytherapy of the prostate with iodine 125]. Strahlenther Onkol 2002;178:548–555.

55. Kwok Y, DiBiase SJ, Amin PP, et al. Risk group stratification in patients undergoing permanent (125)I prostate brachytherapy as monotherapy. Int J Radiat Oncol Biol Phys 2002;53:588–594.

56. Potters L, Fearn P, Kattan M. The role of external radiotherapy in patients treated with permanent prostate brachytherapy. Prostate Cancer Prostatic Dis 2002;5:47–53.

57. Potters L, Fearn P, Kattan MW. External radiotherapy and permanent prostate brachytherapy in patients with localized prostate cancer. Brachytherapy 2002;1:36–41.

58. Shanahan TG, Nanavati PJ, Mueller PW, et al. A comparison of permanent prostate brachytherapy techniques: preplan vs. hybrid interactive planning with postimplant analysis. Int J Radiat Oncol Biol Phys 2002;53:490–496.

59. Stock RG, Stone NN. Importance of post-implant dosimetry in permanent prostate brachytherapy. Eur Urol 2002;41:434–439.

60. Stone NN, Stock RG. Complications following permanent prostate brachytherapy. Eur Urol 2002;41:427–433.

61. Wirth MP, Herrmann T, Alken P, et al. [Recommendations for permanent, interstitial brachytherapy alone in localized prostate carcinoma]. Urologe A 2002;41:369–373.

62. Antolak SJ Jr. Re: permanent interstitial brachytherapy for the management of carcinoma of the prostate gland. Re: health related quality of life in men with prostate cancer. J Urol 2003;170: 2391–2392; author reply 2392.

63. Beyer DC, Thomas T, Hilbe J, et al. Relative influence of Gleason score and pretreatment PSA in predicting survival following brachytherapy for prostate cancer. Brachytherapy 2003;2:77–84.

64. Ellis RJ, Vertocnik A, Sodee B, et al. Combination conformal radiotherapy and radioimmunoguided transperineal [103]Pd implantation for patients with intermediate and unfavorable risk prostate adeno-carcinoma. Brachytherapy 2003;2:215–222.

65. Hakenberg OW, Wirth MP, Hermann T, et al. Recommendations for the treatment of localized prostate cancer by permanent interstitial brachytherapy. Urol Int 2003;70:15–20.

66. Horwitz EM, Mitra RK, Uzzo RG, et al. Impact of target volume coverage with Radiation Therapy Oncology Group (RTOG) 98–05 guidelines for transrectal ultrasound guided permanent Iodine-125 prostate implants. Radiother Oncol 2003;66:173–179.

67. Lee EK, Zaider M. Intraoperative dynamic dose optimization in permanent prostate implants. Int J Radiat Oncol Biol Phys 2003;56:854–861.

68. Lee WR, Moughan J, Owen JB, et al. The 1999 patterns of care study of radiotherapy in localized prostate carcinoma: a comprehensive survey of prostate brachytherapy in the United States. Cancer 2003;98:1987–1994.

69. Li XA, Wang JZ, Stewart RD, et al. Dose escalation in permanent brachytherapy for prostate cancer: dosimetric and biological considerations. Phys Med Biol 2003;48:2753–2765.

70. Merrick GS, Butler WM, Wallner KE, et al. Long-term urinary quality of life after permanent prostate brachytherapy. Int J Radiat Oncol Biol Phys 2003;56:454–461.

71. Merrick GS, Wallner KE, Butler WM. Permanent interstitial brachytherapy for the management of carcinoma of the prostate gland. J Urol 2003;169:1643–1652.

72. Peschel RE, Colberg JW. Surgery, brachytherapy, and external-beam radiotherapy for early prostate cancer. Lancet Oncol 2003;4:233–241.

73. Pinkawa M, Maurer U, Mulhern A, et al. Inverse automated treatment planning with and without individual optimization in interstitial permanent prostate brachytherapy with high- and low-activity [125]I. Strahlenther Onkol 2003;179:417–422.

74. Potters L, Calguaru E, Thornton KB, et al. Toward a dynamic real-time intraoperative permanent prostate brachytherapy methodology. Brachytherapy 2003;2:172–180.

75. Salem N, Simonian-Sauve M, Rosello R, et al. Predictive factors of acute urinary morbidity after iodine-125 brachytherapy for localised prostate cancer: a phase 2 study. Radiother Oncol 2003;66: 159–165.
76. Todor DA, Zaider M, Cohen GN, et al. Intraoperative dynamic dosimetry for prostate implants. Phys Med Biol 2003;48:1153–1171.
77. Bradley EB, Bissonette EA, Theodorescu D. Determinants of long-term quality of life and voiding function of patients treated with radical prostatectomy or permanent brachytherapy for prostate cancer. BJU Int 2004;94:1003–1009.
78. Flam TA, Peyromaure M, Chauveinc L, et al. Post-brachytherapy transurethral resection of the prostate in patients with localized prostate cancer. J Urol 2004;172:108–111.
79. Joseph J, Al-Qaisieh B, Ash D, et al. Prostate-specific antigen relapse-free survival in patients with localized prostate cancer treated by brachytherapy. BJU Int 2004;94:1235–1238.
80. Kupelian PA, Potters L, Khuntia D, et al. Radical prostatectomy, external beam radiotherapy <72 gy, external beam radiotherapy > or = 72 gy, permanent seed implantation, or combined seeds/external beam radiotherapy for stage T1-T2 prostate cancer. Int J Radiat Oncol Biol Phys 2004;58:25–33.
81. McLaughlin PW, Narayana V, Kessler M, et al. The use of mutual information in registration of CT and MRI datasets post permanent implant. Brachytherapy 2004;3:61–70.
82. Merrick GS, Butler WM, Wallner KE, et al. Permanent interstitial brachytherapy in younger patients with clinically organ-confined prostate cancer. Urology 2004;64:754–759.
83. Polo A, Cattani F, Vavassori A, et al. MR and CT image fusion for postimplant analysis in permanent prostate seed implants. Int J Radiat Oncol Biol Phys 2004;60:1572–1579.
84. Potters L, Klein EA, Kattan MW, et al. Monotherapy for stage T1-T2 prostate cancer: radical prostatectomy, external beam radiotherapy, or permanent seed implantation. Radiother Oncol 2004;71:29–33.
85. Reynier C, Troccaz J, Fourneret P, et al. MRI/TRUS data fusion for prostate brachytherapy. Preliminary results. Med Phys 2004;31:1568–1575.
86. Wust P, von Borczyskowski DW, Henkel T, et al. Clinical and physical determinants for toxicity of 125-I seed prostate brachytherapy. Radiother Oncol 2004;73:39–48.
87. Bernard S, Vynckier S. Dosimetric study of a new polymer encapsulated palladium-103 seed. Phys Med Biol 2005;50:1493–1504.
88. Haworth A, Ebert M, St Clair S, et al. Impact of selection of post-implant technique on dosimetry parameters for permanent prostate implants. Brachytherapy 2005;4:146–153.
89. McAleese J, O'Sullivan JM. Monotherapy for stage T1-T2 prostate cancer: radical prostatectomy, external beam radiotherapy, or permanent seed implantation. Radiother Oncol 2005;75:121.
90. Merrick GS, Butler WM, Wallner KE, et al. The impact of radiation dose to the urethra on brachytherapy-related dysuria. Brachytherapy 2005;4:45–50.
91. Narayana V, Troyer S, Evans V, et al. Randomized trial of high- and low-source strength (125)I prostate seed implants. Int J Radiat Oncol Biol Phys 2005;61:44–51.

Index